THE CANCER CHEMOTHERAPY HANDBOOK

Cover Illustration

"Peripheral blood smear of a 13 year old white male with a mediastinal mass and a high white blood cell count. The bone marrow was extensively involved with similar cells and there were some in the spinal fluid. Based on morphology alone, this was called a lymphosarcoma cell leukemia by the hematologist/pathologist in 1979. Today, it would be classified as a leukemia/lymphoma based on cell size and morphology, whether it has T or B cell markers, its immunoglobulin (Ig) cell surface markers, the mix of CD (cluster designation) receptors as characterized by monoclonal antibodies, chromosomal abnormalities and oncogene rearrangements."

Sixth
Edition

THE CANCER CHEMOTHERAPY HANDBOOK

David S. Fischer, MD
Clinical Professor of Medicine (Oncology)
Yale University School of Medicine
Yale Comprehensive Cancer Center
Attending Physician
Yale-New Haven Hospital
New Haven, Connecticut

M. Tish Knobf, RN, PhD, FAAN, AOCN
American Cancer Society Professor of Oncology Nursing
Yale School of Nursing
Oncology Clinical Nurse Specialist
Yale-New Haven Hospital
New Haven, Connecticut

Henry J. Durivage, PharmD
Director, Clinical Research Services
The Cancer Institute of New Jersey
University of Medicine and Dentistry of New Jersey
New Brunswick, New Jersey

Nancy J. Beaulieu, RPh, BCOP
Oncology Clinical Pharmacy Specialist
Oncology Services
Yale-New Haven Hospital
New Haven, Connecticut

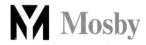

An Affiliate of Elsevier

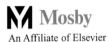

An Affiliate of Elsevier

The Curtis Center
Independence Square West
Philadelphia, Pennsylvania 19106

THE CANCER CHEMOTHERAPY HANDBOOK   ISBN 0-323-01890-4
**Copyright © 2003, 1997, 1993, 1989,
1983, 1980, Mosby, Inc. All rights reserved.**

NOTICE

Library of Congress Cataloging-in-Publication Data
The cancer chemotherapy handbook/David S. Fischer ... [et al.]. – 6th ed.
    p. ; cm.
    Rev. ed. of: The cancer chemotherapy handbook/David S. Fischer, M. Tish Knobf,
Henry J. Durivager. 5th ed. c1997.
    Includes bibliographical references and index.
    ISBN 0-323-01890-4
    1. Cancer–Chemotherapy–Handbooks, manuals, etc. 2. Antineoplastic
agents–Handbooks, manuals, etc. I. Fischer, David S. II. Fischer, David S. Cancer
chemotherapy handbook.
    [DNLM: 1. Neoplasms–drug therapy–Handbooks. 2. Antineoplastic
Agents–Handbooks. QZ 39 F533c 2003]
RC271.C5K58 2003
616.994061–dc21   2003048791

Acquisitions Editor: Dolores Meloni

Printed in the United States of America
Last digit is the print number: 9   8   7   6   5   4   3   2

PREFACE

The goal of the sixth edition of *The Cancer Chemotherapy Handbook* is to continue the previous edition's practical value to clinicians while incorporating large amounts of new data. We have maintained the original format for individual drugs and combination regimens so that the book will continue to serve as a practical reference and resource to all oncology professionals.

Two important additions to the current edition include a new author, Nancy J. Beaulieu, a board certified oncology pharmacist, and a new chapter on the safety and prevention of chemotherapy medication errors. Chapters on pain management and ethics have been maintained because of their direct relevance to the care of patients and professional practice. All other chapters have been updated and expanded to include current state of the art information on both FDA-approved and investigational chemotherapy drugs, biotherapy, and molecular targeted agents. Safety remains a critical element in the process of prescribing and administering chemotherapy. We strongly encourage each clinician to always check the original reference of the listed combination regimens. If there is any question about an individual drug, consult the package insert or investigational drug brochure.

It has been a privilege to have the support of the oncology community to continue with revisions of this book since its inception in 1979, when it was initially created as an in-house handbook for fellows and nurses at Yale New Haven Hospital.

David S. Fischer
M. Tish Knobf
Henry J. Durivage
Nancy J. Beaulieu

ACKNOWLEDGMENTS

In preparing this edition of *The Cancer Chemotherapy Handbook*, we are grateful to many people for their assistance, but the authors take full responsibility for any errors of fact or judgment. We acknowledge the help of Dennis Cooper, MD, for his careful review of the chapter on High-Dose Chemotherapy with Stem Cell Support; Susan Fisher, RN, EdD, C-NP, for her critique on the Chemotherapy Administration chapter; and for the contribution of Edward Snyder, MD, who wrote the Blood Transfusion chapter in the last edition. It has been a pleasure to work with Dolores Meloni, our editor, and we thank her for her support in preparing this edition. Finally, we wish to thank our respective spouses and children for putting up with the temporary neglect that is always a consequence of extensively revising this book.

David S. Fischer
M. Tish Knobf
Henry J. Durivage
Nancy J. Beaulieu

CONTENTS

CANCER CHEMOTHERAPY AND PHARMACOLOGY

An adequate understanding of cancer and its treatment must begin with an appreciation of the fact that cancer is not a single disease but at least 100 different diseases, each with its own characteristics and natural history (DeVita & Chu, 2002; Boyd, 1992). For example, choriocarcinoma is very different from basal cell carcinoma of the skin, and both differ substantially from melanoma, lung, or breast cancer. Even within a "single malignancy," such as breast cancer, major biological and histological differences usually exist. The nature of the neoplastic process is the product of a complex tissue microenvironment in which protein interactions are taking place among the cancer cells, organ parenchymal cells, stroma, blood vessels, and the extracellular matrix (Paweletz et al, 2001). The cancer cells are continuously adapting and evolving. The process is thought to be potentially reversible and comprises an imbalance of regulatory factors that allow certain cells to proliferate, invade, and metastasize. It is important for professionals to know this and counsel patients as to the nature of cancer, modern methods of therapy, and the importance of clinical research as a way to improve the treatment of future patients.

There is no single definition that describes all the malignancies. In general, cancer is a group of relatively normal cells growing without the controls that usually prevent cells from growing beyond their intended size, site, and nutritional base. Cancer can be characterized by a "tip" of the apoptotic balance (i.e., inhibition of apoptosis). Cancer cells have the capacity to extend beyond a capsule or other barrier, to invade normal tissues locally, and to metastasize via blood or lymphoid vessels to distant sites where they may take up residence and proliferate. Thus cancer cells overgrow normal cells, compete with them for space and nutrition, and ultimately cause their death and eventually that of the host.

The causes of cancer are diverse and multifactorial. Epidemiologic studies provide some known links to certain causes, which include genetic traits, environmental and lifestyle factors, viruses, and occupational exposure to chemicals or biological agents (Cole & Rodu, 2001). There is no single cause for all cancers. However, cigarette smoking is the single most important identified cause of cancer in the United States. It is responsible for more than 100,000 deaths yearly from lung cancer, as well as additional morbidity and mortality from cancers of the oral cavity, pharynx, larynx, esophagus, pancreas, bladder, and pleura.

CELLULAR KINETICS

Most cancer cells are not characterized by rapid growth. For example, breast, lung, and colon cancer cells may take up to 100 days to double their population. The growth and division of normal and neoplastic cells occur in a sequence of events called the cell cycle. The cell cycle is divided into several different phases (Figure 1-1). Many of the antineoplastic drugs have been and many continue to be classified based on whether their activity is cell cycle specific or nonspecific.

Synthesis of ribonucleic acid (RNA) and protein occurs during the G_1 phase. When cells are in G_1 for prolonged periods of time, they are often said to be in a resting phase, referred to as G_0. Synthesis of DNA occurs during the S phase. During G_2, DNA synthesis halts, and RNA and protein synthesis continue. The final steps of

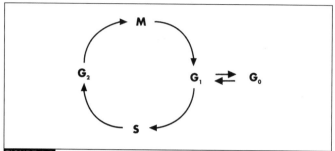

FIGURE 1-1

Phases of the cell cycle. G_0, resting phase (nonproliferation of cells); G_1, pre-DNA synthetic phase (12 hours to a few days); S, DNA synthesis (usually 2 to 4 hours); G_2, post-DNA synthesis (2 to 4 hours; cells are tetraploid in this stage); M, mitosis (1 to 2 hours).

chromosome replication and segregation occur during the mitotic or M phase. The cell undergoes cell division and produces two daughter cells. The rate of RNA and protein synthesis slows during this phase as the genetic material is transferred into the daughter cells. Also located within the cell cycle of normal cells are check points. These are biochemically designated areas that can be activated during the cell cycle process. They prevent the cell from moving forward from one phase to the next if adverse genetic conditions have occurred in the previous phase (Kastan & Skapek, 2001). Many cancer cells have lost these check points.

Drugs that exert their cytotoxic effects during a specific phase of the cell cycle (i.e., phase-specific agents) are usually not effective against cells that are predominantly in a dormant phase (G_0). In contrast, non-phase-specific agents are theoretically more likely to be effective against a tumor population that is not in a state of rapid division.

CANCER CHEMOTHERAPY

Since the first dose of cytotoxic chemotherapy was given in 1942, hundreds of thousands of chemical and biological agents have been tested for their activity in destroying cancer cells. Relatively few of these drugs reach the stage of clinical testing in animals, and fewer still are found to be safe and effective enough to be tested in humans. A small number of those drugs that have been tested in humans are found to be useful for the treatment of patients with cancer. Since it is difficult for clinicians to have at their fingertips all the properties, modes of action, indications, doses, interactions, and toxicities, this book provides information taken from several sources to aid healthcare professionals in the day-to-day care of patients with cancer.

For anticancer drug treatment to be effective, several features must be present. The drug must reach the cancer cells, sufficiently toxic amounts of the drug (or its active metabolite) must enter the cells and remain there for a long enough period of time, the cancer cells must be sensitive to the effects of the drug, and all this must occur before resistance emerges (Chabner, 1990). In addition, the patient must be able to withstand the adverse effects of treatment. Combination chemotherapy, dose, dose intensity, and optimal scheduling are important variables in the effective treatment of some cancers. For the more responsive malignancies (e.g., testicular cancer), it is important that "full doses" of chemotherapy be given "on schedule" for a short period of time.

Low doses of single agent chemotherapy given over a prolonged period of time favors the emergence of drug resistance.

DRUG RESISTANCE

The development of resistance to chemotherapeutic drugs by neoplastic cells is one of the major obstacles to the cure of many malignancies. Malignant cells may be intrinsically resistant or they may adapt after therapy by using various detoxification pathways to acquire resistance to cytotoxic agents (Moscow & Cowan, 1988; DeVita, 1990). The emerging understanding of the resistance process has revealed numerous complex mechanisms that may occur simultaneously or sequentially in cancer cells. Recent research has uncovered one common process that may cause resistance to virtually all chemotherapy agents, despite drug class or mechanism of action (Kaufman & Chabner, 2001). This resistance is referred to as suppression or inactivation of cell-damage-induced apoptosis or loss of the apoptotic pathway (Kaufman & Chabner, 2001; Elstrom & Thompson, 2001).

A full understanding of the myriad of known and potential mechanisms of drug resistance could not be adequately described in full detail in this book. Four resistance processes are described to illustrate how cancer cells acquire resistance. Further references should be consulted for an in-depth understanding of this topic.

INACTIVATION OF THE p53 SUPPRESSOR GENE

The p53 suppressor gene is responsible for triggering cells to begin programmed cell death, or apoptosis. When the p53 gene is functioning, the DNA damage caused by many chemotherapy agents is a signal to the p53 suppressor gene to send the damaged cell through the apoptotic pathway resulting in cell death. If this gene becomes inactivated, despite the genetic damage inflicted by the chemotherapy, the cells continue to survive, replicate, and develop resistance. This resistance mechanism is not drug class specific, but may affect all chemotherapeutic agents that exert their effect through DNA/RNA damage (Kaufman & Chabner, 2001).

ROLE OF THE B-CELL LYMPHOMA (Bcl-2) PROTEINS

The Bcl-2 proteins are regulators of apoptosis. Bcl-2 is concentrated in cellular mitochondria where it regulates the release of substances (e.g., cytochrome C) involved in effecting cell death. In general, Bcl-2 blocks the release of these substances from the mitochondria thereby promoting the survival of cancer cells by slowing or preventing cell death. Resistance to chemotherapy has, on several occasions, been shown to correlate with the overexpression of the Bcl-2 protein.

MULTIDRUG RESISTANCE

Overexpression of the MDR-1 gene enhances the production of the transmembrane glycoprotein (referred to as P-170, Pgp, or P-glycoprotein). P-170 is present in many cells that are resistant to vinca alkaloids, dactinomycin, epipodophyllotoxins, and other natural products. The hallmark of multidrug resistance is cross-resistance to several drugs after exposure to a single drug such as a vinca alkaloid, dactinomycin, or an anthracycline, but not to an alkylating agent, bleomycin, or an antimetabolite. Evidence suggests that P-170 may contribute to drug resistance clinically in multiple myeloma, pediatric sarcomas, non-Hodgkin's lymphoma, and acute nonlymphocytic leukemia (Kaufman & Chabner, 2001).

P-170 functions as a pump that is capable of ejecting cytotoxic agents from the cell (Moscow & Cowan, 1988). The activity of P-170 is under the influence of other cellular substances and is similar to bacterial peristaltic transport proteins. In the laboratory, several compounds have been tested for their ability to reverse or block the effects of the P-glycoprotein pump. Some of these drugs have been tested clinically. Examples include verapamil, cyclosporine, cyclosporine analogues, and phenothiazines (Ford & Hait, 1990). Thus far the results are inconclusive (Kaufman & Chabner, 2001) primarily because cancer cells have the ability to develop more than one form of resistance.

ATYPICAL MULTIDRUG RESISTANCE, TOPOISOMERASES

DNA is attached to the nuclear matrix at regular intervals. The sites where DNA is fixed to the nuclear matrix are called domains. During replication, the two DNA molecules and their domains are wound together like interlocked circles. For cell division to occur, separation and resealing of the DNA molecules must occur. This function and others are performed by DNA topoisomerase enzymes (Bender et al, 1990).

Several antineoplastic drugs exert their effects by inhibition of topoisomerase enzymes (Liu, 1989; Sinha, 1995). Alterations in topoisomerase enzyme activity have been shown in cells resistant to topoisomerase inhibitors. Resistance to amsacrine, doxorubicin, teniposide, and etoposide may be acquired via decreased drug access to the enzyme, alteration of enzyme structure (and activity), or by other mechanisms.

GLUTATHIONE AND GLUTATHIONE S-TRANSFERASE ISOENZYMES

Glutathione (GSH) is a thiol that accounts for the majority of the intracellular nonprotein sulfhydryl content of most cells. It is regulated by other cellular processes and is essential for the synthesis of DNA precursors. GSH enzymes play important roles in detoxifying toxins, scavenging free radicals, and repairing DNA damage.

Glutathione S-transferase (GST) joins toxins with glutathione, forming a less toxic metabolite. Increased amounts of GST have been found in cancers of the head and neck, lung, and colon, but not in surrounding normal colon mucosa.

GST and GSH probably play some role in resistance to nitrogen mustard, melphalan, cisplatin, and nitrosoureas via inactivation of the drugs, through direct binding, increased metabolism, detoxification, and/or DNA repair (Ford & Hait, 1990). O^6-Benzylguanine is being evaluated as a drug that can interrupt DNA repair mechanisms following treatment with alkylating agents, such as carmustine and melphalan.

ANTINEOPLASTIC DRUGS

The original use of the first cytotoxic chemotherapeutic agent, mechlorethamine, occurred at the New Haven Hospital. Studies began when two young investigators at Yale University, Goodman and Gilman, investigated a wartime agent with the code designation HN2. Investigation of this agent revealed that the drug caused depression of the white blood cell and platelet counts. Goodman and Gilman suggested to the thoracic surgeon, Lindskog, that this might be a useful drug for cancer treatment. A patient with inoperable and radiation-resistant lymphosarcoma was treated with HN2, subsequently known as nitrogen mustard, or mechlorethamine, and had a dramatic reduction of tumor size (Gilman, 1963). Although the response was brief and the patient relapsed shortly thereafter, it established the principle that drugs could shrink tumors and indicated the need for further research. Subsequent studies took place in this area with the progress that is now well known. We have chosen to assign the drugs into groups based on their presumed primary mechanism of action.

ALKYLATING AND DNA CROSS-LINKING AGENTS

Alkylating agents are highly reactive compounds that easily attach to DNA and cellular proteins. The primary mode of action for most alkylating drugs is via cross-linking of DNA strands. They can be classified as either monofunctional alkylating agents, implying reactions with only one strand of DNA, or bifunctional alkylating agents, which cross-link two strands of DNA. Replication of DNA and transcription of RNA are prevented by these cross-links (Tew et al, 2001).

Many alkylating agents have been developed (Table 1-1). Although these drugs have similar mechanisms of action, there are major differences in spectrum of activity, pharmacokinetic parameters, and toxicity. Alkylating agents play a significant role in the treatment of lymphoma, Hodgkin's disease, breast cancer, multiple myeloma, and other malignancies. In addition to conventional chemotherapy, the linear dose-response curve of alkylating agents expands their role for incorporation into transplant regimens.

ANTITUMOR ANTIBIOTICS

Antineoplastic drugs that are derived from micro-organisms are called antitumor antibiotics (Table 1-2) (Verweij et al, 1990; Myers & Chabner, 1990). Included in this class are: anthracyclines, bleomycins, dactinomycin, mitomycin C, and plicamycin.

TABLE 1-1
ALKYLATING AGENTS: MECHANISMS OF ACTION

Drug	Mechanisms
Altretamine	DNA cross-linking, binding to microsomal proteins
Amsacrine	DNA intercalation, inhibition of topoisomerase II
Busulfan	DNA cross-linking, alkylation of cellular thiols
Carboplatin	DNA cross-linking
Carmustine	DNA cross-linking; DNA polymerase repair, RNA synthesis inhibition
Chlorambucil	DNA cross-linking, alkylation of cellular thiols
Cisplatin	DNA cross-linking, intercalation, DNA precursor inhibition, alteration of cellular membranes
Cyclophosphamide	DNA cross-linking
Dacarbazine	DNA methylation, alkylation
Ifosfamide	DNA cross-linking and chain scission
Lomustine	DNA cross-linking; DNA polymerase repair, RNA synthesis inhibition
Mechlorethamine	DNA cross-linking
Melphalan	DNA cross-linking, alkylation of cellular thiols
Oxaliplatin	DNA cross-linking
Procarbazine	DNA alkylation, inhibits methyl group incorporation into RNA
Streptozocin	DNA cross-linking, inhibits DNA repair enzyme guanine-O^6-methyl transferase
Temozolomide	DNA methylation, alkylation
Thiotepa	DNA cross-linking
Tirapazamine	Produces radical anions that cause strand breaks in DNA. Appears to be more toxic to hypoxic tumor cells compared to aerobic cells

Several of these drugs interfere with DNA through intercalation, a reaction whereby the drug inserts itself between DNA base pairs. Some of the antitumor antibiotics have other mechanisms to exert antitumor effects, such as inhibition of topoisomerase enzymes, antimitotic effects, and alteration of cellular membranes. Most of the antitumor antibiotics appear to be cell-cycle-nonspecific agents.

TABLE 1-2
NATURAL PRODUCTS: MECHANISMS OF ACTION

Drug	Mechanisms
Arsenic trioxide	DNA fragmentation, degradation of APL-associated fusion protein
Asparaginase	Hydrolyzes the amino acid asparagine
Bleomycin	DNA strand scission by free radicals
Bryostatin-1	Inhibition of protein kinase C. May down-regulate the multidrug-resistant (MDR) gene and induce differentiation of myeloid, lymphoid, and leukemic cell lines
Dactinomycin	DNA intercalation, inhibition of topoisomerase II
Daunorubicin	DNA intercalation, preribosomal DNA and RNA inhibition, alteration of cell membranes, free radical formation
Docetaxel	Promotes microtubule assembly, stabilizes tubulin polymers resulting in formation of nonfunctional microtubules
Doxorubicin	DNA intercalation, preribosomal DNA and RNA inhibition, alteration of cell membranes, free radical formation
Epirubicin	DNA intercalation, preribosomal DNA and RNA inhibition, alteration of cell membranes, free radical formation
Etoposide	Inhibition of topoisomerase II
Flavopiridol	Inhibition of cyclin-dependent kinases (CDK) and vascular endothelial growth factor (VEGF), may induce apoptosis by down-regulation of Bcl-2
Homoharringtonine	Inhibits synthesis of protein, DNA, and RNA by inhibiting chain initiation
Idarubicin	DNA intercalation, preribosomal DNA and RNA inhibition, alteration of cell membranes, free radical formation
Irinotecan	Inhibition of topoisomerase I
Mitomycin	DNA cross-linking and depolymerization, free radical formation
Mitoxantrone	DNA intercalation, inhibition of topoisomerase II
Nitrocamptothecin	Inhibition of topoisomerase I
Paclitaxel	Promotes microtubule assembly, stabilizes tubulin polymers resulting in formation of nonfunctional microtubules
Plicamycin	DNA intercalation and adlineation, osteoclast inhibition
Teniposide	Inhibition of topoisomerase II
Topotecan	Inhibition of topoisomerase I
Valrubicin	Interferes with DNA topoisomerase II
Vinblastine	Tubulin binding. Inhibition of microtubule assembly, dissolution of mitotic spindle
Vincristine	Tubulin binding. Inhibition of microtubule assembly, dissolution of mitotic spindle
Vindesine	Tubulin binding. Inhibition of microtubule assembly, dissolution of mitotic spindle
Vinorelbine	Tubulin binding. Inhibition of microtubule assembly, dissolution of mitotic spindle

PLANT ALKALOIDS AND NATURAL PRODUCTS

Topoisomerase Inhibitors

As mentioned earlier in this chapter, topoisomerases are enzymes that break and reseal DNA strands (Bender et al, 1990; Sinha, 1995). The plant alkaloid camptothecin and its analogues (e.g., topotecan, irinotecan, 9-nitrocamptothecin) are non-classic enzyme inhibitors of topoisomerase I. These agents are no longer referred to as inhibitors but instead classified as topoisomerase I targeting agents or topoisomerase I poisons (Takimoto & Arbuck, 2001). Etoposide, teniposide, and drugs from other classes, such as amsacrine, doxorubicin, mitoxantrone, and daunorubicin, are inhibitors of topoisomerase II (Table 1-2). These drugs form a stable complex by binding to DNA and topoisomerase enzymes, resulting in DNA damage that interferes with replication and transcription.

Mitotic Inhibitors

A group of mitotic inhibitors (e.g., vinblastine, vincristine, vinorelbine) exert their cytotoxic effects by binding to tubulin. This inhibits formation of microtubules, causing metaphase arrest (Bender et al, 1990). Their mechanisms of action and metabolism are similar, but the antitumor spectrum, dose, and clinical toxicities of vincristine, vinblastine, and vinorelbine are very different. Paclitaxel and docetaxel are also mitotic inhibitors. However, they differ from the vinca alkaloids by enhancing microtubule formation. As a result, a stable and nonfunctional microtubule is produced.

Enzymes

L-Asparaginase is an enzyme product that acts primarily by inhibiting protein synthesis by depriving tumor cells of the amino acid asparagine. Cells that have the ability to form their own asparagine, such as many normal cells, are not affected by L-asparaginase. L-Asparaginase is a foreign protein, is antigenic, and can cause serious hypersensitivity reactions. Included in this category are the long-acting pegylated asparaginase and Erwinia-derived asparaginase, both similar in mechanism to L-asparaginase.

ANTIMETABOLITES AND TARGETED THERAPIES

A variety of agents interfere with the synthesis of DNA and RNA by mechanisms other than those described previously. Many of these drugs are called antimetabolites (Table 1-3) because they exert their effects largely in the synthetic phase of the cell cycle. Some antimetabolites are structural analogues of normal metabolites essential for cell growth and replication. This property allows them to be incorporated into DNA or RNA so that a false message is transmitted. Other antimetabolites inhibit enzymes that are necessary for the synthesis of essential compounds. More recently, compounds have been developed (e.g., imatinib, tipifarnib, erlinotib, gefitnib) that disrupt or interfere with specific target enzymes, growth factor receptors, genes (e.g., retinoids), or signal transduction pathways. The antimetabolites traditionally are divided into the cytidine analogues (e.g., 5-azacitidine, cytarabine) (Garcia-Carbonero et al, 2001), fluorinated pyrimidines (e.g., fluorouracil, floxuridine, tegafur) (Grem, 2001), purine analogues (e.g., mercaptopurine, thioguanine) (Hande, 2001), ribonucleotide reductase inhibitors (e.g., hydroxyurea), adenosine deaminase inhibitors (e.g., pentostatin), and the folic acid antagonists or antifolates (e.g., methotrexate, pemetrexed) (Messmann & Allegra, 2001).

TABLE 1-3

ANTIMETABOLITES AND TARGETED THERAPIES: MECHANISMS OF ACTION

Drug	Mechanisms
Azacitidine	Competes for incorporation into nucleic acids, blocks production of cytidine and uridine. Inhibitor of DNA methylation agent at low doses
Bcl-2 antisense oligonucleotide (Genasense®), G3139	Antisense compound that binds to mRNA and blocks Bcl-2 production
Bexarotene	Selectively binds and activates retinoid X receptors, which regulate gene expression that controls cellular proliferation and differentiation
Capecitabine	Inhibition of thymidylate synthase, an enzyme involved in conversion of deoxyuridylic acid to thymidylic acid
Cladribine	Deoxyadenosine analogue that accumulates in cells and blocks RNA synthesis
Cytarabine	Competitive inhibition DNA polymerase, an enzyme involved in conversion of cytidine to deoxycytidine, blocks DNA repair
Decitabine	Pyrimidine nucleoside analogue. Inhibitor of DNA methylation
Endostatin	Inhibition of angiogenesis
Erlinotib (OSI-774)	Inhibitor of epidermal growth factor receptor (EGFR) activation and signaling via inhibition of EGFR tyrosine kinase
Floxuridine	Inhibition of thymidylate synthesis
Fludarabine	Inhibition of DNA polymerase and ribonucleotide reductase
Fluorouracil	Inhibition of thymidylate synthase, an enzyme involved in conversion of deoxyuridylic acid to thymidylic acid
Gefitnib (Iressa®)	Inhibitor of epidermal growth factor receptor (EGFR) activation and signaling via inhibition of EGFR tyrosine kinase
Gemcitabine	Inhibits ribonucleotide reductase, competes with cytidine triphosphate for incorporation into DNA
Hydroxyurea	Inhibition of ribonucleoside reductase (inhibits conversion of ribonucleosides to deoxyribonucleosides), thymidine incorporation into DNA and DNA repair
Imatinib (STI571)	Induces apoptosis in BCR-ABL cells. Inhibits BCR-ABR protein, c-kit and other protein kinases
ISIS 3521	Antisense inhibition of protein kinase C-alfa (PKC-alfa). ISIS 3521 binds to a messenger RNA sequence that is specific to PKC-alfa
Mercaptopurine	Competes with ribotides for enzymes responsible for conversion of inosinic acid to adenine and xanthine ribotides (inhibits purine synthesis)
Methotrexate	Inhibits dihydrofolate reductase, thereby halting thymidylate and purine synthesis
Nolatrexed	Antifolate. Inhibition of thymidylate synthase
Pemetrexed	Inhibition of folate-dependent enzymes including: thymidylate synthase, dihydrofolate reductase, and glycinamide ribonucleotide formyltransferase
Pentostatin	Inhibits adenosine deaminase, an enzyme that is important for the metabolism of purine nucleosides

cont'd

TABLE 1-3

ANTIMETABOLITES AND TARGETED THERAPIES: MECHANISMS OF ACTION
(continued)

Drug	Mechanisms
PS-341	Proteasome inhibitor. Induces apoptosis in cells that overexpress Bcl-2. Also inhibits angiogenesis, IL-6-mediated cell growth, and cellular adhesion molecules
Raltitrexed	Thymidylate synthase inhibition
Tegafur	Converted to fluorouracil which inhibits thymidylate synthase
Thalidomide	Inhibitor of angiogenesis
Thioguanine	Competes with guanine in nucleotide (purine) synthesis pathways
Tipifarnib (R115777)	Inhibition of Ras oncogene farnesylation (activation)
Trimetrexate	Inhibits dihydrofolate reductase, thereby halting thymidylate and purine synthesis

1

OTHER AGENTS

Endocrine therapies such as selective estrogen receptor modulators or SERMS, aromatase inhibitors, estrogens, androgens (e.g., fluoxymesterone), corticosteroids (e.g., prednisone, dexamethasone), progestins (megestrol acetate), and other drugs (e.g., tamoxifen, leuprolide, goserelin, flutamide) have been used for many years. The mechanisms of these and other drugs are discussed in Chapter 4. Biological response modifiers, growth factors, and monoclonal antibody mechanisms are discussed in Chapter 5.

DRUG INTERACTIONS WITH ANTINEOPLASTIC AGENTS

A drug interaction is defined as a reaction that occurs when the effects and/or pharmacokinetics of a drug are altered by the prior use or co-administration of another drug. How quickly the reaction occurs varies. Acute-onset reactions (i.e., within 24 hours) may require immediate attention, whereas "slow" interactions may not require immediate action.

The outcomes of a drug interaction may be diverse and costly. Drug interactions may be beneficial or adverse. A drug interaction may lead to a net increase or decrease in the anticipated pharmacological response, new effects may develop, toxicity may increase, or there may be no clinical changes despite changes in pharmacokinetic parameters. In many cases, such interactions may not be predictable. This is especially true for newer agents that have limited data on outcomes when used with other drugs. A review of general principles of drug interactions is provided here.

THE NATURE OF THE PROBLEM

Drug interactions account for a large percentage of adverse drug events that cost the healthcare system billions of dollars per year. Drug interactions are estimated to account for approximately 7% to 22% of all adverse drug reactions (Cramer et al, 1992). As the number of drugs taken by a patient increases, so does the likelihood of a drug interaction (May, 1977). In patients taking 10 or more drugs, the prevalence of drug interactions may exceed 20%.

The outcome of a drug interaction is dependent on many factors. Some drug interactions may be clinically significant only if the patient has renal dysfunction or some other abnormality. Other drug interactions (e.g., allopurinol and mercaptopurine) require that a drug (e.g., mercaptopurine) be given orally, rather than intravenously (Coffey et al, 1972).

Most drug interactions that have been reported are not of major clinical significance. However, antineoplastic agents and a few other drugs have a narrow therapeutic index. In the oncology patient population, there should be a heightened awareness that a drug interaction may be clinically significant due to the complex and toxic drug therapy that oncology patients receive.

The detection of an adverse drug interaction, however, may be difficult in oncology patients. Some degree of toxicity is expected from every antineoplastic drug; increased toxicity as a result of a drug interaction may be hard to detect. Evidence that a drug interaction reduces the effectiveness of an antineoplastic drug may be difficult to detect, especially when the treatment is effective in a minority of the patient population.

SPECIFIC DRUG INTERACTIONS

A brief description of some of the mechanisms of drug interactions follows. This revised edition has incorporated the more significant individual drug interactions within the drug monograph sections in Chapters 4 and 5. The more obvious additive drug interactions (e.g., additive nephrotoxicity with cisplatin, streptozocin, and other nephrotoxins; overlapping myelosuppression, etc.) are not included. The interaction of live-virus vaccines (e.g., Measles-Mumps-Rubella, Live, attenuated typhoid, BCG vaccine, oral polio, and Yellow Fever) administered to the immunocompromised patient may cause viral replication and should therefore be avoided (Center for Disease Control and Prevention, 1993). For recommendations on the use of vaccines and immune globulins in persons with altered immunocompetence the reader is referred to Recommendations of the Advisory Committee on Immunization Practices (Center for Disease Control and Prevention, 1993).

Oncology patients who are on chronic therapy with drugs known to have narrow therapeutic windows (e.g., phenytoin, warfarin, digoxin, and theophylline) should have levels of the chronic agent monitored regularly once chemotherapy has begun.

The understanding of drug interactions is enhanced with an increased knowledge of the mechanisms by which they can occur. There are three classes of drug interactions: pharmaceutical, pharmacokinetic, and pharmacodynamic (Ciummo & Katz, 1995).

Pharmaceutical Interactions

These are considered chemical or physical interactions and take into account the physical drug properties. They incorporate physical incompatibilities in terms of whether or not drugs can be combined in solution, acid and base interactions (e.g., protamine antagonizes the effects of heparin), and adsorbent effects (e.g., charcoal and cholestyramine decreasing absorption).

Pharmacokinetic Interactions

These involve interference with absorption, distribution, metabolism, or excretion of one or more drugs. Altered absorption can occur by several mechanisms, reducing absorbing surface area and circulation site of absorption (e.g., chemotherapy and oral digoxin), reduction of gastrointestinal flora, (e.g., oral aminoglycosides can increase absorption of methotrexate), change in gastrointestinal pH, and formation of chelation complexes that prevent absorption. Extent of absorption interactions tends to be of greater clinical signficance than rate of absorption interactions (May, 2000).

Protein-binding interactions are usually of the displacement type and account for distribution interactions. One drug is displaced from the protein-binding site by a second agent (e.g., aspirin and other agents displace warfarin, methotrexate, and others). These types of interactions can be of significance depending on the extent of displacement of a drug that is protein-bound, the effect the displaced drug exerts on the body (e.g., antineoplastic displacement can cause increased toxicity), and the drug affinities for plasma proteins.

Alteration of drug metabolism usually involves the hepatic microsomal enzyme cytochrome P450 system. A three-tier classification system (family, subfamily, and gene) individualizes the 30-plus isoenzymes that are involved in metabolism. The most prominent pathways include CYP 3A4, CYP 2D6, CYP 1A2, and the 2C subfamily (May, 2000). The isoenzymes of this system are primarily located in the liver, but can also be found in the lungs, brain, kidneys, and small intestine. These enzymes can be either induced or inhibited. Knowledge of the drugs and their metabolic class as a substrate, inducer, or inhibitor of the P450 enzyme system aids in predicting the risk of potential drug interactions (Box 1-1) (May, 2000).

Induction of hepatic microsomal enzymes by drugs (e.g., phenytoin, barbiturates, polycyclic hydrocarbons, rifampin, etc.) may increase the metabolism of drugs to inactive compounds (e.g. irinotecan, quinidine, estrogens, methadone, etc.). The second alternative is the induction of metabolism of drugs to active compounds (e.g., cyclophosphamide) or toxic metabolites (e.g., meperidine).

Drugs that inhibit cytochrome P450 enzymes may reduce the metabolism of certain agents, resulting in increased toxicity. Drugs that inhibit cytochrome P450 enzymes may also reduce the activation of prodrugs to active compounds resulting in decreased therapeutic effectiveness.

Substrates of the cytochrome P450 system are drugs whose metabolism is dependent on the P450 isoenzyme system and can be affected by agents that either induce or inhibit a P450 isoenzyme. Some common antineoplastic substrates and their pathways include: irinotecan (CYP 3A4), cyclophosphamide (CYP 2B6, 3A4), doxorubicin (CYP 3A4), etoposide (CYP 3A4), vinblastine (CYP 3A4), tamoxifen (CYP 1A2, 2A6), ifosfamide (CYP 2B6), paclitaxel (CYP 2C8) (May, 2000).

Alteration of drug excretion or elimination may occur as a result of interactions that affect renal or hepatic function. Drug toxicity can occur when the kidneys do not excrete the toxic compounds at an expected rate of elimination (e.g., decreased elimination of ifosfamide).

Pharmacodynamic Interactions

These involve inhibitory reactions, synergistic reactions, additive reactions, and potentiation reactions. Inhibitory reactions include antagonistic or agonist reactions such as the combination of opiod analgesics and naloxone, whereby one drug inhibits or reverses the effect of the other.

Additive reactions occur when the combined effect of two or more drugs is equal to the sum of each individual drug alone (Klaassen, 1996). This principle is employed with the use of combination chemotherapy regimens – synergistic reactions whereby one drug potentiates the effects of a second drug leading to a combined effect greater

BOX 1-1

CYTOCHROME P450 SUBSTRATES, INHIBITORS AND INDUCERS
SUBSTRATES, INHIBITORS AND INDUCERS OF CYP 3A4

SUBSTRATES

Amitriptyline (Elavil®)
Benzodiazepines
  -Bupropion (Wellbutrin®)
  -Alprazolam (Xanax®)
  -Triazolam (Halcion®)
  -Midazolam (Versed®)
Calcium channel blockers
Carbamazepine (Tegretol®)
Cisapride (Propulsid®)
Dexamethasone (Decadron®)
Erythromycin
Ethinyl estradiol (Estraderm®, Estrace®)
Glyburide (Glynase®, Micronase®)
Irinotecan (Camptosar®)
Imipramine (Tofranil®)

Ketoconazole (Nizoral®)
Lovastatin (Mevacor®)
Nefazodone (Serzone®)
Terfenadine (Seldane®)
Astemizole (Hismanal®)
Verapamil (Calan®, Isoptin®)
Sertraline (Zoloft®)
Testosterone
Theophylline
Venlafaxine (Effexor®)
Protease inhibitors
  -Ritonavir (Norvir®)
  -Saquinavir (Invirase®)
  -Indinavir (Crixivan®)
  -Nelfinavir (Viracept®)

INHIBITORS

Antidepressants
  -Nefazodone (Serzone®)
  -Fluvoxamine (Luvox®)
  -Fluoxetine (Prozac®)
  -Sertraline (Zoloft®)
  -Paroxetine (Paxil®)
  -Venlafaxene

Azole antifungals
  -Itraconazole (Sporanox®)
  -Ketoconazole (Nizoral®)
  -Fluconazole (Diflucan®)
Cimetidine (Tagamet®)
Clarithromycin (Biaxin®)
Dilfiazem
Erythromycin
Protease inhibitors

INDUCERS

Carbamazepine (Tegretol®)
Dexamethasone
Phenobarbital
Phenytoin (Dilantin®)
Rifampin (Rifadin®, Rimactane®)

NOTE: Unless the substrate is a prodrug, inhibitors will decrease metabolism of substrates and generally lead to increased drug effect and inducers will increase metabolism of substrates and generally lead to decreased drug effect.

Modified from URL:http://www.utmed.com/wmanuel/psyc/p450.html

than the sum of the individual effects of each agent alone (Klaassen, 1996). The antineoplastic combination of fluorouracil and leucovorin utilizes the synergy principle for therapeutic benefit. Potentiation reactions are the increased effect of a toxic agent acting simultaneously with a nontoxic one (Klaassen, 1996).

DRUGS PRESENTED

In this revision, over 100 antineoplastic drugs, targeted therapies, hormonal agents, monoclonal antibodies, biological response modifiers, and other therapeutic agents are discussed. We have continued to list drugs and hormones alphabetically by their current generic name (if known) in Chapter 4. Biotherapy and monoclonal antibodies are listed alphabetically in Chapter 5.

REFERENCES

Bender RA, Hamel E, Hande KR. Plant alkaloids. In Chabner BA, Collins JM, eds. Cancer Chemotherapy, Principles and Practice. Philadelphia, JB Lippincott, 1990:pp253–275.

Boyd NF. The epidemiology of cancer: principles and methods. In Tannock IF, Hill RP, eds. The Basic Science of Oncology, 2nd ed. New York, McGraw-Hill, 1992:pp7–22.

Center for Disease Control and Prevention. Use of vaccines and immune globulins in persons with altered immunocompetence: Recommendations of the Advisory Committee on Immunization Practices (ACIP). MMWR 42(No. RR-4):1–18, 1993.

Chabner BA. Cytidine analogues. In Chabner BA, Collins JM, eds. Cancer Chemotherapy, Principles and Practice. Philadelphia, JB Lippincott 1990:pp154–179.

Ciummo PE, Katz NL. Interactions and drug metabolizing enzymes. Am Pharm 35(9): 41–53, 1995.

Coffey JJ et al. Effect of allopurinol on the pharmacokinetics of 6-mercaptopurine (NSC 755) in cancer patients. Cancer Res 32: 1283–1289, 1972.

Cole P, Rodu B. Analytic epidemiology: cancer causes. In DeVita VT Jr, Hellman S, Rosenberg SA, eds. Principles and Practice of Oncology, 6th ed. Philadelphia, Lippincott Williams and Wilkins, 2001.

Cramer RL et al. Drug interaction monitoring program in a community hospital. Am J Hosp Pharm 49: 627–629, 1992.

DeVita VT Jr. The problem of resistance. In DeVita VT Jr, Hellman S, Rosenberg SA, eds. Principles and Practice of Oncology. PPO Updates 4: 1–12, 1990.

DeVita VT Jr, Chu E. Principles of cancer chemotherapy. In Chu E, DeVita VT Jr, eds. Physicians' Cancer Chemotherapy Drug Manual 2002. Sudbury, MA, Jones and Bartlett, 2002:pp1–30.

Elstrom R, Thompson CB. Influencing the apoptotic mechanisms in cancer treatment. In DeVita VT, Hellman S, Rosenberg S, eds. Progress in Oncology 2001. Sudbury, MA, Jones and Bartlett, 2001:pp72–90.

Ford JM, Hait WN. Pharmacology of drugs that alter multidrug resistance in cancer. Pharmacol Rev 42: 155–199, 1990.

Garcia-Carbonero R, Ryan DP, Chabner BA. Cytidine analogs. In Chabner BA, Longo DL, eds. Cancer Chemotherapy and Biotherapy, Principles and Practice. Philadelphia, Lippincott Williams and Wilkins, 2001:pp265–294.

Gilman A. The initial clinical trial of nitrogen mustard. Am J Surg 105: 574–578, 1963.

Grem JL. Fluorinated pyrimidines. In Chabner BA, Longo DL, eds. Cancer Chemotherapy and Biotherapy, Principles and Practice. Philadelphia, Lippincott Williams and Wilkins, 2001:pp185–264.

Hande KR. Purine antimetabolites. In Chabner BA, Longo DL, eds. Cancer Chemotherapy and Biotherapy, Principles and Practice. Philadelphia, Lippincott Williams and Wilkins, 2001:pp295–314.

Kastan M, Skapek S. Molecular biology of cancer: the cell cycle. In DeVita VT Jr, Hellman S, Rosenberg SA, eds. Principles and Practice of Oncology, 6th ed. Philadelphia, Lippincott Williams and Wilkins, 2001.

Kaufman DC, Chabner BA. Clinical strategies for cancer treatment: the role of drugs. In Chabner BA, Longo DL, eds. Cancer Chemotherapy, Principles and Practice. Philadelphia, Lippincott Williams and Wilkins, 2001:pp1–16.

Klaassen CD. Principles of toxicology and treatment of poisoning. In Hardman JG, Limburd LE, eds. Goodman and Gilman's The Pharmacological Basis of Therapeutics, 9th ed. New York, McGraw-Hill, 1996:pp63–75.

Liu LF. DNA topoisomerase poisons as antitumor drugs. Ann Rev Biochem 58: 351–375, 1989.

May FE, Stewart RB, Cluff LE. Drug interactions and multiple drug administration. Clin Pharmacol Ther 22: 322–328, 1977.

May SK. Significant drug–drug interactions with antineoplastics. Hosp Pharm 35: 1207–1217, 2000.

Messmann RA, Allegra CJ. Antifolates. In Chabner BA, Longo DL, eds. Cancer Chemotherapy and Biotherapy, Principles and Practice. Philadelphia, Lippincott Williams and Wilkins, 2001:pp139–184.

Moscow JA, Cowan KH. Multidrug resistance. J Natl Cancer Inst 80: 14–20, 1988.

Myers CE, Chabner BA. Anthracyclines. In Chabner BA, Collins JM, eds. Cancer Chemotherapy, Principles and Practice. Philadelphia, JB Lippincott, 1990:pp356–382.

Paweletz C et al. Gene analysis using DNA microassays. In DeVita VT, Hellman S, Rosenberg S, eds. Progress in Oncology 2001. Sudbury, MA, Jones and Bartlett, 2001:pp1–15.

Sinha BK. Topoisomerase inhibitors, a review of their therapeutic potential in cancer. Drugs 49: 11–19, 1995.

Takimoto CH, Arbuck SG. Topoisomerase I targeting agents: the camptothecins. In Chabner BA, Longo DL, eds. Cancer Chemotherapy and Biotherapy, Principles and Practice. Philadelphia, Lippincott Williams and Wilkins, 2001:pp579–646.

Tew KD, Colvin OM, Chabner BA. Alkylating agents. In Chabner BA, Longo DL, eds. Cancer Chemotherapy and Biotherapy, Principles and Practice. Philadelphia, Lippincott Williams and Wilkins, 2001:pp374–414

Verweij J, den Hartigh J, Pinedo HM. Antitumor antibiotics. In Chabner BA, Collins JM, eds. Cancer Chemotherapy, Principles and Practice. Philadelphia, JB Lippincott, 1990:pp382–396.

CLINICAL TRIALS – PRINCIPLES AND APPLICATIONS

A clinical trial is a scientific study designed to answer important clinical and biological questions and is carried out by protocol, a written guideline for the study. The protocol, if properly followed, insures that the study is carried out consistently between investigators and between study sites. Good clinical practice (GCP) is an international quality standard for the design, conduct, recording, analysis, and reporting of clinical trials that provides assurance that the data and reported results are accurate (FDA, 1997). The protocol defines the essential elements of the study and how it will be conducted. In the treatment of cancer, clinical trials provide the only scientific mechanism to test the effectiveness of new therapies and are a necessary corollary to laboratory research. This chapter focuses on clinical oncology research, drug development in the United States, and the implementation and conduct of a clinical trial.

Conducting clinical trials requires an evidenced-based approach in order to make informed decisions. Such informed decisions can only be made if patients are approached about participation in clinical trials, if patients agree to participate in clinical trials, and the clinical trials are completed. The chance of discovering successful anticancer therapies and building on current knowledge without the use of clinical trials is very unlikely. Rapid improvement in the treatment of patients with cancer will only be achieved through the widespread participation of physicians and patients in clinical trials. Treatment of patients with nonstandard or modified standard regimens (i.e., "ad hoc" treatments) does not contribute useful information about the safety or effectiveness of the treatment (Hanks, 1984). Furthermore, some would consider these practices to be potentially dangerous because the patients are not monitored as they would be if participating in a study; quality assurance measures are not in place; and data safety monitoring does not occur as it does with a clinical trial.

PATIENT ENROLLMENT TO CLINICAL ONCOLOGY TRIALS

In the United States, the enrollment of adult patients to clinical oncology trials remains at an unacceptably low level. Over a decade ago it was estimated that no more than 3% of all cancer patients were enrolled to a clinical trial (Gelber & Goldhirsch, 1988; Hunter, 1987; Wittes & Friedman, 1988). The percentage of patients enrolled has not changed much since then (Lichter et al, 1999). In the United States the majority of patients with cancer receive their treatment outside of a cancer center/university setting. The initial data from the National Cancer Institute (NCI) on the Community Clinical Oncology Program (CCOP) showed that approximately 19% of the patients for whom there is a clinical trial were enrolled onto the study (Hunter, 1987).

Currently, 45% of the approximately 20,000 patients enrolled in Cooperative Group studies were enrolled through the NCI-funded CCOP (Scott et al, 2000). Over the years cooperative oncology groups have enrolled approximately 10% to 30% of potentially eligible patients for whom there is a clinical trial (Wittes & Friedman, 1988). Participation rates are especially low among the socially disadvantaged and racial/ ethnic minority groups (Giuliano et al, 2000). African American men enrolled to a prostate cancer prevention trial represented 4% of the total randomized population compared to the goal of 8% (Moinpour et al, 2000).

A survey, conducted by the American Society of Clinical Oncology (ASCO), indicated that 80% of those who responded to the survey participated in clinical research (i.e., enrolled a patient to a clinical trial in the previous three years) (Lichter et al, 1999). One-third of the survey respondents worked at an academic center and 80% of all respondents were affiliated with a national oncology cooperative group (e.g., ECOG, SWOG, etc.). The respondents indicated that approximately 20% of their patients were eligible for an available clinical trial; one-half of these patients were approached for enrollment and one-half of the patients agreed and were enrolled to a clinical trial (i.e., 5% of the patient population). "Lack of protected time for clinical research" was most often cited as a reason for not enrolling a patient to a clinical trial, followed by restrictive eligibility criteria and availability of nurses and data managers. Respondents indicated that managed care did not have much of an influence on the enrollment of patients.

Of 276 assessable patients from an academic medical center in the United States, approximately 62% of the patients were considered for enrollment to a clinical trial (Lara et al, 2001). A clinical trial was available to approximately one-half of the patients who were considered for enrollment (i.e., one-third of all patients seen). Approximately 75% of patients for whom a trial was available were eligible for the trial and of these patients, one-half agreed to participate. Thus, of all patients seen at an academic cancer center, 14% of the patients were enrolled to a clinical trial. The most common reason patients gave for declining participation was a desire for a different treatment (70%).

A summary of reasons cited for lack of enrollment of patients onto clinical trials is shown in Box 2-1.

BOX 2-1

REASONS FOR LACK OF PATIENT ENROLLMENT TO ONCOLOGY CLINICAL TRIALS

Lack of protected time for clinical research
Restrictive eligibility criteria
Lack of research nurses and data managers
Poor performance status of the patient
Perception that a clinical trial was not available for the patient
Expense and complexity of monitoring and follow-up
Extra time involved needed to discuss protocol
Practical difficulties with the protocol (e.g., procedures, data collection)
It may harm the doctor-patient relationship
Difficulty with informed consent
Dislike of open discussions about uncertainty
Limited financial support for research activities
Concern with the design of the study
Personal responsibilities if one of the treatments in a comparative trial is
    found to be unequal
Lack of the ability to generalize results
Lack (or perceived lack) of third-party reimbursement
Patient prefers a different treatment
Patient does not live near the study center

PERCEPTIONS ABOUT CLINICAL ONCOLOGY TRIALS

The majority of patients and the public continue to have favorable views regarding the values of clinical research (Cassileth, 1982; Comis et al, 2001; Trauth et al, 2000). Patients participate in clinical trials primarily because they hope to attain direct therapeutic benefit (Daugherty et al, 1995). Patients may participate in clinical trials to help other patients who will develop a similar medical condition in the future, to take advantage of increased monitoring as a part of a clinical study, to obtain a second opinion about their disease, and for many other reasons. Patients most often refuse to take part in a clinical trial or withdraw from one because of real or perceived factors related to the treatment.

Surveys of the general public (i.e., potential clinical trials participants) reveal that approximately 60% to 80% would be willing to take part in a medical research study focusing on a new treatment for their cancer (Comis et al, 2001; Trauth et al, 2000). In one survey 30% of respondents were undecided and 12% expressed an unwillingness to participate in a clinical trial (Trauth et al, 2000). Respondents who were willing to participate in a clinical trial were more likely to have a relative or friend who has the illness, to be between 35 and 64 years old, to have prior experience with participation in a clinical trial, to have a favorable attitude toward the use of human subjects in medical research, and believe that diverse types of persons participate in clinical trials. Persons who were not willing to participate in a clinical trial were more likely not to have a college degree, not to have a favorable attitude toward the use of humans in medical research, and not to believe that the well-being of participants is the primary concern of researchers.

LOCAL ADVANTAGES OF CLINICAL ONCOLOGY RESEARCH

Advantages of a clinical trials program, from a community hospital perspective, may include improved internal and external marketing of the cancer program, stimulation and education of staff, and improved patient care (Chingos, 2002). The requirements of a successful clinical oncology research program include:

- a "physician champion" who is responsible for the success of the program.
- making wise choices regarding collaborators.
- participation in an NCI-sponsored cooperative oncology group.
- participation in selected pharmaceutical industry trials, which can assist in the funding of the clinical research program.
- wise choices regarding studies to activate (i.e., activating studies that are likely to accrue patients will maximize the efforts that are required in the approval and conduct of clinical trials).
- hiring a clinical data manager who can assist with scheduling of patient visits and evaluations required by the protocols.
- hiring a full-time, nonclinical data manager to complete case report forms and handle administrative aspects of the clinical trials program.

ACCESS TO CLINICAL ONCOLOGY RESEARCH STUDIES

Availability and access to clinical trials by practicing oncologists is a problem that limits the enrollment of patients (Lichter et al, 1999; Scott et al, 2000). Currently, there are many sources where one can access information regarding clinical oncology trials. The NCI's Physician's Data Query (PDQ) system has been available for over 15 years as a major on-line source to locate the availability of clinical trials. Access to the PDQ database is available through the National Cancer Institute's website (see Box 2-2).

BOX 2-2

SELECTED CLINICAL TRIALS WEBSITES

ALL TRIALS

American Society of Clinical Oncology, http://www.ASCO.com

Cancer Links, http://www.CancerLinks.com

Centerwatch, http://www.Centerwatch.com

Food and Drug Administration, Cancer Liaison Program,
    http://www.fda.gov/oashi/home.html

http://www.FDA.gov

National Cancer Institute, http://www.NCI.NIH.gov/clinical_trials
    http://cancertrials.nci.nih.gov/

Physicians Data Query, http://www.PDQ.com

People Living With Cancer, http://www.PLWC.org

CANCER-SPECIFIC TRIALS

American Brain Tumor Association, http://www.abta.org/

Brain Tumor Clinical Trials, http://www.virtualtrials.com

National Brain Tumor Foundation, http://www.braintumor.org/

National Alliance of Breast Cancer Organizations (NABCO),
    http://www.nabco.org/trials/

Colon Cancer Alliance, http://www.ccalliance.org/

National Kidney Cancer Association, http://www.nkca.org/index.stm

The Leukemia & Lymphoma Society, http://www.leukemia-lymphoma.org/

Lymphoma Research Foundation of America, http://www.lymphoma.org/

International Myeloma Foundation, http://www.myeloma.org/

US Too International Inc. Prostate Cancer Support Groups,
    http://www.ustoo.com/ctlist.html

SELECTED NCI DESIGNATED CANCER CENTERS

Alabama, Birmingham: UAB Comprehensive Cancer Center,
        http://www.ccc.uab.edu/

Arizona, Tucson: Arizona Cancer Center, http://www.azcc.arizona.edu/

California, Durate: City of Hope, Beckman Research Institute,
    http://www.cityofhope.org/

California, Los Angeles: Jonsson Comprehensive Cancer Center at UCLA,
    http://www.cancer.mednet.ucla.edu/

California, Los Angeles: USC/Norris Comprehensive Cancer Center,
    http://www.uscnorris.com/

California, Orange: Chao Family Comprehensive Cancer Center,
    http://www.ucihs.uci.edu/cancer/

California, Palo Alto: Stanford University School of Medicine,
    http://cancercenter.stanford.edu/

California, San Francisco: University of San Francisco Cancer Center,
    http://www.cc.ucsf.edu/trials/index.html

Colorado, Denver: University of Colorado Cancer Center,
    http://www.uch.uchsc.edu/uccc/welcome/index.html

Connecticut, New Haven: Yale University School of Medicine Cancer Center,
    http://info.med.yale.edu/ycc/

District of Columbia: Lombardi Cancer Research Center,
    http://www.Lombardi.georgetown.edu/

BOX 2-2

SELECTED CLINICAL TRIALS WEBSITES (*continued*)

SELECTED NCI DESIGNATED CANCER CENTERS (*continued*)

Florida, Tampa: H. Lee Moffitt Comprehensive Cancer Center,
  http://www.moffitt.usf.edu/

Illinois, Chicago: University of Chicago Cancer Research Center,
  http://www.uchospitals.edu/cancer.html

Illinois, Chicago: Robert H. Lurie Cancer Center of Northwestern University,
  http://www.lurie.nwu.edu/

Indiana, Indianapolis: Indiana University Cancer Center, http://www.iucc.iu.edu/

Iowa, Iowa City: Holden Comprehensive Cancer Center at the University of
  Iowa, http://www.uihealthcare.com/depts/cancercenter/

Maryland, Baltimore: Johns Hopkins Oncology Center,
  http://www.hopkinscancercenter.org/

Massachusetts, Boston: Dana–Faber/Harvard Cancer Center,
  http://www.dfci.harvard.edu/

Michigan, Ann Arbor: University of Michigan Comprehensive Cancer Center,
  http://www.cancer.med.umich.edu/

Michigan, Detroit: Barbara Ann Karmanos Cancer Institute,
  http://www.karmanos.org/

Minnesota, Minneapolis: University of Minnesota Cancer Center,
  http://www.cancer.umn.edu/

Minnesota, Rochester: Mayo Clinic Rochester, http://www.mayo.edu/cancercenter/

Nebraska, Omaha: University of Nebraska Medical Center/Eppley Cancer Center,
  http://www.unmc.edu/cancercenter

New Hampshire, Lebanon: Norris Cotton Cancer Center,
  http://www.dartmouth.edu/dms/nccc/index.htm

New Jersey, New Brunswick: The Cancer Institute of New Jersey,
  http://www.cinj.umdnj.edu

New York, Bronx: Albert Einstein Comprehensive Cancer Center,
  http://www.aecom.yu.edu/cancer/default.htm

New York, Buffalo: Roswell Park Cancer Center, http://www.roswellpark.org/

New York, New York: Kaplan Cancer Center, New York University Medical Center,
  http://kccc-www.med.nyu.edu

New York, New York: Memorial Sloan Kettering Cancer Center,
  http://www.mskcc.org/

New York, New York: Herbert Irving Comprehensive Cancer Center,
  http://www.ccc.columbia.edu/

North Carolina, Durham: Duke University Comprehensive Center,
  http://www.canctr.mc.duke.edu/

North Carolina, Winston-Salem: Wake Forest University Comprehensive Cancer
  Center, http://www.bgsm.edu/cancer

Ohio, Cleveland: Ireland Cancer Center, Case Western Reserve University,
  http://www.irelandcancercenter.org/

Ohio, Columbus: Arthur G. James Cancer Hospital & Richard J. Solove
  Research Institute, http:www.jamesline.com/

Oregon, Portland: Oregon Cancer Center, http://www.ohsu.edu/occ/

Pennsylvania, Philadelphia: University of Pennsylvania Comprehensive Cancer
  Center, http://www.oncolink.upenn.edu/

cont'd

BOX 2-2

SELECTED CLINICAL TRIALS WEBSITES (continued)

SELECTED NCI DESIGNATED CANCER CENTERS (continued)

Pennsylvania, Philadelphia: Fox Chase Cancer Center, http://www.fccc.edu/

Pennsylvania, Philadelphia: Kimmel Cancer Center, http://www.kcc.tju.edu/

Pennsylvania, Pittsburgh: University of Pittsburgh Cancer Institute, http://www.upci.upmc.edu/

Tennessee, Nashville: Vanderbilt–Ingram Cancer Center, http://www.mc.vanderbilt.edu/cancer/

Texas, Houston: M.D. Anderson Cancer Center, http://www.mdanderson.org/patients_public/clinical_trials/

Texas, San Antonio: San Antonio Cancer Center, http://www.ccc.saci.org/

Utah, Salt Lake City: Huntsman Cancer Institute, University of Utah, http://www.hci.utah.edu/

Vermont, Burlington: Vermont Cancer Center, University of Vermont, http://www.vtmednet.org/vcc/index.html

Virginia, Charlottesville: Cancer Center, University of Virginia, http://www.med.virginia.edu/medcntr/cancer/home.html

Virginia, Richmond: Massey Cancer Center, Virginia Commonwealth University, http://www.vcu.edu/mcc/

Washington, Seattle: Fred Hutchinson Cancer Research Center, http://www.fhcrc.org/

Wisconsin, Madison: University of Wisconsin Comprehensive Cancer Center, http://www.cancer.wisc.edu/

In addition, advocacy groups have websites for each type of malignancy (e.g., renal cancer, breast cancer, pancreas cancer, etc.), as do all of the comprehensive cancer centers in the United States. Recently, ASCO has launched a website called People Living With Cancer (HYPERLINK http://www.plwc.org). This website is another useful place to locate information regarding clinical trials. The US Food and Drug Administration has recently begun an initiative whereby it provides information on active clinical trials for patients with life-threatening diseases. A listing of several internet sites where clinical trial information can be found is provided in Box 2-2.

COSTS ASSOCIATED WITH CLINICAL ONCOLOGY RESEARCH

Studies conducted at the Mayo Clinic in Rochester, Minnesota (Wagner et al, 1999), at the Kaiser-Permanente in California (Fehrenbacher et al, 1999), and in Chicago (Bennett et al, 2001) indicate that the patient care costs associated with a clinical trial are similar to the costs for patients who do not participate in a clinical trial. In the study conducted in California, the average patient care cost for study participants was approximately $17,000 per year; for nonparticipants the average patient care cost was approximately $16,500 per year.

The costs to the institution that conducts clinical oncology research are considerable. In the survey by ASCO, respondents indicated that a total of approximately 4,000 hours was needed to enroll and follow 20 patients on a clinical trial (i.e., 200 hours per patient or 2 full-time equivalents for a 20-patient study) (Lichter et al, 1999). For all studies, direct labor costs were estimated to be $2,000 per patient. However, twice as much in monitoring activities and telephone time was associated with studies sponsored by pharmaceutical companies compared to government-sponsored (i.e., cooperative group) trials. Respondents felt that $6,000 to $7,000 was reasonable reimbursement for a pharmaceutical company-sponsored study. The effort required of clinical research staff has been confirmed by a multicenter study of the National Cancer Institute of Canada (Roche et al, 2002). Sponsor and phase of the study were strong predictors of workload, with pharmaceutical company-sponsored and phase I studies requiring the greatest amount of effort from the clinical research staff.

CLINICAL ONCOLOGY RESEARCH AND INSURANCE REIMBURSEMENT

The US Institute of Medicine released a report that recommended that Medicare reimburse "routine care for patients in clinical trials in the same way it reimburses for routine care of patients not in clinical trials" (Aaron & Gelband, 2000). Over the years, reimbursement policies of insurance companies, health maintenance organizations (HMOs), and Medicare have adversely affected physician and patient participation in clinical trials (Friedman & McCabe, 1992; Lara et al, 2001; McCabe & Friedman, 1989). Refusal to reimburse for the clinical care costs of clinical trial participants is a shortsighted approach that suppresses patient recruitment to clinical trials and slows the advancement of the field of oncology. Practitioners who find that insurance company or HMO policies impede their ability to enroll patients onto a study should notify the principal investigator. Efforts to remedy the situation should be undertaken by the principal investigator and appropriate cancer center/university personnel. Although it appears that most clinical care costs are reimbursed (Lichter et al, 1999), there is evidence that insurance reimbursement policies are still a problem that needs to be corrected (Goldman et al, 2001; Lara et al, 2001). It is also possible that changes in government administrations could roll back Medicare reimbursement policies that currently support reimbursement for the routine costs of care for patients participating in most cancer clinical trials (Anon, 2002; Du et al, 2002). It is recommended that third-party payers reimburse for the costs associated with the clinical care of all cancer clinical trials.

WHAT CAN BE DONE TO IMPROVE PATIENT PARTICIPATION IN CLINICAL ONCOLOGY TRIALS?

Today, more than ever before, patients are more informed about their disease and the available treatment options. Consequently, patients take a more active role in their treatment. Patients should know the importance of clinical trials and be more educated regarding the clinical trial process. Patients who are educated to the clinical trials process are more likely to participate in a randomized clinical trial (Ellis et al, 2001). The availability of clinical trials to the community-based oncologist needs to expand. Clinical trials need to be easier to conduct. Patient selection criteria need to contain only the essential elements and not be overly restrictive. Support (i.e., data management support) for community-based clinical oncologists needs to be improved dramatically. The potential benefits of increasing patient accrual in clinical trials are expansion of the number of trials, rapid completion of the trials, and rapid transfer of results from the investigational stage to routine practice. The National Cancer Institute has initiated several programs to increase patient enrollment to clinical trials including, but not limited to, broadening access to clinical trials, providing education regarding clinical trials, streamlining protocol development and submission procedures, reducing data capture requirements, and automating data systems. The reader is referred to the

NCI website (HYPERLINK http://www.nci.nih.gov/) for additional information regarding these initiatives.

Institutions should strive to improve their contribution to clinical trials. Institutions should evaluate the reasons why they have not been successful at enrolling patients onto clinical trials and develop strategies for overcoming these shortcomings. Priority should be given to invigorating the enthusiasm of previously and/or presently active physicians. Increased patient accrual from noninstitutional practitioners may be enhanced through awareness, availability, applicability, and collaboration. Several methods may be useful in enhancing public awareness of the studies available, primarily through mailings, news media, public appearances (e.g., tumor boards, grand rounds), and telephone calls. Principal investigators need to take an active role in insuring that their studies are completed on time. Increased public relations efforts should be directed at surgeons and primary care physicians who refer patients with cancer for further treatment.

Studies should be made as applicable and as practical as possible (George, 1996). Elimination of extraneous testing procedures, reduction of the number of eligibility criteria, and elimination of nonessential data collection can make clinical trials more palatable to all participants and increase accrual to the clinical trial (Joseph, 1994). Reducing the number of eligibility criteria has been cited as a method for increasing patient enrollment, allowing broader generalizations of study results, and reducing the complexity and costs of patient participation (George, 1996). Relaxation of unnecessary restrictions on treating patients at the cancer center should be done if medically and logistically possible, provided that the quality of the data can be ensured. Institutions interested in increasing patient accrual from community participants should critically evaluate studies that require that patients be treated and/or evaluated solely at the main institution. Those who participate in a clinical trial need to be informed of its progress. Regular meetings among collaborators and frequent updates can be positive influences on patient accrual to clinical trials.

DRUG DEVELOPMENT AND THE PHASES OF CLINICAL TRIALS

In the United States, Canada, the European Union, and other countries, drugs and biological agents become commercially available only after preclinical testing (i.e., studies on animals and laboratory models) followed by clinical trials in man. Major efforts have been made to standardize (or harmonize) the requirements of these stages of drug development (FDA, 1997). In the following section this process is briefly described.

PRECLINICAL EVALUATION OF DRUGS FOR THE TREATMENT OF CANCER

The aim of preclinical testing is to evaluate the effectiveness and toxicity of a drug or biological agent before it is administered to humans. The drug-development program of the NCI has changed from the traditional test system of in vivo animal screening to a panel of tumor cell lines derived from human malignancies. Cell line screening helps identify new drugs but also allows targeted testing of drugs for patients with a particular tumor type. Acceleration of the testing of treatments through large-scale national trials in specific cancers is the goal of these efforts. In addition, as the data accumulate on the biochemical and genetic features of drug resistance, new cell lines with those features are added to the screening process. Development of cytostatic and "targeted" agents will involve preclinical studies to determine the concentration needed to inhibit the target.

Preclinical toxicology studies are also done in at least two species (usually mouse or rat and dog). These studies are performed to determine dose-limiting toxicities, the extent of various toxicities, and the LD10 (i.e., dose of drug that is lethal to 10% of the animals). These studies are essential because they allow for an estimation of a safe starting dose for human studies (Grieshaber & Marsoni, 1986).

For additional information regarding the screening of drugs and biological agents the reader is referred to the NCI's website (http://www.fda.gov) and the FDA's website (http://www.fda.gov).

PHASE I TRIALS OF CYTOTOXIC AGENTS

The major endpoints of a phase I trial are to evaluate acute toxicity, establish the dose-limiting toxicity (DLT), establish the maximum tolerated dose (MTD), and utilize pharmacological data to guide the design of future studies. These endpoints need to be attained for each dosing schedule (e.g., once every three weeks, once daily for five days every three weeks, etc.). Because of their narrow therapeutic index, phase I trials of the heretofore "traditional" antineoplastic drugs differ from the phase I testing of drugs intended for other conditions by virtue of the fact that patients must be used instead of normal volunteers. With the advent of drugs that exert antitumor effects through mechanisms that do not involve DNA or RNA damage (e.g., EGFR inhibitors), some of these early trials have been conducted in normal volunteers. In the field of oncology, it is desirable that phase I trials in patients conducted with therapeutic intent. It has been recognized that approximately 60% of the patients do not receive a biologically active dose with the use of the original phase I study designs (i.e., modified Fibonacci design) (Smith, 1996). Objective responses are uncommon (i.e., overall response rate is approximately 4%), and the majority of responses occur at or near the dose recommended for evaluation in future studies (Smith, 1996). Because of this, phase I trial designs have been modified with the intent of maximizing the number of patients who receive a therapeutic dose. The initial drug dose is traditionally one-tenth of the murine LD10. Current phase I designs utilize a rapid (or accelerated) escalation of the dose until a clinically significant adverse event is observed (Eisenhauer et al, 2000). Typically, one patient is enrolled to each dose level until a grade 2 (or in some designs a grade 3) adverse event is observed. When clinically significant toxicity is observed, at least three patients will be enrolled to all subsequent dose levels. When a dose-limiting toxicity (DLT) occurs in one of three patients, up to six patients are enrolled to the dose level. When two patients develop dose-limiting toxicity at a particular dose level, the trial is stopped. The dose level prior to the level that caused DLT is the MTD (i.e., the dose used for phase II studies). One of the accelerated phase I dose escalation schemes is shown in Table 2-1. Other methods by which to select a safe starting dose and to evaluate different treatment schedules for phase I trials have been proposed and/or evaluated (Eisenhauer et al, 2000).

PHASE I TRIALS OF CYTOSTATIC AGENTS

Several cytostatic agents have undergone initial evaluation using the "typical" phase I design that is used for cytotoxic agents. The wisdom of this approach has been questioned because the maximum toxic dose may not be necessary to elicit response (Korn et al, 2001). In addition, response may not be the ultimate objective with the use of these agents. Certain agents, such as vaccines (which are unlikely to produce many adverse events), probably do not need to be evaluated for toxicity in a dose-escalating phase I study (Simon et al, 2001). In addition, cytostatic drugs are more likely to be administered over a long period of time, in contrast to cytotoxic agents.

TABLE 2-1

PHASE I DOSE ESCALATION, ONE (OF SEVERAL) ACCELERATED METHODS

Dose Level	Patient Enrolled	Outcome
1 = 1n (e.g., 1 mg/kg);	1	No toxicity
2 = 2n (e.g., 2 mg/kg)	1	No toxicity
3 = 4n (e.g., 4 mg/kg)	1	No toxicity
4 = 8n (e.g., 8 mg/kg)	1	Grade 2 toxicity
5 = 16n (e.g., 16 mg/kg)	1	Grade 3 toxicity
(DLT). Expand Dose Level 5	2	No DLT
6 = 16n x 1.4 (40% increase) (e.g., 22.4 mg/kg)	3	DLT in one patient
Expand Dose Level 6	Up to 3	If one additional DLT, dose level 5 is the MTD. If no additional DLT, continue enrollment at Dose Level 7.

DLT = dose-limiting toxicity
MTD = maximum tolerated dose
Modified from: Eisenhauer EA, O'Dwyer PJ, Christian M, et al: Phase I clinical trial design in cancer drug development. J Clin Oncol 18: 684–692, 2000.

Alternative phase I study designs (such as the use of well-defined biological endpoints) have been proposed and/or are under evaluation (Korn et al, 2001).

PHASE II TRIALS OF CYTOTOXIC AGENTS

Phase II trials are intended to determine antitumor activity, gather information on dose response, and further evaluate the safety of the drug. The chances of detecting an active drug are best when the phase II agent is administered before other treatments have been given. Patients who are eligible for phase II trials are untreated or minimally pretreated patients. Most are patients with malignancies for which chemotherapy has shown little or no benefit, such as renal cell carcinoma, non-small-cell lung cancer, melanoma, or pancreatic cancer. Phase II studies in patients with other malignancies will typically be conducted following failure of the primary (i.e., first-line) treatment. Typically, a phase II study is conducted in two steps. During the first step a pre-defined number of patients are enrolled and each patient is evaluated for antitumor activity. If a 20% response rate were thought to be clinically significant, then at least one response in 15 patients would be necessary to continue the study to the second step. If no responses were observed in the first 15 patients it could be concluded with 95% certainty that the drug has a response rate less than 20%. During the second step, 15 or more patients are enrolled to more precisely define the response rate. Thus, at the end of a phase II trial, specific knowledge regarding tumor activity, as well as administration techniques, precautions, modifications of dose and scheduling, predicted acute toxicity, and the necessary supportive care are more clearly defined, and whether or not the drug is developed further is decided. The precise number of patients to enroll to each step of the study is dependent on other factors and the reader is referred to other sources for this information (Simon, 1997).

PHASE II TRIALS OF CYTOSTATIC AGENTS

Drugs that cause disease stabilization as the "best response" cannot be evaluated in the manner where preliminary antitumor activity is assessed by the presence or absence of objective responses. The endpoint of phase II studies of cytostatic agents could be the 1-year survival rate (Korn et al, 2001). If the 1-year survival rate is not appropriate for the malignancy to be evaluated, alternative endpoints (e.g., clinical benefit, symptom improvement, quality of life, time to progression) have been proposed.

RANDOMIZED PHASE III TRIALS

Randomized phase III trials define the role of a drug in a cancer treatment regimen. For example, the effectiveness of a drug may be studied by comparing it with another treatment or combining it with a standard treatment regimen. In phase III comparative studies, patients are randomized to receive one of the treatments to be evaluated. Evaluation of the drug's impact on survival, assessment of rates of response, duration of response, toxicity, and quality of life are all elements that are used to determine the preferred treatment in a comparative study. The primary endpoint has traditionally been survival. However, more recently in the US anticancer drugs have been approved for several other endpoints (Johnson et al, 2002). When the study has been completed, it should be known whether the treatment is equal to or better than the standard therapy, whether it produces equivalent or less toxicity, and whether it has a significant positive effect on the quality of life.

PHASE IV TRIALS

Phase IV trials are post-marketing studies. Their endpoints are often aimed at defining new uses, dosing schedules, treatment combinations, and additional information about the long-term safety of a commercially available drug or biological agent.

CONDUCTING A CLINICAL TRIAL

"If clinical trials are worth doing, then they are worth doing well" (Wittes, 1986). Clinical trials are experiments that are no less important than a laboratory experiment. Thus to protect data quality, clinical trials must be designed and conducted with many of the same assurances that occur in the design and conduct of a laboratory experiment (Ungerleider & Ellenberg, 1997). This is often referred to as good clinical practice, for which guidelines have been established (FDA, 1997). A clinical trial has many components, including, but not limited to, the following:

- planning and development
- patient enrollment and treatment
- maintenance of source documentation
- data collection and management
- prospective monitoring
- assessment of response
- assessment and reporting of adverse events
- data and safety monitoring
- analysis and reporting of results.

Quality assurance mechanisms at every step are needed to insure that potential problems do not interfere with the progress of the study or the integrity of the data (Begg, 1997). Obviously, documentation of events in the medical record and data retrieval are vital components of clinical research. Most problems with data quality arise from lack of attentiveness, failure to maintain adequate source documentation (e.g., tumor measurements, adverse drug reactions, performance status, patient-administered drug therapy), and lack of adherence to protocol guidelines (Zepp & Mackintosh, 1996).

The quality of data generated from investigators who enroll small numbers of patients is occasionally inferior to that of participants who enroll a large number of patients. The investigators who enroll a significant number of patients acquire experience and familiarity with the treatment and study procedures. Thus, it is generally recommended that participants be required to enroll a predetermined number of patients to pharmaceutical-sponsored clinical trials. There is general agreement among investigators, however, that data quality can be maintained through clearly written, unambiguous protocols, strict adherence to patient selection criteria, close communication with the administrative center, effective pre-study orientation of participants, minimal patient eligibility criteria, and a well-trained research team. A discussion follows of some of the more important elements of the conduct of a clinical trial. For a more detailed discussion of clinical trials, see additional sources (Begg, 1997; FDA, 1997; Mulay, 2001; Simon, 1997; Spilker, 1991).

PROTOCOL DEVELOPMENT

Once the need for conducting a study has been established, the specific aims have been enumerated, and it has been determined that adequate resources are available, a plan for conducting the study must be written. There are many important issues to consider when writing a protocol, including, but not limited to:

- eligibility criteria
- definitions of response
- identification of study parameters
- details of treatment, including modifications and duration of treatment.

In addition, data forms, data retrieval schedules, communication, and orientation with participating investigators should be part of the usual study development procedures. As indicated earlier in this chapter, data collection is a detriment to clinical trial participation. The data to be collected should be essential to the evaluation of the safety and efficacy of the treatments. The FDA has published a "Guidance for Industry" which describes what it considers essential data for an investigational drug study (FDA, 2000). A data safety monitoring plan should be a part of every protocol document. Data safety monitoring is required for US government-sponsored clinical trials, and is discussed in more detail later in this chapter (NCIDEA, 2001). A protocol review checklist (Box 2-3) describes many of the questions that should be addressed when writing or reviewing a protocol.

BOX 2-3

PROTOCOL REVIEW CHECKLIST

PROTOCOL SECTION AND ISSUES TO BE ADDRESSED

SCHEMA

Can you tell what the research plan is from the schema?

Does the information provided coincide with information in other protocol sections?

INTRODUCTION AND RATIONALE

Does the introduction and background information provide convincing evidence that the study is worth doing?

Has information been provided concerning preclinical studies and previous clinical trials in humans?

Is the information provided accurate, current, and consistent with study objectives?

BOX 2-3

PROTOCOL REVIEW CHECKLIST (continued)

PROTOCOL SECTION AND ISSUES TO BE ADDRESSED (continued)

OBJECTIVES

Are the objectives of the study clearly stated? (i.e., what are the study endpoints?)

Do the objectives seem to be clinically relevant?

Do the objectives coincide with the background?

PATIENT SELECTION

Are the selection criteria clearly stated? (e.g., if patients with positive HIV serology are not to be enrolled, does this mean patients who are known to be HIV positive or does it mean that HIV serology will be evaluated in all patients?

Similarly, if patients with CNS metastasis are excluded, does this have to be documented by a pre-study CT/MRI of the brain in all patients or does it mean that patients with symptoms suggestive of CNS metastasis are evaluated by CT/MRI?)

Are unnecessary criteria excluded (e.g., life expectancy requirements and other subjective evaluations, obtaining pre-study tests within a particular time frame)?

PATIENT REGISTRATION

Is it clear how patient registration will be handled?

How are patients entered onto the study?

How is dose/treatment assignment handled?

Where applicable, are randomization procedures clearly described?

TREATMENT PLAN AND DRUG DOSE MODIFICATIONS

Is the drug treatment schedule clear and concise?

For drugs administered over consecutive days (e.g., daily for five days), is the daily dose clearly described?

Are drug administration guidelines provided to include route of administration, infusion solutions and concentrations, rate of infusion, and concomitant medications/hydration?

Are guidelines provided for dose calculation in obese patients?

Are dose-rounding guidelines provided?

Are other treatments (radiotherapy, surgery) clearly described? (i.e., can you discern the sequence of therapies given?)

Are there guidelines that detail procedures to follow when a drug is administered at a "satellite" institution or clinic?

Are criteria for the use of colony-stimulating factors (e.g., G-CSF, GM-CSF) necessary/included and, if included, are the guidelines appropriate for the treatment regimen?

Would sample drug orders be useful for clarifying drug administration guidelines and if so, are they available?

For double-blind studies, are there procedures for breaking the blind?

Can you modify drug doses with certainty based on the criteria given? (i.e., if dose modification is based on nadir blood counts, are nadir blood counts always obtained?)

If dose modification is based on toxicity grading, is the potential toxicity routinely assessed?

Are dose modifications required for adverse events thought to be unrelated to the treatment?

Should additional criteria be added?

Should any criteria be deleted?

cont'd

BOX 2-3

PROTOCOL REVIEW CHECKLIST *(continued)*

PROTOCOL SECTION AND ISSUES TO BE ADDRESSED *(continued)*

TREATMENT PLAN AND DRUG DOSE MODIFICATIONS *(continued)*

What should be done when no criterion is listed for a particular toxicity?

Are investigators allowed to administer an additional course of treatment after an initial assessment of response that may indicate progressive disease?

DATA SAFETY MONITORING AND ADVERSE EVENT REPORTING

Is there a data safety monitoring section in the protocol?

Are monitoring and reporting guidelines included and are they appropriate for the study phase?

If this is a phase III study, is there an independent data safety monitoring board (DSMB)? Are the procedures of the DSMB described?

Are adverse drug reaction (i.e., serious adverse event) reporting requirements included and are they consistent with current NCI or FDA policies?

MEASUREMENT OF EFFECT/DEFINITIONS OF RESPONSE

Are the response criteria clearly described?

Do the response definitions apply to the patients under study?

Are response assessments made at times that coincide with the definitions of response? (e.g., if two assessments two months apart are required for response categorization, are these assessments made as described?)

STUDY PARAMETERS

Is it clear when all the tests are due?

Are all tests required for eligibility determination listed as being due "pre-study"?

Are some tests unnecessary?

Is the frequency of testing excessive for certain parameters (e.g., CT scans every four to six weeks)?

Does the testing schedule coincide with the treatment plan, or does it complicate matters?

Are the required tests listed in one section of the protocol?

DRUG INFORMATION

Is the information necessary for investigational drug procurement provided (e.g., dosage forms, availability)?

Is the pharmaceutical information complete? (e.g., is information provided on storage requirements, admixture stability in dry form and in solution, and compatibility/incompatibility?)

Is there an omission of new drug information, such as drug interactions, that should be provided in the protocol?

Is the drug information provided complete and accurate?

Is the drug information provided applicable to this particular protocol?

STATISTICAL CONSIDERATIONS

Is a summary of the statistical analysis plan provided?

Are the primary and secondary endpoints of the study clearly defined?

Is it clear how many patients are to be accrued to achieve the study endpoint(s)?

Is information provided concerning handling of dropouts, ineligible patients, stopping rules, and interim analyses?

Including the time necessary for follow-up, how long will it take to complete this study?

BOX 2-3

PROTOCOL REVIEW CHECKLIST (*continued*)

PROTOCOL SECTION AND ISSUES TO BE ADDRESSED (*continued*)

DATA COLLECTION FORMS/RECORDS TO BE KEPT

Are the data collection forms (i.e., case report form) described?

Is the case report form (CRF) present for review?

Is there a manual that describes how the CRF pages are to be completed?

What are the expectations regarding CRF completion and submission to the
   sponsor?

If a patient diary would be useful in documenting compliance with patient
   self-administered medications, is one available?

Is the patient diary too complex, or is it designed in a way to minimize omissions?

REFERENCES

Are the references current and complete?

Should any references not listed be included?

Are all the references cited in the protocol listed?

CONSENT FORM

Are all essential elements present?

Are all the adverse events provided by the sponsor or NCI described in
   the consent form?

Are the study procedures (i.e., evaluations, visits, etc.) described in the consent
   form and are they the same as those described in the protocol?

THE RESEARCH TEAM

Before initiation of patient enrollment, the principal investigator needs to have a group
of individuals who will plan a strategy for collection of data and monitoring the study
(Begg, 1997; Spilker, 1991). This group, the research team, should review the protocol, all the activities required to carry out the study, and define the responsibilities of
each member (Box 2-4). In addition, the protocol team should develop strategies for
monitoring and correcting unplanned situations, such as severe adverse drug reactions, protocol modifications and deviations, slow accrual, and so on. As discussed
later, the research team should meet regularly during the time frame of the study to
monitor data, and discuss potential problems and other matters in order to keep the
study time lines on track.

Formal patient registration procedures (i.e., eligibility checks) and data-collection
procedures must be firmly established before study activation. Principal investigators
must be actively involved in their studies by reviewing information on patient enrollment, reviewing patient data regularly, and getting involved in problem solving. In
addition, quality assurance guidelines (i.e., reviewing response data, recording tumor
measurements) must be clearly established before enrollment of patients begins.

PATIENT ENROLLMENT

Most cancer centers and universities involved in the conduct of clinical trials have
established a data-coordinating center whose responsibility is overseeing patient enrollment and managing the data from clinical trials. In smaller centers, data managers may
be employed but there may be no central data office. Whatever the case, there should
be a designated group of people whose task it is to conduct eligibility review of potential
study patients, enroll patients to the studies, and handle data-collection activities.

BOX 2-4

RESPONSIBILITIES OF THE CLINICAL TRIALS TEAM

PRINCIPAL INVESTIGATOR

Overall responsibility for the set-up and conduct of the study at his/her site/ network

Protocol development (in collaboration with a biostatistician)

Analyzing and reporting study results (in collaboration with a biostatistician)

ALL PHYSICIAN INVESTIGATORS

Assisting in protocol development and/or review

Patient assessment

Documentation of all interactions with patients in the medical record

Documentation in the medical record of the reasons for any deviation from the protocol (e.g., reasons for dose delays, dose modifications, reason off-study, etc.)

Recording tumor measurements and assessments of disease status in the medical record

Reporting adverse drug reactions

RESEARCH NURSES AND STUDY COORDINATORS

Assisting in protocol development and/or review

Screening patients before registration

Education of patients regarding study procedures, appointments, completion of diaries, etc.

Administration and collection of quality-of-life questionnaires

Review of physician's prescription

Ensuring protocol is followed

Reschedule tests, if necessary

Patient assessment and treatment

Documentation of all interactions and assessment of patients in the medical record and research records

Prospective monitoring and data retrieval

Coordination of specimen collection for pharmacokinetic or laboratory research studies

Completion of Sponsor's case report forms

Assistance with Sponsor's clinical research associate/monitor

ONCOLOGY/INVESTIGATIONAL DRUG PHARMACISTS

Assisting in protocol development and/or review

Proper receipt, storage, and dispensing of investigational drugs and biologics

Maintenance of drug accountability (dispensing) record forms

Insuring proper calculation of doses by rechecking the physician's prescription

Obtaining medication histories from "new" patients

Assistance with patient compliance efforts for drugs self-administered by patients

Education of patients regarding the investigational drug or biologic

SPONSORS OF CLINICAL TRIALS AND CLINICAL RESEARCH ORGANIZATIONS WHO EXECUTE AND/OR MONITOR THE TRIAL

Protocol development

Development of case report form and study manuals

Eliminating barriers to patient enrollment

   -Maximizing participation at the investigator's meeting

   -Collection of essential data on the case report form

BOX 2-4

RESPONSIBILITIES OF THE CLINICAL TRIALS TEAM (*continued*)

SPONSORS OF CLINICAL TRIALS AND CLINICAL RESEARCH ORGANIZATIONS WHO EXECUTE
AND/OR MONITOR THE TRIAL (*continued*)

  -Minimizing repeated telephone contact to obtain extraneous information not essential to the conduct of the study
  -Issuing timely data query requests (that assist in the proper recording of data on the case report form)
  -Minimizing data query requests for "self-evident" information (e.g., date of a CT scan that is a few days late)
  -Providing patient teaching materials and study aids
Training of investigators and their research teams
Patient registration/randomization
Monitoring (verifying case report form entries with the source documents)
Providing a clear definition of "clean patient data"
Assistance with purchase of study-specific items (e.g., drug administration sets if unique for the sponsor's drug)
Minimizing double work (e.g., use of a central laboratory for routine clinical laboratory assessments)

Their responsibilities should include the development and conduct of patient registration and quality control guidelines. Before activating a clinical trial, it is important to develop an eligibility checklist (i.e., a list of specific questions asked when patients are registered to clinical trials) to maximize the ratio of eligible to entered patients. Exceptions to eligibility criteria should not be necessary or allowed. The protocol should be amended if certain eligibility or exclusion criteria are found to be unnecessary. As each patient is enrolled onto the study, an eligibility check must be performed before treatment assignment is given or therapy is begun. In addition, the signed informed consent form should be retrieved and reviewed by the data-coordinating center, and documentation of on-study parameters (i.e., laboratory reports) should be reviewed before initiation of treatment. Review of the signed, informed consent form is intended to insure that the patient and investigator have signed and dated the form, that the most up-to-date version of the form has been used, and, where applicable (i.e., mandated by the IRB), the form has been signed and dated by a witness and/or parent/guardian.

Data-coordinating centers should maintain research (or shadow) charts that are separate from the medical record for all patients enrolled onto clinical trials. Elements of the research chart should include the completed eligibility checklist and copies of the source documents that verify patient eligibility. The research chart should also include registration (or randomization) information, a copy of the signed consent form, operative/pathology reports, study flow sheets, patient diaries, other critical study data (e.g., applicable physician and nurse progress notes, laboratory and radiology reports), and tests. The completed case report forms should also be maintained by the data-coordinating center.

SOURCE DOCUMENTS

As stated in the US Code of Federal Regulations (CFR), "An investigator is required to prepare and maintain adequate and accurate case histories that record all observations and other data pertinent to the investigation on each individual administered the investigational drug or employed as a control in the investigation" (CFR 312.62, 2001). Source documents are defined as original documents and records kept at the pharmacy, laboratories, and medical or technical departments involved in the clinical trial (CFR 312.62, 2001; FDA, 1997; Zepp & Mackintosh, 1996). Source documents may include progress notes, laboratory records, memoranda, patient diaries or evaluation checklists, pharmacy dispensing records, microfiches, photographic negatives, x-ray films, radiology reports, and microfilm or magnetic media. The use of flow sheets is generally not considered to be adequate source documentation unless the flow sheets are signed, dated, and accepted as a part of the official institutional medical record. Source documents contain clinical trial information that allows its accurate reporting, interpretation, and verification. Source documents support the accuracy of the data recorded on case report forms and reported to the sponsor of the clinical trial. Thus, case report forms should not be used as the primary place where source document information is recorded.

With regard to documenting administration of drugs utilized in a clinical trial, the investigator is required to include information on each patient's exposure to the drug, including the date (and time if relevant) of each administration and the quantity administered (FDA, 1997; Zepp & Mackintosh, 1996). In addition, documentation of drug administration should be independent of the flow sheet. Documentation of each dose of an oral or injectable medication self-administered by the patient at home, is often insufficient unless methods are in place to capture this information. In general, pharmacy dispensing records do not provide sufficient information to verify drug administration. Many institutions have found success in documenting patient self-administered medications by using patient diaries and frequent (i.e., weekly) communication with the patients that is documented in the medical record.

DATA COLLECTION AND MANAGEMENT

Although data retrieval will often be retrospective in nature, every attempt should be made to retrieve data on a prospective basis (i.e., at the end of the day the patient is in the clinic or shortly thereafter). Infrequent review of medical records does not lend itself to rapid dissemination of up-to-date information, prevention of future errors in protocol adherence, and maintenance of adequate source documentation.

Data retrieval and quality control are key elements in the conduct of a clinical trial. If the clinician obtains the required study parameters, administers treatment on schedule, and documents adverse effects of treatment, assessment parameters, and all protocol deviations in the medical record, the elements for an assessable patient are in place. When problems with the documentation of events and protocol adherence arise, retrospective chart reviews will not correct the problem. In many centers, prospective monitoring and data retrieval have been put in place to prevent this deficiency.

PROSPECTIVE MONITORING

Participation in clinical research must be made as painless as possible. Consideration should be given to methods that improve protocol adherence and source documentation, and simplify the clinician's efforts. Difficulties following study parameters may be decreased by using protocol-oriented computer systems, protocol-specific flow sheets, study calendars, and/or road maps. Protocol-specific flow sheets and/or study calendars should highlight the tests and procedures to obtain, and when to obtain them. Methods that improve documentation of events in the medical record should be devised. Standardizing the medical dictation format, utilizing patient diaries to collect information on self-administered medications, and including nurses and pharmacists on the protocol team can help improve prospective monitoring and data retrieval. All of the methods described should be implemented via direct communication between cancer center or university personnel (e.g., protocol managers and principal investigator) and the participating clinicians and his or her staff. Prospective monitoring and data retrieval can become a reality at off-site institutions through the use of facsimile machines. Investigators at these sites can send data (e.g., flow sheets and reports) as they are generated (i.e., before treatment decisions are made). As a result, questions regarding eligibility criteria and other elements of the protocol can be answered before problems arise.

REPORTING ADVERSE DRUG REACTIONS AND SERIOUS ADVERSE EVENTS

Adverse drug reactions (ADRs) and serious adverse events (SAEs) occur frequently in patients receiving cancer chemotherapy. Federal regulations and Institutional Review Board policies mandate prompt reporting of SAEs that occur as part of an investigational drug study or a study approved by the NCI or FDA. What constitutes an SAE may vary slightly from study to study. The current FDA definition of an SAE is an event that results in death, is life-threatening, results in hospitalization or prolongation of a hospital stay, is permanently disabling, results in a congenital anomaly, or results in a second malignancy. Adverse events are usually graded according to a five-point scale, with "0" being no adverse event, to "4" being a life-threatening adverse event. Fatalities are grade "5" events. The NCI Common Toxicity Criteria scale or modifications of it are often used to grade adverse events (http://ctep.cancer.gov/forms/ CTCManual_v4_10-4-99.pdf).

For studies sponsored by the NCI, the "NCI Guidelines for Reporting Adverse Drug Reactions" will apply (http://ctep.info.nih.gov/handbook/HandbookEPF.htm).

For all studies, an SAE that is unexpected (i.e., previously unreported) and is possibly, probably, definitely, or of undetermined relationship to the study agent must be reported promptly to the NCI (for NCI-sponsored studies) or to the FDA. The definition of "prompt" is usually within one to three working days of becoming aware of the event. Specific details regarding SAE reporting must be included in the protocol. If the study involves DNA molecules (i.e., gene transfer), additional reporting requirements apply. Investigators involved in this type of research must adhere to NIH Guidelines for Research Involving Recombinant DNA Molecules (HYPERLINK "http://grants.nih.gov/grants/policy/recombinantdnaguidelines.htm").

DATA AND SAFETY MONITORING

Mechanisms need to be in place to ensure that the clinical trial is going smoothly and to assess patient safety on a regular basis. Regular review should also insure that required data are being retrieved and properly recorded on the case report forms. The research team should meet regularly during the course of a clinical trial to make sure that these goals are accomplished. For a phase I study, regular meetings of the research team are often held on a weekly basis to assess patient enrollment, dose-limiting toxicities, and enrollment of patients to subsequent (escalated) dose levels. For phase II studies, less frequent meetings would be appropriate. It is mandatory that all phase III trials that are supported by the NCI be conducted with the oversight of an independent Data Safety Monitoring Board (DSMB) (Smith et al, 1997). In addition, all NCI-funded cancer centers are required to have an institutional Data Safety Monitoring Plan to insure that patient safety is protected for all clinical oncology trials (NCIDEA, 2001). Components of a data safety monitoring plan are described in Box 2-5.

2

CONDUCTING A CLINICAL TRIAL

BOX 2-5

COMPONENTS OF A DATA SAFETY MONITORING PLAN (DSMP)

Requirements (e.g., all protocols must have a DSMP, specific requirements for phase I, phase II, and phase III studies)

Elements (e.g., oversight responsibilities, description of processes)

Clinical trials organization (e.g., membership and responsibilities)

Committee(s) responsible for data safety monitoring (e.g., membership, reporting responsibilities, policies and procedures)

Adverse event reporting (e.g., policies/requirements for sponsors and for local IRB)

Data quality control (e.g., internal and/or external audits, independent review of response assessments)

Conflict of interest (e.g., identify, plan, or manage potential conflicts of interest through university/hospital policies)

ANALYSIS AND REPORTING OF STUDY RESULTS

Upon completion of the study the results should be analyzed and submitted for publication within a reasonable time frame, regardless of the outcome of the study. This is most relevant for post-marketing studies where the desired result is a publication that is positive. For phase III studies that are used to support a marketing application, the results are often submitted to the FDA prior to publication in a medical journal. Recently, concern has been raised that "negative" cancer trials were less likely to be published in a medical journal or their publication was significantly delayed when compared to cancer trials with positive results (Krzyzanowska et al, 2002). Most would consider this practice, if deliberate, to be unethical. A typical time frame for reporting of clinical trial results is analysis completed within four to six weeks of datalock and final report (or manuscript) completed six to eight weeks thereafter.

SUMMARY

Further advancement in the field of oncology will only be obtained by increasing the number of patients enrolled onto clinical studies. Poor patient enrollment and/or the provision of poor data jeopardize the scientific merit of the study. Ineligible patients, major protocol violations, and failure to obtain vital information render the data of a patient's clinical trial experience meaningless, and can be considered a breach of informed consent. There is general agreement among investigators, however, that data quality can be maintained by use of clearly written protocols and analysis plans, close communication with the administrative center, pre-study orientation of participants, strict and clear patient selection criteria, and a well-trained research team.

REFERENCES

Aaron HJ, Gelband H, eds. Extending Medicare reimbursement in clinical trials: Committee on Routine Patient Care Costs in Clinical Trials for Medicare Beneficiaries. Washington, DC, National Academy Press, 2000.

Anon. Medicare may cut support for cancer trials subjects. App Clin Trials 11(4): 24, 2002.

Begg CB. Research data management. In DeVita VT Jr, Hellman S, Rosenberg SA, eds. Cancer Principles and Practices of Oncology, 5th ed, vol. 1. Philadelphia, JB Lippincott, 1997: pp528–534.

Bennett CL et al. Clinical trials: are they a good buy? J Clin Oncol 19: 4330–4339, 2001.

Cassileth BR. Attitudes toward clinical trials among patients and the public. JAMA 248: 968–970, 1982.

Chingos JC. Seven steps to a successful clinical trials program. Oncol Issues 17: 22, 2002.

Code of Federal Regulations: Investigator record keeping and record retention. Title 21 CFR 4.01.01: §312.62 (b).

Comis R et al. Public attitudes about clinical trials. Proc Am Soc Clin Oncol 20: 243a, 2001.

Daugherty C et al. Perceptions of cancer patients and their physicians involved in phase I trials. J Clin Oncol 13: 1062–1072, 1995.

Du W, Gadgeel SM, Peters WP. Economic analysis of lung cancer clinical trial participation demonstrates cost-effectiveness but disparities by insurance coverage and race. Proc Am Soc Clin Oncol 21: 307a (abstract 1224), 2002.

Eisenhauer EA. Phase I clinical trial design in cancer drug development. J Clin Oncol 18: 684–692, 2000.

Ellis PM et al. Randomized clinical trials in oncology: understanding and attitudes predict willingness to participate. J Clin Oncol; 19: 3554–3561, 2001.

Fehrenbacher L et al. The cost of care in cancer clinical trials – a matched, controlled analysis of participation in selected national cooperative group trials. [ASCO website abstract No. 1610]. Available at: http://www.asco.org/prof/me/html/99abstracts/f_toc.htm

Food and Drug Administration, Guidance for Industry, E6 Good Clinical Practice: Consolidated Guideline. Fed Regist 62(90): 25691–25709, 1997. Also available on the FDA website (http://www.fda.gov).

Food and Drug Administration, Guidance for Industry, Cancer Drug and Biological Products – Clinical Data in Marketing Applications, 2000. (http://www.fda.gov/guidance/4332fnl.htm).

Friedman MA, McCabe MS. Assigning care costs associated with therapeutic oncology research: a modest proposal, J Natl Cancer Inst 84: 760–763, 1992.

Gelber RD, Goldhirsch A. Can a clinical trial be the treatment of choice for patients with cancer? J Natl Cancer Inst 80: 886–887, 1988.

George SL. Reducing patient eligibility criteria in cancer clinical trials. J Clin Oncol 14: 1364–1370, 1996.

Giuliano AR et al. Participation of minorities in cancer clinical trials. Ann Epidemiol 10: S22–34, 2000.

Goldman DP et al. Measuring the incremental cost of clinical cancer research. J Clin Oncol 19: 105–110, 2001.

Grieshaber CK, Marsoni S. Relation of preclinical toxicology to findings in early clinical trials. Cancer Treat Rep 70: 65–72, 1986.

Hanks GE. The dangers of ad hoc protocols. J Clin Oncol 2: 1177–1178, 1984.

Hunter CP. Selection factors in clinical trials: results from the Community Clinical Oncology Program physician's log. Cancer Treat Rep 71: 559–565, 1987.

Johnson JR, Williams G, Richard P. Endpoints for FDA approval of oncology drugs. Proc Am Soc Clin Oncol 21: 255a (abstract 1018), 2002.

Joseph RR. Viewpoints and concerns of a clinical trial participant. Cancer 74: 2692–2693, 1994.

Korn EL et al. Clinical trial designs for cytostatic agents: are new approaches needed? J Clin Oncol 19: 265–272, 2001.

Krzyzanowska MK, Pintilie M, Tannock I: Burying of unwanted results: a survey of more than 500 large randomized clinical trials presented at ASCO meetings to determine the probability and causes of failure to publish. Proc Am Soc Clin Oncol 21: 244a (abstract 973), 2002.

Lara PN Jr et al. Accrual patterns in cancer trials: identifying potential barriers. J Clin Oncol 19: 1728–1733, 2001.

Lichter AL, Schnipper L, Emanuel E. Presidential symposium: report of the Clinical Trials Subcommittee [ASCO virtual meeting/lecture website]. May 16, 1999. Available at: www.asco.org.

McCabe M, Friedman MA. Impact of third-party reimbursement on cancer clinical investigations: a consensus statement coordinated by the National Cancer Institute. J Natl Cancer Inst 81: 1585–1586, 1989.

Moinpour CM et al. Minority recruitment in prostate cancer prevention trial. Ann Epidemiol 10: S85–S91, 2000.

Mulay M: A Step-by-Step Guide to Clinical Trials. Sudbury, MA, Jones and Bartlett, 2001.

NCIDEA: Data and Safety Monitoring of Clinical Trials. Policy of the National Cancer Institute for Data and Safety Monitoring of Clinical Trials, March 11, 2001. http://deaninfo.nci.nih.gov/grantspolicies/datasafety.htm

2

REFERENCES

Roche K et al. Factors affecting workload of cancer clinical trials: results of a multi-center study of the National Cancer Institute of Canada Clinical Trials Group. J Clin Oncol 20: 545–556, 2002.

Scott J, Cooper M, Larson T. Making clinical trials financially viable. Oncol Issues 15: 14–16, 2000.

Simon RM. Design and analysis of clinical trials. In DeVita VT Jr, Hellman S, Rosenberg SA, eds. Cancer Principles and Practices of Oncology, 5th ed., vol. 1. Philadelphia, JB Lippincott, 1997: pp513–521.

Simon RM et al. Clinical trial designs for the early clinical development of therapeutic cancer vaccines. J Clin Oncol. 19: 1848–1853, 2001

Smith MA et al. Role of independent data-monitoring committees in randomized clinical trials sponsored by the National Cancer Institute. J Clin Oncol 15: 2736–2743, 1997.

Smith TL: Design and results of phase I cancer trials: three-year experience of the MD Anderson Cancer Center. J Clin Oncol 14: 287–295, 1996.

Spilker B. Guide to Clinical Trials. New York, Raven Press, 1991.

Trauth JM et al. Public attitudes towards medical research studies. J Health Soc Policy 12: 23–43, 2000.

Ungerleider RS, Ellenberg SS. Cancer clinical trials: design, conduct, analysis, and reporting. In Pizzo PA, Poplack DG, eds. Principles and Practice of Pediatric Oncology, 3rd ed. Philadelphia, Lippincott-Raven, 1997:pp385–406.

Wagner JL et al. Incremental costs of enrolling cancer patients in clinical trials: a population-based study. J Natl Cancer Inst 91: 847–853, 1999.

Wittes RE. How we know what we (think we) know. J Clin Oncol 4: 827–829, 1986.

Wittes RE, Friedman MA. Accrual to clinical trials. J Natl Cancer Inst 80: 884–885, 1988.

Zepp VO, Mackintosh DR. Source documentation: a key to GCP compliance in clinical trials. App Clin Trials 5: 42–45, 1996.

CHEMOTHERAPY MEDICATION SAFETY

Medication safety has positioned its way into the spotlight in the delivery of healthcare within the last decade. In 1995, the foundation of oncology practice was rocked with the fatal event that occurred at a major cancer center in Boston, Massachusetts. The national media coverage of a fourfold chemotherapy overdose that resulted in the death of a well-known health reporter affected all disciplines involved in the delivery of care to the oncology patient. The publication of that error and others that followed has brought to the forefront of our daily activities the ultimate responsibility of incorporating safe medication practices into every aspect of the care we deliver.

Safe environments reduce the risk of adverse events. Ensuring patient safety therefore involves the establishment of operational systems and processes in the environment, which increase the reliability of patient care. In 1999, the Institute of Medicine (IOM) published a report that contained staggering statistics, estimating that up to 98,000 people die annually secondary to medical errors. Outpatients are more likely to die from medication errors than hospitalized patients and fatal errors are on the rise. The financial burden of medication errors is enormous; the total national cost of preventable medication errors is estimated to be between 17 and 29 billion dollars, of which half are healthcare costs (IOM, 1999). Medication error prevention is a relevant issue that needs prompt attention by all disciplines of the healthcare team.

The nationally profiled document published by the Institute of Medicine provides numerous recommendations including changes in error prevention, detection, and reporting, but the ultimate recommendation was to create safety systems via implementation of safe practices at the level at which care is being delivered. This chapter is designed to provide practical guidelines for practices and systems that should be considered for all oncology settings (i.e., hospital inpatient and outpatient, homecare, clinics, and private practices) to aid in the prevention and reduction of chemotherapy medication errors. Additionally, information regarding medication use reporting and analysis methods will be discussed.

MEDICATION ERRORS

A discussion of medication errors requires an understanding of the terminology commonly used. An error is a mistake or wrong action. The Institute of Medicine report defines an error of execution as the failure of a planned action to be completed as intended, or an error of planning as the use of the wrong plan to achieve an aim. An adverse event is an injury resulting from a medical intervention and not due to the underlying condition of the patient; an adverse drug event is an injury resulting from a medical intervention relating to a drug (Bates et al, 1997). Medication errors are a subset of adverse events, in that not all adverse events are medication errors. A medication error is defined as any preventable event that may lead to inappropriate medication use or patient harm while the medication is in the control of the healthcare professional, patient, or consumer (Cohen, 1998).

Medication errors can occur in the processes of prescribing, dispensing, and administering. The error types can include the wrong dose, wrong time, wrong drug, wrong patient, wrong route of administration, incorrect product preparation, and errors of omission. Research estimates that approximately 50% of medication errors are preventable (Rogers, 1999) and at least one death per day can be attributed to a medication error (FDA.gov).

CHEMOTHERAPY RISK FACTORS

All medications have inherent risks associated with their use; however, the nature of oncology treatments sets them apart from most other medications. Antineoplastic drugs, like certain other medications (phenytoin, aminophylline, digoxin), possess a narrow therapeutic range. Dosing errors above the range can cause patient harm or even death, while dosing errors below the therapeutic range can result in ineffective treatment. The risk associated with increased morbidity and mortality in oncology practice includes:

- the toxic potential of the drugs involved
- the variability in standard doses that are related to the disease state being treated
- combination regimens with variable schedules
- increased treatment of the elderly population
- many newer agents being used.

Changes in the practice of oncology over the last decade have also placed oncology patients at a greater risk for medication errors. These changes include:

- availability of many supportive care measures that allow oncologists to push dosing limits far beyond those of the past
- the complexity of oncology research protocols
- increased dose intensity
- the flux to outpatient or homecare of high dose therapy stem cell and bone marrow transplant patients
- oncology nurse staffing shortages.

Results of a mailed survey to oncology nurses reported that the most common chemotherapy errors included under- and overdosing, scheduling and timing, infusion rates, wrong drugs, omission of drugs, improper preparation, and drugs administered to the wrong patient (Schulmeister, 1999). A poor working environment also plays a role in chemotherapy errors. Environmental stressors that cause excessive noise, interruptions, and distractions set the stage for medication errors (ASHP, 1993). Understaffing, stress, and unclear orders have been identified as prime factors for nurses, related to potential or actual errors in chemotherapy administration (Schulmeister, 1999).

A SAFE SYSTEM

System issues are largely responsible for medication errors (Allard et al, 2002; Boyle et al, 2002). Safety literature speaks to working within a safe system, a system of multiple checks and balances. Errors reach patients through one or more series of system failures (Rogers, 1999). Examples include personnel in the system who did not follow the check and balance procedures as instructed, completely bypassing the system, or inadequate checks and rechecks. The treatment of an oncology patient may take place in a hospital, outpatient clinic, physician office, or by a homecare agency, and it is vital that the same level of quality, system checks, and oversight applies to any venue where drugs are stored, prepared, dispensed, or administered (ISMP Safety Alert, 2001b).

Multidisciplinary participation is critical to a successful chemotherapy process. The reduction of medication errors through standardized systematic methods has been recommended by the American Medical Association, the American Nurses Association, and the American Society of Health-System Pharmacists (ASHP). ASHP guidelines state:

> Medication errors are episodes in drug misadventuring that should be preventable through effective system controls involving pharmacists, physicians, and other prescribers, nurses, risk management personnel, legal counsel, administrators, patients and others in the organizational setting, as well as regulatory agencies and the pharmaceutical industry. This allows for safe, accurate, and efficient care of the oncology patient from all aspects of the healthcare team.

The term "collaborative practice" implies that the responsibility for safe chemotherapy delivery lies within the hands of the healthcare team including the physician, nurse, pharmacy personnel, and the patient. The goal for drug administration of chemotherapy and other medications is to administer the right drug to the right patient, in the right dose and dosage form at the right time (Cohen et al, 1996). One must not underestimate the importance of multidisciplinary communication upon safe and effective chemotherapy practice. Legible written communication between the physician and those who interpret the orders, communication between the entities that provide diagnostic information, and clear communication to the patient and families who are embarking upon chemotherapy are mandatory. The days of information dissemination on a need-to-know basis are over; those who are providing care must have all the information and tools necessary to perform within a safe system.

Safety does not reside in a person, device, or department, but emerges from the interactions of components of a system (IOM, 1999). The following discussion focuses on oncology issues and the daily processes that are employed to keep our patients and healthcare professionals protected.

In the realm of medication errors, the system comprises key areas that need to be assessed and constructed to be fail-safe for the chemotherapy process. These areas include drug procurement, education, prescribing, verification, compounding, dispensing, and administration.

DRUG PROCUREMENT

There are numerous steps that occur prior to any drug reaching a consumer; these steps involve the pharmaceutical company, the Food and Drug administration (FDA), and other regulatory agencies. They are responsible for identifying any drugs that become available with inherent error potential built-in due to name similarity or poor labeling/packaging design. Many errors have occurred due to nomenclature problems with similar-sounding drug names, for example, vincristine and vinblastine, mithramycin and mitomycin, and the term platinum compounds that includes both cisplatin and carboplatin, of which the dosing is very different.

Proper labeling avoids drug error risks. There have been at least three documented vinorelbine overdoses due to poor labeling (Cohen, 1995). While investigational, vinorelbine was distributed as a 10 mg per 1 mL and a 50 mg per 5 mL vial size. The drug label of both vials indicated a concentration of 10 mg per mL using a very prominent "10", without highlighting the total volume of 5 mL in the larger vial. As a result, there were numerous assumptions that each vial contained 10 mg when in fact the total drug component was 50 mg in a 5 mL vial. The labeling on this drug has since been changed.

The Institute for Safe Medication Practices (ISMP) collects these types of errors, along with all others, and brings them to the attention of all other practitioners, and the regulating bodies that can play a role in decreasing error risk. One major change in labeling occurred due to errors involved with the fatal administration of intrathecal vincristine. It has been mandated that all manufacturers of this product provide, along with the drug vial, an outerwrap packaging that states the following: "Do not remove covering until moment of injection. Fatal if given intrathecally. For intravenous use only." Another ISMP success is the warning printed on the top of cisplatin vials to call the physician if the dose is >100 mg/m^2/cycle (Attilio, 1996).

Pharmacy personnel who are responsible for drug ordering and distribution must be involved with the safety process (Wong & Ignoffo, 1996). They need to inform staff members of the availability and/or purchase of different vial sizes, different concentrations, and manufacturer changes. Oral chemotherapy products should be stored separately from other medications and clearly labeled.

EDUCATION

A common component recognized in most error prevention literature is the importance of appropriate education for all healthcare providers (Cohen et al, 1996; ONS, 2001). Appropriately trained, knowledgeable, and qualified personnel caring for the oncology patient are of benefit to the chemotherapy process. Each educational experience will differ, respective to the discipline and individual responsibility within the chemotherapy drug process (prescribing, compounding, dispensing, administering). The physicians who prescribe chemotherapy should be board-certified or board-eligible oncologists/hematologists, with a working knowledge of the chemotherapy drug profiles. Physicians in acute care hospitals who prescribe chemotherapy for diagnoses outside of cancer (i.e., multiple sclerosis, arthritis) should have specific indications, drugs, and dose ranges within their prescribing authority and this information must be shared with all involved (Fischer et al, 1996). It is also recommended that an attending physician co-sign orders of first-year oncology fellows and advanced practice registered nurses (if the practice act in that state grants prescriptive authority) until competency is determined. Nurses should have experience in the care of oncology patients, with the motivation to become oncology certified nurses. Nurses administering chemotherapy need to demonstrate competency. They should be initially certified by the institution and re-certified annually (Frank-Stromborg & Christensen, 2001). Such a certification process is particularly vital when chemotherapy is being administered sporadically on nononcology units or to nononcology patients.

Ideally, hospital pharmacists who monitor oncology patients should be dedicated personnel with extensive education in the field of oncology therapeutics (Wong & Ignoffo, 1996). A board certification oncology specialty exam is offered and pharmacists practicing in oncology should be encouraged to pursue this certification. Most institutional pharmacies maintain a 24-7 schedule and therefore all pharmacists should be appropriately trained to evaluate, compound, and dispense chemotherapy in off-hours situations. The pharmacy technicians who are compounding chemotherapy need to prove competency, and be re-evaluated periodically. Certification courses should be developed to validate individual knowledge based on practitioner responsibility.

Level of experience and risk of medication error are related, with risk of error greater for inexperienced physicians, nurses, and pharmacists (Allard et al, 2002). Fellowship programs in oncology need to provide physicians with baseline education on cancer pharmacology, safety in order writing and prescribing, unique aspects of investigational drug delivery, and issues related to drug therapy for patients on clinical trials. Ongoing continuing education is also essential. Pharmacy, nursing, and physician personnel should all participate in educational sessions regarding novel drug therapies, investigational protocols, new guidelines for drug use, and reimbursement issues for high cost therapy. Annual interdisciplinary education is strongly recommended (Boyle et al, 2002), which can be used as a documented re-certification program for each discipline. Medication error and error prevention data must also be shared with staff. Collection of this data is only useful if it reaches those who use the system in which the improvement must be made. This also reinforces the fact that collection of error data is vital for positive change.

Healthcare provider education must be coupled with complete, concise, and comprehensible patient education. Patients and their family members provide an additional check in the system when they are appropriately informed. Patients should know the names of their medications and have them easily accessible, they should know when their treatments are going to take place, and maintain calendars of treatment dates. Patients enrolling in trials should have complete and understandable consent forms. All patients should be given a significant amount of time to understand and absorb the information given to them by their healthcare team prior to receiving treatment. Patients and family members should be encouraged to ask questions regarding any aspect of the treatment of their disease.

Education alone is not sufficient and one should not rely on memory (Rogers, 1999). Easy access to resources is essential for safe practice. All personnel should have access to up-to-date reference texts, on-line resources, and institutional protocols. The availability of these resources cannot be located in only one area. Oncology floors, nursing stations, pharmacy satellites, outpatient clinics, and physician practice areas all need easy access to educational and patient information resources.

PRESCRIBING

One strategy to reduce medication errors is to clearly, unambiguously, and uniformly describe orders for cancer chemotherapy (Kohler et al, 1998; NCI, 1997). Inconsistent use of prescribing nomenclature is a major cause of medication errors (Cohen et al, 1996). The information displayed on an order must be complete to allow verification against a published regimen or investigational protocol by all healthcare providers.

Orders generally begin with the name of the drug; it is recommended that chemotherapy should be prescribed in full generic name, avoiding use of any abbreviations, former investigational designations (e.g., VP-16, CPT-11, VM-26), or brand names (NCI, 1997). All medication orders should be clearly expressed and description of treatment regimens should have as much information as possible. Avoid the acceptance of verbal orders. It is generally recommended that initial chemotherapy orders must be entered into a computerized system or written. Some settings may have policies accepting verbal orders only for select changes in an existing order. If verbal orders are to be used in any circumstance, one practice to ensure auditory accuracy is to verify the order with an additional third party listening to the prescriber. The order is then repeated back to the prescriber as given, documented, and then signed by both listeners. Utilize preprinted order sets or computer-generated order sets (Opfer et al, 1999; Schulmeister, 1999; Wong & Ignoffo, 1996). For any orders that are handwritten, poor legibility is a factor that can increase the risk of drug errors. Guidelines related to refusal to accept illegible orders are useful to practitioners, and examples of problematic handwriting of orders can be used for quality improvement purposes (Boyle et al, 2002).

Utilize computer systems and technology to its fullest. All computer entries should be cross-checked for accuracy similar to the written order. One benefit of utilizing computer-based ordering systems is that maximum doses of chemotherapy agents can be programmed in to avoid overdoses. Include all pertinent information, patient name and identification number (if applicable), patient height, weight, body surface area, any weight modifications, diagnosis, regimen, literature reference, cycle number, or protocol number (if enrolled). Ascertain that the patient weight is recent and correct. The institution or practice should adopt standardized formulas for body surface area and body weight calculations (see dosing, Chapter 6).

Be consistent with units of measure, do not switch back and forth between milligrams (mg) and grams (gms), and always write out the word units. A capital U has been previously mistaken for a zero, causing tenfold overdose. Never write a trailing zero, such as vincristine 2.0 mg; the decimal place can be overlooked and a tenfold overdose can occur. Try to round doses to the nearest whole number, this avoids the use of decimal points that can be overlooked. Always use a leading zero when writing for a dose less than 1, for example, dactinomycin should be written as 0.5 mg, not .5 mg.

The orders that have historically been ambiguous are those that include a total dose to be given over a set number of days. It is vital that prescribers write orders that indicate the dose in $mg/m^2/day$, the actual daily dose, and the number of days to be treated, and some recommend including the total dose per cycle at the end of the order.

For example: Fluorouracil 4,000 mg/m^2 over four days should be written as Fluorouracil 1,000 $mg/m^2/day$ in 500 mL normal saline administered intravenously as a continuous infusion on days 1,2,3,4 (total dose = 4,000 mg/m^2 over 96 hours).

Prescribers should always sign and date their orders and write a pager or phone number where they can be reached if someone has a question regarding the order. New orders should be written with each new cycle, dose reduction, or change in the order content. Avoid crossing out on original orders.

Prescribers should maintain professional courtesy to any other member of the healthcare team who may question or need to clarify an order that was written. Conflict resolution training may be useful for nursing staff to help them to deal with occasional intimidating or confrontational behavior (Boyle et al, 2002). Nursing and pharmacy staff always have the right to refuse to carry out medication orders if there are questions about any aspect or appropriateness of the order.

VERIFICATION

Order verification is a systematic methodology that provides double-checks of all information required to safely treat a patient with chemotherapy. The first step in order verification is access to patient information. Nurses, pharmacists, and others require all pertinent information to appropriately verify that a prescribed order is acceptable to act upon. This information should be accessible on the patient order form. Access to the patient's charts, computerized records, laboratory data, and clinical protocols are required along with multidisciplinary discussions of the treatment plan. In an order verification process, specific roles must be defined to maintain consistency in the checking system. The system will define the process and therefore remove interpersonal variability as long as the steps in the process are followed.

- The oncology nurse and pharmacist who receive an order need to verify the patient's height, weight, and body surface area, and calculate adjusted weight if necessary.
- Verify that the diagnosis matches the treatment regimen and that a copy of the treatment regimen or reference is provided for verification purposes. Non-standard treatment regimens should be placed in the patient's charts.

- Verify that the drug name (generic preferred), dosage (i.e., mg/m^2 or mg/kg), total dose to be given, route, frequency of administration, rate of administration, and treatment days are all correct.
- Additional information for the oncology nurse and pharmacist are laboratory values. The responsibility for obtaining this information must be identified by the individual practice area, and treatment monitoring values should be provided directly on the chemotherapy order by the physician. Depending on the drug being administered, certain pertinent values are required prior to compounding and treatment. For example, if doxorubicin is to be administered, all involved should know the patient's left ventricular ejection fraction, bilirubin values, and total cumulative dose of anthracyclines the patient has already received.

DISPENSING/COMPOUNDING

The dispensing process includes drug compounding, labeling, and dispensing to the nurse. Chemotherapy compounding must be performed in a certified biological safety cabinet (BSC) segregated from high traffic areas (see Chapter 6, Table 6-1). Appropriate chemotherapy safety apparel must be worn and the environment should be free from chaos, interruptions, excessive noise, and unnecessary personnel.

Site-of-service-specific verification checklists can be used for compounding to assign responsibility for each step that needs to be checked. Compounding of chemotherapy needs to include verification that the correct drug is being mixed with the correct amount and choice of diluent. All calculations of concentrations and volumes to be administered should be performed by both the pharmacist and technician involved in the preparation. Any parenteral product for patient administration that is compounded should be sterile, stable, free from particulates, and appropriately labeled. Pharmacists should verify the actual amount of drug being placed into the final container; this can be done via observation of the amount drawn up, or by utilizing an electronic balance scale system. When compounding cytotoxic agents, only one product should reside in the BSC at any one time, and once a drug is administered to the final container, it should be labeled. Products for intrathecal administration should be designated as such, and clearly distinguished from intravenous chemotherapy.

Once the final product is complete, a label should be affixed to it. The label should be easily readable, clear, and complete. The label must contain:

- the patient's full name and identifier (i.e., medical record number)
- the preparation date
- the drug name
- the drug amount per dose (to be administered over a 24-hour period)
- the total drug amount in the final container (if excess is added for overfill purposes).

Also included are:

- the name of the diluent
- the volume of diluent to administer and the final total volume
- the administration guidelines including route of administration
- duration of infusion
- rate of administration
- expiration dating.

Ancillary information relating to stability and storage is also recommended. Practice guidelines should require a comparison of the final product to the actual order, cross-checking each segment of information to insure accuracy. The product should be delivered to the administration site and segregated from other intravenous infusions until the time of administration.

ADMINISTRATION

The administration step takes into account the five rights:

- right patient
- right drug
- right dose
- right route
- right time.

Each of these five rights has the potential for error. Prior to actual administration, the nurse administering the drug should check the chemotherapy product with another staff member. The correct patient must receive the correct drug. Policies should be in place for verification of patient identification. In most hospital settings, the drug label is compared to the patient's identification band number. In some ambulatory settings, a patient identification label (i.e., similar to a name tag on clothing) may be used. While these policies are strongly recommended, if they are not in place, verbal authorization with the patient or family member, or patient birth date, might be considered for identification purposes. Show the labeled final product to the patient and/or family member for verification, prior to administration of the drug. The labeled medication must be compared to the original order and read by an oncology certified nurse and another staff member to assure accuracy.

Ascertain that the treatment date and time are correct, the drug is correct, the dose is correct, the volume of drug is correct, the route of administration is specified, and the rate is determined. Ambulatory infusion pumps may vary in rate for administration settings (i.e., mL/min, mL/hour) and therefore the calculations involved in programming these pumps must be double-checked. Once the chemotherapy has been administered, documentation in the patient's medical record is essential and the product container should be disposed of utilizing chemotherapy waste policy.

The variability factor is removed if the administration policy and procedures are standardized for all sites of service within an institution. Included in administration is the monitoring component of treatment; this includes immediate monitoring for adverse events, as well as short- and long-term monitoring of complications due to treatments. Errors that have gone unnoticed can be uncovered by listening to the patient's symptomatic complaints. If these symptoms appear unusual or severe, they may indicate potential overdosage (Bourret, 1996). Monitoring the oncology patient requires astute nursing assessment skills, well-educated patients, and the ability to listen and decipher patient symptoms.

MEDICATION ERROR REPORTING/ERROR RECOVERY

One of the essential components in preventing medication errors is an understanding of the risk factors that contribute to the error or the potential error, referred to as near miss, error recovery, or prevented error. Error recovery is most common during the prescribing and dispensing phases, and results in avoidance of significant harm to the patient (Allard et al, 2002). The collection of near miss or prevented errors is as important as those errors that reach the patient, because they identify faults in the delivery system, and personnel tend to be more open in discussing potential errors than actual ones (Leape, 1994).

The actual reporting process must be quick and efficient or it will not be utilized to its fullest. If medication errors or prevented errors are not documented easily, with details, there is little hope of collecting data to improve the system in which the error occurred. It is common knowledge that medication errors are underreported; the reasons for underreporting vary, but may include minimizing the error, feelings of guilt, coworker disapproval, and fear of punishment. In general, employees do not like to report mistakes in an environment in which punitive action may be enacted. High reporting rates exist in the nonpunitive and anonymous reporting environment that focuses on the overall system and problem resolution, not the personnel involved (Upton & Cousins, 1995). Employees can be made aware that useful information regarding the system may be derived from an error that caused no patient harm and may prevent a serious future medication error.

In addition to individual institution error reporting, systems exist at the national level for medication error or adverse event reporting. These programs are designed to collect information and share it so that everyone can learn from prior mistakes irrespective of where they may have occurred. The FDA has a program entitled MED WATCH; this program is accessible on line and is mainly focused on post-marketing surveillance of adverse drug reactions (Rogers, 1999). The United States Pharmacopoeia has a program referred to as MERP, medication error reporting program. MERP allows practitioners to report potential or actual medication errors in a confidential and anonymous fashion if desired, or they have the option to identify themselves. This information is coordinated by the ISMP. MedMARx is the third national database medication error prevention and reduction reporting program; it is also internet accessible. This program offers anonymous reporting and standard format tracking of medication errors. MedMARx allows for medication error documentation and then furthers its usefulness by providing risk management solutions and medication error trends (USP, 1999).

The Institute of Safe Medication Practice (ISMP) is a nonprofit organization that works with healthcare professionals, practitioners, institutions, regulatory agencies, pharmaceutical companies, and professional organizations to provide education about medication errors, adverse drug effects, and error prevention (Vaida & Ellis, 2002). They detail a four-pronged error analysis that includes identifying and segregating individual medication errors, hospital specific data, data from prevented (or near miss) errors, and collective data from other similar institutions. The ISMP publishes and distributes a bulletin that highlights reported medication errors from across the country in the hopes that it will enlighten other institutions and healthcare professionals in an attempt to correct potential problems.

ROOT CAUSE ANALYSIS

Investigation into medication errors allows for an uncovering of the underlying root causes that have played a role in either system failures due to faulty design or faulty implementation (Leape, 1994). Root cause analysis is a reactive process that is undertaken after a documented error has occurred (ISMP Safety Alert, 2001a). This is an investigative process that is designed to identify underlying causes of errors through a process of questions. Root cause analysis tends to uncover pieces of information that initially would not have been thought to play a role in the error. There is rarely one specific root cause of any medication error. The sources of medication errors tend to be multidisciplinary and multifactorial (ASHP, 1993) and thus provide us with multiple opportunities to improve the system. Root cause analysis is often used in institutional-based settings with support from the organizational structure. It is

3

MEDICATION ERROR REPORTING/ERROR RECOVERY

recommended, in any environment where an error may have occurred, to evaluate the error and factors that may have played a role, and to reduce the risk of repeat errors.

FAILURE MODE AND EFFECTS ANALYSIS (FMEA)

Unlike root cause analysis, failure mode and effects analysis is a process that occurs before an actual error happens (ISMP Safety Alert, 2001c). It is an evaluation of a new drug product, new equipment, new service or process that looks for areas of vulnerability. This procedure allows for evaluation before any actual use or change comes into action. Interdisciplinary committees can utilize this procedure to determine the potential for error of new products. For example, if the new product were a drug, the use of a product would be evaluated, from procurement to administration. Potential failure modes would be discussed (i.e., is it a drug with a name that can be mistaken for something else?). Then, what is the chance of this error happening and if an error occurred, what would be the consequences? A discussion of systems processes to detect this error prior to it happening would occur. Finally, if this product had failure modes that could potentially cause significant harm, systems would need to be installed to prevent them, prior to the product ever being used. (i.e., limiting those that could prescribe it, or storing the product separately, etc.) (ISMP Safety Alert, 2001c; Rogers, 1999).

CONCLUSION

The fifth leading cause of death in the United States may be medication errors (Hayward & Hofer, 2001). This fact alone challenges the healthcare system to improve its patient safety initiatives. A total of 50 million dollars has been allocated by the US Department of Health and Human services to fund projects, grants, and contracts focusing on medication error reduction and patient safety issues (Patient Safety Alert, 2002). These programs should reveal relevant information that will help us all to improve all of our systems.

The reduction of medication errors and improving patient safety are critical issues that need to be incorporated into the everyday practice of oncology. As healthcare professionals, it is imperative that the safety checks, double-checks, and redundancies be performed without deviation. Utilization of appropriately educated staff, prescribing guidelines, verification processes, good manufacturing and compounding practices, and administration and monitoring techniques are the only ways to assure that patients are kept safe and free from medication errors in the oncology practice.

SAFETY WEBSITES

http://books.nap.edu/books/0309068371/html/index/html
IOM REPORT ONLINE
http://www.quic.gov/index.htm
MULTIPLE LINKS-"DOING WHAT COUNTS FOR PATIENT SAFETY," The Report to the President, February 2000.
http://www.ismp.org
INSTITUTE FOR SAFE MEDICATION PRACTICES

REFERENCES

Allard J et al. Medication errors, causes, prevention and reduction. Br J Haematol 116: 255–265, 2002.

American Society of Hospital Pharmacists. ASHP guidelines on preventing medication error in hospitals. Am J Hosp Pharm 50: 305–314, 1993.

Attilio RM. Caring enough to understand. The road to oncology medication error prevention. Hosp Pharm 31: 17–26, 1996.

Bates DW et al. The costs of adverse drug events in hospitalized patients. JAMA 277: 307–311, 1997.

Bourret JA. Medication use review process and information systems utilized for oncology chemotherapy quality improvement. Pharm Pract Manage Q 16: 1–17, 1996.

Boyle DA et al. Medication misadventure in cancer care. Semin Oncol Nurs 18: 109–120, 2002.

Cohen MR. Cancer chemotherapy needs improved quality assurance. Hosp Pharm 30: 258–259, 1995.

Cohen MR, Institute for Safe Medication Practices. Health Insight's meeting on adverse drug events: reducing medication errors in Utah. Current Issues in Medication Safety. Salt Lake City, UT, Health Insight: February 18, 1998.

Cohen MR et al. Preventing medication errors in cancer chemotherapy. Am J Health-Syst Pharm 53: 737–746, 1996.

FDA.gov/cder/handbook/mederror.htm.

Fischer D et al. Improving the cancer chemotherapy use process. J Clin Oncol 14: 3148–3155, 1996.

Frank-Stromborg M, Christensen A. Legal issues in chemotherapy administration. In: Gullatee MM, ed. Clinical Guide to Antineoplastic Therapy: A Chemotherapy Handbook. Pittsburgh, PA, Oncology Nursing Society 2001:pp281–295.

Hayward RA, Hofer TP. Estimating hospital deaths due to medication errors: prevention is in the eye of the reviewer. JAMA 286: 415–420, 2001.

Institute of Medicine. To Err is Human: Building a Safer Health System. Washington, DC, Academy Press, 1999.

ISMP Medication Safety Alert, Aug. 8, 2001a.

ISMP Medication Safety Alert, Aug. 22, 2001b.

ISMP Medication Safety Alert, Oct. 17, 2001c.

Kohler DR et al. Standardizing the expression and nomenclature of cancer treatment regimens. Am J Health-Syst Pharm 55: 137, 1998.

Leape LL. Error in medicine. JAMA 272: 1851–1857, 1994.

National Cancer Institute, Division of Cancer Treatment and Diagnosis. Guidelines for Treatment Regimens, Expression and Nomenclature, September 19, 1997.

Oncology Nursing Society. Position paper: Preventing and reporting medication errors. Oncol Nurs Forum 28:15–16, 2001.

Opfer KB, Wirtz DM, Farley K. A chemotherapy standard order form for preventing errors. Oncol Nurs Forum 26: 123–128, 1999.

Patient Safety Alert. Healthcare Benchmarks. 9(1): suppl 3–4, 2002.

Rogers, B. Preventing and detecting cancer chemotherapy drug errors. In Hubbard SM, Goodman M, Knobf MT, eds. Oncol Nurs Updates, 6(1): 1–12, 1999.

Schulmeister, L. Chemotherapy medication errors: descriptions, severity and contributing factors. Oncol Nurs Forum, 26: 1033–1042, 1999.

Upton DR, Cousins DH. Avoiding drug errors. Reporting of errors should be free of recrimination. BMJ 311: 1367, 1995.

USP Updates New Version of MedMARx. http://www.usp.org/aboutusp/releases/1999/pr_0010.htm

Vaida AJ, Ellis WM. Institute for Safe Medication Practices: creating a safer health care environment. J Am Pharm Assoc 42: 126, 2002.

Wong WM, Ignoffo RJ. If there are expert systems and dose checks, why do we still need the clinical pharmacist? Pharm Pract Manage Q 16: 50–58, 1996.

CHEMOTHERAPY DRUGS AND DRUGS USED IN THE TREATMENT OF CANCER

More than 120 drugs are discussed in this edition. Several drugs have been removed and many new investigational drugs have been added. All drug monographs have been updated to include new information, including adverse events, dosing and administration, drug interactions, and storage and stability. Chapter 5 is devoted to biotherapy and monoclonal antibodies. Targeted therapy agents can be located in both Chapters 4 and 5. Those targeted drugs listed in Chapter 5 will display either biotherapy or monoclonal antibody therapy properties. All drugs and biologicals are listed alphabetically by their current generic name or the United States Adopted Name.

Separate chapters are devoted to the management of the more common side effects, such as gastrointestinal toxicity, dermatological toxicity, and myelosuppression. Some aspects of toxicity are highlighted in the discussion of specific drugs. For example, renal toxicity appears in the discussion of cisplatin, cardiac toxicity and its evaluation with left ventricular ejection fraction (LVEF) appear in the doxorubicin section.

Each drug monograph is divided into several subsections. The following general guidelines were followed in the preparation of each monograph:

1. **Classification**. Drugs are categorized based primarily on their mechanisms of action (e.g., antimetabolites) or derivation (e.g., plant alkaloids). Unless the drug has mechanisms of action that have not been previously discussed in Chapter 1, they will not be discussed in detail in this chapter.

2. **Indications**. The indications listed for each commercially available drug are from the manufacturer's package insert or one of the compendia used to determine Medicare reimbursement (i.e., United States Pharmacopeia, American Hospital Formulary Service [AHFS] Drug Information), or from the primary literature. In some instances, indications will be listed for the investigational drugs and these were taken from the primary literature. The compendia can be accessed via the following website: **www.accc-cancer.org**

3. **Dose.** Commonly used doses are listed, along with some dose regimens recently published. In all cases, consult the specific protocol and/or the manufacturer for doses and dose-adjustment guidelines. The issues regarding dose calculations based upon body surface area (BSA) or other methods are controversial (see Chapter 6). The doses presented are those that have been published and/or those that are approved by the US Food and Drug Administration. It is anticipated that better methods of dose calculation will be devised that take into account patient variability in drug pharmacokinetics and pharmacodynamics. Calculation of dose in obese patients is worthy of mention here. Studies have been conducted suggesting that calculation of dose based upon actual weight does not lead to additional toxicity. The Southwest Oncology Group (SWOG) requires all patients enrolled in a SWOG study to have their initial dose calculated using actual body weight. The SWOG policy (number 38) is available at their website.

4. **Administration.** Routes of administration that have been used are listed, and recommended routes may be described. In all cases, consult the specific protocol and/or the manufacturer for guidelines.

5. **Toxicity.** Adverse drug reactions are listed by organ system. Effects that are dose-limiting or rare are usually noted as such. The incidence figures cited refer to the incidence of toxicities that have been reported (regardless of relationship to the drug) after the use of recommended doses and routes of administration. Where possible, we have attempted to include toxicities thought to be possibly, probably, or definitely related to the drug. In addition, unless otherwise indicated, the incidence of toxicities noted herein includes all grades (i.e., mild, moderate, severe, and life-threatening) of the particular toxicity. With all drugs, especially those that are investigational, unexpected effects may occur.

6. **Drug/Food Interactions.** Information includes well-documented interactions and some potential drug interactions. Interactions with homeopathic drugs or natural products are not included, unless the interaction is well documented. The use of live virus vaccines in immunocompromised patients can result in severe, sometimes fatal infections and is generally not recommended. This is not specifically listed under each drug entry, as the caution applies to all immunosuppressive drugs. The severity of each interaction is not specifically addressed. Further detail on the general mechanisms of drug interactions can be found in Chapter 1. With all drugs, especially those that are investigational, unexpected drug interactions may occur.

7. **Storage and Stability.** Information may include data that are not part of the official labeling of marketed drugs but have been described in the literature. In all cases, the expiration date on the drug container should be observed unless the clinician has been officially notified that the expiration date has been extended as a result of stability testing. Stability studies are ongoing for many investigational drugs. For parenteral drugs that do not contain a preservative, the customary recommendation is to discard any unused solution after 8 to 24 hours. It is suggested that each institution follow its own policy regarding products that may be chemically stable for longer periods of time.

8. **Preparation.** Methods for reconstitution and dilution are described. In some cases, methods of preparation will be discussed that are not a part of the official drug label but have been described in the literature. For investigational drugs the recommendations regarding reconstitution and further dilution may change and one should always consult the protocol or investigational drug brochure for the most up-to-date recommendations.

9. **Incompatibilities and Compatibilities**. Mixtures that should be avoided or are known to be compatible or incompatible are described. In general, the compatibility information included in this chapter is brief and only notes information where chemical compatibility has been assayed. It is recommended that admixtures not be prepared unless stability is known and that a pharmacist be consulted for detailed information.

10. **Availability.** Sources of the drugs are listed. For commercially available drugs, a pharmacist should be consulted for manufacturers or wholesalers. Most investigational drugs are obtained from the National Cancer Institute (NCI) or the manufacturer.

11. **References (Selected Readings).** Each drug monograph of the investigational drugs is followed by one or two references from the primary literature. A reference has not been provided for all of the drugs that are commercially available in the United States. We refer the reader to readily available sources, which are listed at the end of this chapter.

AE-941

Other names
Neovastat®; NSC-706456.

Indications
AE-941 is an investigational agent in the United States and Canada. It is undergoing evaluation as a treatment for patients with renal cell carcinoma, non-small-cell lung cancer, breast cancer, and other malignancies.

Classification and Mechanisms of Action
AE-941 is an antiangiogenic agent. AE-941 is a matrix metalloproteinase inhibitor that is derived from shark cartilage. AE-941 has been shown to inhibit vascular endothelial growth factor (VEGF-R2).

Dose
120 mL twice daily. AE-941 is administered in conjunction with chemotherapy, such as cisplatin and gemcitabine for non-small-cell lung cancer. AE-941 has also been administered in combination with radiation therapy.

Administration
AE-941 is administered by mouth on an empty stomach. The dose must be shaken well prior to administration.

Toxicity
Gastrointestinal. Nausea occurs in approximately 10% of the patients, vomiting in 5%, diarrhea in 5%, anorexia in 2%. Hiccups and taste alterations have been reported.
Dermatological. Skin rash and pruritus have been reported in 2% of the patients.
Other. Weakness. Hypoglycemia (rare).

Storage and Stability
AE-941 is stored in the freezer (i.e., −10° to −30°F). The solution is stable at room temperature for at least 12 hours. After thawing, the solution may be returned to the freezer. No more than one "freeze-thaw" cycle is recommended.

Preparation
The solution is removed from the freezer and allowed to thaw in hot tap water for less than 1 hour. Thawing by microwave is not recommended. Within the next 12 hours the dose must be administered. The solution must be mixed (by shaking), then immediately ingested.

Availability
AE-941 is an investigational agent in the United States that is available as an oral solution from the manufacturer or the National Cancer Institute.

Selected Readings
Riviere M et al. AE-941 (Neovastat), an inhibitor of angiogenesis: phase I/II cancer clinical trial results. Cancer Invest 17(suppl 1): 16–17, 1999.
Riviere M et al. Phase I/II lung cancer clinical trial results with AE-941 (Neovastat), an inhibitor of angiogenesis. Clin Invest Med (suppl): S14, 1998.

ALTRETAMINE

Other names
Hexalen®; Hexastat®; hexamethylmelamine; HMM; HXM; NSC-13875.

Indications
FDA approved as a single agent for the treatment of persistent or recurrent ovarian carcinoma. Altretamine may be a useful treatment for patients with non-Hodgkin's lymphoma and cancers of the lung, endometrium, and cervix.

Classification and Mechanisms of Action
Alkylating agent. Altretamine is activated by the liver to metabolites that are thought to bind with nucleic acids or microsomal proteins. Altretamine inhibits DNA and RNA synthesis by inhibiting their uptake into cells.

Pharmacokinetics
Well absorbed (75% to 89%) by mouth and reaches peak plasma levels 0.5 to 3 hours after dosing. Extensively metabolized in the liver (by microsomal enzymes) on first pass. Methylated metabolites appear to accumulate in the central nervous system. Elimination half-life is 4 to 13 hours. The pharmacokinetics of altretamine are not altered in patients with ascites. Less than 1% is eliminated in the urine as unchanged drug.

Dose
The approved dose for advanced ovarian carcinoma is 260 mg/m^2/day in four divided doses for 14 to 21 days of a 28-day treatment cycle. When altretamine is combined with other myelosuppressive drugs, a dose of 150 mg/m^2/day for 14 days is commonly administered. Oral dosage ranges from 4 to 12 mg/kg/day in four divided doses for periods up to 3 to 6 weeks have been utilized. Higher doses (240 to 320 mg/m^2/day for 21 days) have been administered every 6 weeks.

Administration
Oral, usually taken after a meal.

Toxicity
Hematological. Leukopenia and thrombocytopenia are common (20% to 40% incidence) but usually mild. Nadir blood counts usually occur 3 to 4 weeks after beginning treatment, and recovery occurs 2 to 3 weeks thereafter. Anemia occurs frequently.
Gastrointestinal. Nausea and vomiting are common and occasionally dose-limiting. These toxicities may worsen with continued therapy. Taking the drug with food or at bedtime may lessen these effects. Abdominal cramps, anorexia, and diarrhea occur occasionally.
Neurological. Reversible peripheral neuropathy (31%), other neurological adverse effects occur infrequently and may include paresthesias, hyperesthesia, hyperreflexia, motor weakness, decreased sensory sensations, decreased proprioceptive sensations, agitation, anxiety, hallucinations, confusion, lethargy, depression, or coma.
Other. Weight loss, hepatic toxicity, cystitis, skin rash, pruritus, and alopecia are uncommon. Second malignancies (leukemia) have been reported.

Drug Interactions
Drug compounds that induce or inhibit the cytochrome P450 system can alter elimination of altretamine.

ALTRETAMINE *(continued)*

Phenobarbital could enhance the metabolism of altretamine, resulting in decreased therapeutic effect.

Cimetidine could slow the metabolism of altretamine, resulting in increased toxicity.

Altretamine may potentiate orthostatic hypotension if administered with monoamine oxidase inhibitors.

Storage and Stability

Altretamine capsules should be stored in tightly sealed bottles at room temperature. Each bottle bears an expiration date.

Availability

Commercially available in 50-mg capsules.

Selected Readings

Foster BJ et al. Hexamethylmelamine: a critical review of an active drug. Cancer Treat Rev 13: 197–217, 1986.
Hansen LA, Hughes TE. Altretamine, DICP. Ann Pharmacother 25: 146–152, 1991.

AMIFOSTINE

Other names

Ethyol®; WR-2721; ethiofos; ethanethiol; 2-[(3-aminopropyl)amino]-dihydrogen phosphate (ester); gammaphos; NSC-296961.

Indications

Amifostine is FDA approved as a treatment to reduce the nephrotoxicity of cisplatin in patients with ovarian carcinoma and non–small-cell lung cancer. Also approved for use concurrently with radiation therapy in cancer of the head and neck, whereby the parotid gland is in the field of radiation, to reduce the incidence of xerostomia. Other uses include prevention or reduction of toxicity secondary to radiation therapy, cyclophosphamide, cisplatin or paclitaxel-induced neuropathies, and bone marrow toxicity.

Classification and Mechanisms of Action

Amifostine is an organic sulfhydryl compound that protects (in laboratory animals) normal tissues against the cytotoxicity of radiation and alkylating agents. The mechanism by which this occurs appears to be in part related to the differential absorption of amifostine in normal and malignant tissues.

Pharmacokinetics

Amifostine is 30% to 40% absorbed by mouth (in experimental animals). The drug is preferentially distributed to normal tissues (such as bone marrow, gastrointestinal mucosa, and skin) but not to tumor tissue. Amifostine is almost totally metabolized and is undetectable in the plasma approximately 6 minutes after IV administration. Approximately 0.7% to 2.5% of a dose is excreted in the urine unchanged.

Dose

For the prevention/reduction of renal toxicity. The recommended dose of amifostine is 910 mg/m^2 starting 30 minutes before initiating treatment with a cisplatin-containing chemotherapy regimen. If this full dose is not tolerated, subsequent cycles can be initiated at 740 mg/m^2.

For the prevention/reduction of xerostomia. The recommended dose of amifostine is 200 mg/m^2/day administered 15 to 30 minutes prior to each radiation treatment.

Administration

Amifostine has been given as an IV infusion over a 15-minute period. Longer infusions increase the likelihood of hypotension and vomiting.

Toxicity

Gastrointestinal. Nausea and vomiting may be severe. Antiemetic premedication is recommended. The manufacturer suggests the use of dexamethasone (20 mg IV) and a 5-HT$_3$ receptor antagonist before administration of amifostine.
Neurological. Somnolence.
Cardiovascular. Transient hypotension, usually asymptomatic; concomitant administration of drugs that could exacerbate the hypotensive effects of amifostine (e.g., benzodiazepines) should be avoided. The manufacturer recommends monitoring blood pressure every 5 minutes during the 15-minute IV infusion and 5 minutes after completion of the infusion. If the systolic blood pressure drops below a threshold level defined below, the infusion should be stopped, the patient should be placed in the Trendelenburg position, and hydration with normal saline should be initiated. If blood pressure returns to normal within 5 minutes, the infusion of amifostine may be resumed; if it does not, treatment with amifostine should be discontinued. The infusion of amifostine should be interrupted if the baseline systolic blood pressure is:

- 100 mm Hg and decreases by 20 mm Hg or more
- 100 to 119 mm Hg and decreases by 25 mm Hg or more
- 120 to 140 mm Hg and decreases by 30 mm Hg or more
- 140 to 179 mm Hg and decreases by 40 mm Hg or more
- equal to or greater than 180 mm Hg and decreases by 50 mm Hg or more.

Other. Sneezing, hypocalcemia (rare), flushing.

Drug Interactions

Antihypertensive therapy should be temporarily discontinued 24 hours prior to amifostine administration due to potential exacerbation of the hypotensive side effects of amifostine therapy.

Storage and Stability

Amifostine vials are stable at room temperature, vials bear expiration dates. Reconstituted and dilute solutions of amifostine (5 to 40 mg/mL) are stable for at least 5 hours at room temperature and at least 24 hours in the refrigerator.

Preparation

The 500-mg vial is reconstituted with 9.7 mL of normal saline to yield a 50 mg/mL solution. The desired dose is further diluted with normal saline to a concentration of 5 to 40 mg/mL.

Compatibilities

Normal saline is the preferred solution for further dilution, the use of other solutions is not recommended.

Availability

Amifostine, 500 mg per vial, is commercially available.

AMIFOSTINE *(continued)*

Selected Readings
Hensley ML et al. American Society of Clinical Oncology clinical practice guidelines for the use of chemotherapy and radiotherapy protectants. J Clin Oncol 17: 3333–3335, 1999.

Kemp G et al. Amifostine pretreatment for protection against cyclophosphamide-induced and cis-platin-induced toxicities: results of a randomized control trial in patients with advanced ovarian cancer. J Clin Oncol 14: 2101–2112, 1996.

AMINOGLUTETHIMIDE

Other names
Cytadren®; Elipten®; BA-16038; NSC-330915.

Indications
FDA approved for the treatment of breast cancer and suppression of adrenal function in selected patients with Cushing's syndrome. Aminoglutethimide may also be useful in the treatment of prostate and adrenal cortical carcinoma and ACTH-producing tumors.

Classification and Mechanisms of Action
Aminoglutethimide is an aromatase inhibitor. It inhibits aromatase enzymes necessary for conversion of androgens to estrogens. Aminoglutethimide also blocks adrenal steroid biosynthesis by interfering with the enzymatic conversion of cholesterol to delta-5 pregnenolone. The onset of adrenal suppression occurs 3 to 5 days after initiation of therapy; recovery occurs within 1.5 to 3 days after discontinuing the drug.

Pharmacokinetics
Aminoglutethimide is well absorbed (90%) by mouth and reaches peak serum concentrations approximately 1.5 hours after dosing. Approximately 20% to 25% of the drug is bound to plasma proteins. The drug is metabolized by the liver to at least eight metabolites and excreted in the urine primarily as unchanged drug (35% to 50%) and metabolites. aminoglutethimide has an elimination half-life of approximately 7 to 9 hours. The half-life is longer (13 hours) at the start of treatment.

Dose
Treatment is occasionally begun with a lower dose of aminoglutethimide (250 mg twice daily) and a higher hydrocortisone dose (100 mg/day) for 2 weeks before initiating full doses. The usual dose is 250 mg 4 times per day in combination with hydrocortisone, 40 mg/day in three divided doses (i.e., 10 mg in the morning, 10 mg at noon, and 20 mg at bedtime). Occasionally, a mineralocorticoid is also needed (e.g., fludrocortisone 0.1 mg/day). When aminoglutethimide therapy is discontinued, there is no need to taper the corticosteroid dose.

Administration
Aminoglutethimide is given orally in divided fractions 4 times a day.

Toxicity
Hematological. Leukopenia, agranulocytosis, and pancytopenia are rare.
Gastrointestinal. Mild nausea, vomiting, anorexia.
Dermatological. Frequently (33%) transient erythematous maculopapular eruptions are associated with fever. Both of these toxicities remit within 3 to 4 days without

stopping administration of the drug. Pustular psoriasis, desquamation, and oral ulceration have been reported.

Neurological. Lethargy (40%), fatigue (common, transient), ataxia (10%), dizziness, nystagmus, drowsiness. Lethargy usually resolves slowly (after 4 to 6 weeks of treatment).

Other. Adrenal insufficiency. Postural hypotension and hyponatremia (caused by decreased aldosterone secretion). Virilization, myalgia, fever, weight gain, facial fullness, leg cramps. Rarely: hypothyroidism, a systemic syndrome resembling lupus erythematosus with cholestatic jaundice and hepatic enzyme elevations. Possible elevated serum cholesterol levels in patients with breast cancer may predispose to atherosclerosis, but the great variation in levels among patients returns to normal level within a few weeks after therapy is stopped.

Drug Interactions

Aminoglutethimide has been shown to increase the metabolic elimination of warfarin by as much as 90%, decreasing its therapeutic effect.

Aminoglutethimide also increases metabolism of theophylline, dexamethasone, digitoxin, medroxyprogesterone, and tamoxifen, and may lead to decreased therapeutic effect of these drugs. Increased dose adjustments may need to be considered.

Aminoglutethimide and sedatives can result in additive CNS depression.

Storage and Stability

Aminoglutethimide tablets are stored at room temperature and protected from light. Each bottle bears an expiration date.

Availability

Aminoglutethimide is commercially available as 250-mg tablets.

Selected Reading

Cocconi G et al. Low-dose aminoglutethimide with and without hydrocortisone replacement as first-line endocrine treatment in advanced breast cancer: a prospective randomized trial of the Italian Oncology Group for Clinical Research. J Clin Oncol 10: 984–989, 1992.

AMSACRINE

Other names

m-AMSA; AMSA P-D®; Amsidine®; Amsidyl®; 4'-(9-acridinylamino) methanesulfon-m-anisidide; AMSA; acridinylanisidide; NSC-249992.

Indication

In the United States amsacrine is a Group C (investigational) agent for the treatment of acute nonlymphocytic leukemia. In Canada and in the United Kingdom amsacrine is approved for the treatment of acute nonlymphocytic leukemia.

Classification and Mechanisms of Action

Amsacrine is an intercalating agent that also inhibits topoisomerase II.

Pharmacokinetics

Amsacrine is poorly absorbed by mouth. After IV administration it is metabolized by the liver and excreted in the bile (80% as unchanged drug and metabolites) and urine (2% to 10% as unchanged drug). Plasma protein binding is approximately 98%. Approximately 2% of amsacrine reaches the cerebrospinal fluid. The drug has an elimination half-life of 2 hours. The elimination half-life is approximately 17 hours in patients with severe liver dysfunction and hyperbilirubinemia > 34 micromol/L (2 mg/dL).

AMSACRINE *(continued)*

Dose

For leukemia (adults), the induction dose is 75 to 125 mg/m^2/day for 5 days. For children with leukemia the induction dose is 75 to 150 mg/m^2/day for 5 days. Maintenance doses are reduced by 50% and administered every 4 to 8 weeks. The dose for the NCI Group C protocol is 120 mg/m^2/day for 5 days. The manufacturer recommends a 40% decrease in the dose for patients with a serum bilirubin between 26 and 51 micromol/L (1.52 to 3 mg/dL) and that the dose be further reduced or omitted if the serum bilirubin is > 51 micromol/L (> 3 mg/dL).

Administration

Slow IV infusion in 250 to 500 mL of 5% dextrose over a period of 60 to 90 minutes. Do not use chloride-containing solutions. Make sure that the potassium level is normal before administering amsacrine. For children, amsacrine may be diluted in 150 to 250 mL of 5% dextrose and administered over 1 to 2 hours.

Toxicity

Hematological. Leukopenia (dose-limiting), thrombocytopenia (usually mild), anemia. Nadir leukocyte and platelet counts usually occur within 11 to 13 days with recovery by days 21 to 28.
Gastrointestinal. Nausea (30%), vomiting (30%), stomatitis (10%), diarrhea (10%), abdominal pain (10%).
Dermatological. Phlebitis, pain at injection site. Slowing the infusion rate, further dilution of amsacrine and/or a cold pack at the injection site may be necessary. Urticaria, skin rash, and erythema are rare.
Hepatic. Elevation of liver function tests (bilirubin, transaminases, alkaline phosphatase) are uncommon and transient.
Neurological. Rarely: seizures, neuropathy, headache, dizziness, central nervous system depression.
Cardiovascular. Congestive heart failure (rare), ventricular arrhythmias (incidence 30% in hypokalemic patients). Cardiac arrests have been reported in a few cases, while the drug was infusing, usually in the presence of hypokalemia.
Other. Orange urine (common). Rarely, allergic reactions (urticaria, skin rashes, anaphylaxis).

Storage and Stability

Unopened vials are stored at room temperature. After preparation, the combined solution is stable for at least 48 hours at room temperature with room lighting. Further diluted in 500 mL of 5% dextrose its stability at room temperature is 7 days; however, the manufacturer recommends that diluted solutions be administered within 24 hours of preparation.

Preparation

Add 1.5 mL from the ampule containing amsacrine, 50 mg/mL, to the vial containing 13.5 mL of diluent, 0.035 M L-lactic acid. The resulting orange-red combined solution contains 5 mg/mL of amsacrine. Dilute the combined solution in 500 mL of 5% dextrose. Generally plastic syringes are not recommended but a plastic syringe may be used to transfer amsacrine to the diluent, but only if the solution remains in the syringe for less than 15 minutes.

Incompatibilities

Amsacrine should not be mixed with a sodium chloride injection or any sodium chloride-containing solutions, including those often found in evacuated containers. This may cause precipitation.

Availability

In the United States the drug is available from the National Cancer Institute in 75 mg/1.5 mL ampules with 13.5 mL of 0.035 M lactic acid diluent.

Selected Readings

Hornedo J, Van Echo DA. Amsacrine (m-AMSA): a new antineoplastic agent. Pharmacology, clinical activity and toxicity. Pharmacotherapy 5: 78–90, 1985.

Miller RP, Pyesmany AF, Wolff LJ. Successful reinduction therapy with amsacrine and cyclocytidine in acute nonlymphoblastic leukemia in children. Cancer 67: 2235–2240, 1991.

ANAGRELIDE

Other names

Agrylin®; anagrelide hydrochloride; BMY26538-01; BL4126A.

Indications

Anagrelide is FDA approved for patients with myeloproliferative disorders for the treatment of life-threatening thrombocythemia that is no longer responsive to standard treatment. Anagrelide may also be a useful treatment for patients with myelodysplastic syndromes, polycythemia vera, and chronic myelogenous leukemia.

Classification and Mechanisms of Action

Anagrelide inhibits platelet aggregation and suppresses platelet concentration.

Pharmacokinetics

Anagrelide is readily absorbed from the gastrointestinal tract with a peak concentration approximately one hour after ingestion. Anagrelide is extensively metabolized by the liver, with 72% to 90% excreted via the kidneys and up to 18% excreted in the feces.

Dose

The usual starting dose is 2 mg/day taken in four equally divided doses (i.e., 0.5 mg 4 times a day) or 1 mg twice daily for a minimum of 7 days. Doses are adjusted in increments of 0.5 mg/day every 5 to 7 days to maintain platelet counts at a particular level. It has been recommended that platelet counts be quickly reduced to a level less than 600,000/mm^3 and maintained within 150,000 and 450,000/mm^3. The daily dose of anagrelide should not exceed 10 mg. Individual doses should not exceed 2.5 mg. It is recommended that the starting dose be reduced by 50% for patients with abnormal liver or renal function (i.e., 0.5 mg twice daily). It is recommended that patients with a cardiac history that puts them at risk for developing severe toxicity begin treatment with 0.5 mg/day.

Administration

Oral, with or without food.

Toxicity

Hematological. Mild anemia (36%), thrombocytopenia, ecchymosis, thrombotic episodes, rarely.

ANAGRELIDE *(continued)*

Gastrointestinal. Nausea (15%), vomiting (7%), gas or bloating, pain or gastric distress. Diarrhea has been reported in approximately 24% of patients, and it has been observed that a lactase supplement can prevent diarrhea in the majority of patients. Pancreatitis has been reported in a few patients.

Dermatological. Rash (infrequent), pruritus, hyperpigmentation of lower extremities.

Hepatic. Elevation of hepatic transaminase levels has been reported rarely.

Neurological. Headache (43%). Headache usually occurs within the first two weeks of treatment and can be controlled with acetaminophen. Dizziness has been reported in 8% of the patients and is usually mild or moderate in severity. Asthenia, malaise, and parathesias are also reported.

Cardiovascular. Hypotension, palpitations (27%), and/or tachycardia, angina, fluid retention, or edema congestive heart failure, atrial fibrillation (rare). Deaths possibly related to treatment with anagrelide have occurred, predominately in patients with known coronary artery disease.

Pulmonary. Dyspnea (11%), pharyngitis, and cough. Pulmonary hypertension, pulmonary hypotension, and pulmonary infiltrates, which improve after treatment with corticosteroids, have been reported.

Other. Anagrelide is contraindicated in pregnant women.

Drug Interactions

Sulcralfate may reduce the absorption of anagrelide.

Storage and Stability

Anagrelide tablets are stored at room temperature and protected from light. Each bottle bears an expiration date.

Availability

Commercially available in 0.5-mg and 1-mg tablets.

Selected Reading

Anagrelide Study Group. Anagrelide, a therapy for thrombocythemic states: experience in 577 patients. Am J Med 92: 69–76, 1992.

ANASTROZOLE

Other names

Arimidex®; NSC-719344.

Indications

Anastrozole is FDA approved as first-line therapy in locally advanced or metastatic breast cancer patients with hormone receptor-positive disease or hormone receptor status unknown. Also used for the treatment of advanced breast cancer in post-menopausal women who have previously received tamoxifen therapy. Patients with estrogen receptor-negative disease and patients whose tumor did not respond to tamoxifen, rarely benefit from treatment with anastrozole.

Classification and Mechanisms of Action

Anastrozole is a nonsteroidal aromatase inhibitor. The drug produces its antitumor effects by significantly reducing serum estradiol levels. It does not affect the formation of adrenal corticosteroids or aldosterone. Corticosteroid replacement therapy is not required for patients taking anastrozole.

Pharmacokinetics

Anastrozole is well absorbed (85%) after oral administration. Food does not appear to affect the absorption of anastrozole. Approximately 40% of the drug is bound to plasma proteins. Most of the drug is metabolized by the liver, and its major metabolite is inactive. Approximately 11% of a dose eliminated into the urine as unchanged drug. The elimination half-life is approximately 50 hours.

Dose

The usual dose is 1 mg daily. Adjustment of dose for patients with renal and hepatic function impairment is not necessary.

Administration

Oral.

Toxicity

Hematological. Mild leukopenia and anemia were rarely observed.
Gastrointestinal. Nausea (16%), vomiting (9%), diarrhea (8%), constipation (7%), abdominal pain (7%), anorexia (7%), xerostomia (5%).
Dermatological. Rash (5%); pruritus and thinning hair (rare).
Hepatic. Rare elevations of hepatic serum enzyme levels.
Neurological. Headache (13%), dizziness (6%), depression (5%), and paresthesia (4%). Insomnia, anxiety, nervousness, confusion, and somnolence were rarely observed.
Cardiovascular. Vasodilation (25%), peripheral edema (5% to 10%); hypertension and thrombophlebitis occurred in less than 4% of the patients treated with anastrozole.
Pulmonary. Dyspnea (9%).
Other. Asthenia (16%), hot flushes (12%), pain (10%), back pain (10%), bone pain (6%), pelvic pain (5%), chest pain (5%), vaginal hemorrhage (2%), diaphoresis (1.5%), and weight gain (1.5%). Flu-like symptoms, fever, neck pain, breast pain, malaise, myalgia, arthralgia, infection, and weight loss were rarely observed.

Drug Interactions

No significant drug interactions have been reported.

Storage and Stability

Anastrozole tablets are stored at room temperature. Each bottle bears an expiration date.

Availability

Commercially available in 1-mg tablets.

Selected Reading

Goss PE, Strasser K. Aromatase inhibitors in the treatment and prevention of breast cancer.
 J Clin Oncol 19: 881–894, 2001.

ARSENIC TRIOXIDE

Other names

Trisenox®; As_2O_3; AS203; NSC-706363.

Indications

FDA approved for use in adults and children over the age of 5 years who have refractory or relapsed acute promyelocytic leukemia (APL) or APL with the presence of the t (15;17) translocation or PML/RAR alfa gene expression.

ARSENIC TRIOXIDE *(continued)*

Classification and Mechanisms of Action
Antineoplastic and antiangiogenic. Arsenic trioxide may induce differentiation of APL cells.

Pharmacokinetics
Arsenic trioxide distributes into the blood and is highly bound to hemoglobin (96%). The drug is not detected in the cerebral spinal fluid, but accumulates in nails, hair, and bone marrow due to their high content of sulfhydryl groups. Concentrations were also detected in the heart, liver, lungs, and kidney. The distribution half-life is 0.9 hours, with an approximate 4-liter volume of distribution. Liver metabolism occurs via the enzyme arsenate reductase, followed by a series of conversions. Methyltransferases further break down trivalent arsenic to dimethylarsenic acid. Unchanged arsenic trioxide is minimally renally excreted (approximately 8%) and extensively excreted in bile. The metabolite trivalent arsenic is methylated and mostly excreted in the urine. The elimination half-life after a 10-mg intravenous dose is 12 hours.

Dose
For the treatment of acute promyelocytic leukemia induction is accomplished with 0.15 mg/kg/day. Treatment is continued until bone marrow remission is observed, but not to exceed 60 doses. Consolidation therapy, 0.15 mg/kg/day for 25 doses, begins 3 to 6 weeks after induction therapy has ended. Dose modification may be necessary for patients with renal insufficiency.

Administration
Arsenic trioxide is given as a 1 to 2 hour intravenous infusion, via central or peripheral venous access. Extending the infusion time to 4 hours may be necessary if patients experience acute vasomotor symptoms, such as hypotension, flushing, or tachycardia.

Toxicity
Hematological. Leukocytosis occurs in up to 50% of patients and can be observed up to one week after the start of therapy. Other hematological effects include anemia (20%), thrombocytopenia (19%), and neutropenia (10%), with a 14 to 21-day nadir, and febrile neutropenia (13%). A less common, but severe reaction may include disseminated intravascular coagulation and hemorrhage.
Gastrointestinal. Abdominal pain occurs in up to 58% of patients. Nausea, vomiting and diarrhea are common. Anorexia and constipation have been reported. Severe gastrointestinal toxicity has prevented the use of oral arsenic trioxide.
Dermatological. Most common: pruritus, dermatitis, and ecchymosis. Up to 20% of patients experience urticaria, dry skin, petechiae, hyperpigmentation, injection site reactions, swelling of the eyelids, and exfoliation of the skin. Rash due to hypersensitivity occurs in less than 5% of patients.
Genitourinary. Vaginal hemorrhage and breakthrough bleeding.
Hepatic. Elevated hepatic transaminase levels.
Neurological. Headache, fever, and fatigue are reported in up to 60% of patients. Also common are depression, dizziness, insomnia, rigors, paresthesias, and anxiety. Somnolence and tremors occur less frequently.
Cardiovascular. Tachycardia (55%). Commonly seen is the prolongation of the QT interval, premature ventricular contractions, and the potentially fatal Torsades-de-Pointes

ventricular arrhythmia. For QT intervals > 500 msec, correct other risk factors and reassess risk versus benefit of continuing or suspending therapy. For irregular heartbeats, tachycardia, or syncope, reassess and discontinue therapy with arsenic trioxide until the QT interval is < 460 msec. Hypertension and hypotension, flushing, pericardial effusion, edema (40%), and weight gain have been reported.

Cardiopulmonary. "Retinoic acid syndrome" occurs in up to 31% of patients treated with arsenic trioxide. Symptoms can occur within 2 to 3 weeks after initiation of treatment, and can be fatal. High fever, dyspnea, respiratory distress, pulmonary infiltrates, and pericardial and/or pleural effusion have been characteristic of this syndrome. Some patients have required intubation and mechanical ventilation. Initiation of treatment with corticosteroids at the first sign of dyspnea has been recommended (i.e., for adults intravenous dexamethasone 10 mg for 3 days or more until symptoms resolve).

Pulmonary. Dyspnea, cough, and sore throat are common. Also reported are tachypnea, wheezing, pleural effusions, hypoxia, and epistaxis.

Ocular. Blurred vision, dry and/or red eyes.

Other. Arthralgias, myalgias, weakness, and bone pain. Earache and ringing in the ears have been reported. Electrolyte imbalances, commonly: hypomagnesemia, hypokalemia, and hyperglycemia; less commonly: hypocalcemia, hyperkalemia, and hypoglycemia.

Drug Interactions

Arsenic trioxide, when administered with antiarrhythmics or other medications that prolong the QT interval (e.g., amphotericin B), can increase the risk of arrhythmias.

Arsenic trioxide therapy alone can increase or decrease blood glucose levels. Patients on insulin or antidiabetic agents (e.g., sulfonylureas, glyburide, chlorpropamide, glipizide) should be frequently monitored.

Storage and Stability

Store at room temperature. Undiluted solution in the original ampule should be used within 24 hours of opening. Further diluted solutions in 5% dextrose and water or normal saline are stable for 24 hours at room temperature or 48 hours refrigerated.

Preparation

The desired dose should be withdrawn from the ampule and passed through a filter needle before further dilution in 100 or 250 mL of 5% dextrose and water or normal saline.

Incompatibilities

Do not mix with any other medications.

Availability

Commercially available as a 1 mg/mL preservative-free solution in 10-mL ampules.

Selected Readings

Shen ZX et al. Use of arsenic trioxide (As2O3) in the treatment of acute promyelocytic leukemia (APL): II. Clinical efficacy and pharmacokinetics in relapsed patients. Blood 89: 3354–3360, 1997.

Soignet SL et al. United States multicenter study of arsenic trioxide in relapsed acute promyelocytic leukemia. J Clin Oncol 19: 3852–3860, 2001.

ARZOXIFENE

Other names
LY 353381.

Indications
Arzoxifene is an investigational agent in the United States that is being evaluated as a treatment for patients with breast cancer and other malignancies.

Classification and Mechanisms of Action
Arzoxifene is a selective estrogen receptor modifier (SERM). The drug does not have uterine agonist activity.

Pharmacokinetics
The pharmacokinetics of arzoxifene are linear, maximum concentrations occur within 2 to 6 hours after oral administration. The elimination half-life is approximately 30 hours.

Dose
20 mg daily.

Administration
Oral. In clinical studies the drug has been administered on an empty stomach.

Toxicity
Hematological. Leukopenia (grade 1, less than 8%) and anemia (grade 1, less than 5%).
Gastrointestinal. Nausea (21%), vomiting occurs less frequently.
Dermatologic. Skin rash (10%), pruritus.
Hepatic. Grade 1 to 3 elevation of liver transaminase levels is reported in less than 5% of the patients. Grade 3 hyperbilirubinemia has been rarely reported.
Other. Mild to moderate hot flushes are common (50%). Asthenia (5%), vaginal bleeding (less than 2%), dizziness (less than 2%), and headache have been reported.

Storage and Stability
Room temperature.

Availability
Arzoxifene is an investigational agent in the United States that is available as a 20-mg tablet from the manufacturer.

Selected Readings
Münster PN et al. Phase I study of a third generation selective estrogen receptor modulator, LY353381.HCl, in metastatic breast cancer. J Clin Oncol 19: 2002–2009, 2001.

Buzdar AU et al. Preliminary results of a randomized double-blind phase II study of the selective estrogen receptor modulator (SERM) arzoxifene (AZ) in patients (pts) with locally advanced or metastatic breast cancer (MBC). Proc Am Soc Clin Oncol 20: 45a, 2001.

ASPARAGINASE

Other names
Escherichia coli-derived: Elspar; L-Asparaginase®; NSC-109229.
Erwinia carotovora-derived: Erwinia asparaginase; Erwinase®; Porton asparaginase; NSC-106977.
PEG-modified (*E. coli*-derived): Oncaspar®; PEG-asparaginase; pegaspargase; NSC-624239.

Indications

E. coli and PEG-modified asparaginase are FDA approved for the treatment of acute lymphocytic leukemia. Asparaginase has also been used for the treatment of patients with acute nonlymphocytic leukemia, chronic lymphocytic leukemia, chronic myelogenous leukemia, soft-tissue sarcoma, and Hodgkin's and non-Hodgkin's lymphoma. Erwinia asparaginase is an investigational (Group C) agent that may be used in acute lymphocytic leukemia patients who are sensitive to *E. coli* L-asparaginase.

Classification and Mechanisms of Action

Enzyme. Asparaginase hydrolyzes the amino acid asparagine. The drug is believed to inhibit protein synthesis by depriving tumor cells of asparagine. Tumor cells that require asparagine are most affected by asparaginase.

Pharmacokinetics

Asparaginase is not absorbed by mouth and undergoes metabolic degradation. After intramuscular (IM) injection, peak plasma levels occur within 14 to 24 hours. Approximately 30% of the drug is protein-bound. The *E. coli* formulation of asparaginase has an elimination half-life of 40 to 50 hours. PEG-asparaginase has an elimination half-life of 3 to 5 days. Only trace amounts of the drug are excreted in the urine.

Dose

Test dose. The manufacturer of the *E. coli*-derived preparation recommends that a 2-IU intradermal test dose be given with the first treatment and with subsequent treatments if more than 1 week separates successive doses. Observation of the patient for 1 hour before administering the full dose is also recommended. Presence of a wheal or erythema at the intradermal test site indicates a positive skin reaction. Patients with negative skin tests are not precluded from developing hypersensitivity reactions.

As a single agent, 200 IU/kg intravenously daily for 28 days has been used. A commonly used dose regimen is 6,000 to 10,000 IU/m^2 via IM injection for nine injections, given every 3 days after cytotoxic therapy. PEG-asparaginase is administered at a dose of 2,500 IU/m^2 every 14 days in children whose body surface area (BSA) is greater than 0.6 m^2 and 82.5 IU/kg every 14 days for whose BSA is less than 0.6 m^2.

Administration

All preparations of asparaginase may be given intramuscularly, subcutaneously, or by IV infusion. The recommended route of administration is IM. For IV administration, an infusion in 50 to 100 mL normal saline or 5% dextrose over a 30-minute period is preferred. It is recommended that PEG-asparaginase be given intramuscularly or by IV in 100 mL of normal saline or 5% dextrose over a period of 1 to 2 hours. The test dose, if desired, is usually administered as an intradermal injection. The following precautions should be taken when the drug is administered:

- Avoid giving the drug at night
- Medical professionals (i.e., a registered nurse and a physician) must be directly accessible
- Have a running IV infusion in place
- Have syringes of epinephrine (adrenalin) (1:1,000, 1 mg), diphenhydramine (50 mg), and hydrocortisone (100 mg) readily available
- Monitor the patient's blood pressure every 15 minutes for 1 hour.

ASPARAGINASE *(continued)*

Toxicity

Hematological. Prolonged thrombin, prothrombin times. Decrease in protein synthesis (decreased fibrinogen and depression of clotting factors, in particular antithrombin III), resulting in thrombosis and/or pulmonary embolism. Myelosuppression is not common.

Gastrointestinal. Nausea and vomiting are common (50% to 60%) but usually controlled with antiemetics. Anorexia, abdominal cramps, weight loss (25%), diarrhea (rare), mucositis, and malabsorption. Pancreatitis has been observed in up to 15% of patients, monitor serum amylase and lipase levels regularly.

Hepatic. Hepatotoxicity (i.e., elevations in liver enzyme and alkaline phosphatase levels; depression of serum albumin levels, cholesterol, and/or plasma fibrinogen levels) is very common (50% to 100%), but rarely severe.

Neurological. EEG changes, depression, somnolence, lethargy, fatigue, seizures, coma, headache, confusion (25%), irritability, agitation, dizziness, and hallucinations, ranging from mild to severe.

Hypersensitivity reactions. Most hypersensitivity reactions occur within 30 minutes of an IV dose, usually longer than 30 to 60 minutes after an IM dose. Some clinicians believe the intradermal test dose is not predictive of who will develop a hypersensitivity reaction. Manifestations of a hypersensitivity reaction may include urticarial eruptions (may be controlled with antihistamines), laryngeal constriction, hypotension, diaphoresis, edema, asthma, and loss of consciousness. The most serious hypersensitivity reactions occur after several doses have been administered, but reactions have been reported after the first dose. The risk of developing a hypersensitivity reaction is greatest when:

- patients are **not** receiving prednisone or other concomitant steroid
- a one-month or greater period of time has elapsed since the last dose was given
- the IgG3 level exceeds 100 AU
- the drug is given by IV infusion rather than intramuscular or subcutaneous injection.

Patients who have had reactions to the *E. coli* product may be able to tolerate Erwinia or PEG-asparaginase. Approximately 30% of patients who developed a hypersensitivity reaction to the *E. coli* preparation will develop a reaction to PEG-asparaginase.

Renal. Azotemia (68%), usually prerenal; renal failure (rare).

Other. Hyperglycemia, chills, fever (25%), hyperthermia (rare).

Drug Interactions

Asparaginase pretreatment antagonizes the effects of methotrexate. Administration of asparaginase and methotrexate should be separated by at least 24 hours.

Asparaginase administered prior to or with vincristine may cause increased toxicity, due to decreased elimination of vincristine. Administer vincristine 12 to 24 hours prior to asparaginase dosing.

Asparaginase can cause decreased synthesis of clotting factors and antithrombin III and therefore should be used with caution in patients taking warfarin, aspirin, nonsteroidal anti-inflammatory agents, and heparin.

Storage and Stability

Intact vials of all asparaginase preparations are refrigerated. Reconstituted solutions of the *E. coli* and Erwinia formulations and those further diluted are stable for 8 hours at room temperature and 14 days in the refrigerator. Cloudy solutions should not be used. Erwinia asparaginase is incompatible with the rubber stopper on the vial;

therefore the reconstituted solution should be used within 15 minutes. PEG-asparaginase should be used immediately and the remainder of the vial discarded. PEG-asparaginase must not be frozen as this destroys its activity.

Preparation

To the *E. coli* formulation, add 1 to 5 mL of sterile water or sodium chloride injection without preservative to each 10,000-IU vial of drug. This results in a concentration of 10,000 to 2,000 IU/mL, respectively. Vigorous shaking of the vial may cause excessive foaming. A small number of gelatinous fiber-like particles that occasionally develop may be removed using a 0.5-micron filter. The desired dose may be further diluted in normal saline or 5% dextrose.

Reconstitute the 10,000-IU vial of Erwinia preparation with 2 mL normal saline without preservative to yield a 5,000 IU/mL solution. PEG asparaginase is packaged as a liquid formulation.

Incompatibilities

Use of a 0.2-micron filter results in a loss of potency.

Availability

Available in 10,000-IU vials as lyophilized cake material from two natural sources. The *E. coli* preparation is commercially available. Erwinia asparaginase (10,000 IU/vial) is an investigational Group C agent available from McKesson BioServices located in Rockville, MD. PEG-asparaginase is commercially available in 5-mL vials that contain 3,750 IU (750 IU/mL).

Selected Reading

Evans WE et al. Anaphylactoid reactions to *Escherichia coli* and *Erwinia* asparaginase in children with leukemia and lymphoma. Cancer 49: 1378–1383, 1982.

AZACITIDINE

Other names

5-azacitidine; ladakamycin; AZAC; AZA-CR; 5-AZC; NSC-102816.

Indications

Group C (investigational) agent for the treatment of refractory acute non-lymphocytic leukemia. Azacitidine is an active agent for myelodysplastic syndromes.

Classification and Mechanisms of Action

Antimetabolite (cytidine analogue). At doses lower than those used in the treatment of acute leukemia, azacitidine acts as a demethylating agent.

Pharmacokinetics

The drug is activated to azacytidine triphosphate and deaminated by the liver to 5-azauridine. Approximately 90% of the drug and its metabolites are excreted in the urine (20% as unchanged drug) in 24 hours. Azacitidine has an elimination half-life of 3 to 6 hours.

Dose

For the treatment of acute leukemia, doses are 150 to 300 mg/m^2/day for 5 days, repeated every 3 weeks, and 150 to 200 mg/m^2 twice weekly for 2 to 8 weeks. Azacitidine, 750 mg/m^2/week, has also been given. Low-dose regimens of azacitidine, 25 mg/m^2 for 14 days, have been used for the treatment of myelodysplastic syndromes.

AZACITIDINE *(continued)*

Administration

Usually administered as a continuous infusion. Has also been given as an IV bolus (in 50 mL or more of 5% dextrose or normal saline), as a short infusion over a period of 10 to 30 minutes, and by subcutaneous injection. Because of its short stability in solution, "fresh bags" must be prepared every 2 to 3 hours for long infusions.

Toxicity

Hematological. Leukopenia, dose-related and dose-limiting, occasionally prolonged; thrombocytopenia, less common; anemia.

Gastrointestinal. Nausea and vomiting, severe and dose-limiting when given as an IV bolus but less common with continuous infusions, diarrhea (50%), stomatitis (infrequent).

Dermatological. Alopecia; rash (rare), pruritus (occasional). Local injection site reactions may occur after subcutaneous injection.

Hepatic. Elevations of liver enzyme, bilirubin, and/or alkaline phosphatase levels. Because of hepatic coma, some have warned against its use in patients with hypoalbuminemia (i.e., less than 3 g/dL).

Neurological. Progressive lethargy, confusion, and coma have been reported.

Cardiovascular. Hypotension after an IV bolus (rare).

Genitourinary. Azotemia (transient and reversible), renal tubular acidosis (rare), proteinuria (rare).

Other. Hypophosphatemia, sometimes with myalgia, muscle weakness, restlessness, insomnia, fatigue, rhabdomyolysis (rare), conjunctivitis, fever.

Storage and Stability

The vials are stored in the refrigerator. It is stable for at least 3 years when stored at room temperature and for 4 years when refrigerated. After reconstitution or upon further dilution the drug rapidly decomposes. It is recommended that azacitidine be administered within 30 minutes of preparation. Its stability in solution is concentration and fluid dependent. On further dilution to a concentration of 2 mg/mL, 10% of its potency is lost in 2.4 hours (normal saline), 3 hours (5% dextrose or Normosol-R), and 2.9 hours (lactated Ringer's solution). At a concentration of 0.2 mg/mL the drug loses 10% of its potency within 1.9 hours (normal saline, lactated Ringer's solution, or Normosol-R) and 0.8 hours (5% dextrose).

Preparation

The 100-mg vial is reconstituted with 19.9 mL sterile water to yield a 5 mg/mL solution. It may be further diluted in an appropriate fluid.

Incompatibilities

Electrolytes have a destabilizing effect and should not be added to azacitidine solutions.

Availability

Available as an investigational agent from the National Cancer Institute in 100-mg vials of lyophilized powder.

Selected Reading

Verbeek W, Ganser A. Evolving treatment options of myelodysplastic syndromes. Ann Hematol 80: 499–509, 2001.

BEXAROTENE

Other names
Targretin®; LDG-1069.

Indications
FDA approved for the treatment of refractory cutaneous T-cell lymphoma (CTCL).
May be useful in the treatment of AIDS-related Kaposi's sarcoma, non-small-cell lung cancer, and renal cell cancer. The topical product is approved for refractory early-stage CTCL lesions, and may be useful in Kaposi's sarcoma.

Classification and Mechanisms of Action
Retinoid. Selective activator of retinoid X receptors.

Pharmacokinetics
Bexarotene is well absorbed with a fat-containing meal. Peak plasma concentrations occur 2 to 4 hours after administration. The drug is almost completely plasma protein-bound and active oxidative metabolites are formed in the liver by the cytochrome P450 3A4 pathway. The elimination half-life of bexarotene ranges from 1 to 7 hours, with less than 1% renal excretion.

Dose
The starting dose is 300 mg/m^2/day orally as a single daily dose. The dose may be increased to 400 mg/m^2/day if, after 8 weeks of therapy, there is no response. Dose adjustments are recommended for patients with liver disease, liver toxicity, neutropenia, and non-responsive hypertriglyceridemia.

Topical Administration
Bexarotene gel is applied to each lesion once every other day for one week. Thereafter the dose is increased incrementally by weekly intervals to daily applications, twice a day applications, three times a day applications, and lastly four times a day applications as clinically indicated.

Administration
Oral. Capsules should be taken with a meal. Topical gel formulation. Use generously on each lesion.

Toxicity
The toxicities listed below are those that have been reported following systemic (oral) therapy, unless otherwise noted.
Hematological. Leukopenia occurs within 2 to 4 weeks of starting therapy and is the most frequent hematological effect. Mild anemia has been reported, thrombocytopenia is uncommon.
Gastrointestinal. Nausea (15%) and vomiting (7%), diarrhea, abdominal pain and anorexia.
Dermatological. Following oral administration: diffuse maculopapular rash (16%), dry skin (10%), exfoliative dermatitis (9%), pruritus, and facial flushing several hours after administration. Rash, pruritus, skin disorder, and pain have been observed following topical administration.
Hepatic. Increased liver function tests and hyperbilirubinemia. Reported rarely, pancreatitis, which may be associated with hypertriglyceridemia.

BEXAROTENE *(continued)*

Lipid abnormalities. These are prominent and include hyperlipidemia and hypercholesteremia. An increase greater than 2.5 times the upper limit of normal in fasting triglycerides has been observed. Utilize antihyperlipidemic therapy; however, not gemfibrizol (see drug interactions) and monitor lipid levels frequently.

Neurological. Headache and asthenia are commonly observed.

Cardiovascular. Peripheral edema (13%).

Other. Myalgias, infection, cataracts, hypercalcemia, hypothyroidism (28%), fever, chills, dryness of mucous membranes, fetal abnormalities and/or fetal malformation. Do not administer to pregnant women, classified as a pregnancy category X drug.

Drug Interactions

Bexarotene administered concomitantly with hypoglycemic agents, including oral sulfonylureas and insulin, may cause an exaggerated hypoglycemic effect. Dose adjustments may be necessary.

Bexarotene administered concomitantly with gemfibrizol can increase bexarotene levels and this combination is not recommended.

Bexarotene elimination may be reduced and toxicity increased by concomitant administration of agents that inhibit the cytochrome P450 3A4 isoenzymes. These agents include but are not limited to itraconazole, calcium channel blockers, gemfibrozil, cimetidine, and macrolides.

Bexarotene elimination may be increased and efficacy reduced by agents that induce the cytochrome P450 3A4 isoenzymes. These agents include but are not limited to phenytoin, rifampin, and phenobarbital.

Bexarotene administered concomitantly with oral contraceptives may decrease their effectiveness by decreasing concentrations. Other nonhormone methods of birth control should be utilized.

Bexarotene administered concomitantly with tamoxifen may decrease levels of the tamoxifen.

It is suggested that other vitamin A-containing supplements be limited or avoided while using bexarotene.

Storage and Stability

Store at room temperature, protected from light and moisture. Each bottle bears an expiration date.

Availability

Bexarotene is commercially available as a 75 mg oral gelatin capsule and commercially available as a 60-gram tube of 1% topical gel.

Selected Reading

Duvic M, Hymes K, Heald P. Bexarotene is effective and safe for the treatment of refractory advanced-stage cutaneous T-cell lymphoma: multinational phase II-III trial results. J Clin Oncol 19: 2456–2471, 2001.

BICALUTAMIDE

Other names
Casodex®; ICI 176,334; NSC-722665.

Indications
FDA approved for the treatment of patients with advanced cancer of the prostate in combination with a luteinizing hormone-releasing hormone (LHRH) analogue (e.g., leuprolide, goserelin).

Classification and Mechanisms of Action
Nonsteroidal antiandrogen. Bicalutamide inhibits the effects of androgens by preventing their binding to cellular androgenic receptors. The drug may also inhibit androgen uptake in the pituitary gland.

Pharmacokinetics
Bicalutamide is slowly absorbed after oral administration and reaches peak plasma concentrations approximately 30 hours after administration. Food does not affect the absorption of bicalutamide from the gastrointestinal tract. The drug is metabolized in the liver to inactive metabolites and the elimination half-life is approximately 6 days. Use with caution in patients with moderate to severe hepatic dysfunction. The elimination of bicalutamide does not appear to be affected by renal impairment.

Dose
Bicalutamide is administered as a daily dose of 50 mg in combination with an LHRH analogue.

Administration
Oral, at the same time each day. Bicalutamide may be administered with meals or on an empty stomach.

Toxicity
Hematological. Anemia (7%), leukopenia (rare).
Gastrointestinal. Nausea (11%), vomiting (3%), anorexia, constipation (7% to 17%), diarrhea (10%), flatulence, xerostomia; rectal bleeding and melena occur rarely.
Dermatological. Rash (6%), diaphoresis (6%), dry skin, pruritus, alopecia (5%).
Hepatic. Increased liver enzyme levels (6%). Severe hepatotoxicity is rare.
Neurological. Dizziness (7%), paresthesia (6%), insomnia (5%), anxiety, headache (4%), depression, decreased libido, hypertonia, confusion, neuropathy, somnolence, nervousness (5%).
Cardiovascular. Hypertension (5%), angina pectoris, peripheral edema (8%), congestive heart failure (5%).
Pulmonary. Dyspnea, cough, pharyngitis, bronchitis, pneumonia, rhinitis, lung disorder (5%). Rarely, interstitial pneumonitis and pulmonary fibrosis have been reported.
Endocrine. Hot flushes (49%), breast pain (39%), gynecomastia (38%). Impotence and diabetes mellitus have occurred in patients receiving bicalutamide and an LHRH analogue.
Genitourinary. Nocturia (9%), hematuria (7%), urinary tract infection (6%), impotence (5%), urinary incontinence (2%), urinary frequency, impaired urination, dysuria, urinary retention, urinary urgency, increased BUN and creatinine levels.
Musculoskeletal. Myasthenia, arthritis, myalgia, leg cramps, pathological fractures (5%).

BICALUTAMIDE *(continued)*

Other. Generalized pain (27%), back pain (15%), pelvic pain (13%), asthenia (15%), infection (10%), flu-like symptoms (4%), fever, chills, weight loss (4%), hyperglycemia (5%).

Drug Interactions

Bicalutamide may displace coumarin anticoagulants from protein-binding sites and lead to prolongation of prothrombin times.

Storage and Stability

Bicalutamide tablets are stored at room temperature. Each bottle bears an expiration date.

Availability

Commercially available as a 50-mg tablet.

Selected Reading

Wirth M et al. Bicalutamide (Casodex) 150 mg as immediate therapy in patients with localized or locally advanced prostate cancer significantly reduces the risk of disease progression. Urology 58: 146–151, 2001.

BLEOMYCIN

Other names

Blenoxane®; BLM; NSC-125066.

Indications

FDA approved for the treatment of squamous cell carcinoma (head and neck, skin, penis, cervix, vulva), Hodgkin's and non-Hodgkin's lymphoma, reticulum cell sarcoma, lymphosarcoma, and testicular carcinoma (embryonal cell, choriocarcinoma, teratocarcinoma). Bleomycin has been used as a sclerosing agent for pleural and pericardial effusions and may be useful in the treatment of Kaposi's sarcoma, soft-tissue sarcoma, osteosarcoma, melanoma, and cancers of the bladder, kidney, endometrium, esophagus, ovary, and thyroid.

Classification and Mechanisms of Action

Antitumor antibiotic.

Pharmacokinetics

Bleomycin is poorly absorbed by mouth. Approximately 45% is absorbed into the systemic circulation after intracavitary administration. Less than 1% is bound to plasma proteins. The kidneys excrete approximately 50% to 70% of the drug as unchanged drug that cannot be removed by hemodialysis. The remaining drug is metabolized by intracellular aminopeptidase (hydrolysis). Bleomycin has an elimination half-life of 2 to 5 hours in patients with normal renal function and up to 30 hours in patients with renal failure. The dose should be reduced in patients with reduced creatinine clearance (e.g., a 25% reduction for a creatinine clearance of 10 to 50 mL/min and a 50% to 100% reduction for a creatinine clearance less than 10 mL/min).

Dose

Common doses include:

- 10 to 20 units/m^2 weekly or twice weekly via IM injection, intravenously, or subcutaneously.

- a continuous infusion over a period of 3 to 7 days at 15 to 20 units/m^2/day has also been used.
- the intrapleural dose is usually 60 units.

Test dose. Because anaphylactoid reactions can occur in patients with lymphoma (1% to 8% incidence), it has been recommended that a 2-unit test dose be given before the first treatment. The test dose is usually given intravenously (in 50 mL 5% dextrose or normal saline over 15 minutes) and followed by an observation period of 1 to 2 hours, although some advocate 6 to 24 hours before administering the full dose.

Total lifetime dose. Until predictive methods are available for the diagnosis of impending pulmonary damage, the total lifetime dose of bleomycin should never exceed 400 units. Many physicians limit the total dose to 300 units.

Administration

Bleomycin may be given via IM injection, by slow IV push over at least 10 minutes, by IV infusion in 50 to 100 mL of normal saline or 5% dextrose over 15 minutes or longer, intra-arterially, intratumorally, by bladder instillation, subcutaneously, or intra-cavitarily. The intrapleural dose is usually dissolved in 50 mL of normal saline and left in the pleural space for 8 to 24 hours.

Toxicity

Hematological. Myelosuppression is uncommon and mild.

Gastrointestinal. Anorexia is common. Mucositis occurs occasionally and mild nausea and/or vomiting are unusual.

Dermatological. Skin reactions are common (50%) and may include striae, pruritus, hyperpigmentation, hyperkeratosis (mainly on the palms and fingers), edema, erythema, and thickening of nail beds. Skin peeling (especially on the fingertips), skin tenderness, urticaria, rash, and alopecia may also occur.

Pulmonary. Up to 10% of patients treated with bleomycin may experience pulmonary toxicity. Interstitial pneumonitis and pulmonary fibrosis are related to the total cumulative dose; doses greater than 400 units must be avoided. Signs and symptoms include dyspnea, cough, fine rales, radiographic findings resembling pneumonia, and altered pulmonary function status (e.g., reduced carbon monoxide diffusing capacity).

Hypersensitivity. Anaphylactoid reactions occur in about 1% (up to 8% in some series) of lymphoma patients and are often associated with a severe febrile reaction. Deaths have been reported.

Other. Fever with or without chills is common (25%), frequently occurs within 4 to 10 hours after administration, and lasts 4 to 12 hours or longer. The incidence may decrease with subsequent doses. Preventive treatment with acetaminophen (e.g., 650 mg every 4 to 6 hours for three to four doses) is recommended. Hypotension, pain at the injection site, phlebitis, headache, Raynaud's phenomenon, lethargy, and unusual taste sensations have also been reported.

Drug Interactions

Patients on chronic digoxin or phenytoin therapy could experience a decrease in serum levels of these medications if bleomycin is administered.

Cisplatin has been shown to inhibit renal elimination of bleomycin.

Prior radiation to the chest and use of high oxygen concentrations may increase the risk of bleomycin-induced pulmonary toxicity.

Storage and Stability

Bleomycin is stored in the refrigerator. After reconstitution the solution is stable for at least 28 days if refrigerated or for 14 days at room temperature.

BLEOMYCIN (continued)

Preparation

One to 5 mL of normal saline is added to the 15-unit vial to result in concentrations of 15 to 3 units/mL, respectively. A standard dilution of 5 mL (to yield 3 units/mL) is recommended. It may be further diluted in normal saline or 5% dextrose.

Incompatibilities

Bleomycin should not be mixed with solutions containing divalent or trivalent cations (especially copper) because of chelation. It is inactivated by hydrogen peroxide, methotrexate, mitomycin, and ascorbic acid.

Compatibilities

Reconstituted bleomycin in 5% dextrose solution with 100 to 1,000 units/mL of heparin is stable for 24 hours at room temperature. Bleomycin is compatible with cyclophosphamide, doxorubicin, mesna, vinblastine, and vincristine. A pharmacist should be consulted for more information.

Availability

Commercially available in 15-unit vials as a lyophilized powder.

Selected Reading

Comis RL. Detecting bleomycin pulmonary toxicity: a continued conundrum. J Clin Oncol 8: 765–767, 1990.

BRYOSTATIN-1

Other names

Bryostatin; BMY-45618; NSC-339555.

Indications

Bryostatin-1 is an investigational agent in the United States. Brytostatin-1 may have activity in non-Hodgkin's lymphoma, non-small-cell lung cancer, head and neck cancer, and other malignancies. Bryostatin-1, in combination with paclitaxel, has an orphan product designation for the treatment of esophageal cancer.

Classification and Mechanisms of Action

Bryostatin-1 is an inhibitor of protein kinase C that is derived from a marine bryozoan. The drug has also been shown to down-regulate the multidrug-resistant (MDR) gene and induce differentiation of myeloid, lymphoid, and leukemic cell lines.

Pharmacokinetics

Bryostatin-1 is rapidly distributed throughout the body following administration. In animals the drug is distributed to the heart, liver, lung, lymph nodes, and adipose tissues. Using a competition bioassay, the half-life is 44 minutes.

Dose

As a single agent: 40 microg/m^2/day as a continuous infusion for 3 days (i.e., 120 microg/m^2 administered over 72 hours). Treatment is repeated every 2 weeks. Bryostatin-1, 25 microg/m^2 as a 24-hour continuous infusion, has been used in combination with paclitaxel 80 mg/m^2 as a 1-hour infusion, with both drugs repeated weekly for 3 weeks followed by 1 week of rest. On this schedule paclitaxel is administered on day 1 and bryostatin-1 on day 2. Sequential use of bryostatin-1 followed by vincristine 2 mg has been evaluated.

Administration

Bryostatin-1 is administered IV, usually as a continuous infusion over 24 to 72 hours.

Toxicity

Hematological. Mild and transient neutropenia, thrombocytopenia, and anemia have been observed. These effects may be more severe in patients with bone marrow involvement (e.g., patients with multiple myeloma).

Gastrointestinal. Nausea and vomiting (grade 3) has been reported in up to 15% of courses when bryostatin-1 is administered as a weekly 24-hour infusion for 3 consecutive weeks. These symptoms have been reported less frequently following bryostatin-1 administration as a 72-hour infusion every 2 weeks. Diarrhea has been reported.

Dermatological. Skin rash has been reported in up to 40% of patients receiving a 72-hour infusion every 2 weeks. Generalized bronzing of the skin has been observed in some patients following several courses of therapy. Mild hyperpigmentation in sun-exposed areas has also been reported. Phlebitis is a common toxicity when bryostatin-1 is administered through a peripheral vein. Alopecia is rare.

Hepatic. Elevations of alkaline phosphatase, bilirubin, and transaminases have been observed.

Renal. Elevations of serum creatinine have occurred infrequently.

Neurological. Headache, primarily grade 1 or 2, is reported in approximately up to 33% of the patients.

Cardiovascular. Sinus bradycardia, usually occurring during the infusion. Phlebitis, usually superficial.

Pulmonary. Dyspnea (grade 2) was observed in approximately 50% of the patients who received bryostatin-1 and paclitaxel. A few patients had severe pulmonary symptoms.

Musculoskeletal. Myalgia is a dose-limiting toxicity and tends to increase in severity with cumulative doses of bryostatin-1. Myalgia (grade 2) has been reported in up to 50% of patients. Attenuation of dose has been used to delay the onset of severe symptoms. Acetaminophen or non-steroidal anti-inflammatory drugs are helpful in most cases, but opioid analgesics have been necessary in many cases.

Other. Fatigue, which has been dose-limiting in some studies, is reported in 45% to 80% of the courses. Fatigue (grade 3) appears to be more common with the 72-hour infusion (20% incidence). Fever and infection have been reported in up to 25% of the courses of bryostatin-1 administration as a 72-hour infusion. The incidence appears to be more common if the drug is administered every week, compared to every 2 weeks. Hyponatremia has been reported in approximately 25% of the patients enrolled to one study. Eye pain and/or photophobia were dose-limiting in pediatric patients who received weekly 1-hour infusions of bryostatin-1. Eye pain usually occurred within a few days of the second or third week of treatment. The symptoms usually resolved within a week. Eye pain has also been reported in adults, but this has not been a dose-limiting toxicity. Infusion reactions (flushing, dyspnea, hypotension, and bradycardia) have been reported infrequently.

Storage and Stability

Intact vials of bryostatin-1 are to be stored in the refrigerator. Solutions of 1 to 10 microg/mL in preserved normal saline are stable at room temperature for up to 14 days.

BRYOSTATIN-1 *(continued)*

Preparation

Add 1 mL of PET special diluent to the 0.1-mg vial to yield a concentration of 100 microg/mL. This dose is further diluted with 9 mL of normal saline to yield a concentration of 10 microg/mL. Bryostatin-1 may be further diluted with normal saline or 5% dextrose in water to a concentration of 0.15 to 0.75 microg/mL in a glass or polyolefin container.

Incompatibilities

Bryostatin-1 is not compatible with polyvinylchloride (PVC); plasticizer leaching occurs.

Availability

Bryostatin-1 is an investigational agent in the United States that is available as a lyophilized powder (0.1 mg/vial) with a special diluent called PET (NSC 641159) from the National Cancer Institute.

Selected Reading

Brockstein B et al. Phase II studies of bryostatin-1 in patients with advanced sarcoma and advanced head and neck cancer. Invest New Drugs 19: 249–254, 2001.

BUSULFAN

Other names

Myleran®; Busulfex®; BSF; NSC-750.

Indications

FDA approved for the treatment of chronic myelogenous leukemia, and as part of a conditioning regimen prior to peripheral blood stem cell or bone marrow transplants. Busulfan has also been used in the treatment of acute nonlymphocytic leukemia, polycythemia vera, myelofibrosis, and severe thrombocytosis.

Classification

Alkylating agent.

Pharmacokinetics

Well absorbed by mouth with peak plasma levels occurring 0.5 to 2 hours after administration. Busulfan distribution includes the cerebrospinal fluid. The intravenous formulation is completely bioavailable and extensively liver metabolized through a conjugation reaction with glutathione followed by liver oxidation. The drug is metabolized to several metabolites that are excreted into the urine. Approximately 25% to 35% of a dose is eliminated via the kidneys as methanesulfonic acid. Busulfan has an elimination half-life of approximately 2.5 hours.

Dose

The usual oral adult dose for induction therapy is 4 to 12 mg/day. Maintenance doses are usually 1 to 3 mg/day but have ranged from 2 mg/week to 4 mg/day.

Transplant Preparative Regimens

Consult specific transplant protocols. Intravenous busulfan in a dose of 0.8 mg/kg is generally considered equivalent to 1 mg/kg of the oral preparation.

Administration

Oral or intravenous infusion over 2 hours.

Toxicity

Hematological. Prolonged myelosuppression with slow recovery and severe thrombocytopenia; anemia, agranulocytosis (rare). Following oral administration nadir blood counts occur in 11 to 30 days. Following IV administration nadir blood counts occur within 4 to 17 days.

Gastrointestinal. Nausea and vomiting are mild to moderate with standard doses but are moderate to severe with the doses used for patients undergoing bone marrow transplantation. Diarrhea is uncommon, anorexia; moderate to severe mucositis with accompanying diarrhea can occur with high-dose therapy.

Dermatological. Hyperpigmentation (diffuse brown, bronze, dusky), dryness of skin and mucous membranes, alopecia, rashes, melanoderma, urticaria.

Hepatic. Abnormalities in hepatic enzymes, cholestatic jaundice, hepatic veno-occlusive disease (transplant doses).

Neurological (associated with high-dose therapy). Dizziness, blurred vision, confusion, seizures.

Cardiovascular. Hypertension (36%), tachycardia (44%), thrombosis (33%), vasodilation (25%), hypotension (11%). Uncommonly, ECG abnormalities may occur with the IV formulation. Hypotension has been reported (rare).

Pulmonary. "Busulfan lung" (interstitial pulmonary fibrosis) with persistent cough, fever, rales, dyspnea, and respiratory insufficiency. Pulmonary fibrosis is rare and most often occurs after chronic therapy.

Other. Occasional gynecomastia, hyperuricemia, hyperuricosuria, Addison-like syndrome, asthenia, fatigue, impairment of fertility, cheilosis, impotence (rare), amenorrhea, hemorrhagic cystitis (rare), endocardial fibrosis (rare), cataracts, second malignancy. Hypomagnesemia, hyperglycemia, hypokalemia, hypercalcemia, and edema have occurred with the IV formulation.

Preparation

The prescribed dose is withdrawn from the glass ampule using the provided filter needle. Change to a standard needle and add the busulfan to dextrose 5% or normal saline to achieve a final concentration of approximately 0.5 mg/mL.

Drug Interactions

Acetaminophen administered within 72 hours of busulfan may cause decreased busulfan clearance and increased toxicity.

Itraconazole administered concomitantly with busulfan may cause decreased busulfan clearance by 25% and increased toxicity.

Chronic phenytoin therapy increases metabolism and clearance of busulfan by phenytoin's induction of glutathione-S-transferase.

Busulfan administration concomitantly with long-term thioguanine therapy may cause an increase in hepatotoxicity and occurrence of esophageal varices.

Storage and Stability

Tablets are stored at room temperature. Busulfan injection is stored in the refrigerator. Containers bear expiration dates.

Availability

Busulfan is commercially available in 2-mg scored tablets and in 10-mL ampules as a sterile 6 mg/mL injectable solution (5-micron filter provided).

Selected Reading

Buggia I et al. Busulfan, DICP. Ann Pharmacother 28: 1055–1062, 1994.

CAPECITABINE

Other names

Xeloda®; Ro 09-1978/000; NSC-712807.

Indications

FDA approved for the treatment of metastatic breast cancer patients who no longer benefit from paclitaxel- and anthracycline-based regimens or in patients who cannot continue anthracycline therapy. Also approved for use in combination with docetaxel in the treatment of metastatic breast cancer patients who no longer benefit from anthracycline-containing regimens. Capecitabine is also approved for use in the treatment of metastatic colorectal cancer, as a single agent. Capecitabine is a prodrug of fluorouracil and, as such, is likely to be active in malignancies that respond to 5-fluorouracil.

Classification

Fluoropyrimidine antimetabolite.

Pharmacokinetics

Capecitabine is an oral systemic prodrug that is metabolized to fluorouracil. It is well absorbed orally. Peak plasma concentrations of capecitabine occur 1.5 hours after administration and peak plasma levels of fluorouracil occur 30 minutes later. If taken with food, both the rate and extent of absorption are decreased. Less than 60% of capecitabine is plasma protein-bound, with approximately 35% of the drug bound to albumin. The elimination half-life is 45 minutes for the capecitabine and fluorouracil components. Greater than 90% of capecitabine and its metabolites are recovered in the urine.

Dose

The recommended starting dose is 2,500 mg/m^2/day. The total daily dose is administered orally in two divided doses, approximately 12 hours apart, for 2 consecutive weeks followed by a week of no treatment. Treatment cycles are repeated every 21 days. Elderly (> 80 years of age) patients may experience increased toxicity, adjust dose as required. Capecitabine should not be used in patients with severe renal dysfunction, and it should be dose reduced by 25% in patients with moderate renal dysfunction (i.e., creatinine clearance = 30 to 50 mL/min). There are no specific dose reductions for hepatic toxicity.

Administration

Oral. Take capecitabine with water immediately after a meal.

Toxicity

Hematological. Neutropenia and thrombocytopenia occur in approximately 20% of patients, while anemia is observed in approximately 14%.

Gastrointestinal. Diarrhea is common (50%), may be severe and require clinical management (e.g., hydration, electrolyte replacement). Other gastrointestinal side effects include nausea (40%), vomiting, stomatitis, constipation, abdominal pain, dyspepsia, anorexia, and dehydration.

Dermatological. Hand and foot syndrome (i.e., palmar-plantar erythrodysesthesia or acral erythema) occurs in up to 50% of patients. Signs and symptoms include numbness, dysesthesia/paresthesia, tingling, painless or painful swelling, erythema, desquamation, blistering, and pain. If grade 2 or 3 toxicity occurs, it is recommended that treatment be discontinued until symptoms resolve to at least grade 1.

Hepatic. Hyperbilirubinemia (17%), increased alkaline phosphatase, increased hepatic transaminases.
Neurological. Paresthesias, headache, dizziness, and insomnia are most common. Less commonly observed are confusion, ataxia, encephalopathy, and altered state of consciousness.
Cardiovascular. EKG changes, myocardial infarctions, angina pectoris, cardiomyopathy, hypotension, hypertension. These side effects are more commonly seen in patients with a previous cardiac history.
Other. Eye irritation, fatigue, edema, fever, muscle aches.

Drug Interactions

Capecitabine administered concomitantly with chronic warfarin therapy can cause coagulation abnormalities, bleeding, and increased INR and PT. Deaths have been reported. Monitor coagulation parameters frequently and adjust dose per clinical judgment.

Capecitabine may inhibit the hepatic isoenzyme CYP 2C9 and therefore decrease the metabolism of phenytoin; monitor levels frequently when used concurrently.

Capecitabine should not be administered with aluminum- or magnesium-containing antacids.

Similar to fluorouracil, administration of leucovorin before capecitabine can cause a synergistic effect with increased activity and toxicity.

Storage and Stability

Capecitabine tablets are stored at room temperature. Each bottle bears an expiration date.

Availability

Capecitabine is commercially available as 150- and 500-mg tablets.

Selected Readings
Blum JL et al. Multicenter, phase II study of capecitabine in taxane-pretreated metastatic breast carcinoma patients. Cancer 92: 1759–1768, 2001.
Poole C et al. Effect of renal impairment on the pharmacokinetics and tolerability of capecitabine (Xeloda) in cancer patients. Cancer Chemother Pharmacol 49: 225–234, 2002.
Van Cutsem E et al. Capecitabine, an oral fluoropyrimidine carbamate with substantial activity in advanced colorectal cancer: results of a randomized phase II study. J Clin Oncol 18: 1337–1345, 2000.

CARBOPLATIN

Other names
Paraplatin®; CBDCA; carboplatinum; JM-8; NSC-241240.

Indications
FDA approved for the treatment of ovarian carcinoma. Carboplatin has also been found to be useful in the treatment of non-small-cell and small-cell lung cancer, neuroblastoma, refractory leukemias, non-Hodgkin's and Hodgkins' lymphomas, melanoma, and cancers of the bladder, brain, breast, testes, head and neck, endometrium, esophagus, kidney, and cervix.

Classification
Heavy metal alkylating-like agent.

CARBOPLATIN *(continued)*

Pharmacokinetics

After IV administration, carboplatin disappears rapidly from the bloodstream. It has an elimination half-life of approximately 2.5 to 6 hours. Carboplatin crosses the blood-brain barrier. At least 60% to 70% of the drug is eliminated unchanged in the urine, necessitating dose attenuation in patients with impairment of renal function when dosing does not take into account renal function.

Dose

The dose of carboplatin is commonly based upon a desired (or targeted) area under the [pharmacokinetic] curve (AUC), using the following formula:

$$\text{Dose (total mg)} = \text{Target AUC} \times (\text{GFR} + 25).$$

The patient's creatinine clearance, in mL/minute, is often used in place of GFR. The creatinine clearance can be obtained from a 24-hour urine collection, or an estimated value utilizing mathematical formulas (e.g., Cockcroft-Gault or Jeliffe methods). A target AUC of 6 to 7 is often used depending on the patient's prior therapies and drug(s) that will be used in combination with carboplatin. A target AUC of 4 to 6 may be appropriate for patients who have received extensive prior treatment, and a higher target AUC may be appropriate for previously untreated patients. A lower AUC of 1.5 to 2 has also been used in conjunction with radiation therapy on a weekly basis. The numeric value of 25 in this formula is a constant value that represents nonrenal clearance of carboplatin.

Other carboplatin doses have been used. A common IV dose is 360 to 400 mg/m^2 every 4 weeks. Doses of 400 to 550 mg/m^2 have been given by the intraperitoneal route. Consult transplant protocols for specific doses.

Administration

Usually by IV infusion in 50 to 250 mL of 5% dextrose or normal saline over 15 to 30 minutes. Carboplatin has also been given intraperitoneally and intra-arterially (intrahepatic and intracarotid). Concomitant hydration is not necessary.

Toxicity

Hematological. Thrombocytopenia is dose-limiting (nadir, within 2 to 3 weeks; recovery, 1 to 2 weeks thereafter). Neutropenia occurs frequently but is usually not dose-limiting. When doses are calculated based on mg/m^2, patients with impaired renal function will experience more pronounced myelosuppression unless the dose is attenuated. Clinically significant anemia is uncommon after treatment with carboplatin but may be cumulative.

Gastrointestinal. Nausea and vomiting occur frequently but are less severe when compared with cisplatin and usually preventable with antiemetic treatment. Symptoms usually begin 6 to 12 hours after administration and may last for 24 hours. Anorexia, constipation, and diarrhea have been reported.

Dermatological. Rash, urticaria, alopecia, mucositis (8%).

Hepatic. Abnormal liver function values occur in 20% to 30% of patients and are generally mild and transient. Hepatic veno-occlusive disease has been reported after high-dose carboplatin therapy before bone marrow transplantation.

Neurological. Peripheral neuropathy is infrequent and more common in patients older than 65 years of age. This toxicity may be cumulative, especially in patients who have received prior treatment with cisplatin. Ototoxicity occurs in approximately 12% of patients.

Renal. Elevations in serum creatinine and BUN levels and significant electrolyte loss (i.e., hypomagnesemia, hyponatremia, hypokalemia) are uncommon; hematuria is rare.
Other. Pain at the site of injection, asthenia (44%), blurred vision, flu-like syndrome, optic neuritis, hyperamylasemia.

Drug Interactions

Carboplatin, if given prior to paclitaxel, causes an increase in hematological toxicity due to decreased paclitaxel clearance. Carboplatin should be administered after paclitaxel.

Carboplatin can cause a decrease in phenytoin levels due to decreased absorption and/or increased phenytoin metabolism.

Storage and Stability

Carboplatin vials are stored at room temperature and protected from light. The reconstituted solution and 1 mg/mL solutions are stable for at least 24 hours at room temperature and 5 days in the refrigerator. When further diluted in glass or polyvinyl plastic to a concentration of 0.5 mg/mL, solutions have the following stability: in normal saline, 8 hours at room temperature, 24 hours in the refrigerator; in 5% dextrose (when reconstituted in sterile water), 24 hours at room and refrigeration temperatures.

Preparation

Add 5, 15, or 45 mL sterile water, normal saline, or 5% dextrose to the 50-, 150-, or 450-mg vial, respectively. The resulting solution contains 10 mg/mL. The desired dose is further diluted, usually in 5% dextrose.

Incompatibilities

Forms a precipitate when in contact with aluminum.

Compatibilities

Carboplatin (0.3 mg/mL) and etoposide (0.4 mg/mL) are chemically compatible in normal saline or 5% dextrose for at least 24 hours at room temperature.

Availability

Commercially available as a lyophilized powder in 50-, 150-, and 450-mg vials.

Selected Reading

Calvert AH et al. Carboplatin dosage: prospective evaluation of a simple formula based on renal function. J Clin Oncol 7: 1748–1756, 1989.

CARBOXYPEPTIDASE

Other names

Carboxypeptidase-G2; CPDG2; NSC-641273.

tIndications

Carboxypeptidase is an investigational agent in the United States. Emergency access to carboxypeptidase-G2 for high-dose methotrexate-induced renal dysfunction is available for intravenous administration through a "compassionate-use protocol" from the Cancer Therapy Evaluation Program (CTEP) of the National Cancer Institute.

Classification and Mechanisms of Action

Carboxypeptidase is an enzyme that converts greater than 98% of methotrexate into 2,4-diamino-N10-methylpteroic acid (DAMPA). DAMPA is not cytotoxic and is

CARBOXYPEPTIDASE *(continued)*

eliminated by nonrenal mechanisms. Administration of carboxypeptidase leads to a rapid reduction in methotrexate concentrations from the cerebrospinal fluid following intrathecal administration, or plasma following intravenous administration.

Dose

The intrathecal dose of carboxypeptidase is 2,000 units. The intravenous dose is 50 units/kg. Patients with plasma methotrexate concentrations greater than 100 microM immediately prior to carboxypeptidase administration are to be given a second dose 48 hours after the first dose. Calcium leucovorin is to be continued.

Administration

Carboxypeptidase is administered IV over 5 minutes. The intrathecal dose is also administered over 5 minutes with the drug diluted in an amount of saline that is appropriate for the age of the patient.

Toxicity

Hematological. Anemia.
Dermatological. Skin rash.
Other. Hypersensitivity reactions.

Storage and Stability

Intact vials are stored in the freezer ($-20°C$ to $-10°C$). The drug is stable for 24 hours at room temperature. Reconstituted solutions are stable for at least 8 hours at room temperature.

Preparation

Add 1 mL of normal saline to the 1,000-unit vial to yield a concentration of 1,000 units/mL. Doses are usually further diluted in normal saline.

Availability

Carboxypeptidase is an investigational agent in the United States that is available as a lyophilized powder (1,000 units/vial) from the National Cancer Institute.

Selected Readings

Widemann B et al. Carboxypeptidase-G2, thymidine, and leucovorin rescue in cancer patients with methotrexate-induced renal dysfunction. J Clin Oncol 15: 2125–2134, 1997.

Widemann B et al. Rescue with carboxypeptidase-G2 (CPDG2) and leucovorin (LV) for patients with high-dose methotrexate (HDMTX) induced renal failure. Proc Am Soc Clin Oncol 1998; 17: 222a.

CARMUSTINE

Other names

BCNU; BiCNU®; bis-chloronitrosourea; NSC-409962 Carmustine wafers; Gliadel®; NSC-714372.

Indications

Carmustine injection is FDA approved for the treatment of brain tumors, multiple myeloma, Hodgkin's disease, and non-Hodgkin's lymphoma. Carmustine may also be a useful treatment for melanoma, cutaneous T-cell lymphoma, and cancers of the colon, rectum, stomach, and liver.

Carmustine wafers (Gliadel®) are FDA approved for implantation during surgical resection of glioblastoma multiforme.

Classification
Alkylating agent of the nitrosourea class.

Pharmacokinetics
Carmustine rapidly distributes into the tissues after IV injection. Significant amounts of carmustine and/or its metabolites, some of which are active, penetrate into the cerebrospinal fluid (up to 70% of plasma concentrations). Carmustine metabolites also distribute into breast milk. The drug is metabolized by the liver (microsomal enzymes may play a significant role), and approximately 80% of the drug and its metabolites are eliminated via the kidneys. Carmustine has a half-life of approximately 15 to 20 minutes; metabolites have longer half-lives. Carmustine is not hemodialyzable.

The chemical components of carmustine wafers biodegrade at a variable rate in the brain tissue. There is limited data on the pharmacokinetics of the wafer.

Dose
Carmustine injection. The usual dose as a single agent is 150 to 200 mg/m^2 every 6 weeks as a single dose or divided over a period of 2 days. As a preparative agent before bone marrow transplantation, consult Chapter 10.
Carmustine wafers. Up to 8 carmustine wafers should be implanted in the brain tumor area of surgical resection.

Administration
Usually administered in 100 mL or more of 5% dextrose or normal saline as a 1- to 2-hour intravenous infusion. Do not infuse over longer than 2 hours because of incompatibility with the IV tubing. Carmustine has also been given intra-arterially, topically as a 0.2% solution or 0.4% ointment, and intratumorally as a biodegradable polymer (Gliadel® wafer).

Toxicity
Carmustine Injection
Hematological. Leukopenia and thrombocytopenia occur within 25 to 35 days, may last 60 days, and are cumulative. Anemia may also occur after treatment with carmustine.
Gastrointestinal. Nausea and vomiting are common but preventable with antiemetics. Diarrhea, anorexia, esophagitis, and dysphagia are infrequent side effects.
Dermatological. Alopecia, brown discoloration of the skin (more common with topical administration), skin rash, pruritus. Burning at the injection site and along the vein is common and can be lessened by the application of a cold compress above the site and/or by slowing the rate of the infusion.
Hepatic. Reversible elevation of liver enzyme levels (25%), hyperbilirubinemia, veno-occlusive disease after transplantation doses.
Neurological. Dizziness and ataxia have been reported following IV use. Severe retinal toxicity, blindness, and seizures have been reported when given by intracarotid artery.
Cardiovascular. Hypotension (from rapid or concentrated infusion).
Pulmonary. Infiltrates and/or fibrosis, especially with prolonged therapy and higher doses. Pulmonary damage may not become evident until years after treatment has been discontinued. It has been recommended that a cumulative dose of 1,400 mg/m^2 not be exceeded.
Renal. Azotemia, decrease in kidney size, and renal failure with large cumulative doses.
Other. Impotence, testicular damage causing infertility, facial flushing, and second malignancies have also been reported.

CARMUSTINE (continued)

Carmustine Wafers
Neurological. Seizures, convulsions, headaches, somnolence, confusion, brain edema, intracranial infection, and obstructive hydrocephalus. Brain herniation has been associated with wafer implantation.
Other. Surgical healing abnormalities, fever, pain.

Storage and Stability

Carmustine vials are stored in the refrigerator and protected from light. If exposed to heat, the powder becomes an oily liquid, and should be discarded. The reconstituted solution is stable for 48 hours if refrigerated and 14 hours at room temperature when protected from light. After further dilution to 1 mg/mL or less in normal saline or 5% dextrose, it is stable for 16 hours in glass or polyolefin containers when protected from light at room temperature and for 48 hours when refrigerated.

Carmustine wafers should be maintained in their foil pouches and stored in the freezer. The temperature must remain at or below −20°C. The wafers may be kept at room temperature for no longer than 6 hours.

Drug Interactions (Carmustine Injection)

Cimetidine may slow the metabolism of carmustine, presumably by decreasing liver blood flow, resulting in enhanced myelosuppression.

Carmustine administered concomitantly with digoxin may cause a decrease in digoxin plasma levels.

Carmustine administered concomitantly with phenytoin may cause a decrease in phenytoin plasma levels.

Preparation

Each vial is reconstituted with 3 mL of the provided alcohol. After complete dissolution, 27 mL of sterile water is added to yield a concentration of 3.3 mg/mL. The desired dose is further diluted in 100 to 250 mL of 5% dextrose or normal saline in a glass or polyolefin container. A stock solution of carmustine for topical administration may be prepared by dissolving 100 mg of carmustine in 50 mL of 95% ethanol. A 5-mL portion of the stock solution is diluted with 60 mL of tap water just before topical administration.

Incompatibilities

Incompatible with polyvinyl chloride infusion bags and with sodium bicarbonate.

Availability

Carmustine injection is commercially available as a duopak containing a 100-mg vial of carmustine and a 3-mL vial of absolute alcohol. Carmustine wafers are commercially available as a single dose treatment box containing 8 individually foil-wrapped wafers (7.7 mg/wafer).

CELECOXIB

Other names

Celebrex®; NSC-719627.

Indications

Celecoxib is FDA approved for use in adults to relieve the signs and symptoms of osteoarthritis and rheumatoid arthritis. Celecoxib has a role in the treatment of patients with familial adenomatous polyposis (FAP), in combination with standard of care. Celecoxib has been shown to reduce the number and size of adenomatous colorectal polyps. Celecoxib, and similar agents, are being evaluated as an adjunctive treatment for patients with advanced malignancies.

Classification and Mechanisms of Action

Celecoxib is a nonsteroidal anti-inflammatory drug (NSAID) that inhibits the enzyme cyclooxygenase-2 (Cox-2). Similar to other NSAIDs, celecoxib possesses anti-inflammatory, antipyretic, and analgesic properties. Celecoxib inhibits Cox-2, which in turn prevents prostaglandin synthesis. When Cox-2 is stimulated, prostaglandin synthesis is activated in both inflammatory tissues and malignant tissues. Inhibition of Cox-2 prevents the production of prostaglandins and prostanoids, potentially causing decreased tumor growth, antiangiogenic effects, apoptotic effects, and potential stimulation of immune function.

Pharmacokinetics

Celecoxib is absorbed after oral administration. Peak plasma levels occur approximately 3 hours after a dose. Food affects the absorption of celecoxib. High-fat meals cause a 1- to 2-hour delay in absorption but an increase in the total amount absorbed. The half-life of celecoxib is approximately 11 hours. The drug exhibits extensive protein binding (i.e., approximately 97%) and distributes extensively into tissues. Celecoxib is metabolized via the hepatic isoenzyme cytochrome P450 2C9 pathway, resulting in three inactive metabolites. The majority of celecoxib is eliminated via the liver. Less than 3% of the unchanged drug is found in the feces or urine.

Dose

The usual dose of celecoxib for familial adenomatous polyposis (FAP) is 400 mg twice a day. The usual dose of celecoxib for osteoarthritis is 100 mg twice a day or 200 mg daily. The usual dose of celecoxib for rheumatoid arthritis is 100 to 200 mg twice a day. As an adjunctive treatment for patients with advanced malignancies, in combination with chemotherapy, celecoxib is administered as 400 mg twice a day. Adjustment of dose for patients with mild to moderate renal and hepatic dysfunction is not necessary. Celecoxib is not recommended for patients with severe hepatic dysfunction.

Administration

Oral. Take with food.

Toxicity

The toxicities listed below are published data from controlled arthritis trials.
Hematological. Rarely anemia is observed (< 1%).
Gastrointestinal. There is a risk of gastrointestinal bleeding during NSAID therapy. Patients should be informed of signs and symptoms. Dyspepsia was reported in almost 9% of patients, other reported gastrointestinal toxicities were observed in less than 6% of patients and include: abdominal pain, diarrhea, flatulence, and nausea.
Dermatological. Rash (2.2%).
Neurological. Headache is reported in up to 15% of patients, insomnia in 2.3%, dizziness in 2%, and nervousness, somnolence, and depression in less than 2%.
Hepatic. Elevated liver transaminases are reported infrequently following NSAID therapy. Rarely reported hepatic toxicities include: hepatitis, jaundice, liver necrosis, and hepatic failure.
Cardiovascular. Palpitations, tachycardia, and peripheral edema were observed in less than 2% of patients.

CELECOXIB *(continued)*

Pulmonary. Upper respiratory tract infections were reported in 8% of patients, sinusitis in 5%, pharyngitis and rhinitis in less than 3%. Use with caution in asthma patients secondary to potential bronchospasm.

Renal. Chronic NSAID therapy can cause renal dysfunction or renal papillary necrosis.

Hypersensitivity. NSAIDs can cause anaphylactoid-type reactions and rare anaphylactic cases have been reported following celecoxib administration.

Other. Back pain and accidental injury were reported in less than 3% of patients.

Drug Interactions

Celecoxib is metabolized through the hepatic isoenzyme cytochrome P450 2C9 pathway. Medications that inhibit this pathway should be used with caution (e.g., fluconazole significantly increases celecoxib plasma concentrations). Celecoxib is also an inhibitor of hepatic isoenzyme cytochrome P450 2D6, medications metabolized by this pathway may be affected.

The antihypertensive effect of angiotensin-converting enzymes may be inhibited by celecoxib.

Due to inhibition of renal prostaglandin synthesis, celecoxib may decrease the effectiveness of thiazide diuretics and furosemide.

Celecoxib can increase lithium plasma levels by up to 17%.

Celecoxib should be used with caution in patients on chronic warfarin therapy. Increased prothrombin times and bleeding events have been reported in post-marketing surveillance.

Storage and Stability

Celecoxib capsules are stored at room temperature. Each bottle bears an expiration date.

Availability

Celecoxib is commercially available in 100-mg and 200-mg capsules.

Selected Readings

Bresalier RS. Chemoprevention comes to clinical practice: COX-2 inhibition in familial adenomatous polyposis. Gastroenterology 119: 1797, 2000.

Thun MJ, Henley SJ, Patrono C. Nonsteroidal anti-inflammatory drugs as anticancer agents: mechanistic, pharmacologic, and clinical issues. J Natl Cancer Inst. 94: 252–266, 2002.

CHLORAMBUCIL

Other names

Leukeran®; NSC-3088.

Indications

FDA approved for the treatment of chronic lymphocytic leukemia and malignant lymphomas (including lymphosarcoma, giant follicular lymphoma, and Hodgkin's disease). Chlorambucil may also be a useful treatment for Waldenström's macroglobulinemia, breast cancer, hairy-cell leukemia, multiple myeloma, and ovarian, testicular, and trophoblastic neoplasms.

Classification
Alkylating agent.

Pharmacokinetics
Chlorambucil is well absorbed (85% to 90%) following oral administration. Maximum plasma concentrations occur approximately 1 hour after administration. Concomitant administration with food slows the rate of oral absorption but does not affect overall bioavailability. Chlorambucil is almost entirely metabolized by the liver (to some active metabolites) and has an elimination half-life of 1 to 2 hours. Less than 1% of the drug is eliminated via the kidneys as unchanged chlorambucil or phenylacetic acid mustard, the primary active metabolite. Chlorambucil and phenylacetic acid mustard are not dialyzable.

Dose
Chlorambucil has been given in various dose schedules, including:
- 0.1 to 0.2 mg/kg/day for 3 to 6 weeks (leukemia induction)
- 0.4 mg/kg as a single dose every 2 to 4 weeks
- 16 mg/m^2/day for 5 days every 4 weeks (lymphoma).

Maintenance therapy has been given at:
- 0.03 mg/kg/day up to 0.1 mg/kg/day or
- 2 mg to 4 mg orally once a day, depending on blood counts.

Administration
Oral.

Toxicity
Hematological. Leukopenia and thrombocytopenia are dose-related. Cumulative, dose-limiting myelosuppression has been observed in some patients. Anemia occurs infrequently.
Gastrointestinal. Nausea, vomiting, anorexia, and diarrhea are relatively uncommon.
Dermatological. Alopecia and mucositis are uncommon. Dermatitis, rash, pruritus, urticaria, erythema multiforme, epidermal necrolysis, and Stevens–Johnson syndrome are rare.
Hepatic. Increased liver enzyme levels occur but are usually mild and transient.
Pulmonary. Cumulative pulmonary fibrosis (rare).
Neurological. Seizures (more common in patients with impaired renal function), confusion, agitation, tremors, ataxia, and peripheral neuropathy are rare side effects.
Ocular. Diplopia, papilledema, retinal hemorrhage, and keratitis are rare.
Other. Sterility (amenorrhea, azoospermia, oligospermia), possible secondary malignancy (i.e., leukemia), cystitis (rare), drug fever (rare).

Storage and Stability
Chlorambucil tablets are stored at room temperature. Each bottle bears an expiration date.

Availability
Chlorambucil is commercially available in 2-mg sugar-coated tablets.

CISPLATIN

Other names
Platinol-AQ®; Platinol®; cis-platinum; cisdiamminedichloroplatinum (II); CDDP; DDP; platinum; NSC-119875.

Indications
FDA approved for the treatment of testicular carcinoma, ovarian cancer, and transitional cell bladder cancer. Cisplatin may be a useful treatment for cancers of the brain, adrenal cortex, breast, cervix, uterus, endometrium, head and neck, esophagus, lung, skin, prostate, and stomach; non-Hodgkin's lymphoma; osteosarcoma; and trophoblastic neoplasms.

Classification
Heavy metal alkylating-like agent.

Pharmacokinetics
Approximately 50% to 100% of cisplatin is absorbed into the systemic circulation after intraperitoneal administration. After IV administration, cisplatin rapidly distributes into tissues, including breast milk. Approximately 90% of the platinum compound is bound to plasma proteins (i.e., albumin, transferrin and gamma-globulin) within 2 to 4 hours of dosing. The kidneys account for up to 90% of excretion of platinum with approximately 10% to 40% of the drug excreted in the urine within 24 hours. Although only 10% of cisplatin is measured in the plasma 1 hour after a dose, cisplatin has a long terminal half-life (i.e., 60 to 90 hours). Cisplatin is not hemodialyzable within 1 to 1.5 hours after administration because of its extensive protein binding.

Dose
Doses vary from:
- 20 to 40 mg/m²/day for 3 to 5 days every 3 to 4 weeks or
- 20 to 120 mg/m² given as a single dose every 3 to 4 weeks
- intraperitoneal doses of 100 to 270 mg/m² have been given in combination with IV sodium thiosulfate.

It has been recommended that doses be reduced by 25% and 50% in patients with a creatinine clearance of 10 to 50 mL/min and less than 10 mL/min, respectively. Many physicians avoid using cisplatin when the creatinine clearance is less than 40 mL/min.

Administration
Usually administered by IV infusion in 100 to 500 mL of normal saline, over 30 minutes or longer. Many believe that drug infusions should not exceed 1 mg/min. The drug has also been given intra-arterially, intraperitoneally, by intravesical instillation, and by isolated limb perfusion.
Hydration. Concomitant hydration is necessary when doses of 40 mg/m² or greater are given as a short infusion. Prehydration with 1 to 2 L of normal saline (plus 20 mEq KCl and 8 mEq MgSO₄ per liter) is commonly given. Mannitol, 12.5 to 25 g, may be given before cisplatin but is not necessary if the patient is voiding. Furosemide or a similar diuretic may be added to increase diuresis, but most believe that it should not be used except to prevent fluid overload. In general, hydration should be adequate to maintain a urine output of 100 to 150 mL/hour before administration of the drug. Post-cisplatin hydration with 1 to 2 L of the same fluids is common. Treatment of

testicular cancer patients with cisplatin, 20 mg/m^2/day for 5 days, requires only 1 L of hydration per day.

Toxicity

Hematological. Leukopenia and thrombocytopenia occur, but are rarely dose-limiting. Anemia occasionally occurs after several treatments. Coombs-positive hemolytic anemia has been reported.

Gastrointestinal. Nausea and vomiting are common and may persist for up to 24 to 96 hours. Aggressive antiemetic treatment is required during the first 24 hours and for the next 4 days. Anorexia and diarrhea are common.

Dermatological. Alopecia and rash are uncommon.

Hepatic. Elevated hepatic enzyme levels (uncommon).

Cardiovascular. Rarely reported cardiovascular toxicities include bradycardia, bundle branch block, congestive heart failure, and Raynaud's phenomenon.

Neurological. Peripheral sensory neuropathies are common and dose-limiting when the cumulative cisplatin dose exceeds 400 mg/m^2. Symptoms may become apparent after the administration of 210 mg/m^2. Treatment should be discontinued when numbness and tingling of the fingers and/or toes become bothersome, as continued dosing can be disabling. Symptoms may begin and/or progress after discontinuing therapy. The toxicity is reversible, but may take many months to resolve. Other neurological toxicities occur infrequently but may include seizures (possibly caused by hyponatremia or hypomagnesemia), dizziness, loss of taste, tetany, agitation, disorientation, paranoia, Lhermitte's sign, aphasia, and cortical blindness.

Renal. Nephrotoxicity (elevated serum creatinine and BUN levels) is dose-related and relatively uncommon with adequate hydration and diuresis. This can be cumulative, and careful assessment of kidney function is essential before each dose. Each patient should have BUN and serum creatinine levels, and, when practical, a 24-hour urine creatinine clearance evaluated before treatment. Concomitant use of nephrotoxic drugs such as aminoglycosides, methotrexate, or amphotericin B should be undertaken with great caution.

Otic. Ototoxicity, manifested initially by high-frequency hearing loss and/or tinnitus, occurs occasionally. It occurs more commonly in patients receiving higher doses of cisplatin (i.e., greater than 100 mg/m^2) by rapid infusion and may also be associated with high cumulative doses. Significant hearing loss occurs commonly when a single dose of cisplatin exceeds 150 mg/m^2.

Other. Hypomagnesemia is common, can be severe, and is difficult to correct in some patients. It is not known whether prophylactic magnesium supplementation during each treatment, as a part of the hydration regimen, is helpful at preventing this adverse effect. Other toxicities may include hyperuricemia, hypocalcemia, hyponatremia, syndrome of inappropriate antidiuretic hormone (SIADH), hypophosphatemia, vein irritation, papilledema (rare), retrobulbar neuritis (rare), blurred vision (rare), myalgia, fever, altered color perception (rare), anaphylaxis (rare), and fatigue (common).

Drug Interactions

Concomitant use of nephrotoxic drugs such as aminoglycosides, methotrexate, or amphotericin B should be undertaken with great caution due to the risk of additive renal toxicity.

Concomitant use of loop diuretics such as furosemide may increase the risk of cisplatin-induced ototoxicity. Increased ototoxicity has also been observed in patients receiving combination chemotherapy with cisplatin and high-dose cytarabine.

CHEMOTHERAPY DRUGS

CISPLATIN *(continued)*

Cisplatin may decrease phenytoin levels due to decreased absorption or increased phenytoin metabolism.

Cisplatin if given prior to paclitaxel causes an increase in hematological toxicity due to a decreased paclitaxel clearance. Cisplatin administration should always be administered after paclitaxel.

Storage and Stability

Vials of cisplatin are stored at room temperature and protected from light. The cisplatin solution for injection (Platinol AQ®) is stable for 28 days after the vial has been entered, if protected from light. If the solution is not protected from light (i.e., is left under fluorescent light) at room temperature it is stable for 7 days. Reconstituted solutions of cisplatin are stable at room temperature for 72 hours. When further diluted to less than 0.6 mg/mL with normal saline, it is stable for 96 hours at room or refrigerator temperatures; protect from light. Refrigeration may result in precipitation of solutions greater than 0.6 mg/mL.

Preparation

Cisplatin solution for injection, 1 mg/mL, can be further diluted. Cisplatin lyophilized powder, 10- and 50-mg vials, should be reconstituted with 10 and 50 mL of sterile water, respectively, to yield a 1 mg/mL solution. The desired dose is often further diluted with 250 mL or more of 0.45% NaCl and 5% dextrose, normal saline, or 3% sodium chloride. Do not use 5% dextrose alone.

Incompatibilities

Cisplatin is less stable in solutions that do not contain chloride ions (i.e., 5% dextrose). Cisplatin may react with the aluminum found in some syringe needles or IV sets to form a black precipitate. Cisplatin is incompatible with metoclopramide, sodium bicarbonate, sodium thiosulfate, fluorouracil, and mesna.

Compatibilities

Cisplatin is compatible with mannitol, magnesium sulfate, potassium chloride, carmustine, cyclophosphamide, and etoposide. Consult your pharmacist regarding specific concentrations, containers, and storage conditions.

Availability

Commercially available as a 1 mg/mL solution (50 and 100 mg/vial). The original manufacturer has discontinued the lyophilized powder for injection (10- and 50-mg vials), but these are likely to be available through other suppliers.

CLADRIBINE

Other names

Leustatin®; chlordeoxyadenosine; 2-chlordeoxyadenosine; 2-chloro-2-deoxyadenosine; 2-CdA; CldAdo; NSC-105014.

Indications

FDA approved for the treatment of hairy-cell leukemia. Cladribine may also be useful for the treatment of chronic lymphocytic leukemia, cutaneous T-cell lymphoma, Sézary syndrome, low-grade non-Hodgkin's lymphoma, acute nonlymphocytic leukemia, Waldenström's macroglobulinemia, and autoimmune hemolytic anemia.

CHEMOTHERAPY DRUGS

Classification and Mechanisms of Action

Cladribine is an adenosine deaminase-resistant deoxyadenosine congener. The drug induces DNA strand breaks, prevents repair of DNA single strand breaks, and blocks RNA synthesis. The phosphorylated metabolites of the drug accumulate in cells with high deoxycytidine kinase activity such as lymphocytes. Cellular metabolism is disrupted and this results in cell death.

Pharmacokinetics

Approximately 37% to 55% of an oral dose of cladribine is absorbed. Cladribine rapidly distributes (initial half-life 36 minutes) after IV administration and is approximately 20% protein-bound. The drug has been detected in significant concentrations in the cerebrospinal fluid after doses of 0.15 mg/kg/day. Cladribine has an elimination half-life of approximately 5 to 7 hours.

Dose

Patients with hairy-cell leukemia receive a single 7-day treatment, 0.09 mg/kg/day (4 mg/m^2/day), as a continuous infusion. A second cycle of treatment has been given to some nonresponding patients. Patients with other malignancies have received 0.1 to 0.3 mg/kg/day for 7 days as a continuous infusion repeated every 4 to 5 weeks or the same dose daily for 5 days. Higher doses (0.4 to 0.5 mg/kg/day for 7 to 14 days) have been associated with more adverse effects. Daily doses of cladribine should not exceed 0.3 mg/kg/day. There are no specific dose adjustment recommendations for obese patients. A dose of 0.05 mg/kg/day has been combined with chlorambucil, 10 mg/m^2. A weekly dose has also been used at a dose of 0.15 mg/kg/week.

Administration

Continuous IV infusion over a 7-day period. Outpatients may receive the full 7-day dose in 100 mL of bacteriostatic normal saline; inpatients may receive each daily dose in 500 to 1,000 mL of normal saline. Cladribine has also been given as a 2-hour infusion and by subcutaneous injection.

Toxicity

Hematological. Neutropenia (20% to 43%), lymphopenia (100%), thrombocytopenia (recovery, 7 to 10 days after end of a 7-day infusion), mild anemia. Myelosuppression has been cumulative in some studies. Purpura, petechiae, and epistaxis have been reported in 5% to 10% of patients.

Gastrointestinal. Nausea (18% to 28%) is usually mild and preventable with antiemetic drugs, vomiting (13%), anorexia (17%), diarrhea (10%), constipation (9%), abdominal pain (6%).

Dermatological. Skin reactions (i.e., cellulitis) at catheter site (9% to 18%), phlebitis (2%), rash (28%), pruritus, erythema (6%).

Neurological. Headache (13% to 22%), dizziness (9%), insomnia (7%), motor weakness, paresthesias, paraparesis, and quadriparesis have been reported at high doses.

Cardiovascular. Edema, tachycardia (6%).

Pulmonary. Cough, dyspnea.

Renal. Elevated serum creatinine levels and renal failure have been reported in patients receiving cladribine 0.4 to 0.5 mg/kg/day for 7 to 14 days.

Other. Asthenia (45% to 70%), fever (66%), chills (18%), fatigue (17% to 45%), myalgia (7%), arthralgia (5%), pancreatitis (rare), diaphoresis, malaise, and trunk pain (rare).

CLADRIBINE *(continued)*

Storage and Stability

Cladribine vials are stored in the refrigerator. Diluted in 100 to 500 mL of normal saline, the drug is stable for at least 7 days at room temperature, although it is recommended that cladribine should be administered promptly or stored in the refrigerator for no more than 8 hours. Admixtures are stable for at least 7 days in SIMS Deltec medication cassettes. Freezing has no adverse effects on cladribine. If freezing occurs, the drug should be thawed at room temperature. A precipitate may form during freezing that can be resolubilized by allowing the solution to warm to room temperature or by shaking vigorously. Do not heat or microwave.

Preparation

The desired dose should be passed through the 0.22 micron filter before further dilution in 100 mL of bacteriostatic normal saline (for outpatient continuous infusion) or 500 to 1,000 mL of normal saline (for inpatient administration).

Incompatibilities

Dextrose 5% in water is not recommended as a diluent because it increases cladribine degradation.

Availability

Cladribine is commercially available as a 1 mg/mL solution in 10-mL vials.

Selected Reading

Estey EH et al. Treatment of hairy cell leukemia with 2-chlorodeoxyadenosine (2-CdA). Blood 79: 882–887, 1992.

CYCLOPHOSPHAMIDE

Other names

Cytoxan®; Cytoxan Lyophilized®; Neosar®; Procytox®; Endoxan®; CTX; CPM; NSC-26271.

Indications

FDA approved indications include non-Hodgkin's lymphoma, Hodgkin's disease, myeloma, cutaneous T-cell lymphoma, neuroblastoma, adenocarcinoma of the ovary, and adenocarcinoma of the breast. Other indications may include retinoblastoma, acute leukemias, chronic myelogenous leukemia, Ewing's sarcoma, osteosarcoma, Wilms' tumor, soft-tissue sarcomas, rhabdomyosarcoma, trophoblastic neoplasms, and cancers of the prostate, head and neck, lung, bladder, cervix, stomach, and uterus. Nonneoplastic uses include nephrotic syndrome, multiple sclerosis, and rheumatologic diseases including Wegener's granulomatosis, severe rheumatoid arthritis, and systemic lupus erythematosus.

Classification

Alkylating agent.

Pharmacokinetics

When administered orally at least 75% of cyclophosphamide is absorbed. Peak plasma levels occur approximately 1 hour after oral administration. Maximum plasma concentrations of metabolites occur 2 to 3 hours after an intravenous dose. The drug is activated by P450 hepatic microsomal enzymes. The liver is also involved in metabolizing cyclophosphamide metabolites to inactive compounds that are excreted by the kidney. The drug is distributed into breast milk. Approximately 12% and 50% to 75% of unchanged cyclophosphamide and its metabolites, respectively, are excreted into the urine. Dose reductions are not necessary for patients with severe renal impairment. Cyclophosphamide has an elimination half-life of 3 to 10 hours, and its principal active metabolite (phosphoramide mustard) has a half-life of 8 to 9 hours. Approximately 36% of an IV dose of cyclophosphamide can be removed by hemodialysis (9% per hour for a 4-hour hemodialysis treatment).

Dose

Cyclophosphamide may be given as a single dose or in several divided doses over a period of time. Some common doses are:

- 500 to 1,500 mg/m^2/dose intravenously every 3 weeks
- 50 to 200 mg/m^2/day orally for 14 days of a 28-day treatment cycle
- 400 mg/m^2/day for 4 days every 4 to 6 weeks.

Dose reductions may be required for renal and hepatic dysfunction.

Administration

May be given orally or by IV push or infusion (in 100 mL or more of 5% dextrose; 5% dextrose in 0.9% sodium chloride; 5% dextrose in Ringer's injection, lactated Ringer's injection, or sodium chloride injection [0.45% sodium chloride]; or sodium lactate injection [1/6 molar sodium lactate]) over a 15-minute or longer period. It is generally recommended that doses of cyclophosphamide be given in the morning or early afternoon because of the potential for allowing toxic metabolites to remain in the bladder overnight resulting in hemorrhagic cystitis. It is recommended that patients receiving higher doses (e.g., greater than or equal to 1,000 mg or 500 mg/m^2) of cyclophosphamide receive hydration, 500 mL or more of normal saline.

Toxicity

Hematological. Leukopenia, with nadir counts in 8 to 14 days after administration and recovery 1 to 2 weeks thereafter. Thrombocytopenia occurs but is rarely significant. Anemia occurs occasionally.

Gastrointestinal. Nausea and vomiting are relatively common after administration of larger doses (i.e., > 600 mg/m^2). Symptoms usually begin 6 to 10 hours after administration, which necessitates preventative antiemetic therapy through this time. When the drug is given orally, nausea can be chronic and extremely annoying. Eating small, frequent meals sometimes helps to relieve the nausea. Dividing the dose may also be helpful. Stomatitis, diarrhea, anorexia, and hemorrhagic colitis have occurred in patients receiving treatment with cyclophosphamide.

Dermatological. Alopecia (common), pigmented fingernails and/or skin (19%), dermatitis, rash, hives, pruritus.

Hepatic. Increased liver enzyme levels (uncommon); hepatitis and jaundice (rare).

Neurological. Headache, dizziness.

Pulmonary. Interstitial pulmonary fibrosis (rare).

Cardiovascular. Cardiac necrosis and/or acute myopericarditis with high-dose cyclophosphamide (rare).

Genitourinary. In conventional doses, cyclophosphamide rarely causes hemorrhagic cystitis. When cyclophosphamide is used in extremely high doses (i.e., 50 to 60 mg/kg) as a part of a preparative regimen for bone marrow transplantation, hemorrhagic cystitis is more common and can be severe. Prevention includes hydration and treatment with mesna (see the mesna drug review for specific instructions on its use).

CYCLOPHOSPHAMIDE *(continued)*

Other, less common toxicities include bladder fibrosis (most often after long-term oral therapy), bladder carcinoma, syndrome of inappropriate antidiuretic hormone (SIADH) (more common with single doses greater than 2,000 mg/m^2, especially if saline-poor solutions are used in the hydration regimen).

Other. Metallic taste during injection, nasal congestion and burning, diaphoresis, faintness, facial flushing, type-1 hypersensitivity reactions, blurred vision, cataracts (rare), hypothyroidism, hyperglycemia, testicular atrophy, amenorrhea, fertility impairment; decreased spermatogenesis and oogenesis, anaphylaxis, urticaria, angioedema, fever, secondary neoplasms (i.e., leukemia, bladder cancer).

Drug Interactions

Cyclophosphamide administered concomitantly with allopurinol may cause an increase in myelosuppression.

Cyclophosphamide and warfarin concomitant administration causes an increased anticoagulation effect. Cyclophosphamide administered concomitantly with digoxin may cause a decrease in serum digoxin levels. Cyclophosphamide can decrease the absorption of oral quinolones (e.g., ciprofloxacin, gatifloxacin).

Enzyme inducers such as phenobarbital and phenytoin may cause an increase in the metabolism of cyclophosphamide to active and toxic compounds, which may lead to an increase in toxicity.

Cyclophosphamide administered concomitantly with doxorubicin may lead to increased cardiac toxicity.

Cyclophosphamide inhibits cholinesterase enzyme activity up to 70%, leading to increased neuromuscular blockade and prolonged respiratory depression caused by succinylcholine. These effects are cyclophosphamide dose-dependent and may occur up to several days after cyclophosphamide therapy is discontinued.

Storage and Stability

Cyclophosphamide tablets and injectable powder are stored at room temperature. Containers bear an expiration date.

Preparation

Dissolve the 100-, 200-, 500-, 1,000-, and 2,000-mg vials with 5, 10, 25, 50, and 100 mL, respectively, of sterile water or normal saline to yield a 20 mg/mL solution.

Compatibilities

Cyclophosphamide (6 to 8 mg/mL) and doxorubicin (0.4 to 0.6 mg/mL) are compatible for 7 days at room temperature. Cyclophosphamide is also compatible with dacarbazine, bleomycin, cisplatin, mesna, and other drugs. A pharmacist should be consulted for additional information.

Availability

Commercially available in 25- and 50-mg tablets and as powder for injection in 100-, 200-, 500-, 1,000-, and 2,000-mg vials.

CYTARABINE

Other names

Cytosar-U®; Cytosar®; Tarabine Pfs®; Ara-C; cytosine arabinoside; NSC-63878.
Depocyt®; cytarabine liposome injection; liposomal cytarabine; liposomal Ara-C.

Indications

Cytarabine injection is FDA approved for the treatment of acute nonlymphocytic
leukemia, acute lymphocytic leukemia, non-Hodgkin's lymphoma, and chronic
myelogenous leukemia. Intrathecal cytarabine is approved for the prophylaxis and treatment of meningeal leukemia. Cytarabine may be useful in the treatment of Hodgkin's
and non-Hodgkin's lymphoma.

Cytarabine liposome injection is FDA approved for the intrathecal treatment of
lymphomatous meningitis.

Classification and Mechanisms of Action

Antimetabolite.

Pharmacokinetics

Cytarabine is poorly absorbed by mouth (i.e., 20%). After IV administration, it is rapidly distributed throughout the body and is rapidly deaminated within the bloodstream.
Peak plasma concentrations after subcutaneous or intramuscular administration occur
within 20 to 60 minutes. Within 24 hours up to 80% of the drug is eliminated. Less
than 10% of the drug is eliminated in the urine as unchanged drug. However, one
metabolite, uracil arabinoside (ara-U), has the ability to produce high concentrations
of cytosine arabinoside triphosphate (ara-CTP) in patients with renal insufficiency.
Accumulation of ara-CTP in the central nervous system may result in nervous system
toxicities. Cytarabine has an elimination half-life of 1 to 3 hours.

Cytarabine liposome injection demonstrates peak levels of free cytarabine in the
lumbar sac and ventricles within 5 hours of administration. A biphasic elimination
then occurs with a terminal cerebral spinal fluid half-life of 100 to 263 hours. Due to
low enzyme levels in the CSF, minimal conversion to ara-U occurs.

Dose

Cytarabine injection

Some common doses are as follows:

- 60 to 200 mg/m^2/day as a continuous IV infusion for 5 to 10 consecutive days.
- 100 mg/m^2 intravenously or subcutaneously twice a day for 5 days every 28 days.
- 10 to 30 mg/m^2 intrathecally up to 3 times per week.
- 1,000 to 3,000 mg/m^2 intravenously over a period of 1 to 3 hours every 12 hours
  for 3 to 6 days.
- 10 mg/m^2 subcutaneously every 12 hours for 15 to 21 days.

Cytarabine liposome injection. Induction regimens for lymphomatous meningitis: liposomal cytarabine 50 mg intrathecally every 2 weeks for 2 doses (week 1 and week 3).

Consolidation regimens for lymphomatous meningitis: liposomal cytarabine 50 mg
intrathecally every 2 weeks for 3 doses (i.e., weeks 5, 7 and 9), then another 50-mg
intrathecal dose at week 13.

Maintenance regimen for lymphomatous meningitis: liposomal cytarabine 50 mg
intrathecally every 28 days for 4 doses (i.e., weeks 17, 21, 25 and 29).

CYTARABINE *(continued)*

Administration

Cytarabine injection. Administered by IV push, IV infusion in 50 mL or more of 5% dextrose or normal saline over a 30-minute or longer period. High-dose cytarabine is usually given in 250 to 500 mL of 5% dextrose or normal saline over 1 to 3 hours. The drug has also been given subcutaneously, intrathecally, and intraperitoneally.

Cytarabine liposome. Administered only by intrathecal (directly into lumbar sac) or by intraventricular reservoir administration over a period of 1 to 5 minutes. Concomitant dexamethasone, 4 mg/day IV or orally, for a total of 5 days is recommended, with one dose administered prior to injection. Patients should remain lying in a flat position for an hour if administered via lumbar injection.

Toxicity

Hematological. Leukopenia and thrombocytopenia are expected, with nadir counts occurring in 5 to 7 days and recovery in 2 to 3 weeks. Anemia is common. Hematological toxicity is more severe when cytarabine is given as a prolonged IV infusion versus administration as an IV bolus.

Cytarabine liposome injection can also cause neutropenia, thrombocytopenia, and rarely anemia.

Gastrointestinal. Nausea, vomiting (dose-related, common, and often prevented by antiemetic drugs), anorexia, diarrhea (potentiated with the addition of an anthracycline), metallic taste, dysphagia, stomatitis, severe gastrointestinal ulceration, pancreatitis, peritonitis.

Cytarabine liposome injection can cause mild nausea, vomiting, and constipation.

Dermatological. Transient skin erythema without exfoliation, alopecia (uncommon); rash, cellulitis, and thrombophlebitis are rare.

Hepatic. Transient, usually mild elevations of liver enzyme levels and/or hyperbilirubinemia.

Neurological. A 16% to 40% incidence (7% to 18% severe) with high-dose therapy (i.e., 2,000 to 3,000 mg/m^2 every 12 hours for 12 or more doses). Toxicity is usually cerebellar (i.e., lethargy progressing to confusion, ataxia, nystagmus, slurred speech). Symptoms begin on the fourth or fifth day of treatment and resolve 4 to 7 days thereafter. In most cases toxicity totally resolves, but in some cases it is irreversible or fatal. Toxicity is dose-related. Age (i.e., less than 50 years), renal dysfunction (i.e., creatinine clearance less than 60 mL/min), gender (i.e., men more than women), infusion rate (i.e., 1-hour infusion greater than a 3-hour infusion), and hepatic dysfunction have been implicated as factors that influence the incidence and severity of cerebellar toxicity. Treatment with pyridoxine (vitamin B$_6$) does not prevent neurotoxicity.

Rare neurotoxicities include expressive aphasia, peripheral and sensory neuropathies, brachial plexopathy, bilateral rectus muscle palsy, parkinsonism, dizziness, and somnolence. Dizziness and somnolence appear to be associated with rapid IV infusion. Headache has also been reported.

After intrathecal administration of cytarabine injection, the most common side effects are nausea, vomiting, fever, and headache that are usually mild and self-limiting. Meningism, paresthesia, paraplegia, seizures, blindness, and necrotizing encephalopathy have rarely occurred.

After intrathecal administration of cytarabine liposome injection, the most common side effects are chemical arachnoiditis, which is characterized by headache, nausea, vomiting, fever, neck pain or rigidity (co-administration of dexamethasone with each dose of drug

may prevent or reduce severity of this side effect). Other side effects include: asthenia, confusion, pain, back pain, somnolence, abnormal gait, peripheral edema, urinary incontinence, and metabolic disorders, transient elevation in CSF protein and white blood cells.
Pulmonary. Rare syndrome of sudden respiratory distress, rapidly progressing to pulmonary edema.
Cardiovascular. Rare cardiomegaly, pericarditis with tamponade, thrombophlebitis.
Renal. Urinary retention (rare).
Ocular. Conjunctivitis, keratitis (usually on days 1 to 3 but reduced with prophylactic glucocorticoid eye drops), photophobia.
Other. "Ara-C" syndrome. Bone and muscle pain, chest pain, fever, general weakness, reddened eyes, and skin rash. Generally occurs 6 to 12 hours after administration and may respond favorably to treatment with corticosteroids.

Hemorrhagic cystitis (rare), rhabdomyolysis, and hyperuricemia and hyperphosphatemia if tumor lysis syndrome develops.

Drug Interactions

Nephrotoxic drugs may decrease the elimination of cytosine arabinoside triphosphate (ara-CTP), a neurotoxic metabolite of cytarabine-resulting in neurotoxic sequelae (i.e., confusion, lethargy, ataxia).

Cytarabine may decrease the absorption of oral quinolones (e.g., ciprofloxacin, gatifloxacin).

Cytarabine may decrease the absorption of digoxin.

Previous asparaginase treatment prior to cytarabine therapy may increase the risk of acute pancreatitis.

Storage and Stability

Cytarabine injection vials are stored at room temperature. After reconstitution, the solution is stable for 8 days (15 days in a plastic syringe) at room temperature and 15 days when refrigerated. Cytarabine, 20 to 80 mg/mL, is stable for 28 days in an Infusaid® pump. Solutions with a slight haze should be discarded.

Cytarabine liposome injection is to be kept refrigerated at a temperature of 2° to 8°C. Do not freeze and do not shake aggressively. Each vial bears an expiration date.

Preparation

Cytarabine injection for IV use, reconstitute the 100-mg vial with 5 mL bacteriostatic water for injection to achieve a concentration of 20 mg/mL. Add 10 mL of bacteriostatic water to the 500-mg vial to achieve a concentration of 50 mg/mL. Add 10 and 20 mL of bacteriostatic water to the 1,000- and 2,000-mg vials, respectively, to achieve a concentration of 100 mg/mL. For subcutaneous use, reconstitute the powder with sterile water or normal saline to a concentration of 50 to 100 mg/mL. For intrathecal use, mix with lactated Ringer's solution or normal saline without preservatives.

Cytarabine liposome injection for intrathecal use should be brought to room temperature prior to administration, gently swirl the vial and then withdraw the specified dose. No further dilution is required. Use within 4 hours of drawing it out of the vial into a syringe.

Incompatibilities

Cytarabine is incompatible with carbenicillin, fluorouracil, heparin sodium, oxacillin, penicillin G sodium, and nafcillin.

In-line filters must not be used when administering cytarabine liposome injection.

CYTARABINE *(continued)*

Compatibilities

Cytarabine (0.26 mg/mL), daunorubicin (0.03 mg/mL), and etoposide (0.4 mg/mL) are stable in 5% dextrose and 0.45% NaCl for 72 hours at room temperature. Cytarabine is also compatible with methotrexate, vincristine, hydrocortisone, sodium chloride, potassium chloride, calcium, and magnesium sulfate. Cytarabine and idarubicin are compatible at the "Y"-site. A pharmacist should be consulted for information on concentrations, containers, and storage conditions.

Availability

Cytarabine injection vials are commercially available as a lyophilized powder in 100-, 500-, 1,000-, and 2,000-mg vials and as an injectable 20 mg/mL solution in 100-, 500-, and 1,000-mg vials.

Cytarabine liposome injection is commercially available as a 10 mg/mL opaque preservative-free solution in 5-mL vials.

Selected Readings

Damon LE, Mass R, Linker CA. The association between cytarabine neurotoxicity and renal insufficiency. J Clin Oncol 7: 1563–1568, 1989.

Glantz MJ et al. Randomized trial of a slow release versus a standard formulation of cytarabine for the intrathecal treatment of lymphomatous meningitis. J Clin Oncol 17: 3110–3116, 1999.

DACARBAZINE

Other names

DTIC®; DTIC-Dome; DIC; imidazole carboxamide; dimethyl triazeno imidazole carboxamide; NSC-45388.

Indications

FDA approved for the treatment of metastatic melanoma and Hodgkin's disease. Dacarbazine may also be a useful treatment for soft tissue or bone sarcomas, renal cell carcinoma, neuroblastoma, and islet cell carcinoma.

Classification

Alkylating agent.

Pharmacokinetics

Dacarbazine is poorly absorbed after oral administration. The drug is activated to cytotoxic metabolites by hepatic microsomal enzymes and is not widely distributed throughout the body. Less than 15% penetrates into the cerebrospinal fluid. Approximately 30% to 50% of the active metabolite is excreted unchanged in the urine. Dacarbazine has an elimination half-life of 3 to 5 hours.

Dose

Common doses are:

- 375 mg/m^2 on days 1 and 15 (as a part of the Adriamycin®, bleomycin, vinblastine, and dacarbazine [ABVD] regimen for Hodgkin's disease)
- 5-day course of 150 to 250 mg/m^2/ day repeated every 3 to 4 weeks
- 400 to 500 mg/m^2 by IV push or rapid infusion on days 1 and 2 every 3 to 4 weeks
- 200 mg/m^2 daily as a continuous 96-hour infusion repeated every 3 to 4 weeks
- Single-dose regimen of 650 to 1,450 mg/m^2 repeated every 3 to 4 weeks.

Administration

Usually administered by IV infusion in 100 mL or more of 5% dextrose or normal saline over a period of 30 to 60 minutes. The drug may also be given by IV push or by rapid infusion over a period of 15 minutes, but this may increase venous irritation compared with longer durations of IV infusion. Dacarbazine has also been given as a continuous IV infusion and by the intra-arterial route.

Toxicity

Hematological. Leukopenia and thrombocytopenia are common and may be dose-limiting. Nadir blood counts occur 2 to 4 weeks after treatment; recovery occurs 1 to 2 weeks thereafter. Anemia also occurs after administration of dacarbazine.

Gastrointestinal. Severe nausea and vomiting are common and prevented in some patients with aggressive antiemetic support. These symptoms tend to lessen with each subsequent daily dose. Also reported are anorexia, metallic taste, diarrhea (rare), and stomatitis (rare).

Dermatological. Alopecia (uncommon), facial flushing, skin rash, photosensitivity. Extravasation of the drug may result in severe pain but has not resulted in tissue damage. Rapid IV injection causes pain along the injection site more frequently compared with slower durations of IV infusion.

Hepatic. Increased liver enzyme levels, hepatic vein thrombosis (rare). Hepatic necrosis is a rare and fatal toxicity.

Cardiovascular. Thrombophlebitis.

Neurological. Facial paresthesia, confusion, lethargy, seizures, weakness, headache, polyneuropathy, and blurred vision have been reported.

Renal. Increased serum creatinine and BUN concentrations are rare.

Other. Flu-like syndrome (with fever, malaise, sinus congestion, and myalgia) is rare, occurs about 7 days after treatment, and lasts 1 to 3 weeks. Other rare toxicities include anaphylaxis, fever, and cerebral hemorrhage.

Drug Interactions

Dacarbazine administered concomitantly with interleukin-2 may increase the risk of hypersensitivity reactions characterized by pruritus, erythema, and hypotension.

Storage and Stability

Dacarbazine vials are stored under refrigeration and protected from light. In solution, dacarbazine is stable for 96 hours if refrigerated and for 24 hours at room temperature and protected from light. When further diluted in 500 mL of 5% dextrose or normal saline, it is stable for 24 hours if refrigerated and for 8 hours at room temperature.

Photodegradation. The manufacturer of dacarbazine states that the drug does not decompose when left at room temperature under normal lighting conditions for 8 hours. Dacarbazine should, however, be protected from exposure to sunlight.

NOTE: A change in the color of the solution from pale yellow to pink is indicative of drug decomposition.

Preparation

Dilute the 100- and 200-mg vials with 9.9 and 19.7 mL of sterile water, respectively, to result in a concentration of 10 mg/mL. Discard if solution turns pink or red. The drug can be further diluted in 100 to 500 mL of 5% dextrose or normal saline.

Incompatibilities

Dacarbazine is physically incompatible with allopurinol injection, hydrocortisone, and L-cysteine. Because of pH differences, admixtures containing dacarbazine and sodium

DACARBAZINE *(continued)*

bicarbonate are not recommended. The compatibility of heparin and dacarbazine is dependent on the concentration of heparin.

Compatibilities

Dacarbazine is compatible with cyclophosphamide, doxorubicin, dactinomycin, vinblastine, methotrexate, and other drugs. A pharmacist should be consulted for additional information.

Availability

Commercially available as a lyophilized powder in 100- and 200-mg vials.

Selected Reading

Del Prete SA et al. Combination chemotherapy with cisplatin, carmustine, dacarbazine and tamoxifen in metastatic melanoma. Cancer Treat Rep 68:1403–1405, 1984.

DACTINOMYCIN

Other names

Actinomycin-D; ACT-D; Actinomycin-C; Cosmegen®; NSC-3053.

Indications

FDA approved for the treatment of Wilms' tumor, rhabdomyosarcoma, testicular carcinoma, choriocarcinoma, carcinoma of the uterus, Ewing's sarcoma, and sarcoma botryides. Dactinomycin may be a useful treatment for acute nonlymphocytic leukemia, Kaposi's sarcoma, melanoma, osteosarcoma, trophoblastic neoplasms, and cancers of the endometrium and ovary.

Classification

Antitumor antibiotic.

Pharmacokinetics

Dactinomycin is poorly absorbed after oral administration. After IV administration, dactinomycin is widely distributed throughout the body, but only negligible amounts of drug penetrate into the cerebrospinal fluid. Dactinomycin is metabolized by the liver and eliminated in the bile (up to 50%) and urine (6% to 31%) as unchanged drug. Dactinomycin has an elimination half-life of 30 to 40 hours.

Dose

Common doses are:

- 1 to 2 mg/m^2 every 3 weeks
- 0.25 to 0.6 mg/m^2/day for 5 days every 3 to 4 weeks for adults
- 12 microg/kg/day for 5 consecutive days as a single agent for gestational trophoblastic neoplasia
- 15 microg/kg/day (maximum dose intensity per 2-week cycle) for 5 consecutive days for Wilm's tumor, rhabdomyosarcoma, and Ewing's sarcoma, usually in various regimens and combinations
- 0.25 to 0.5 mg/m^2/day for 5 consecutive days (not to exceed 0.5 mg each day) for children
- As an isolated perfusion for solid tumors, dactinomycin has been administered at doses of 50 microg/kg (lower extremity) and 35 microg/kg (upper extremity).

Administration

With extravasation precautions, dactinomycin is given over a period of 2 to 3 minutes, preferably into the tubing of a free-flowing IV infusion of 5% dextrose or normal saline. Dactinomycin has been given by IV infusion in 50 mL of 5% dextrose or normal saline over a period of 20 to 30 minutes. The drug has been administered by isolated perfusion.

Toxicity

Hematological. Leukopenia and thrombocytopenia are expected and occur approximately 1 to 2 weeks after treatment, with the nadir at 3 weeks and recovery 1 to 2 weeks thereafter. Anemia occurs occasionally.

Gastrointestinal. Nausea and vomiting (often worsening with successive daily doses) occur about 1 hour after a dose and may last several hours. Mucositis, with ulcerative sores often under the tongue, occurs occasionally. Dysphagia, proctitis, cheilitis, anorexia, and diarrhea occur infrequently.

Dermatological. Acneiform changes, erythema, hyperpigmentation (especially in previously irradiated areas), rash, alopecia (may not be limited to scalp hair). Extravasation may result in severe pain, swelling, and necrosis.

Hepatic. Ascites, hepatomegaly, hepatitis, and elevated liver enzyme levels are rare toxicities.

Other. "Radiation recall" (skin irritation or even necrosis in previously irradiated areas) has been reported. Rarely reported toxicities include anaphylaxis, hypocalcemia, fever, fatigue, lethargy, and secondary neoplasms.

Storage and Stability

Intact dactinomycin vials are stored at room temperature and protected from light. Reconstituted solutions are chemically stable for 2 months at room temperature.

Preparation

Add 1.1 mL preservative-free sterile water for injection to the 0.5-mg vial. The final concentration is 0.5 mg/mL (500 microg/mL).

Incompatibilities

Diluents containing preservatives. It has been shown that significant binding of dactinomycin occurs with 0.2-micron cellulose ester (Millex OR®) and polytetrafluoroethylene (Millex-GV®) filters.

Compatibilities

Dactinomycin is compatible with dacarbazine.

Availability

Commercially available in vials containing 500 microg (0.5 mg) lyophilized powder, with 20 mg of mannitol.

DAUNORUBICIN

Other names

Cerubidine®; daunomycin; DNR; rubidomycin; NSC-82151.
Daunorubicin citrate liposomal (liposomal formulation of daunorubicin): DaunoXome®; NSC-697732.

Indications

Daunorubicin for injection is FDA approved for the treatment of acute nonlymphocytic leukemia (adults), acute lymphocytic leukemia (adults and children). Daunorubicin

DAUNORUBICIN *(continued)*

may also be a useful treatment for erythroleukemia, neuroblastoma, non-Hodgkin's lymphomas, and chronic myelogenous leukemia.

Liposomal daunorubicin citrate injection is FDA approved for the first-line treatment of HIV-associated Kaposi's sarcoma.

Classification

Anthracycline antitumor antibiotic.

Pharmacokinetics

Daunorubicin is widely distributed throughout the body after IV administration, and extensively plasma protein bound. Daunorubicin does not cross the blood-brain barrier. The drug is extensively metabolized by the liver to several metabolites, including the active metabolite daunorubicinol. Approximately 40% of the drug is eliminated by the biliary route. Approximately 15% to 25% is eliminated via the urine. Daunorubicin and daunorubicinol have elimination half-lives of 18 to 20 hours and 25 to 30 hours, respectively. Dose reductions may be indicated for severe renal or hepatic insufficiency.

Dose

Daunorubicin for injection is usually given as a single IV injection or split into a 3- to 5-day schedule. A common regimen for induction treatment of acute leukemia uses 45 mg/m^2/day for 3 days. Pediatric dosing will vary. A lesser dose may be necessary in patients greater than 60 years of age. Specific dosing will also vary depending on the combination of antineoplastic therapy.

Liposomal daunorubicin citrate injection is administered at a dose of 40 mg/m^2 intravenously every 2 weeks.

Administration

Daunorubicin for injection is administered using extravasation precautions; inject into a recently established patent IV site through the sidearm of a running IV over 2 to 5 minutes.

Liposomal daunorubicin citrate injection is administered intravenously over 60 minutes and has not been associated with severe tissue reactions after extravasation.

Toxicity

Hematological. Leukopenia is expected (nadir between 1 and 2 weeks, recovery 2 to 3 weeks thereafter); thrombocytopenia and anemia also occur. Liposomal daunorubicin, at the doses recommended for the treatment of Kaposi's sarcoma, induces grades 3 and 4 neutropenia in 36% and 15% of patients, respectively.

Gastrointestinal. Nausea and vomiting commonly occur 1 hour after a dose and may last for several hours but are usually prevented by antiemetics. Diarrhea (uncommon) and stomatitis (common) may also occur. Liposomal daunorubicin is associated with an 18% incidence of moderate to severe nausea and 13% incidence of moderate to severe vomiting. Diarrhea is reported to occur in 38% of patients treated with liposomal daunorubicin.

Dermatological. Rash, urticaria, alopecia (common), chemical thrombophlebitis or local necrosis if extravasation occurs, pigmentation of fingernails. Alopecia occurs in approximately 8% of patients treated with liposomal daunorubicin.

Hepatic. Transient elevations in serum bilirubin and liver enzyme levels.

Neurological. Neuropathies have been reported to occur in 13% of patients receiving liposomal daunorubicin.

Cardiovascular. Arrhythmias, usually asymptomatic and transient, congestive cardiomyopathy (incidence becomes unacceptable after a total dose of 500 to 600 mg/m^2 has been given). See doxorubicin drug review for additional information. Cumulative cardiotoxicity after administration of liposomal daunorubicin at doses above 600 mg/m^2 is rare. However, the manufacturer of liposomal daunorubicin recommends monitoring of the left ventricular ejection fraction after administration of cumulative doses of 320 mg/m^2 and 480 mg/m^2, and every 160 mg/m^2 thereafter.

Other. Fever, chills, hyperuricemia, red urine (expected), anaphylaxis (rare). Within the first 5 minutes of an IV infusion of liposomal daunorubicin, 14% of patients experienced back pain, flushing, and chest tightness. Interruption of the infusion and readministration at a slower rate tend to ameliorate these symptoms.

Drug Interactions
Daunorubicin can decrease the absorption of oral quinolones such as ciprofloxacin and gatifloxacin.

Storage and Stability
Daunorubicin for injection vials are stored at room temperature. Reconstituted solutions are stable for 72 hours when refrigerated and 48 hours at room temperature.

Liposomal daunorubicin vials are stored in the refrigerator. Diluted to a concentration of 1 mg/mL with 5% dextrose, liposomal daunorubicin is stable for at least 6 hours at room temperature.

Preparation
Daunorubicin for injection 20-mg vials are reconstituted with 4 mL of sterile water to give a final concentration of 5 mg/mL. The desired dose is drawn into a syringe containing 10 to 15 mL of normal saline.

Liposomal daunorubicin citrate formulation is diluted to a concentration of 1 mg/mL with preservative-free 5% dextrose.

Incompatibilities
Heparin sodium, 5-fluorouracil, and dexamethasone sodium phosphate. Liposomal daunorubicin citrate formulation is incompatible with any solution other than preservative-free 5% dextrose. In-line filters should not be used when administering liposomal daunorubicin.

Compatibilities
Daunorubicin (0.03 mg/mL), cytarabine (0.26 mg/mL), and etoposide (0.4 mg/mL) are stable in 5% dextrose in 0.45% sodium chloride for 72 hours at room temperature.

Availability
Daunorubicin for injection is commercially available in 20-mg vials of lyophilized drug. Liposomal daunorubicin citrate is available at a concentration of 2 mg/mL in vials containing 50 mg.

Selected Reading
Fassas A et al. Safety and efficacy assessment of liposomal daunorubicin (DaunoXome) in adults with refractory or relapsed acute myeloblastic leukaemia: a phase I-II study. Br J Haematol 116: 308–315, 2002.

DECITABINE

Other names

5-azadeoxycytidine; DAC; 5-aza-2'-deoxycytidine; 5-Aza-CdR; NSC-127716.

Indications

Decitabine is an investigational agent in the United States that may be an effective treatment for myelodysplastic syndrome, chronic myelogenous leukemia, and/or acute myelogenous leukemia.

Classification and Mechanisms of Action

Decitabine is a pyrimidine nucleoside analogue that is believed to exert its antineoplastic effect in a manner similar to cytarabine. In addition, decitabine has been shown to be an inhibitor of DNA methylation and may be able to restore sensitivity of cancer cells that have become resistant to therapy with various agents.

Dose

Several dosing regimens have been evaluated, including:

- 75 mg/m^2 every 8 hours times three doses, repeated every 5 to 8 weeks
- 30 to 50 mg/m^2/day for 3 consecutive days, repeated every 6 to 8 weeks
- 150 to 300 mg/m^2/day for 5 consecutive days, alone and in combination with idarubicin or amsacrine
- 5 to 10 mg/m^2/day for 5 to 20 days, repeated every 28 days.

Administration

Decitabine is administered IV in normal saline or 5% dextrose and water over 1 to 8 hours. Decitabine has been administered as a 72-hour continuous infusion.

Toxicity

Hematological. At dose of 45 mg/m^2/day for 3 consecutive days, in patients with myelodysplastic syndromes, grade 3 to grade 4 hematological toxicities are: neutropenia (12%), thrombocytopenia (5%), anemia (11%). Infection (grade 3 or 4) was documented in 20% and sepsis in 11% of these patients.
Gastrointestinal. Abdominal pain and cramping, diarrhea, nausea, vomiting, stomatitis, peritonitis
Dermatological. Alopecia.
Hepatic. Hyperbilirubinemia, elevations of hepatic transaminase levels.
Other. Fatigue. Case reports of seizures, creatinine elevation, and atrial fibrillation have been published.

Storage and Stability

Intact vials are stable at room temperature for at least 1 year and at refrigeration temperatures for at least 2 years. Reconstituted solutions lose approximately 10% of their potency after 12 hours at 25°C or 24 hours at 4°C. The National Cancer Institute recommends that doses be prepared just prior to administration.

Preparation

Add 10 mL of sterile water to the 50-mg vial to yield a concentration of 5 mg/mL. Doses are usually further diluted to a concentration between 1 mg/mL and 0.1 mg/mL in normal saline, 5% dextrose and water, or lactated Ringer's solution.

Availability

Decitabine is an investigational agent in the United States that is available as a lyophilized powder (50 mg/vial) from the manufacturer or the National Cancer Institute.

Selected Readings

Cheson BD et al. Novel therapeutic agents for the treatment of myelodysplastic syndromes. Semin Oncol 27: 560–577, 2000.

Wijermans P et al. Low-dose 5-aza-2'-deoxycytidine, a DNA hypomethylating agent, for the treatment of high risk myelodysplastic syndrome: a multicenter phase II study in elderly patients. J Clin Oncol 18: 956–968, 2000.

DEXAMETHASONE

Other names

Decadron®; Hexadrol®; Dexone®; DXM; NSC-34521.

Indications

FDA approved for the treatment of brain metastases with edema, breast cancer, acute and chronic lymphocytic leukemia, multiple myeloma, non-Hodgkin's lymphoma, autoimmune hemolytic anemia, immunothrombocytopenia, rheumatic disorders, allergic disorders, dermatological rashes, and inflammation (intra-articularly). It is also frequently used as an antiemetic, with a 5-HT3-serotonin blocker, before cancer chemotherapy, and post-chemotherapy for delayed nausea and vomiting.

Classification and Mechanisms of Action

Dexamethasone is a potent adrenal corticosteroid that affects almost every body system. It has anti-inflammatory, immunosuppressant, antineoplastic, and antiemetic properties and very little mineralocorticoid activity. As an antineoplastic agent, dexamethasone may bind to specific proteins within the cell, forming a steroid-receptor complex. Binding of the receptor-steroid complex with nuclear chromatin alters mRNA and protein synthesis within the cell.

Pharmacokinetics

Approximately 75% to 80% of dexamethasone is absorbed by mouth. The drug is metabolized by the liver to inactive metabolites and has an elimination half-life of 3 to 4 hours.

Dose

For multiple myeloma, 40 mg/day on days 1 to 4, 9 to 12, and 17 to 20 of each 28-day cycle is often administered as part of the vincristine, Adriamycin®, dexamethasone (VAD) regimen.

For neurological syndromes, 10 to 100 mg is used initially, followed by 4 to 8 mg every 6 to 12 hours.

Antiemetic doses: 10 to 20 mg intravenously before chemotherapy for prevention of acute nausea and vomiting and 4 mg to 8 mg orally twice a day for delayed nausea and vomiting (see Chapter 11, Box 11-3).

Administration

Orally whenever possible; also slow IV push or as a short IV infusion in 50 to 100 mL of 5% dextrose or normal saline over 10 to 20 minutes. Dexamethasone may also be administered topically, intra-ocularly, intranasally, and by intramuscular, intra-articular, and intralesional injection.

DEXAMETHASONE *(continued)*

Toxicity

Hematological. Leukocytosis.

Gastrointestinal. Nausea, vomiting, anorexia, increased appetite, weight gain, pancreatitis, aggravation of peptic ulcers.

Dermatological. Rash, skin atrophy, acne, facial erythema, ecchymoses, poor wound healing, hirsutism.

Neurological. Insomnia, euphoria, headache, vertigo, psychosis, depression, seizures, muscle weakness.

Cardiovascular. Fluid retention and edema, hypertension; rarely, thrombophlebitis and thromboembolism.

Genitourinary. Menstrual changes (amenorrhea, menstrual irregularities).

Ocular. Cataracts, increased intraocular pressure, exophthalmos.

Metabolic. Hyperglycemia, decreased glucose tolerance, aggravation or precipitation of diabetes mellitus, adrenal suppression (with Cushinoid features), hypokalemia, sodium and fluid retention.

Other. Osteoporosis (and resulting back pain); aseptic necrosis of the femoral head; appearance of serious infections, including herpes zoster, varicella zoster, fungal infections, *Pneumocystis carinii*, and tuberculosis; muscle wasting; delayed wound healing; suppression of reactions to skin tests.

Drug Interactions

Dexamethasone administered concomitantly with nonsteroidal anti-inflammatory agents or aspirin may result in an increased risk of stomach irritation and/or ulceration.

Aluminum- or magnesium-based antacids may decrease the oral absorption of the dexamethasone.

The elimination of dexamethasone may be increased by agents that induce the cytochrome P450 enzymes. These agents include, but are not limited to, phenytoin, rifampin, and phenobarbital. The concentrations and efficacy of dexamethasone may be decreased.

Storage and Stability

Dexamethasone tablets and injection are stored at room temperature in a dry place. When the injection is further diluted in 5% dextrose or normal saline it is stable for at least 24 hours at room temperature.

Preparation

The injection may be further diluted in 50 to 100 mL of 5% dextrose or normal saline.

Availability

Commercially available in 0.25-, 0.5-, 0.75-, 1-, 1.5-, 2-, 4-, and 6-mg tablets; 0.5 mg/5 mL and 0.1 mg/mL oral solution or syrup; and 4, 10, 20, or 24 mg/mL solution for injection (dexamethasone sodium phosphate). It is also available as inhalers, ophthalmic solution, and dexamethasone acetate suspension for injection.

Selected Reading

Krzakowski M et al: Clinical report. A multicenter, double-blind comparison of i.v. and oral administration of ondansetron plus dexamethasone for acute cisplatin induced emesis. Anti-Cancer Drugs 9: 593–598, 1998.

DEXRAZOXANE

Other names
Zinecard®; ADR-529; ICRF-187; NSC-169780.

Indications
Dexrazoxane is FDA approved as a protective agent for doxorubicin-induced cardiotoxicity in patients with metastatic breast cancer. The drug is approved for use in patients who have already received a total cumulative doxorubicin dose of 300 mg/m^2. Dexrazoxane has also been used as a cardioprotectant along with other anthracycline therapy.

Classification and Mechanisms of Action
Dexrazoxane is an intracellular chelating agent that prevents iron from combining with doxorubicin to form free oxygen radicals.

Pharmacokinetics
After IV administration, dexrazoxane is rapidly distributed throughout the body. Only 2% to 3% of dexrazoxane is bound to plasma proteins. The drug is metabolized by the liver, approximately 35% to 50% is eliminated in the urine unchanged, and the elimination half-life is 2 to 4 hours.

Dose
Dexrazoxane is to be dosed at 10 mg/m^2 for every 1 mg/m^2 of doxorubicin (10:1 ratio). A dose of dexrazoxane 500 mg/m^2 would be required for a dose of doxorubicin 50 mg/m^2. The drug is to be administered 30 minutes before administration of doxorubicin.

Administration
Dexrazoxane is given by slow IV push or IV infusion in 50 to 100 mL of 5% dextrose or normal saline over 15 to 30 minutes. Investigational clinical trials have included infusions of 8 and 48 hours.

Toxicity
In randomized studies dexrazoxane has been shown to enhance leukopenia slightly when administered with doxorubicin. The incidence and severity of all other toxicities were no different in patients receiving doxorubicin-containing chemotherapy compared with patients receiving chemotherapy plus dexrazoxane. Listed below are the toxicities reported in phase I and II trials of dexrazoxane.
Hematological. Leukopenia. Thrombocytopenia and anemia are uncommon.
Gastrointestinal. Mild nausea and vomiting, anorexia, stomatitis.
Dermatological. Alopecia, urticaria.
Hepatic. Elevated liver enzyme levels, hyperbilirubinemia.
Cardiovascular. Hypotension, deep venous thrombosis.
Other. Phlebitis, pain at injection site, mild, transient elevation of serum amylase levels, elevated serum triglyceride levels, fatigue, fever, seizure, respiratory arrest.

Drug Interactions
Dexrazoxane prevents cardiotoxicity when administered with doxorubicin, and potentially other anthracycline therapy. Myelosuppression may be increased when administered with chemotherapy agents.

Storage and Stability
Intact vials are stored at room temperature. Containers bear expiration dates. Reconstituted dexrazoxane and solutions further diluted to 1.3 to 1.5 mg/mL in

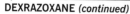

DEXRAZOXANE (continued)

5% dextrose or normal saline are stable for at least 6 hours at room and refrigeration temperatures.

Preparation

Add 50 mL of the diluent provided (preservative-free M/6 sodium lactate injection) to the 500-mg vial of dexrazoxane to yield a 10 mg/mL solution. The drug may be further diluted to a concentration of 1.3 to 5 mg/mL in normal saline or 5% dextrose.

Availability

Dexrazoxane is commercially available as a lyophilized powder in 250- and 500-mg vials.

Selected Reading

Levien T, Baker DE, Ballasiotes AA. Reviews of dexrazoxane and thalidomide. Hosp Pharm 31: 487–510, 1996.

DOCETAXEL

Other names

Taxotere®; RP 56976; NSC-628503.

Indications

FDA approved for the treatment of locally advanced or metastatic breast and non-small-cell lung cancer. The drug also may be useful in the treatment of ovarian, pancreatic, esophageal, bladder, prostate, gastric, head and neck cancers, and other malignancies.

Classification and Mechanisms of Action

Antimicrotubule agent. Docetaxel promotes the assembly of tubulin and inhibits microtubule depolymerization. Bundles of microtubules accumulate and interfere with cell division.

Pharmacokinetics

After administration, docetaxel exhibits a triphasic elimination profile with an elimination half-life of approximately 11 hours. Docetaxel is extensively protein-bound (94% to 97%), is metabolized in the liver, and is eliminated from the body primarily in the feces. Less than 10% of a dose of the drug is eliminated unchanged in the feces. Docetaxel pharmacokinetics do not appear to be influenced by age or gender or pretreatment with dexamethasone. Although there is considerable inter-patient variation concerning docetaxel elimination, patients with elevated hepatic transaminase and/or alkaline phosphatase levels tend to eliminate the drug more slowly than patients with normal liver function tests. The manufacturer does not recommend treatment with docetaxel in patients with hepatic transaminase levels greater than 1.5 times the upper limit of normal concurrent with alkaline phosphatase levels greater than 2.5 times the upper limit of normal.

Dose

For the treatment of advanced breast cancer the initial recommended dose is 60 to 100 mg/m^2 every 3 weeks. For patients dosed at 100 mg/m^2 who experience febrile neutropenia or other severe toxicities (e.g., peripheral neuropathy), a reduction in the dose to 75 mg/m^2 is recommended. If the toxicity continues, then a dose of 55 mg/m^2 can be used or treatment discontinued.

Weekly doses of docetaxel up to 40 mg/m^2/week for 6 weeks followed by a 2-week rest have been used.

For the treatment of advanced non-small-cell lung cancer the initial recommended dose is 75 mg/m^2 every 3 weeks. For patients who experience febrile neutropenia or other severe toxicities (e.g., peripheral neuropathy) a reduction in the dose to 55 mg/m^2 is recommended, once toxicity resolves. Discontinue docetaxel therapy if grade 3 peripheral neuropathy occurs.

Weekly doses of docetaxel up to 36 mg/m^2/ week for 6 weeks followed by a 2-week rest have also been evaluated in advanced non-small-cell lung cancer.

Other doses have been evaluated, including:

- 12 mg/m^2/day for 5 days repeated every 3 weeks
- 100 mg/m^2/ week for 2 doses repeated every 3 weeks
- 90 mg/m^2 as a 24-hour IV infusion repeated every 3 weeks.

Administration

Docetaxel is administered by IV infusion over 1 hour. The drug is usually diluted in 250 mL of 5% dextrose or normal saline, to produce a final concentration of 0.3 to 0.74 mg/mL. Longer durations of IV infusion, including continuous infusion, have been administered. It is recommended that a 3-day course of dexamethasone be administered, starting one day before administration of docetaxel, to lessen the severity and likelihood of fluid retention and hypersensitivity reactions. Dexamethasone, 8 mg twice daily (16 mg/day), administered orally has been recommended. For weekly docetaxel an abbreviated 3-dose course of dexamethasone, 8 mg every 12 hours for 3 doses starting the night before treatment, has been used.

Toxicity

The toxicities listed are those observed in patients with normal liver function tests receiving docetaxel at a dose of 100 mg/m^2 every 3 weeks. Patients with elevated liver function tests (i.e., transaminase levels greater than 1.5 times the upper limit of normal and alkaline phosphatase levels greater than 2.5 times the upper limit of normal) have been shown to experience a significantly higher incidence of certain toxicities (e.g., myelosuppression, fluid retention, stomatitis). Weekly scheduled docetaxel is well tolerated with the most common reported toxicities being neutropenia and fatigue.

Hematological. Neutropenia, often severe, is the primary dose-limiting toxicity. Grade 4 neutropenia has been reported to occur in 80% to 94% of patients receiving doses of 75 to 100 mg/m^2, respectively. Grade 4 thrombocytopenia is rare, and anemia (hemoglobin less than 11 g/dL) has been reported in over 90% of patients receiving doses of 75 to 100 mg/m^2. Febrile neutropenia was observed in 22% of patients receiving 100 mg/m^2.

Gastrointestinal. Mucositis (56%, severe in 9%), nausea, vomiting, dysguesia, anorexia, and diarrhea have been reported. Taste alterations are rare. Severe nausea, vomiting, and diarrhea are uncommon.

Dermatological. Alopecia is expected and total. Severe (grade 3) skin rashes have been reported to occur in approximately 10% of patients and may include desquamation after a localized pruriginous maculopapular eruption and erythema with edema. Extravasation reaction (erythema, swelling, tenderness, pustules), reversible peripheral phlebitis, hand-foot syndrome, and nail changes (hypopigmentation or hyperpigmentation) have been reported.

Hepatic. Increased liver enzyme levels, hyperbilirubinemia, hepatic failure (rare).

DOCETAXEL *(continued)*

Neurological. Reversible dysesthesia or paresthesia (7%), peripheral neuropathy (13%), mild or moderate lethargy or somnolence, headache, seizure (rare).

Cardiovascular. Fluid retention (edema, pericardial effusion, pleural effusion, peripheral edema, ascites) occurs in 41% to 70% of patients (severe in 3.4% to 10%) receiving docetaxel and the recommended premedications. Fluid retention may first appear as progressive weight gain followed by lower-extremity edema. Fluid retention is dose-related and cumulative. In one study the median time to significant fluid retention was 15 to 20 weeks, the median cumulative dose of docetaxel was 705 mg/m^2. Up to 80% of patients who received five or more courses of docetaxel developed significant fluid retention. Fluid retention slowly resolves over a median period of 16 weeks. A 3-day course of dexamethasone, beginning the day before administration of docetaxel, appears to be useful in delaying the onset of this toxicity. Hypotension requiring treatment has been reported in approximately 3% of patients.

Pulmonary. Dyspnea with restrictive pulmonary syndrome, pleural effusions.

Hypersensitivity. Local or generalized rash, flushing, pruritus, drug fever, chills and rigors, low back pain; severe anaphylactoid reactions (flushing with hypotension or hypertension, with or without dyspnea). Hypersensitivity reactions have been reported in approximately 12% to 29% of patients. Severe hypersensitivity reactions have been reported to occur in up to 2.8% of patients receiving the recommended 3-day course of dexamethasone.

Other. Fatigue, asthenia (63% to 80%, severe in 11%), conjunctivitis, arthralgia, myalgia (12% to 35%), and myopathy have been reported.

Drug Interactions

Docetaxel is metabolized by cytochrome P450 3A4. Drugs that induce or inhibit this enzyme may adversely affect the metabolism of docetaxel and lead to enhanced toxicity or decreased efficacy. Drugs that may interact with docetaxel include cyclosporine, terfenadine, ketoconazole, erythromycin, and troleandomycin.

Storage and Stability

Docetaxel is stored at room temperature and protected from bright light. The solvent vials may be stored at room or refrigeration temperatures. The reconstituted 10 mg/mL solution is stable at room or refrigeration temperatures for at least 8 hours.

Preparation

Vials of docetaxel should be at room temperature for 5 minutes prior to reconstitution. The entire contents of the diluent is added to the vial of docetaxel. The resulting solution contains 10 mg/mL of docetaxel. The desired dose of docetaxel is further diluted in 5% dextrose or normal saline to a maximum concentration of 0.9 mg/mL. Non-PVC-containing intravenous infusion bags and administration sets should be used to avoid patient exposure to the plasticizer DEHP.

Availability

Docetaxel is commercially available as a concentrated solution (40 mg/mL) in 20- and 80-mg vials.

Selected Readings

Burstein HJ et al. Docetaxel administered on a weekly basis for metastatic breast cancer. J Clin Oncol 18: 1212–1219, 2000.

Cortes JE, Pazdur R. Docetaxel. J Clin Oncol 13: 2643–2655, 1995.

DOXORUBICIN

Other names

Adriamycin®; Rubex®; Adriamycin RDF®; Adriamycin PFS®; Adriamycin MDV®; Adria;
hydroxydaunorubicin; hydroxydaunomycin; NSC-123127.
Doxorubicin hydrochloride liposomal injection (Doxil®); Pegylated liposomal
doxorubicin; NSC-712227.

Indications

FDA approved for the treatment of acute nonlymphocytic leukemia, acute lymphocytic
leukemia, Wilms' tumor, neuroblastoma, soft-tissue and bone sarcomas, breast carcinoma, ovarian carcinoma, transitional-cell bladder carcinoma, thyroid carcinoma,
Hodgkin's disease, non-Hodgkin's lymphoma, gastric carcinoma, and small-cell lung
cancer. Doxorubicin may also be a useful treatment for multiple myeloma, chronic
lymphocytic leukemia, Ewing's sarcoma, Kaposi's sarcoma, rhabdomyosarcoma,
trophoblastic neoplasms, and cancers of the cervix, endometrium, liver, esophagus,
head and neck, islet cells, pancreas, prostate, and testes. The liposomal formulation
of doxorubicin is approved for the treatment of AIDS-related Kaposi's sarcoma, and in
ovarian cancer patients in whom both platinum and paclitaxel therapy has failed. The
liposomal formulation may also have a role in the treatment of breast cancer patients.

Classification

Anthracycline antitumor antibiotic.

Pharmacokinetics

Doxorubicin is poorly absorbed (5%) by mouth. After IV administration doxorubicin is
widely distributed throughout the body, including breast milk. Approximately 70% of the
drug is bound to plasma proteins. Doxorubicin does not penetrate into the cerebrospinal
fluid. The drug is extensively metabolized by the liver to several metabolites, including
the active metabolite doxorubicinol. Approximately 40% to 50% of doxorubicin and doxorubicinol is eliminated by the biliary route, and 4% to 5% is eliminated via the urine.
Doxorubicin and doxorubicinol have elimination half-lives of 18 to 30 hours.

Dose

Doxorubicin injection. The usual dose is 60 to 75 mg/m^2 as a bolus injection or
continuous infusion over 2 to 4 days, repeated every 3 to 4 weeks. Higher bolus
doses (80 to 90 mg/m^2) have also been used.

Other dosage schedules are 20 mg/m^2 weekly and 30 mg/m^2/day for 3 days,
repeated every 3 to 4 weeks.

It has been recommended that patients with serum total bilirubin levels of 1.2 to
3 mg/dL should receive 50% of the usual dose and that patients with total bilirubin
levels greater than 3 mg/dL should receive 25% of the usual dose.
Liposomal doxorubicin injection. The dose of liposomal doxorubicin is 20 mg/m^2 every
3 weeks for Kaposi's sarcoma, and for ovarian cancer the dose is 50 mg/m^2 every
4 weeks.

Administration

Doxorubicin injection. Intravenously, either as a bolus injection (using extravasation
precautions into a free-flowing IV line over 2 to 5 minutes) or as a continuous infusion
in 50 mL or more of 5% dextrose or normal saline through a central venous line.
Doxorubicin has also been given intra-arterially to the liver, intravesicularly, and
intraperitoneally.

DOXORUBICIN *(continued)*

Liposomal doxorubicin injection. Liposomal doxorubicin is not a vesicant. Doses of 20 mg/m^2 are administered over 30 minutes. Doses greater than 20 mg/m^2 are administered at an initial rate of 1 mg per minute to minimize the risk of infusion-related reactions. If the patient tolerates the initial rate, then the rate can be incrementally increased to complete the administration of the remaining drug over 1 hour. No more than 90 mg should be diluted in 250 mL of 5% dextrose.

Toxicity

Hematological. Leukopenia (dose-limiting), also thrombocytopenia and anemia. Nadir blood counts occur in 10 to 14 days, recovery in 21 days. In more than 700 patients with AIDS-associated Kaposi's sarcoma, the following hematological toxicities have been reported after treatment with liposomal doxorubicin: grade 3 neutropenia (50%), anemia (20%), thrombocytopenia (10%).

Gastrointestinal. Nausea and vomiting, sometimes severe, is dose-related and largely preventable with antiemetic prophylaxis. Anorexia, diarrhea, mucositis (especially with the 3 times daily schedule, 10% incidence after doses of 60 to 75 mg/m^2); ulceration and necrosis of the colon have also been reported. In more than 700 patients with AIDS-associated Kaposi's sarcoma, the following gastrointestinal toxicities have been reported after treatment with liposomal doxorubicin: nausea (17%), vomiting (8%), diarrhea (8%), stomatitis (7%), oral moniliasis (5.5%).

Dermatological. Alopecia is usually total when doxorubicin is administered as a bolus injection every 3 to 4 weeks. Weekly injections of 10–20 mg/m^2 are associated with minimal or no hair loss. Hyperpigmentation of nail beds and dermal creases and radiation recall reactions occur occasionally. In more than 700 patients with AIDS-associated Kaposi's sarcoma, the following dermatological toxicities have been reported after treatment with liposomal doxorubicin: palmar-plantar erythema (i.e., hand-foot syndrome, 3.4%), alopecia (9%). Rare toxicities of liposomal doxorubicin include: rash, skin ulcer, dermatitis, skin discoloration, erythema multiforme, psoriasis, urticaria, and skin necrosis.

Local effects. Vesicant if extravasated, flush along vein, facial flush, urticaria. Liposomal doxorubicin does not appear to be a vesicant.

Cardiovascular. Arrhythmias, ECG changes, rare sudden death. Congestive heart failure caused by cardiomyopathy is related to the total cumulative dose. The risk of developing significant cardiomyopathy is greatest when total doses exceed 550 mg/m^2 (7% incidence at 550 mg/m^2, 15% at 600 mg/m^2, 30% to 40% at 700 mg/m^2). Other risk factors include mediastinal irradiation, pre-existing cardiac disease, and old age. The risk of developing this serious toxicity is reduced by giving the drug on a weekly schedule or as a continuous infusion or concomitant administration of dexrazoxane. Serial monitoring of left ventricular ejection fraction (LVEF) by equilibrium radionuclide angiocardiography (ERNA) is mandatory. A baseline ERNA is done before beginning treatment and is repeated when the total dose of doxorubicin exceeds 250 to 300 mg/m^2 and again after 450 mg/m^2 has been given. If criteria for dose-limiting cardiotoxicity are not met, ERNA is repeated before each or every other subsequent treatment. Doxorubicin is discontinued when there is an absolute decrease in the LVEF of 10% or more that is associated with a decline to a level less than 50%. Reports of cardiomyopathy occurring years after discontinuing therapy suggest that the LVEF may give a false sense of security when doses exceed 550 mg/m^2. In over 700 patients with AIDS-related Kaposi's sarcoma who received treatment with liposomal doxorubicin, chest pain, hypotension, and tachycardia have been reported in 1% to 5%. Cardiomyopathy after liposomal doxorubicin treatment has occurred in less than

1% of patients. However, experience is limited with long-term treatment of liposomal doxorubicin.

Other. Red urine, fever, chills, muscle weakness, lacrimation, conjunctivitis, anaphylactoid reaction; may enhance cyclophosphamide cystitis or mercaptopurine hepatotoxicity. Infusion-associated reactions have occurred in approximately 7% of the patients treated with liposomal doxorubicin. These reactions resolve within a day of the infusion and may consist of flushing, chills, dyspnea, facial swelling, headache, back pain, chest or throat tightness, and/or hypotension.

Storage and Stability

Rubex® or Adriamycin RDF® vials are stored at room temperature. Doxorubicin injection in liquid form is stored in the refrigerator. Liposomal doxorubicin is stored in the refrigerator.

Preparation

Doxorubicin powder for injection: add 5, 10, 25, 50, or 75 mL of preservative-free normal saline to the 10-, 20-, 50-, 100-, or 150-mg vials, respectively, to produce a solution containing 2 mg/mL.

Liposomal doxorubicin for injection should be admixed in 250 mL 5% dextrose. The maximum amount of drug per 250 mL is 90 mg.

Incompatibilities

Physically incompatible with heparin, fluorouracil, aminophylline, cephalothin, methotrexate, dexamethasone, sodium phosphate, diazepam, hydrocortisone sodium succinate, or furosemide.

Compatibilities

Stable with vincristine in normal saline for at least 5 days at room temperature and 7 days in the refrigerator. The manufacturer states that doxorubicin (1.4 mg/mL) and vincristine (0.33 mg/mL) in normal saline are chemically stable for 14 days at room temperature. Also compatible in solution with cyclophosphamide, dacarbazine, bleomycin, vinblastine, and other drugs. A pharmacist should be consulted for additional information.

Availability

Doxorubicin for injection is commercially available as a powder for injection in 10-, 20-, 50-, 100-, and 150-mg vials, and as 2 mg/mL solution for injection in 10-, 20-, 50-, and 200-mg vials. Liposomal doxorubicin is available as a 2 mg/mL solution in a 10-ml vial (20 mg/vial).

Selected Reading

Gordon AN et al. Recurrent epithelial ovarian carcinoma: a randomized phase III study of pegylated liposomal doxorubicin versus topotecan. J Clin Oncol 19: 3312–3322, 2001.

EFAPROXIRAL SODIUM

Other names

RSR13; NSC-722758.

Indications

Efaproxiral is an investigational agent in the United States. Efaproxiral is being evaluated as an enhancer of radiation therapy for primary and metastatic central nervous system malignancies.

EFAPROXIRAL SODIUM *(continued)*

Classification and Mechanisms of Action

Efaproxiral is a radiation therapy enhancer. The drug is an allosteric modifier of hemoglobin. Efaproxiral crosses into red blood cells, binds to hemoglobin, decreases hemoglobin-oxygen binding affinity, thereby increasing the release of oxygen into the bloodstream. These effects increase the oxygenation of hypoxic cells.

Pharmacokinetics

There is no accumulation of efaproxiral with the 10-day regimen. Measurement of the oxygen half-saturation pressure of hemoglobin (P50) has been shown to correlate with concentrations of efaproxiral in red blood cells.

Dose

Efaproxiral is administered at a dose of 75 to 100 mg/kg/day for 10 days in combination with radiation therapy. In patients with primary brain tumors, efaproxiral has been administered daily for 30 to 32 days in combination with a 6- to 7-week course of radiation therapy.

Administration

Efaproxiral is administered IV over 30 to 90 minutes. Supplemental oxygen, 4 L/minute, is administered with efaproxiral. Radiation therapy is delivered within 30 minutes after administration of efaproxiral.

Toxicity

Renal. Elevation of serum creatinine has been observed.

Other. Transient persistent hypoxemia and cerebral edema were reported in a patient with glioma who was receiving high-dose corticosteroids. In one study, grade 3 or 4 hypoxemia was observed in 16% of patients with lung cancer who received 32 days of combined efaproxiral and radiation therapy.

Storage and Stability

Room temperature and protected from light. Do not refrigerate or freeze efaproxiral.

Preparation

Efaproxiral is diluted to a concentration of 10 mg/mL in normal saline.

Availability

Efaproxiral is an investigational agent in the United States that is available as a 20 mg/mL injectable solution (2,000 mg/100 mL vial and 10,000 mg/500 mL vial) from the manufacturer.

Selected Reading

Kleinberg L et al. Phase I trial to determine the safety, pharmacodynamics, and pharmacokinetics of RSR13, a novel radio enhancer, in newly diagnosed glioblastoma multiforme. J Clin Oncol 17: 2593–2603, 1999.

EPIRUBICIN

Other names
Ellence®; 4'-epidoxorubicin; 4'-epiadriamycin; NSC-256942.

Indications
Epirubicin is FDA approved for use in breast cancer. Epirubicin has been shown to be a useful treatment for patients with acute nonlymphocytic leukemia, soft-tissue sarcomas, ovarian carcinoma, non-Hodgkin's lymphoma, and small-cell lung cancer.

Classification
Anthracycline antitumor antibiotic.

Pharmacokinetics
The drug is widely distributed in tissues. Excretion is primarily via the biliary route; approximately 10% is eliminated via the urine. Epirubicin has an elimination half-life of approximately 30 to 40 hours.

Dose
For the treatment of breast cancer: 100 mg/m^2/day on day 1, repeated every 21 days, or 60 mg/m^2/day on days 1 and 8, repeated every 28 days. Epirubicin 90 mg/m^2 produces a degree of myelosuppression equivalent to doxorubicin, 60 mg/m^2.

Administration
Intravenously, either as a bolus injection (using extravasation precautions into a free-flowing IV line over 2 to 5 minutes) or as a continuous infusion through a central venous line. Epirubicin is a vesicant.

Toxicity
Hematological. Leukopenia is dose-limiting and expected (nadir at 10 to 14 days). Thrombocytopenia and anemia occur less commonly.
Gastrointestinal. Nausea and vomiting are usually prevented with antiemetics. Anorexia, diarrhea (rare), and mucositis have been reported.
Dermatological. Alopecia is common but less pronounced than with doxorubicin. Hyperpigmentation of nail beds and dermal creases, dermatitis, and radiation recall occur frequently.
Local effects. If extravasated, epirubicin will cause local tissue damage, flush along vein, facial flush, urticaria, and phlebitis.
Cardiovascular. Arrhythmias and ECG changes occasionally occur but are rarely clinically significant. Congestive heart failure caused by cardiomyopathy may occur and is related to total cumulative dose (i.e., risk increases significantly when the total dose exceeds 900 mg/m^2, or 650 mg/m^2 for patients who have received previous mediastinal radiation). Mediastinal irradiation, pre-existing cardiac disease, and advanced age increase risk; weekly or continuous infusion regimens decrease risk.
Other. Red urine (common), fever, anaphylactoid reactions, paresthesias, fatigue, headache.

Drug Interactions
Epirubicin administered concomitantly with cimetidine can cause an increase in serum concentrations of epirubicin and increase the risk of additional toxicity.

EPIRUBICIN *(continued)*

Storage and Stability
Epirubicin is stored in the refrigerator and protected from light. The reconstituted 2 mg/mL solution should be used within 24 hours of penetrating the vial.

Incompatibilities
Heparin can cause epirubicin to precipitate, lines must be flushed with a heparin-free solution. Fluorouracil is chemically incompatible with epirubicin.

Availability
Epirubicin is commercially available as a preservative-free solution for injection in 25- and 100-mL vials, at a concentration of 2 mg/mL.

ERLINOTIB

Other names
Tarceva®; OSI-774; CP-358774; NSC-718781.

Indications
Erlinotib is an investigational agent in the United States. It is undergoing evaluation and has been shown to have activity in non-small-cell lung cancer, esophageal cancer, head and neck cancers, renal cell cancer, and other malignancies.

Classification and Mechanisms of Action
Erlinotib is an inhibitor of epidermal growth factor receptor (EGFR) activation and signaling. Erlinotib is thought to exert its primary antineoplastic effects by inhibiting signal transduction pathways within cancer cells by blocking the activity of epidermal growth factor receptor (EGFR) tyrosine kinase. EGFR is found in varying amounts in cells from colon, lung, head and neck, and other malignancies.

Pharmacokinetics
Erlinotib is well absorbed (80%) following oral administration. Peak serum levels occur within 2 hours of administration. The drug is metabolized by the P450 microenzyme CYP1C to an active metabolite (OSI-420). Drug accumulation does not occur at 150 mg/day. The mean elimination half-life is approximately 24 hours.

Dose
Erlinotib has been administered as a single daily dose of 100 mg to 150 mg. Erlinotib, 100 mg/day, has been administered in combination with docetaxel, 60 mg/m². Dose-limiting febrile neutropenia was observed when docetaxel, 75 mg/m², was administered. Erlinotib, 100 to 150 mg/day, is being evaluated in combination with gemcitabine, paclitaxel, carboplatin, and other drugs.

Administration
Erlinotib is administered by mouth on an empty stomach.

Toxicity
Gastrointestinal. Diarrhea is a common side effect (30%), is usually mild to moderate in severity but may be dose-limiting in some patients. The onset of symptoms usually occurs by the third or fourth week of treatment. Diarrhea is usually dose-limiting when daily doses exceed 150 mg. Nausea (20%), vomiting (20%), and oral pain/stomatitis

(25%) are common, usually mild. Dysphagia, dyspepsia, and taste alterations have been reported.

Dermatological. An acneiform rash is a common adverse event that occurs in approximately 60% to 75% of patients. The rash appears as a diffuse erythematous eruption or a papulopustular dermatitis that involves the face, scalp, trunk, and arms. The rash usually appears within 8 to 10 days of initiation of treatment, reaches a maximum intensity in the second week of treatment, and resolves slowly while treatment is continued. There are usually no symptoms associated with the rash. In those patients whose rash did not resolve on treatment, it did so following treatment discontinuation. Treatment of the rash (e.g., corticosteroids, retinoids, etc.) has not been effective. Pruritus and dry skin are reported to occur in approximately 20% to 25% of patients.

Hepatic. Transient elevations of transaminase enzymes and bilirubin have been reported.

Other. Headache. Corneal toxicities (e.g., corneal edema), observed in preclinical studies, have been rare.

Storage and Stability
Room temperature.

Availability
Erlinotib is an investigational agent in the United States that is available in an oral formulation (25 mg, 100 mg, and 150 mg/tablet) from the manufacturer.

Selected Reading
Hidalgo M et al. Phase I and pharmacologic study of OSI-774, an epidermal growth factor receptor tyrosine kinase inhibitor, in patients with advanced solid malignancies. J Clin Oncol 19: 3267–3279, 2001.

ESTRAMUSTINE

Other names
Estramustine phosphate; Emcyt®; Estracyt®; NSC-89199.

Indications
FDA approved for the treatment of advanced prostate cancer. It may also be useful for metastatic renal cell carcinoma.

Classification and Mechanisms of Action
Estramustine has been classified as a hormone but may also be an antimicrotubule agent. Estramustine elicits some pharmacological effects that are similar to those of estrogens. Estramustine has been shown to bind to microtubule-associated proteins and disrupt the normal cytoskeletal structure of cells by depolymerizing microtubules. Distribution studies with radioactive estramustine have shown that the drug accumulates in cells that contain a binding site called estramustine-binding protein (EMBP). EMBP levels have been found to be increased in prostatic carcinoma, a disease for which estramustine is an active therapy.

Pharmacokinetics
Estramustine is well absorbed (75%) by mouth, is metabolized by the liver, and has an elimination half-life of approximately 20 hours. The majority of the drug is excreted in the feces as metabolites.

ESTRAMUSTINE *(continued)*

Dose

The usual oral daily dose of estramustine for the treatment of prostate cancer is 14 mg/kg in three or four divided doses. A range of doses from 10 mg/kg/day to 16 mg/kg/day has been used.

Administration

Orally, at least 1 hour before or 2 hours after a meal. Calcium-rich foods, antacids, milk, and milk products may decrease absorption of estramustine.

Toxicity

Hematological. Leukopenia and thrombocytopenia are rarely clinically significant.
Gastrointestinal. Nausea and vomiting. These symptoms usually lessen with continued dosing. Other gastrointestinal toxicities include anorexia and diarrhea.
Dermatological. Skin rash, alopecia (rare), pruritus, and dry skin.
Hepatic. Increased liver enzyme levels, hyperbilirubinemia, jaundice (rare), increased serum amylase and lipase levels (rare).
Neurological. Headache, lethargy, insomnia, emotional lability.
Cardiovascular. Thromboembolic disorders; cerebrovascular accident; sodium retention resulting in edema, hypertension, and congestive heart failure (rare).
Genitourinary. Decreased libido (20% to 50%), impotence.
Endocrine. Hypercalcemia, decreased glucose tolerance.
Other. Gynecomastia and breast tenderness (up to 60%), phlebitis, lacrimation, leg cramps and edema.

Drug/Food Interactions

Calcium supplements or calcium-rich foods should not be taken with estramustine because calcium binds to estramustine and prevents its absorption.

Storage and Stability

Store intact capsules at refrigeration temperatures. Each bottle bears an expiration date. The drug retains its potency for up to 30 days at room temperature.

Availability

Estramustine is commercially available as 140-mg capsules.

ETOPOSIDE

Other names

VePesid®; Toposar®; VP-16; VP-16-213; EPEG; epipodophyllotoxin; NSC-141540; etoposide phosphate (Etopophos®).

Indications

FDA approved for the treatment of refractory testicular cancers and small-cell lung cancer. Etoposide may be a useful treatment for acute leukemias, Hodgkin's and non-Hodgkin's lymphoma, Kaposi's sarcoma, Ewing's sarcoma, neuroblastoma, trophoblastic neoplasms, brain tumors, and cancers of the breast, lung (small-cell and non-small-cell), adrenal cortex, bladder, stomach, and prostate. In high-dose chemotherapy regimens, the use of etoposide phosphate allows for the administration of etoposide in a smaller volume than would be necessary with etoposide. As a result, etoposide phosphate may shorten the time necessary to administer high-dose chemotherapy and reduce the volume of fluid that would otherwise be necessary.

Classification
Plant alkaloid (topoisomerase II inhibitor).

Pharmacokinetics
Oral absorption of etoposide varies from 25% to 75% (average 50%), and peak plasma levels occur approximately 1 to 1.5 hours after dosing (absorption half-life, 0.44 hours). There is no evidence of first-pass metabolism in the liver after oral administration. Etoposide has been measured in breast milk. Cerebrospinal fluid concentrations of etoposide rarely exceed 5% of the concurrent plasma concentration. The drug is extensively protein-bound (96%), metabolized by the liver, and eliminated in the bile (10% to 15% as unchanged drug) and urine (30% to 40% as unchanged drug). Etoposide is not hemodialyzable. The elimination half-life is 7 to 14 hours. Etoposide phosphate is rapidly converted to etoposide in plasma after IV administration. Etoposide and etoposide phosphate are bioequivalent when administered in molar equivalent doses.

Dose
Common intravenous doses are 50 to 120 mg/m^2/day by IV infusion for 3 to 5 days.

For the treatment of testicular cancer (in combination with cisplatin and bleomycin), the dose is 100 mg/m^2/day for 5 days, repeated every 3 weeks. The oral dose is usually twice the IV dose. Daily oral doses of 50 mg/m^2 for 21 days have been used. Etoposide doses should be reduced if renal function is impaired. A 25% and 50% reduction has been recommended for creatinine clearances of 10 to 50 mL/min, and less than 10 mL/min, respectively. Doses of etoposide should not be reduced for elevated serum bilirubin concentrations. It has been recommended that doses of etoposide be reduced by 33% in patients with a serum albumin less than 3.5 g/dL.

Administration
Etoposide. Slow IV infusion as a 0.2 to 0.4 mg/mL solution in 5% dextrose or normal saline over at least 30 to 60 minutes. Capsules are administered orally.
Etoposide phosphate. IV infusion over a period of 5 minutes or longer. Etoposide phosphate does not require further dilution before administration, although it may be diluted to a concentration as low as 0.1 mg/mL in 5% dextrose or normal saline.

Toxicity
Hematological. Leukopenia, dose-related, primarily granulocytopenia, nadirs within 7 to 14 days and recovery within 20 days of administration; significant thrombocytopenia and anemia are uncommon.
Gastrointestinal. Nausea and vomiting are relatively uncommon after IV dosing, but common with oral dosing. Anorexia occurs in 10% to 13% of patients, and stomatitis is rare with conventional doses (more common and more severe in patients who have received radiation to the head and neck and with high doses). Abdominal pain, diarrhea, aftertaste, parotitis, dysphagia, and constipation occur rarely.
Dermatological. Alopecia is generally mild and reversible and is reported to occur in 20% to 66% of patients, although some patients develop total baldness. Other toxicities include rash (rare), severe pruritus (rare), radiation recall reactions (rare), phlebitis, pain at the injection site, and hyperpigmentation (rare).
Hepatic. Hyperbilirubinemia and increased transaminase levels, usually mild, transient, and more common when high doses are given.

ETOPOSIDE *(continued)*

Neurological. Peripheral neuropathy (1% to 2%), somnolence, fatigue, headache, vertigo, transient cortical blindness (all rare), transient confusion with high doses, perhaps caused by the alcohol-containing vehicle.

Cardiovascular. Transient hypotension associated with rapid administration, transient hypertension (rare), and other cardiovascular events (e.g., congestive heart failure) thought to be related to large amounts of sodium chloride administered with the drug. Rare reports of arrhythmias.

Hypersensitivity. Anaphylactoid reactions (bronchospasm, fever, chills, dyspnea, tachycardia) are rare.

Other. Rarely, fever, muscle cramps, metabolic acidosis, hyperuricemia, second malignancy (acute myeloid leukemia).

Drug Interactions

Etoposide can increase the anticoagulation effects of warfarin.

Storage and Stability

Etoposide solution for injection should be stored at room temperature and the capsules must be refrigerated. Capsules are stable for 24 months when refrigerated. After dilution in normal saline or 5% dextrose to concentrations of 0.2 to 0.4 mg/mL, the drug is chemically stable for 96 and 72 hours at room temperature, respectively. Bristol-Myers data indicate that etoposide may be stable in 5% dextrose or normal saline for 24 hours (0.6 mg/mL), 4 hours (1 mg/mL), and 2 hours (2 mg/mL) at room temperature.

Etoposide phosphate is stored at refrigeration temperatures before reconstitution. After reconstitution or further dilution, etoposide phosphate is stable at room temperature for at least 24 hours.

Preparation

The desired dose of etoposide is usually diluted to a concentration of 0.2 to 0.4 mg/mL in normal saline or 5% dextrose. More concentrated solutions have been used but they have shorter stability (and may precipitate).

Etoposide phosphate: add 5 or 10 mL of 5% dextrose, normal saline, or sterile water to the 100-mg vial to produce a solution containing 20 or 10 mg/mL, respectively. Etoposide phosphate may also be reconstituted with bacteriostatic water or saline containing benzyl alcohol.

Compatibilities

Compatible with cisplatin 0.2 mg/mL in 5% dextrose and 0.45% NaCl or normal saline for 24 hours when protected from light. The addition of mannitol and/or potassium chloride reduces the stability to 8 hours in normal saline, but it remains stable for 24 hours in 5% dextrose and 0.45% NaCl. Also compatible with carboplatin, cytarabine, mesna, and daunorubicin. A pharmacist should be consulted for additional information.

Availability

Etoposide is commercially available as an injection in 100-, 150-, 500-, and 1,000-mg (20 mg/mL) multiple-dose vials and in 50-mg capsules for oral use. Etoposide phosphate is commercially available as a lyophilized powder in 100-mg vials.

Selected Reading

Joel SP et al. Predicting etoposide toxicity: relationship to organ function and protein binding. J Clin Oncol 14: 257–267, 1996.

EXEMESTANE

Other names
Aromasin®; PNU 155971; NSC-713563.

Indications
Exemestane is FDA approved for use in the treatment of advanced breast cancer in postmenopausal women who no longer benefit from tamoxifen therapy. It may also be useful as a first-line agent in postmenopausal breast cancer and in the prevention of prostate cancer.

Classification and Mechanisms of Action
Exemestane is an irreversible steroidal aromatase inhibitor. The drug produces its anti-tumor effects by irreversibly binding to and inactivating the aromatase enzyme. This in turn inhibits the peripheral tissue conversion of androstenedione to estrone and estradiol, thus significantly reducing serum estrogen levels. Exemestane does not affect the formation of adrenal corticosteroids or aldosterone. Corticosteroid replacement therapy is not necessary in patients taking exemestane.

Pharmacokinetics
Exemestane is rapidly and well absorbed after oral administration. Taken with a high-fat meal can increase plasma levels by up to 40%. Exemestane is highly plasma protein-bound (90%) and widely distributed into tissues. The drug is metabolized via oxidation by the liver cytochrome P450 3A4 pathway. The terminal half-life of exemestane is approximately 24 hours. Equal amounts of drug are excreted in the urine and feces, with less than 1% of the drug excreted unchanged in the urine.

Dose
The usual dose of exemestane is 25 mg daily.

Administration
Oral, taken after a meal to enhance absorption.

Toxicity
Gastrointestinal. Nausea (18%) is most common. Vomiting, anorexia, dyspepsia, diarrhea, constipation, abdominal pain, and increased appetite occur occasionally.
Neurological. Headache, dizziness, insomnia, depression and anxiety have been reported.
Cardiovascular. Hypertension was observed in approximately 5% of patients. Chest pain was reported in 2% to 5%.
Pulmonary. Dyspnea, cough.
Other. Fatigue is common (22%), increased sweating (6%), hot flushes (13%), pain, flu-like symptoms, and edema. Arthralgias, back pain, skeletal pain, infections, rhinitis, and alopecia are rare (2% to 5% of patients).

Drug Interactions
Exemestane is extensively metabolized by the cytochrome P450 3A4 pathway and therefore elimination may be reduced and toxicity increased by agents that inhibit the cytochrome P450 3A4 enzymes. These agents include, but are not limited to, itraconazole, calcium channel blockers, gemfibrozil, cimetidine, and macrolides.

Agents that induce the cytochrome P450 3A4 enzymes may increase exemestane elimination. These agents include, but are not limited to, phenytoin, rifampin, and phenobarbital. The concentrations and efficacy of exemestane may decrease if this inhibition occurs.

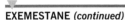

EXEMESTANE *(continued)*

Storage and Stability
Exemestane tablets are stored at room temperature. Each bottle bears an expiration date.

Availability
Exemestane is commercially available in 25-mg tablets.

Selected Reading
Kaufmann M et al. Exemestane is superior to megestrol acetate after tamoxifen failure in post-menopausal women with advanced breast cancer: results of a phase III randomized double-blind trial. The Exemestane Study Group. J Clin Oncol 18: 1399–1411, 2000.

EXISULIND

Other names
Aptosyn™; Prevatac™; sulindac sulfone; FGN-1; NSC-719619.

Indications
Exisulind is an investigational agent in the United States. It is being evaluated as a treatment for familial adenomatous polyposis coli, to prevent or delay disease progression in advanced breast, colon, head/neck cancers, and non-small-cell lung cancer. Exisulind is being evaluated in combination with other drugs, such as docetaxel or capecitabine, in the treatment of patients with breast cancer.

Classification and Mechanisms of Action
Exisulind is a selective apoptotic antineoplastic agent (SAAND). The drug is believed to selectively trigger apoptosis by inhibiting cyclic-GMP phosphodiesterases leading to protein kinase G activation. The drug may also cause down-regulation of androgen receptors. Exisulind does not inhibit COX-1 or COX-2 enzymes, p53, or Bcl-2.

Pharmacokinetics
Peak serum concentrations occur approximately 2 hours after oral administration. The absorption half-life is 0.7 hours and the elimination half-life is 4 to 6 hours. Exisulind does not appear to affect or to be a substrate for cytochrome P450 enzymes.

Dose
As a single agent, exisulind is given as 250 mg twice daily. This continuous dose of exisulind has been administered in combination with 28-day cycles of docetaxel, 30 mg/m^2/week for 3 weeks, followed by one week of no docetaxel treatment.

Administration
Oral.

Toxicity
Gastrointestinal. Dyspepsia, nausea, and vomiting are dose-related. Diarrhea has been reported; cholecystitis and pancreatitis are rare.
Hepatic. Mild to moderate elevation of transaminase levels (approximately 33%) occurs early in the course of treatment, is reversible, and may resolve with dose attenuation. Hyperbilirubinemia is uncommon.
Other. Weakness, asthenia, abdominal or back pain, and viral infection have been reported.

Storage and Stability
Room temperature.

Availability
Exisulind is an investigational agent in the United States that is available as a 250-mg capsule from the manufacturer.

Selected Readings
Prager D et al. Long-term use of exisulind in men with prostate cancer following radical prostatectomy. Proc Am Soc Clin Oncol 21: 184a, 2002.

Von Stolk R et al. Phase I trial of exisulind (sulindac sulfone, FGN-1) as a chemopreventive agent in patients with familial adenomatous polyposis. Clin Cancer Res 6: 78–89, 2000.

FENRETINIDE

Other names
4-hydroxyphenylretinamide; *N*-(4-hydroxyphenyl)retinamide; 4-HPR; NSC-374551.

Indications
Fenretinide is an investigational agent in the United States that is undergoing evaluation as a treatment for patients with cervical cancer, breast cancer, bladder cancer, and other malignancies.

Classification and Mechanisms of Action
Fenretinide is a synthetic retinoid that may induce apoptosis through nonretinoic receptor acid-mediated pathways. The drug may also have antiangiogenesis properties. Fenretinide also modulates insulin growth factor-1.

Pharmacokinetics
Fenretinide is well absorbed by mouth. Absorption is significantly increased if administered with food, especially a high-fat meal. Peak concentrations occur approximately 3 to 9 hours after a dose. The elimination half-life of fenretinide is approximately 18 to 28 hours. In a phase I study, plasma levels did not increase with daily doses greater than 900 mg/m^2, suggesting that absorption mechanisms can be saturated.

Dose
Several doses of fenretinide have been evaluated. In breast cancer prevention studies, a daily dose of 200 mg has been administered. The drug should be administered with food. Dose-limiting toxicities have not been observed with doses as high as 4,800 mg/m^2/day. The maximum tolerated dose in children is reported to be 2,475 mg/m^2/day for 7 days followed by 14 days of rest. The dose-limiting toxicities were elevations of hepatic transaminases and bilirubin.

Administration
Oral.

Toxicity
Gastrointestinal. Dyspepsia (5%), nausea (3%), vomiting (rare), abdominal cramping, and diarrhea have been reported.

Dermatological. Disorders of the skin are the most common side effects of fenretinide, occurring in approximately 18% of patients. These disorders include: skin and/or mucosal dryness, pruritus, urticaria, and dermatitis.

Hepatic. Elevations of transaminase enzymes and bilirubin have been reported. In children, these toxicities were dose-limiting.

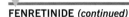

FENRETINIDE *(continued)*

Ocular. Diminished dark adaptation is reported to occur in approximately 19% of patients receiving fenretinide for 5 years. Dryness, lacrimation, and/or conjunctivitis have been reported in approximately 8% of patients.

Other. Hot flushes, dizziness, arthralgia, and headache have been reported.

Storage and Stability

Fenretinide is stored at room temperature.

Availability

Fenretinide is an investigational agent in the United States that is available in 100-mg capsules from the manufacturer or the National Cancer Institute.

Selected Readings

Camerini T et al. Safety of the synthetic retinoid fenretinide: long-term results from a controlled clinical trial for the prevention of contralateral breast cancer. J Clin Oncol 19: 1664–1670, 2001.

Torrisi R et al. Chemoprevention of breast cancer with fenretinide. Drugs 61: 909–918, 2001.

FINASTERIDE

Other names

Proscar®; MK-906.

Indications

FDA approved for the treatment of benign prostatic hypertrophy. Finasteride may also be a useful preventative therapy for patients with early-stage prostate cancer.

Classification and Mechanisms of Action

Finasteride is a 5-alfa-reductase inhibitor. Finasteride inhibits the conversion of testosterone to dihydrotestosterone (DHT) but does not significantly affect serum testosterone levels. Hyperplasia of cells within the prostate is inhibited because DHT stimulates prostate cell growth.

Pharmacokinetics

Finasteride is well absorbed (63%) after oral administration. Absorption is not affected by food and peak plasma levels occur approximately 1 to 2 hours after administration of a single dose. After 2 weeks of dosing, peak plasma levels are approximately 50% higher. Approximately 90% of the drug is bound to plasma proteins. Finasteride is metabolized in the liver to compounds that retain approximately 20% of the potency of the parent compound. Metabolites are eliminated from the body in the feces (57%) and urine (39%). Dose adjustments are not recommended for patients with hepatic or renal dysfunction.

Dose

The FDA-approved dose for benign prostatic hypertrophy is 5 mg/day for 6 to 12 months. The drug can be taken with food. Finasteride tablets may be crushed, if necessary.

Administration

Oral.

Toxicity

Genitourinary. Impotence (3.7%), decreased libido (3.3%), decreased volume of ejaculate (2.8%).

Other. Breast tenderness or enlargement, headache, hypersensivity reactions, dizziness. Finasteride may affect male fetal development if the film coating of the tablets is broken (e.g., crushed). A woman who is or may become pregnant should not handle tablets.

Storage and Stability
Room temperature, protected from light. Containers bear an expiration date.

Availability
Commercially available in 5-mg tablets.

Selected Reading
Thompson I, Feigl P, Coltman C. Chemoprevention of prostate cancer with finasteride. In Devita VT Jr, Hellman S, Rosenberg SA, eds. Principles and Practice of Oncology, PPO Updates 10: 1–18, 1996.

FLAVOPIRIDOL

Other names
HMR 1275; L86-8275; NSC-649890.

Indications
Flavopiridol is an investigational agent in the United States that is being evaluated in a variety of malignancies. Flavopiridol may have activity in non-small-cell lung cancer, non-Hodgkin's lymphoma, and other malignancies.

Classification and Mechanisms of Action
Flavopiridol is a semisynthetic flavone that inhibits cyclin-dependent kinases (CDK). Flavopiridol binds to CDK molecules leading to cell cycle arrest. Flavopiridol has also been shown to inhibit vascular endothelial growth factor (VEGF) and to induce apoptosis by down-regulating Bcl-2.

Pharmacokinetics
Glucuronidation appears to be the major route of metabolism. The terminal half-life of flavopiridol is approximately 10 hours.

Dose
Different doses and regimens have been evaluated:
- as a 72-hour continuous infusion, with concomitant antidiarrheal prophylaxis, the maximum tolerated dose is 78 mg/m^2/day × 3 days
- as a 1-hour infusion, daily × 5 days, the maximum tolerated dose is 52 mg/m^2/day
- as a weekly 24-hour continuous infusion the maximum tolerated dose is 80 mg/m^2
- in combination with paclitaxel, 175 mg/m^2 as a 3-hour infusion on day 1, flavopiridol is given as a 24-hour continuous infusion at a dose of 70 to 80 mg/m^2, beginning on day 2
- as a weekly 24-hour continuous infusion the maximum tolerated dose of flavopiridol is 80 mg/m^2
- when carboplatin, administered at a dose of AUC = 5, is administered with paclitaxel the maximum tolerated dose of flavopiridol is 70 mg/m^2.

Administration
Flavopiridol is administered IV in 100 to 250 mL of 5% dextrose and water over 1 to 72 hours.

FLAVOPIRIDOL *(continued)*

Toxicity

Hematological. Neutropenia is dose-limiting with 1-hour infusion regimens. Thrombocytopenia and anemia are not dose-limiting.

Gastrointestinal. Nausea (all grades, 45%), vomiting (all grades, 30%), dysgeusia, metallic taste and taste disturbances (25%), anorexia (35%), and diarrhea have been reported in patients receiving flavopiridol. Diarrhea (grade 1 to 2) is common and usually well controlled with loperamide. Secretory diarrhea was dose-limiting with a 72-hour continuous infusion schedule.

Dermatological. Alopecia, skin rash, pruritus, and flushing have been reported.

Hepatic. Hyperbilirubinemia, elevations of hepatic transaminases.

Cardiovascular. Hypotension may be dose-limiting with a 72-hour continuous infusion schedule. Hypotension occurs less frequently with shorter infusion regimens. Venous thrombosis at central catheter site following infusion has been reported.

Pulmonary. Dyspnea, nonmalignant pleural effusion.

Other. Fatigue (grade 1 to 2) occurs in approximately 40% of patients. Headache is reported in approximately 25% of patients. Hyperglycemia, weight loss, rigors and chills, myalgia, and altered sense of smell have been reported.

Storage and Stability

Intact vials of the lyophilized powder are stored in the refrigerator. The injectable solution may be stored at room temperature. Reconstituted solutions of flavopiridol are stable for at least 8 hours at room temperature. Flavopiridol concentrations of 0.05 mg/mL to 1.0 mg/mL in PVC bags are stable at room temperature for at least 28 hours. When flavopiridol is reconstituted with preserved normal saline and further diluted to a concentration between 0.25 mg/mL and 2.5 mg/mL in PVC bags, the solution is stable at room temperature for 72 hours.

Preparation

To the lyophilized powder add 2 mL normal saline, 5% dextrose in water, or sterile water to the 10-mg vial or add 10 mL to the 50-mg vial to yield a concentration of 4.5 mg/mL. Doses are usually further diluted in normal saline or 5% dextrose in water.

Compatibilities

Flavopiridol solutions are compatible with CADD administration sets.

Availability

Flavopiridol is an investigational agent in the United States that has been available as a lyophilized powder (10 mg and 50 mg/vial) and more recently as a 5 mg/mL solution for injection (50 mg/vial) from the manufacturer or the National Cancer Institute.

Selected Reading

Schwartz GK et al. Phase I study of the cyclin-dependent kinase inhibitor flavopiridol in combination with paclitaxel in patients with advanced solid tumors. J Clin Oncol 20: 2157–2170, 2002.

FLOXURIDINE

Other names
FUDR®; 5-FUDR; 5-fluoro-2'-deoxyuridine; NSC-27640.

Indications
FDA approved for the treatment of gastrointestinal adenocarcinoma metastatic to the liver, administered by continuous intrahepatic arterial infusion. Floxuridine may also be useful in the treatment of cancers of the breast, ovary, cervix, bladder, kidney, and prostate. Also administered as an intraperitoneal infusion for pseudomyxoma peritonei.

Classification
Pyrimidine antimetabolite.

Pharmacokinetics
Floxuridine is metabolized in the liver to its active metabolite FUDR-MP. Floxuridine is preferred over 5-fluorouracil (5-FU) for intrahepatic therapy because 90% of the drug is metabolized by the liver to inactive metabolites. Approximately 10% to 15% of a dose is eliminated in the urine as unchanged drug. Floxuridine has an elimination half-life of 0.3 to 0.6 hours.

Dose
FDA-approved doses include 0.1 to 0.6 mg/kg/day by intrahepatic arterial infusion. Floxuridine has also been given intravenously in doses up to 60 mg/kg/week.
For pseudomyxoma peritonei a dose of 3 grams per day is administered into the intraperitoneal cavity daily for 3 days; this is generally repeated every 4 weeks as clinically indicated.

Administration
Floxuridine may be administered by intra-arterial or IV infusion. Intra-arterial infusions are usually administered continuously over a period of 7 to 14 days. IV infusions may be given in 100 to 500 mL of normal saline or 5% dextrose over a 15-minute or longer period.

Toxicity
Hematological. Leukopenia and, less commonly, thrombocytopenia. These toxicities are dose- and schedule-related and more frequently observed with IV bolus dose regimens. Anemia occurs infrequently.
Gastrointestinal. Nausea (uncommon), vomiting (uncommon), anorexia, diarrhea (more common with continuous infusion), mucositis (dose-related, more common with continuous IV infusions), gastritis and abdominal cramps (more common with intrahepatic administration), enteritis, and duodenal ulcer.
Dermatological. Alopecia occurs infrequently and is generally mild. Dermatitis, localized erythema, edema, rash, pigmentation, pruritus, excoriation, and maceration are rare toxicities.
Hepatic/biliary. Hyperbilirubinemia, increased transaminase levels, increased alkaline phosphatase levels (occasionally an early indication of biliary toxicity, i.e., biliary sclerosis, stenosis, stricture), jaundice, cholecystitis, cirrhosis (rare), all mild and transient with IV injection, but dose-limiting with intra-arterial infusion to the liver. Adding dexamethasone to intrahepatic floxuridine may decrease biliary toxicity.
Neurological. Rarely: ataxia, blurred vision, fatigue, headache, depression, vertigo, nystagmus, seizures, and hemiplegia.

FLOXURIDINE *(continued)*

Mechanical. A variety of catheter problems may occur, including leakage, ischemia of the artery, occlusion of the catheter, bleeding at the catheter site, thrombosis or embolism, perforation of the vessel, dislodgement of the catheter, or infection. Periodic radionuclide scans can detect alterations in flow distribution.

Other. Fever, dysuria, hiccups, excess lacrimation, lethargy, malaise, and weakness are rare.

Drug Interactions

Concomitant intrahepatic dexamethasone and floxuridine may reduce the hepato-toxicity of floxuridine.

The bioavailability of floxuridine may be increased in patients receiving cimetidine.

Calcium leucovorin may enhance the efficacy and potentiate the toxicity of the floxuridine.

Storage and Stability

Intact vials of floxuridine are stored at room temperature. Reconstituted floxuridine (100 mg/mL) is chemically stable for at least 14 days at refrigeration and room temperatures. Further dilution to 0.5 mg/mL in 5% dextrose or normal saline results in a solution that is stable for at least 7 days at room temperature.

Preparation

Floxuridine lyophilized powder is reconstituted by adding 5 mL of sterile water to the 500-mg vial to yield a 100 mg/mL solution.

Compatibilities

Floxuridine (2.5 to 12 mg/mL) in bacteriostatic 0.9% sodium chloride with heparin (200 units/mL) is chemically stable for at least 14 days in an implantable infusion pump (Infusaid model 400). Floxuridine is also compatible with dexamethasone.

Availability

Commercially available as a lyophilized powder for injection in 500-mg vials and a 500 mg/10 mL preservative-free injection.

Selected Reading

Kemeny N et al. A randomized trial of intrahepatic infusion of fluorodeoxyuridine with dexamethasone versus fluorodeoxyuridine alone in the treatment of metastatic colorectal carcinoma. Cancer 69: 327–334, 1992.

FLUDARABINE

Other names

Fludarabine phosphate; Fludara®; 2-fluoroadenine arabinoside-5-phosphate; 2-fluoro-ara AMP; FAMP; NSC-312887.

Indications

FDA approved for the treatment of relapsed or refractory B-cell chronic lymphocytic leukemia. Fludarabine may also be a useful treatment for low-grade non-Hodgkin's lymphoma, Hodgkin's disease, cutaneous T-cell lymphoma, hairy-cell leukemia, prolymphocytic leukemia, and macroglobulinemic lymphoma. Fludarabine has also been used in peripheral blood stem cell transplant regimens.

Classification
Purine antimetabolite.

Pharmacokinetics
Fludarabine is metabolized to an active metabolite, 2-fluoro-ara-A (2-FLAA). 2-FLAA is extensively bound to body tissues, is eliminated primarily by the kidneys (i.e., urinary elimination 60% [range 24% to 86%]). 2-FLAA has an elimination half-life of 9 to 10 hours. A significant correlation between area under the curve (AUC) and absolute neutrophil count (ANC) has been demonstrated as well as a significant correlation between creatinine clearance and total body clearance (i.e., AUC). Doses need to be modified for renal impairment.

Dose
Fludarabine, 25 or 30 mg/m^2/day for 5 consecutive days every 4 weeks, for chronic lymphocytic leukemia and low-grade non-Hodgkin's lymphomas.

Administration
Usually administered by IV infusion, in 50 to 150 mL of 5% dextrose or normal saline, over 30 minutes or longer.

Toxicity
Hematological. Leukopenia (nadir 13 days), primarily lymphopenia and granulocy-topenia, and thrombocytopenia (nadir 16 days) are dose-related, may be cumulative, and are dose-limiting. Significant anemia occurs less frequently.
Gastrointestinal. Nausea and vomiting (low emetogenic potential) occur and are pre-ventable with standard antiemetic drugs. Anorexia (7% to 34%), stomatitis (rare with conventional doses), diarrhea (13% to 15%), constipation, and abdominal cramps occur infrequently.
Dermatological. Alopecia (uncommon, mild), rash (15%), dermatitis (rare).
Hepatic. Increased hepatic enzyme levels, mild and transient; cholestasis (rare).
Neurological. Somnolence, confusion, weakness, agitation, fatigue (10% to 38%), and peripheral neuropathy (4% to 12%) are usually transient. Delayed demyelinating central nervous system toxicities, including mental status changes, cortical blindness, severe somnolence and coma, have occurred, usually with high doses (e.g., 150 to 200 mg/m^2/day for 5 days); seizures (rare). Visual disturbances and coma have been reported rarely in patients receiving conventional doses of fludarabine.
Cardiovascular. Hypotension (rare), chest pain (rare), edema (8% to 19%).
Pulmonary. Dyspnea and interstitial infiltrates have been reported in a few patients previously treated with chlorambucil. Cough (10% to 44%) and pneumonia (16% to 22%) have been reported.
Other. Fever (60% to 70%), chills (10% to 20%). Increased risk of opportunistic infections secondary to decreased CD4 and CD8 T-cell counts, Co-trimoxazole prophy-laxis may be required. Metabolic acidosis and lactic acidemia caused by rapid tumor lysis; myalgia (4% to 16%); fever (rare).

Drug Interactions
Combined treatment with pentostatin and fludarabine is contraindicated because of the increased risk of fatal pulmonary toxicity.

Storage and Stability
Fludarabine vials are stored in the refrigerator. Each vial bears an expiration date. At a concentration of 25 mg/mL and after dilution in normal saline or 5% dextrose to

FLUDARABINE *(continued)*

a concentration of 1 mg/mL, the drug is chemically stable for at least 16 days at room temperature. Solutions of 0.04 mg/mL in 5% dextrose or normal saline in glass bottles or PVC bags are chemically stable for at least 48 hours at room and refrigerated temperatures.

Preparation

Fludarabine, 50 mg/vial, is reconstituted with 2 mL of sterile water to result in a 25 mg/mL solution. The desired dose is further diluted to concentrations of 0.04 to 1 mg/mL in normal saline or 5% dextrose.

Availability

Fludarabine, 50 mg/vial, is commercially available as a lyophilized powder.

FLUOROURACIL

Other names

5-Fluorouracil; 5-FU; Adrucil®; Efudex®; Fluoroplex®; NSC-19893.

Indications

FDA approved for the treatment of carcinoma of the stomach, colon, rectum, breast, and pancreas. Fluorouracil may also be useful for the treatment of cancers of the bladder, cervix, endometrium, esophagus, head and neck, islet cells, liver, lung, ovary, prostate, and skin (topically).

Classification and Mechanisms of Action

Pyrimidine antimetabolite.

Pharmacokinetics

Fluorouracil is poorly absorbed (25% to 30%) by mouth. After IV administration, the drug is metabolized to active metabolites. Activation is inhibited to some extent by allopurinol. Less than 10% of fluorouracil is protein-bound. Approximately 22% to 45% of a dose of 5-FU is metabolized by the liver and 15% is excreted unchanged into the urine. Fluorouracil has an elimination half-life of 10 to 20 minutes.

Dose

Several regimens have been used, including:

- 300 to 450 mg/m^2/day intravenously for 5 days every 28 days
- 600 to 750 mg/m^2 intravenously weekly or every other week
- 1,000 mg/m^2/day intravenously, infused over a 24-hour period, for 4 to 5 days
- 300 mg/m^2/day, infused intravenously indefinitely

Fluorouracil cream and/or fluorouracil topical solution may be applied twice a day for treatment of actinic keratosis and superficial basal cell carcinoma. This therapy may be required for several months.

Administration

The drug may be given by IV push, by IV infusion in 50 mL or more of 5% dextrose or normal saline over a 10-minute period or longer (i.e., continuous infusion), by arterial infusion, intracavitarily, intraperitoneally, topically, or orally mixed in water, grape juice, or a carbonated beverage.

Toxicity

Toxicities associated with fluorouracil are more common and more severe in patients with dihydropyrimidine dehydrogenase (DPD) deficiency.

Hematological. Leukopenia, thrombocytopenia, anemia, any of which can be dose-limiting, but less common with continuous infusion.

Gastrointestinal. Mucositis, more common with 5-day infusion and is occasionally dose-limiting. Mucositis may occur as small, shallow ulcerations on the inner surface of the lower lip or buccal mucosa and may progress to include a painful, erythematous tongue and generalized mouth sores. Allopurinol mouthwash does not prevent mucositis. Diarrhea, which can be a severe, cholera-like diarrhea when fluorouracil is given with high doses of leucovorin. Life-threatening toxicity and fatalities have resulted from drug-induced diarrhea. Nausea, vomiting, and anorexia occur infrequently.

Dermatological. Dermatitis, nail changes, dry skin, erythema, photosensitivity, hyperpigmentation, pruritic maculopapular skin rash, hand-foot syndrome (paresthesia, erythema, and swelling of the palms and soles) with protracted infusions, alopecia (uncommon).

Hepatic. Hepatitis with hepatic infusion.

Neurological. Rare and more common with high doses: cerebellar syndrome (headache, cerebellar ataxia, nystagmus, confusion).

Cardiovascular. Myocardial ischemia and angina are rare.

Ocular. Eye irritation, nasal discharge, excessive lacrimation caused by tear duct stenosis (10% to 25%), blurred vision, photophobia.

Other. Anaphylaxis (rare), vein pigmentation, fever (rare), thrombophlebitis, epistaxis.

Drug Interactions

Fluorouracil and calcium leucovorin are synergistic in effect.

Allopurinol inhibits activation of fluorouracil to one of its cytotoxic metabolites and may decrease the effectiveness of fluorouracil.

Halogenated antiviral drugs (e.g., sorivudine, netivudine) inhibit dihydropyrimidine dehydrogenase, an important enzyme in the metabolism of fluorouracil. Concomitant administration of sorivudine and fluorouracil significantly increases the toxicity of fluorouracil. Fluorouracil and levamisole concomitant administration may cause an increased risk of hepatotoxicity.

Storage and Stability

Fluorouracil is stable at room temperature if protected from light. Each vial bears an expiration date. Inspect for precipitate; if apparent, agitate vial vigorously or gently heat to a temperature not greater than 140°F in a water bath. Do not allow to freeze. Solutions in 5% dextrose, 10 mg/mL, are stable for at least 16 weeks in the refrigerator.

Preparation

Fluorouracil is available as a ready-to-use injectable solution. The desired dose may be further diluted in 5% dextrose or normal saline.

Incompatibilities

Incompatible with daunorubicin, doxorubicin, idarubicin, cisplatin, cytarabine, and diazepam.

Compatibilities

Fluorouracil is compatible with heparin sodium, vincristine, methotrexate, potassium chloride, and magnesium sulfate. A pharmacist should be consulted for additional information.

FLUOROURACIL *(continued)*

Availability

Commercially available in 500 mg/10 mL vials, and 1,000 mg/20 mL, 2,500 mg/50 mL, and 5,000 mg/100 mL vials. Also available as a 2% and 5% topical solution in 10-mL vials and a 1%, 30-mL topical solution. Fluorouracil cream is available in a 5%, 25-gram tube and a 1%, 30-gram tube.

FLUOXYMESTERONE

Other names

Halotestin®; Ora-testryl®; NSC-12165.

Indications

Fluoxymesterone is used primarily in the treatment of breast cancer and hypogonadism in men (androgen replacement).

Classification and Mechanisms of Action

Androgens are steroidal derivatives of testosterone. The antitumor actions of androgens may be caused by a reduction of or competition with prolactin receptors. Other potential mechanisms include inhibition of estrogen synthesis (by inhibition of adrenal precursors), inhibition at the estrogen receptor, and/or estrogen production in vivo via peripheral conversion of androgenic substances.

Dose

For the treatment of breast cancer the usual dose is 10 to 40 mg/day orally (in two or three divided doses) for at least 2 to 3 months.

Administration

Oral.

Toxicity

Hematological. Erythropoiesis.
Gastrointestinal. Nausea and vomiting occur infrequently.
Dermatological. Patchy alopecia, acne.
Hepatic. Liver function abnormalities, usually reversible when treatment is discontinued; cholestatic jaundice with high doses; peliosis of the liver; hepatocellular carcinoma.
Cardiovascular. Edema caused by sodium retention.
Genitourinary. In women: hirsutism, amenorrhea, clitoral hypertrophy, increased libido, voice deepening, and hoarseness. In men: oligospermia, priapism.
Metabolic. Hypercalcemia may occur, especially in immobilized patients with bony disease.
Other. Gynecomastia occurs in some men at high doses; anaphylactoid reactions are rare.

Storage and Stability

Room temperature; containers bear expiration dates.

Availability

Commercially available in 2-, 5-, and 10-mg tablets.

FLUTAMIDE

Other names
Eulexin®; Euflex®; NSC-147834.

Indications
FDA approved for the treatment of prostate cancer; to be used in combination with a luteinizing hormone-releasing hormone (LHRH) agonist (e.g., leuprolide, goserelin).

Classification and Mechanisms of Action
Flutamide is a nonsteroidal antiandrogen that blocks the activity of testosterone at the androgen-dependent accessory sex structures.

Pharmacokinetics
Flutamide is almost completely absorbed after oral dosing. Peak plasma concentrations of flutamide occur 0.5 to 2 hours after administration. The drug is almost totally metabolized to several metabolites, including 2-hydroxyflutamide, the metabolite principally involved in the action of the drug. 2-Hydroxyflutamide is metabolized by the liver, and approximately 50% is eliminated unchanged in the urine. 2-Hydroxyflutamide has an elimination half-life of 8 to 10 hours. Flutamide is unlikely to be dialyzable because of its extensive protein binding.

Dose
The usual dose is 250 mg 3 times daily, and it is usually given in conjunction with an LHRH agonist or orchiectomy.

Administration
Oral. For patients unable to swallow the capsule, it may be opened and the contents mixed with apple sauce, pudding, or other soft foods. Mixing flutamide in a beverage is not recommended because the drug does not dissolve well in water.

Toxicity
When flutamide was administered in combination with an LHRH agonist, the following side effects were observed:
Hematological. Anemia (6%), thrombocytopenia (1%), leukopenia (3%), and methemoglobinemia have been reported (rare).
Gastrointestinal. Nausea and vomiting occurred in 11% of patients, diarrhea in 12%.
Dermatological. Rash (3%), photosensitivity (rare).
Hepatic. Elevations of hepatic transaminase levels (fourfold or more above upper normal limits) occur in fewer than 1% of patients. Hyperbilirubinemia, elevated alkaline phosphatase and lactic dehydrogenase levels, hepatitis, hepatic necrosis, and hepatic encephalopathy are rare. Hepatic abnormalities usually resolve on discontinuation of flutamide.
Endocrine. Hot flushes (61%), loss of libido (36%), impotence (15% to 33%), galactorrhea. Gynecomastia occurred in approximately 10% of patients and was occasionally associated with breast tenderness.
Other. Myalgia.

Drug Interactions
Flutamide when administered concomitantly with chronic warfarin anticoagulants may lead to prolongation of prothrombin times.

FLUTAMIDE *(continued)*

Storage and Stability
Flutamide capsules are stored at room temperature. Containers bear expiration dates.

Availability
Commercially available as 125-mg capsules.

FULVESTRANT

Other names
Faslodex®; ZD9238; ICI 182780; NSC-719276.

Indications
Fulvestrant is approved by the FDA for the treatment of postmenopausal women with hormone receptor positive metastatic breast cancer who have disease progression following antiestrogen therapy.

Classification and Mechanisms of Action
Fulvestrant is an analogue of estradiol that competes for binding to the estrogen receptor on breast cancer cells. Fulvestrant causes down-regulation of the estrogen receptor. Fulvestrant has no estrogen agonist actions.

Pharmacokinetics
Peak plasma concentrations of fulvestrant occur approximately 7 to 9 days following intramuscular injection. Steady-state plasma levels are usually achieved following 3 monthly doses. Approximately 99% of fulvestrant is protein-bound. The apparent half-life is approximately 40 hours. Drug accumulation has been observed over a 6-month period of treatment. Fulvestrant does not cross the blood-brain barrier. Fulvestrant is liver metabolized to several metabolites. Some of the metabolites are active. Cytochrome P-450 enzyme 3A4 is partially involved in the metabolism of fulvestrant. Less than 1% of the drug is eliminated in the urine.

Dose
250 mg once each month.

Administration
Fulvestrant is administered by intramuscular injection, either as one 5-mL injection or two 2.5-mL injections.

Toxicity
Hematological. Anemia (all grades) has been observed in approximately 13% of patients receiving fulvestrant.
Gastrointestinal. Gastrointestinal disturbances (i.e., nausea, dyspepsia, anorexia) are the most common adverse effects, occurring in up to 50% of patients. These effects are rarely dose-limiting.
Dermatological. Skin rash (all grades) has been reported in approximately 7% of patients.
Local: Injection site reactions (pain and inflammation) have been reported to occur in 7% of European patients following a single 5-mL injection and in 27% of North American women following two 2.5-mL injections.

Neurological. Dizziness (7%), insomnia (7%), paresthesia (6%), depression (6%), anxiety (5%).

Pulmonary. Pharyngitis (16%), dyspnea (15%), cough (10%).

Other. Hot flushes occur in approximately 25% of patients, myalgia (5%), vaginitis (3%), and weight gain (2%). Asthenia (all grades) has been reported to occur in approximately 69% of patients. Pain is reported in 23%, headache in 19%, flu syndrome 7%, fever 6%.

Storage and Stability

Fulvestrant is stored at refrigeration temperatures (2° to 8°C).

Availability

Fulvestrant is available as a 50 mg/mL injectable solution in prefilled syringes (250 mg/5-mL syringe and 125 mg/2.5-mL syringe).

Selected Reading

Curran M, Wiseman L. Fulvestrant. Drugs 61: 807–813, 2001.

GEFITINIB

Other names

Iressa®; ZD1839; NSC-715055.

Indications

Gefitinib has been shown to have activity against non-small-cell lung cancer, colon cancer, head and neck cancer, and other malignancies. The drug does not appear to have activity against tumors that do not stain positively for the epidermal growth factor receptor (EGFR). The drug does not appear to be active against renal cell cancer.

Classification and Mechanisms of Action

Gefitinib is a signal transduction inhibitor that is thought to exert its antitumor effects primarily by preventing activation of tyrosine kinase. Tyrosine kinase is necessary for the function of epidermal growth factor. Thus, gefitinib is thought to exert its primary antineoplastic effects by inhibiting the epidermal growth factor receptor (EGFR). The EGFR is located in varying amounts in cells from colon, lung, head and neck, and other malignancies.

Pharmacokinetics

Peak plasma levels occur 3 to 7 hours after oral administration. The mean terminal half-life is approximately 48 hours. In a healthy volunteer study, food decreased the maximum plasma concentration by 34% and the AUC by 14%. The terminal half-life was not affected by food. Gefitinib is metabolized by CYP 3A4. Inducers of this enzyme will decrease the total AUC (e.g., rifampicin reduced gefitinib AUC by 83%). Inhibitors of CYP 3A4 will increase the AUC (e.g., itraconazole increased the gefitinib AUC by 80%). Although significant biliary elimination occurs, a daily dose of 250 mg appears to be safe in patients with "moderate" hepatic dysfunction (i.e., defined as the sum of the Common Toxicity Criteria scores for AST, total bilirubin, and alkaline phosphatase being 3, 4 or 5). Urinary recovery of gefitinib is less than 0.5%.

Dose

250 to 500 mg as a single daily dose. The drug has also been administered in 28-day courses where the drug is given as a daily dose for 14 days followed by 14 days of no treatment. On this schedule, 700 mg/day was dose-limiting.

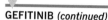

GEFITINIB (continued)

Gefitinib has been administered at doses of 250 to 500 mg/day in combination with antineoplastic agents, including carboplatin, at a dose of AUC = 6 plus paclitaxel 200 mg/m^2.

Administration

Gefitinib is administered orally. The drug has been administered by a G-tube in patients who cannot swallow tablets.

Toxicity

Gastrointestinal. Diarrhea is a common adverse event, with grade 1 to grade 2 diarrhea occurring in up to 42% of patients. In phase I dose-escalation studies, diarrhea was commonly the dose-limiting toxicity. Diarrhea appears to occur less frequently when the drug is administered on an intermittent (versus continuous) basis. Mucositis has occurred in some patients.

Dermatological. An acneiform rash is a common adverse event. In some studies more than 80% of the patients developed a grade 1 to grade 2 acneiform rash that is usually located on the face and upper torso. Grade 3 cellulitis has been observed in some patients. Dry skin and/or erythema are occasionally reported.

Hepatic. Elevations of transaminase levels have been observed.

Ocular. Mild and transient redness and/or itchiness. Corneal erosion has been reported in a few patients, with most of the reactions deemed to be due to causes other than gefitinib.

Other. Facial swelling (grade 4) has been observed in one patient on a phase II NCI-sponsored study. Hypercalcemia has occurred in some patients. Fatigue has also been reported.

Drug Interactions

Gefitinib is metabolized by CYP 3A4. Inducers of this enzyme will decrease the total AUC (e.g., rifampicin reduced gefitinib AUC by 83%). Inhibitors of CYP 3A4 will increase the total AUC (e.g., itraconazole increased the gefitnib AUC by 80%).

Storage and Stability

Gefitinib tablets are stored at room temperature.

Availability

As of this writing (March 2003), gefitinib is an investigational agent in the United States that is available as a tablet for oral use (250 mg/tablet and 500 mg/tablet) from the manufacturer.

Selected Readings

Baselga J, Averbauch SD. ZD1839 (Iressa). Drugs 60 (suppl 1): 33–40, 2000.

Rabin D et al. ZD1839, a selective epidermal growth factor receptor tyrosine kinase inhibitor, alone and in combination with radiation and chemotherapy as a new therapeutic strategy in non-small cell lung cancer. Semin Oncol 29 (suppl 4): 37–46, 2002.

GEMCITABINE

Other names

Gemzar®; gemcitabine hydrochloride; 2',2'-difluorodeoxycytidine; dFdC; 2'-deoxy-2',2'-difluorocytidine monohydrochloride; NSC-613327.

Indications

Gemcitabine is FDA approved for the treatment of advanced carcinoma of the pancreas and locally advanced or metastatic non-small-cell lung cancer (in combination with cisplatin). Gemcitabine may also be a useful treatment for patients with breast cancer, ovarian cancer, bladder, biliary, head and neck, and refractory testicular malignancies.

Classification and Mechanisms of Action

Antimetabolite (nucleoside analogue). Gemcitabine is converted to gemcitabine diphosphate, which inhibits the activity of ribonucleotide reductase and production of cellular nucleotides. Gemcitabine triphosphate inhibits DNA synthesis by competing with cytidine triphosphate for incorporation into DNA.

Pharmacokinetics

Maximum serum concentration of gemcitabine occurs approximately 30 minutes after a short IV infusion. The pharmacokinetics of gemcitabine are influenced by the length of the IV infusion and the age and gender of the patient. Men appear to eliminate the drug from the body more rapidly than women, and younger patients tend to eliminate the drug more rapidly than older patients. The elimination half-life of gemcitabine is reported to range from 42 to 79 minutes in men who are 29 to 79 years of age, respectively. The elimination half-life of gemcitabine in women aged 29 to 79 years is reported as 49 to 94 minutes, respectively. Gemcitabine is not protein-bound to any significant degree, is metabolized primarily to a single inactive metabolite, and is eliminated almost entirely into the urine. Approximately 10% of a dose of gemcitabine is detected in the urine as unchanged drug.

Dose

For the treatment of pancreatic carcinoma, gemcitabine is administered at a dose of 1,000 mg/m^2 once weekly for 7 weeks, followed by one week of rest. Subsequent courses of treatment are administered at a dose of 1,000 mg/m^2/week for 3 weeks, followed by one week of rest.

For the treatment of non-small-cell lung cancer, in combination with cisplatin, gemcitabine is administered at a dose of:

- 1,000 mg/m^2/day on days 1, 8, and 15 of a 28-day cycle or
- 1,250 mg/m^2/day on days 1 and 8 of a 21-day cycle.

Administration

Intravenously over a period of at least 30 minutes. The drug may be administered as the reconstituted solution (38 mg/mL) or may be further diluted with normal saline at a concentration as low as 0.1 mg/mL.

Toxicity

Hematological. Mild to moderate neutropenia, thrombocytopenia, and anemia are common. The incidence of grade 3 or greater hematological toxicity is neutropenia 26%, thrombocytopenia 5% to 10%, and anemia 8% to 11%.

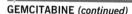

GEMCITABINE (continued)

Gastrointestinal. Mild nausea and vomiting (28% to 66%), severe nausea and vomiting (6% to 20%). Diarrhea (8% to 31%), constipation (6% to 30%), mucositis (7% to 11%).

Dermatological. Rash (10% to 28%), accompanied by pruritus (10%). Skin rashes are usually mild, respond to local therapy, and are rarely dose-limiting. Desquamation, vesiculation, ulceration, and significant alopecia are rare adverse effects.

Hepatic. Elevations of hepatic transaminase levels occur in approximately 66% of patients and are grade 3 or greater in 10% to 17%. Hyperbilirubinemia has been reported in 26% of patients and is grade 3 or greater in 8% to 10%.

Neurological. Somnolence is an uncommon adverse effect, occurring in approximately 10% of patients. Insomnia and paresthesias have been reported.

Cardiovascular. Peripheral edema (30%), mild to moderate facial edema (rare); hypotension, myocardial infarction, congestive heart failure, and arrhythmia have been reported in patients receiving treatment with gemcitabine.

Pulmonary. Mild and transient bronchospasm (less than 1%), but parenteral therapy may be required. Dyspnea (10% to 23%) usually occurs within a few hours of administration and rapidly resolves without treatment. Cough and rhinitis are rare adverse effects.

Renal. Proteinuria (32%), hematuria (23%), elevated levels of BUN (15%) and serum creatinine (6%).

Other. Malaise and diaphoresis are common. Flu-like symptoms (i.e., fever, headache, back pain, chills, myalgia, asthenia) have been reported in approximately 16% to 28% of patients.

Storage and Stability

Unreconstituted vials of gemcitabine are stored at room temperature. Reconstituted solutions are stable at room temperature for at least 24 hours. It is not recommended that reconstituted solutions of gemcitabine be refrigerated because crystallization may occur.

Preparation

Each 200- or 1,000-mg vial is reconstituted with 5 or 25 mL preservative-free normal saline, respectively, to yield a solution containing 38 mg/mL.

Availability

Gemcitabine is available in 200- and 1,000-mg vials of lyophilized powder.

GOSERELIN

Other names

Zoladex®; ICI 118630; NSC-606864.

Indications

FDA approved for the palliative treatment of endometriosis and advanced carcinoma of the prostate. Goserelin may also be a useful treatment for patients with breast cancer.

Classification and Mechanisms of Action

Goserelin is a luteinizing hormone–releasing hormone (LHRH) analogue. In men, administration of pharmacological doses inhibits gonadotropin release, resulting in decreased serum concentrations of luteinizing hormone (LH), follicle-stimulating hormone (FSH), and testosterone (estradiol in women). After 1 to 2 weeks, down-regulation of LHRH receptors occurs, with reduced LH and FSH secretion and castration levels of testosterone or estradiol. With continued goserelin therapy (every 28 days) the concentrations of these hormones can be expected to remain at castration levels for over 2 years. The drug also binds to LHRH receptors in breast cancer tissue.

Pharmacokinetics

Goserelin is slowly released from the implanted pellet over a 28-day period. Peak serum concentrations occur 12 to 15 days after administration. The drug is almost totally eliminated as unchanged goserelin in the urine; its elimination half-life is 4.2 hours. The half-life is prolonged (to approximately 12 hours) in patients with impaired renal function (i.e., creatinine clearance less than 20 mL/min); however, dose adjustments are not necessary.

Dose

Recommended doses are 3.6 mg every 28 days or 10.8 mg every 12 weeks.

Administration

Subcutaneous injection of the depot pellet into abdominal fat after swabbing the site with alcohol. A local anesthetic, such as 0.2 mL of lidocaine 1%, may be administered intradermally before injection.

Toxicity

Gastrointestinal. Infrequent nausea (5%), vomiting, anorexia (5%), diarrhea, and/or constipation.
Dermatological. Local discomfort lasting up to 30 minutes occurs occasionally. Skin rash (7%), diaphoresis (6% men, 45% women). In women, acne (42%), seborrhea (26%), hirsutism (7%).
Hepatic. Elevated serum cholesterol levels.
Neurological. Dizziness (5%), insomnia (5% to 11%), depression (54% in women), lethargy (8%).
Endocrine. Hot flushes (men, 62%; women, 96%), decreased libido (men, 21%), increased libido (women, 12%), impotence (18% to 21%), gynecomastia in men, cessation of menses, spotting, dyspareunia (14%), vaginitis (75%).
Tumor flare. In patients with carcinoma of the prostate or breast, tumor flare (consisting of increased bone pain, spinal cord compression, and other symptoms) may occur in up to 25% of patients. Tumor flare reactions usually occur in the first 2 weeks of treatment and are blocked by antiandrogens (flutamide) in men.
Other. Headache (75% in women), muscle weakness (rare), fatigue (5% to 8%); pituitary adenomas have been reported in rats.

Storage and Stability

Store at room temperature. Each syringe bears an expiration date.

Availability

Commercially available in prefilled syringes containing 3.6 and 10.8 mg of goserelin.

HOMOHARRINGTONINE

Other names
Cephalotaxine; HHT; 4-methyl-2-hydroxy-2-(4-hydroxy-4-methylpentyl)butanedioate ester; NSC-141633.

Indications
Homoharringtonine is an investigational agent that is undergoing evaluation as a treatment for acute and chronic leukemias and myelodysplastic syndromes.

Classification and Mechanisms of Action
Homoharringtonine is a semisynthetic plant alkaloid derived from the *Cephalotaxus* tree. The drug has been shown to inhibit synthesis of protein, DNA, and RNA by inhibition of chain initiation. Homoharringtonine may also induce apoptosis and differentiation and decrease resistance to imatinib (STI-571).

Dose
Doses of 2 to 7 mg/m^2/day for a period of 7 to 14 days by continuous IV infusion have been investigated.

In combination every 4 weeks homoharringtonine 2.5 mg/m^2/day for 5 days by continuous IV infusion and cytarabine 7.5 mg/m^2 twice daily for 5 days by subcutaneous injection has been evaluated.

Administration
Intravenously, usually by continuous infusion.

Toxicity
Hematological. Leukopenia and thrombocytopenia are expected.
Gastrointestinal. Mild nausea, vomiting, anorexia, diarrhea.
Dermatological. Alopecia.
Hepatic. Transient elevations of hepatic transaminase levels.
Neurological. Confusion, lethargy, agitation, depression, headache.
Cardiovascular. Hypotension may be severe and can occur during administration of the drug or up to 12 hours after discontinuation of the IV infusion. Tachycardia and cardiac arrhythmias have been reported.
Other. Hyperglycemia.

Storage and Stability
Intact vials are stable for at least 5 years at room temperature. Reconstituted solutions and solutions further diluted to concentrations of 0.05 mg/mL in normal saline or 5% dextrose in water are chemically stable for at least 96 hours at room temperature.

Preparation
The 5-mg vial is reconstituted with 4.9 mL of normal saline to yield a 1 mg/mL solution. The desired dose is usually further diluted in normal saline or 5% dextrose.

Availability
Homoharringtonine is an investigational drug that is available from the National Cancer Institute as a lyophilized powder in 5-mg vials.

Selected Reading
Kantarjian HM et al. Homoharringtonine: history, current research, and future directions. Cancer 92: 1591–1605, 2001.

HYDROXYUREA

Other names
Hydrea®; hydroxycarbamide; SQ-1089; WR-83799; NSC-32065.

Indications
FDA approved for the treatment of melanoma; resistant chronic myelogenous leukemia; recurrent, metastatic, or inoperable carcinoma of the ovary; and head and neck cancer. Hydroxyurea may also be useful for polycythemia vera, trophoblastic neoplasms, and cancers of the cervix and prostate.

Classification
Antimetabolite (ribonucleotide reductase inhibitor).

Pharmacokinetics
Hydroxyurea is well absorbed (greater than 80%) following oral administration. Peak serum concentrations occur approximately 2 hours after dosing. Hydroxyurea is distributed into breast milk. Approximately 50% of the drug is metabolized by the liver to inactive compounds; the other 50% is excreted unchanged in the urine. Hydroxyurea has an elimination half-life of 2 to 5 hours.

Dose
For the treatment of chronic myelocytic leukemia, a daily dose of 20 to 30 mg/kg has been used.

To control hyperleukocytosis initial doses up to 50 mg/kg may be used.

For the treatment of solid tumors or in combination with radiation therapy for the treatment of patients with cancer of the head and neck, a recommended dose is 60 to 80 mg/kg (or 2,000 to 3,000 mg/m^2) as a single dose every third day, starting 7 days prior to radiation and continuing during and post radiation therapy.

Alternatively, 1,250 mg/m^2 every 8 hours for 5 doses has been given once weekly. It has been recommended that the dose be reduced in patients with renal impairment (i.e., a 50% reduction for a creatinine clearance of 10 to 50 mL/min, a 75% reduction for a creatinine clearance less than 10 mL/min).

Administration
Oral. If the capsules cannot be swallowed, they may be opened and the drug may be dissolved in water. Some of the excipients in the capsules will not dissolve in water. The white powder floating on top of the water may be discarded.

Toxicity
Hematological. Leukopenia is expected and is occasionally dose-limiting. Thrombocytopenia, anemia, and megaloblastic erythropoiesis are frequent occurrences.

Gastrointestinal. Nausea and vomiting are uncommon. Diarrhea, constipation, mucositis, and anorexia are rare.

Dermatological. Maculopapular rash, facial erythema, hyperpigmentation, pruritus, alopecia (rare), radiation recall phenomenon (rare).

Hepatic. Transient elevation of hepatic transaminase levels; jaundice and hepatitis have been rarely reported.

Neurological. Headache, drowsiness, dizziness, disorientation, hallucinations, and seizures are rare events.

HYDROXYUREA *(continued)*

Renal. Hyperuricemia, dysuria, increased BUN and serum creatinine levels, proteinuria.
Other. Pulmonary edema (rare), flu-like syndrome (fever, chills, malaise), acral
erythema (rare). Amenorrhea, gonadal suppression.

Drug Interactions

Hydroxyurea administered concomitantly with antiviral therapy, stavudine, or didanosine
may increase the risk of hepatotoxicity or fatal pancreatitis.

Storage and Stability

Store oral capsules at room temperature. Bottles bear expiration dates.

Availability

Hydroxyurea is commercially available in 500-mg capsules. An injectable formulation
of hydroxyurea is available from the NCI as a 2,000-mg vial.

IDARUBICIN

Other names

Idarubicin hydrochloride; Idamycin®; Zavedos®; 4-demethoxydaunorubicin;
NSC-256439.

Indications

FDA approved for the treatment of acute nonlymphocytic leukemia.

Classification

Anthracycline antitumor antibiotic.

Pharmacokinetics

Idarubicin is poorly absorbed (approximately 20% to 30%) following oral administration.
Idarubicin is metabolized by the liver to several metabolites, including idarubicinol,
which is active. Significantly more idarubicinol is formed compared to the other metabolites. The clinical significance of this observation is uncertain. Some of the drug penetrates into the cerebrospinal fluid (20% idarubicin, 10% idarubicinol). Approximately
25% of the drug is excreted unchanged in the bile, 2% to 3% in the urine. The elimination half-life of idarubicin is 13 to 26 hours; for idarubicinol, it is 38 to 63 hours.

Dose

The usual dose for leukemia induction therapy is 12 mg/m^2/day for 3 days (combined
with cytarabine, 200 mg/m^2/day for 7 days). Single doses of 8 to 15 mg/m^2 every
3 weeks have also been used. Reduce dose for hepatic dysfunction (i.e., 50%
decrease for bilirubin 2.6 to 5 mg/dL, if bilirubin is > 5 mg/dL do not administer
idarubicin). Consider dose modification for serum creatinine > 2.5 mg/dL. Monitor
cardiac function, proposed maximum lifetime dose of idarubicin is 150 mg/m^2.

Administration

Idarubicin is a vesicant and is administered as an IV injection (using extravasation
precautions) over a 1- to 5-minute period.

Toxicity

Hematological. Myelosuppression (leukopenia and thrombocytopenia) is expected.
Leukopenia is usually more severe than thrombocytopenia. Anemia also occurs but is
a less frequent complication.

Gastrointestinal. Nausea and vomiting are common (82%), usually mild to moderate in severity, and preventable with antiemetic treatment. Diarrhea (20% to 73%), mucositis (50%), and enterocolitis may also occur.

Dermatological. Alopecia is common but usually partial; extravasation reactions, hives, urticaria, palmar-plantar erythrodysesthesias, and radiation recall reactions are uncommon.

Hepatic. Transient elevation of hepatic transaminase and bilirubin levels.

Cardiovascular. Transient arrhythmia; cardiomyopathy and congestive heart failure can occur after large cumulative doses have been administered. Idarubicin is less cardiotoxic than daunorubicin and doxorubicin, but the same monitoring criteria apply. At cumulative doses of 150 to 290 mg/m^2, cardiomyopathy occurred in 5% of patients. The results from a retrospective study indicated that the probability of developing a 15% or greater decrease in left ventricular ejection fraction to a level less than or equal to 45% is 7% after a cumulative idarubicin dose of 150 mg/m^2.

Neurological. Headache (20%), peripheral neuropathy (7%), seizures (4%).

Storage and Stability

Idarubicin powder for injection is stored at room temperature. The preservative-free solution (PFS) for injection is stored in the refrigerator. Both products need to be protected from light. The reconstituted solution is stable for 3 days at room temperature and 7 days under refrigeration.

Preparation

Each 5-, 10-, or 20-mg vial is diluted with 5, 10, or 20 mL, respectively, of preservative-free normal saline or sterile water for injection to yield a 1 mg/mL solution. The manufacturer does not recommend the use of diluents that contain preservatives.

Compatibilities

Idarubicin and cytarabine are compatible at the "Y"-site.

Incompatibilities

Idarubicin is incompatible with fluorouracil, etoposide, dexamethasone, heparin, hydrocortisone, methotrexate, vincristine, and other drugs. Idarubicin is deactivated on prolonged contact with alkaline solutions. A pharmacist should be consulted for additional information.

Availability

Commercially available as a lyophilized powder in 5-, 10-, and 20-mg vials and as a 1 mg/mL solution for injection in 5-, 10-, and 20-mL single use vials.

IFOSFAMIDE

Other names

Ifex®; isophosphamide; Mitoxana; Holoxan; Naxamide; NSC-109724.

Indications

FDA approved for the treatment of relapsed testicular carcinoma. Ifosfamide may be useful for Hodgkin's and non-Hodgkin's lymphoma, acute leukemias, Ewing's sarcoma, osteosarcoma, trophoblastic neoplasms, soft-tissue sarcomas, and cancers of the breast, lung, ovary, stomach, and pancreas.

Classification

Alkylating agent.

IFOSFAMIDE *(continued)*

Pharmacokinetics

Similar to cyclophosphamide, ifosfamide must be activated by hepatic microsomal enzymes. However, since less of the drug is activated, higher doses must be given (as compared with cyclophosphamide). The drug is metabolized by the liver to inactive metabolites and approximately 15% to 56% of the drug is excreted unchanged in the urine. The chloroacetaldehyde metabolite of ifosfamide may be responsible for much of the neurotoxic adverse effects. The clearance of this metabolite is slowed in patients with renal dysfunction. Ifosfamide has an elimination half-life of 7 to 15 hours. Ifosfamide is believed to be more efficacious when given daily for 5 days as compared with a single dose. Pharmacokinetic changes between the two dosing schedules (decreased half-life and urinary recovery of unchanged drug associated with the 5-day schedule) suggest that a single dose of drug "activates" microsomal enzyme systems to activate subsequent doses. Ifosfamide has been detected in breast milk.

Dose

Ifosfamide, 1,000 to 1,200 mg/m^2/day, is often given over 5 consecutive days and repeated every 3 to 4 weeks.

Higher doses (e.g., 2,500 to 4,000 mg/m^2/day) have been given over a 2- to 3-day period. Mesna must also be given with ifosfamide. The usual dose of mesna is 20% of the ifosfamide dose, given just before and 4 and 8 hours after ifosfamide (the total mesna dose is 60% of the ifosfamide dose). Mesna may be given orally (double the dose) for patient convenience. Mesna has also been given as a continuous IV infusion concurrently with ifosfamide. For continuous infusion, a total dose of mesna equal to the total dose of ifosfamide is given, preceded by a loading dose of 6% to 10% of the total ifosfamide dose.

Administration

Administered intravenously in 250 mL or more of 5% dextrose or normal saline over 30 minutes or longer. It is recommended that patients receive aggressive concomitant hydration (at least 2 L/m^2/day) during ifosfamide dosing to reduce the incidence of hemorrhagic cystitis. Concomitant uroprotective therapy with mesna, as described above, is required with ifosfamide therapy.

Toxicity

Hematological. Myelosuppression is a major dose-limiting toxicity. The leukopenic nadir usually occurs 7 to 10 days post-treatment. Thrombocytopenia and anemia occur less frequently.

Gastrointestinal. Nausea and vomiting are common (58%), dose-related, and preventable in the majority of patients when antiemetics are used. However, antiemetic regimens that include sedating drugs may mask detection of somnolence sometimes caused by ifosfamide. Anorexia, constipation, diarrhea, salivation, and stomatitis occur occasionally.

Dermatological. Alopecia is common (83%). Rash, urticaria, nail ridging, dermatitis, and hyperpigmentation are uncommon.

Hepatic. Elevated hepatic transaminase levels and hyperbilirubinemia are usually mild, transient, and uncommon.

Neurological. Occasional (12%) episodes of somnolence, lethargy, ataxia, disorientation, confusion, dizziness, malaise, depressive psychosis, and coma have been reported. These toxicities occur more frequently when ifosfamide is given over a 1-day period (versus 5 days), in the presence of impaired renal function (caused by impaired clearance of the toxic metabolite chloroacetaldehyde), in patients with hypoalbuminemia, and when sedatives (e.g., lorazepam, opiates) are administered concomitantly. Intravenous administration of methylene blue 50 mg of a 1% to 2% solution has been shown to reverse neurotoxicity. This dose can be repeated 3 to 4 times per day. Myoclonus and seizures have been rarely reported.

Genitourinary. Ifosfamide-induced hemorrhagic cystitis (more than 4 rbc/hpf) occurs relatively frequently when uroprotective measures are not used. The incidence of hemorrhagic cystitis is dose- and schedule-related (i.e., more common with a single high-dose regimen versus multiple-dose regimens). The use of mesna (greater than 20% of the ifosfamide dose) given before and after each ifosfamide dose greatly reduces the incidence and severity of this adverse effect. Whether mesna reduces the risk of developing secondary bladder carcinoma is not known.

Renal. Elevated serum creatinine levels occur infrequently with standard doses of ifosfamide. However, with higher doses (e.g., 4,000 mg/day for 3 days) renal toxicity may be dose-limiting.

Other. Hyponatremia, hypokalemia, phlebitis, fever, and hypotension or hypertension.

Storage and Stability

Unreconstituted vials are stored at room temperature. Ifosfamide liquefies at temperatures above 35°C. Appropriately reconstituted ifosfamide and ifosfamide further diluted to 16 mg/mL or 0.6 mg/mL in 5% dextrose, 5% dextrose and Ringer's injection, 5% dextrose and normal saline, lactated Ringer's solution, 0.45% sodium chloride, normal saline, or 1/6 M sodium lactate are stable for 7 days at room temperature and 6 weeks under refrigeration. Ifosfamide, 10 to 80 mg/mL in normal saline, is stable for at least 8 days in PVC portable pump infusion cassettes.

Preparation

Reconstitute the 1,000-mg and 3,000-mg vials with 20 and 60 mL of sterile water, respectively, to yield a concentration of 50 mg/mL. Bacteriostatic water for injection may be used to reconstitute ifosfamide.

Compatibilities

Ifosfamide and mesna (in equal concentrations) are chemically stable at room temperature for at least 24 hours in 5% dextrose or lactated Ringer's solution. Ifosfamide (2,600 mg/L) and mesna (1,600 mg/L) are stable for at least 7 hours at room temperature in 5% dextrose or 0.9% sodium chloride. Ifosfamide (500 mg/10 mL) and mesna (400 mg/10 mL) combined in polypropylene syringes are compatible for at least 7 days at room temperature.

Availability

Ifosfamide is commercially available as a lyophilized powder in 1,000- and 3,000-mg vials.

IMATINIB MESYLATE

Other names

Gleevec®; Glivac®; STI 571; CGP57148B; NSC-716051.

Indications

FDA approved for treating chronic myeloid leukemia (CML) that is in blast crisis, accelerated phase, or for patients who no longer benefit from interferon therapy for

IMATINIB MESYLATE *(continued)*

chronic phase CML. FDA approved for gastrointestinal stromal tumors that express the c-kit tyrosine kinase. Imatinib may also be useful in other types of leukemia.

Classification and Mechanisms of Action

Imatinib mesylate is a protein-tyrosine kinase inhibitor. By inhibition of the Bcr-Abl tyrosine kinase, imatinib mesylate can induce apoptosis and inhibit further proliferation of the cell lines that are positive for Bcr-Abl. These cell lines are prominent in Philadelphia chromosome-positive chronic myeloid leukemia.

Pharmacokinetics

Imitinib mesylate is rapidly and well absorbed after oral administration. Maximum concentrations occur 2 to 4 hours after administration. Plasma protein binding, in vitro, is extensive, up to 95% bound to albumin and alfa-1-acid glycoprotein. The half-life of imatinib mesylate is approximately 18 hours and its major metabolite has an elimination half-life of approximately 40 hours. Most of the drug is metabolized by the liver cytochrome P450 3A4 pathway to active metabolites. Within 7 days approximately 68% of a dose is eliminated in the feces and 13% in the urine. Elimination occurs mostly as metabolites, with approximately 25% being the parent compound.

Dose

The starting dose of imatinib mesylate for patients with chronic phase CML is 400 mg per day.

The starting dose of imatinib mesylate for patients with accelerated phase CML or blast crisis is 600 mg per day.

For gastrointestinal stromal tumors doses of 400 mg once or twice a day have been used.

Do not adjust dose based on body weight or age, but based on toxicity exhibited.

Administration

Oral. Take with food and a large glass of water.

Toxicity

Hematological. Neutropenia and thrombocytopenia occur commonly. Grade 3 or 4 hematological toxicity tends to be more prominent in blast crisis and accelerated phase CML in comparison with chronic phase CML. Neutropenia lasted 2 to 3 weeks and thrombocytopenia 3 to 4 weeks. Management can include dose reduction or intermittent discontinuation of therapy. Rarely does therapy need to be stopped permanently. Hemorrhage is observed frequently in accelerated phase and blast crisis, and in less than 15% of chronic phase.

Gastrointestinal. Nausea (all grades) ranged upwards to 68%, with grade 3 nausea reported in 5% of patients. Greater than 30% of patients will experience mild to moderate diarrhea and vomiting. Abdominal pain, anorexia, dyspepsia, and constipation were observed in less than 26% of patients. Overall, grade 3 to 4 gastrointestinal toxicity was reported in less than 5% of patients.

Dermatological. Skin rashes are observed in up to 39% of patients. Also reported are pruritus and petechiae.

Hepatic. Grade 3 to 4 elevated liver function tests, including bilirubin, transaminases, and alkaline phosphatase, is observed in up to 5% of patients. Management can include dose reduction or intermittent discontinuation of therapy. Rarely does therapy need to be permanently discontinued.

Neurological. Headache and rarely hemorrhage in the central nervous system.

Cardiovascular. Edema and/or fluid retention (all grades) were observed in over 60% of patients, with severe pulmonary edema, pericardial effusion, pleural effusion, and ascites reported rarely (less than 3%).

Pulmonary. Dyspnea, cough, nasopharyngitis, pneumonia.

Other. Arthralgias (up to 26%), fatigue (up to 33%), myalgias (up to 18%), fever (up to 38%), night sweats (10%), muscle cramps (up to 46%), musculoskeletal pain (39%), weakness, and hypokalemia.

Drug Interactions

Imatinib mesylate elimination may be reduced, and toxicity increased, by agents that inhibit the cytochrome P450 3A4 enzymes. These agents include, but are not limited to, itraconazole, ketoconazole, calcium channel blockers, gemfibrozil, cimetidine, and macrolides.

Agents that induce the cytochrome P450 3A4 enzymes may increase imatinib mesylate elimination, resulting in decreased concentrations of imatinib mesylate. These agents include, but are not limited to, phenytoin, dexamethasone, carbamazepine, rifampin, phenobarbital, and St. John's Wort. The efficacy of imatinib mesylate may decrease if this inhibition occurs.

Imatinib mesylate administered concomitantly with acetaminophen, or acetaminophen-containing products, may cause an increase in severe hepatotoxicity.

Imatinib mesylate may act as an inhibitor of the metabolism of drugs that are substrates of the cytochrome P450 3A4 enzymes. This could increase the concentrations of certain drugs, including: simvastatin, cyclosporine, pimozide, triazolobenzodiazepines, carbamazepine, dihydropyridine calcium channel blockers (diltiazem, verapamil), fentanyl, tacrolimus, lovastatin, antivirals (e.g., indinavir, ritonavir, saquinavir), warfarin, and other agents. Increased levels may increase toxicity of these agents, particularly those with a narrow therapeutic index.

Imatinib mesylate may act as an inhibitor of the metabolism of drugs that are substrates of the cytochrome P450 2C9 enzymes. This would result in increased concentrations of these drugs, including warfarin, phenytoin, and oral hypoglycemic agents (e.g., glipizide, glimepiride, and glyburide).

Storage and Stability

Imatinib mesylate capsules are stored at room temperature. Each bottle bears an expiration date.

Availability

Imatinib mesylate is commercially available as a 100-mg gelatin capsule. There are 120 capsules in each bottle.

Selected Readings

Drucker BJ et al. Efficacy and safety of a specific inhibitor of the BCR-ABL tyrosine kinase in chronic myeloid leukemia. N Engl J Med 344: 1031–1037, 2001.

Joensuu H et al. Effect of the tyrosine kinase inhibitor STI 571 in a patient with a metastatic gastrointestinal stromal tumor. N Engl J Med 344: 1052–1056, 2001.

IRINOTECAN

Other names

Camptosar®; CPT-11; camptothecin-11; NSC-616348.

Indications

FDA approved for metastatic colorectal carcinoma as initial therapy combined with flu-orouracil and leucovorin. Also approved for second-line treatment in colorectal carci-noma patients who are no longer responding to initial fluorouracil therapy. The drug is also active in carcinoma of the lung, pancreas, ovary, and other malignancies.

Classification and Mechanisms of Action

Topoisomerase I inhibitor.

Pharmacokinetics

Metabolized to 7-ethyl-10-hydroxycamptothecin (SN-38), which is 40 to 200 times as potent as irinotecan. Irinotecan has a triphasic elimination pattern with an elimination half-life of 16 to 18 hours. SN-38 has an elimination half-life of 7 to 14 hours.

Dose

Standard dosing of single agent irinotecan is 125 mg/m^2 intravenously weekly for 4 weeks followed by a 2-week rest, or 350 mg/m^2 intravenously once every 21 days. Adjust dose for hepatic dysfunction (not recommended if serum bilirubin is greater than 2 mg/dL), hematological toxicity, and diarrhea.

When combined with cisplatin, 80 mg/m^2 on day 1 repeated every 4 weeks, the usual dose of irinotecan is 60 mg/m^2/week for 3 weeks (days 1, 8, and 15).

Irinotecan has been evaluated utilizing other dosing schedules and regimens.

Administration

Irinotecan is given by IV infusion in 500 mL of 5% dextrose or normal saline over 60 to 90 minutes or longer.

Toxicity

Hematological. Neutropenia is dose-limiting, and there is a 25% incidence of grade 3 or greater neutropenia with 100 mg/m^2/week. With the weekly for 3 weeks schedule, nadir blood counts occur around day 30 and recover by day 35. Other hematological toxicities include eosinophilia (30%), anemia (15%), and thrombocytopenia.

Gastrointestinal. Diarrhea is dose-limiting, occasionally severe and unpredictable. In some studies a 15% to 25% incidence of grade 3 or 4 diarrhea occurred with irinote-can administered at a dose of 100 mg/m^2/week. Early-onset diarrhea begins within 24 hours of an irinotecan infusion; administration of atropine 0.25 mg to 1 mg may be administered to alleviate this side effect. Late-onset diarrhea, beginning 24 hours after an irinotecan infusion, is treated with loperamide. An aggressive regimen of lop-eramide should be initiated at the first sign of diarrhea (e.g., first loose stool or episode of two or more bowel movements in one day). The recommended loperamide dose is 4 mg at the first sign of diarrhea followed by 2 mg every 2 hours (4 mg every 4 hours during the night) until there are no signs of diarrhea for a period of at least 12 hours. This exceeds standard over the counter loperamide labeling. Prophylactic use of loperamide is not recommended.

Moderate to severe nausea and vomiting occurs in 20% to 25% of patients. Other gastrointestinal toxicities include anorexia (63%), abdominal pain (19%), mucositis

(4%), constipation (13%), bloating, and heartburn. Flushing, cramping, and diarrhea were reported to be significantly reduced by premedication with ondansetron and diphenhydramine with or without atropine.

Dermatological. Alopecia (40% to 56% overall, 4% significant), sweating, skin rash (rare), hives, pigmentation.

Hepatic. Elevated liver enzyme levels (7% to 20%).

Neurological. Headache, dizziness, insomnia.

Cardiovascular. Thromboembolic complications have been reported.

Pulmonary. Dyspnea on exertion and pulmonary infiltrates (3%). The onset of symptoms occurs in approximately 60 days (range 40 to 175 days) after beginning treatment with irinotecan. Pneumonitis has also been reported.

Renal. Elevated serum creatinine levels and hematuria are rare.

Other. Fever (7%), chills, diaphoresis, fatigue (25%), salivation (35%), lacrimation (26%), bradycardia (13%), elevated serum amylase levels.

Drug Interactions

Inducers of cytochrome P450 3A4 (e.g., phenobarbital, phenytoin, etc.) will increase the elimination of irinotecan. Higher doses of irinotecan will be necessary to achieve the same therapeutic effect in these patients.

In patients who are taking warfarin, an increase in prothrombin times has been observed after treatment with irinotecan.

Common laxatives or laxative-like agents must be avoided in patients receiving irinotecan.

Irinotecan administered concurrently with the herbal supplement St. John's Wort resulted in significantly decreased levels of irinotecan (up to 40% less bioavailable). It is unclear as to the amount of time a patient has to be off the herbal supplement in order to prevent this drug interaction, but it is longer than a 24-hour time frame. St. John's Wort may affect other chemotherapy agents in a similar manner.

Metoclopramide and irinotecan used concomitantly can increase diarrhea and the combination should be avoided.

Prochlorperazine use should be avoided within the first 24 hours after receiving irinotecan, there is an increased incidence of akathesia if used concomitantly.

Storage and Stability

Irinotecan is stored at room temperature, each vial bears an expiration date. Mixed in glass bottles or plastic containers containing 500 mL of 5% dextrose or normal saline, the drug is stable at room temperature for at least 24 hours. Solutions of irinotecan should not be refrigerated; precipitation may occur.

Preparation

Irinotecan is further diluted in 250 to 500 mL of 5% dextrose (preferred) or normal saline. The final concentration should be 0.12 to 2.8 mg/mL.

Availability

Irinotecan is available as a 20 mg/mL solution in 2- and 5-mL vials.

Selected Reading

Saltz LB et al. Irinotecan plus fluorouracil and leucovorin for metastatic colorectal cancer. N Engl J Med 343: 905–914, 2000.

IROFULVEN

Other names

MGI-114; 6-hydroxymethylacylfulvene; HMAF; NSC-683863.

Indications

Irofulven is an investigational agent in the United States undergoing evaluation in patients with carcinoma of the pancreas, prostate, ovarian cancer, and other malignancies.

Classification and Mechanisms of Action

Irofulven is an acylfulvene, a semisynthetic compound derived from a cytotoxic mushroom metabolite. Irofulven induces caspase-8 and caspase-9-mediated apoptosis. Irofulven is active against several multidrug-resistant cell lines. The cytotoxic effects of irofulven do not appear to be related to p53 or Bcl-2 expression.

Pharmacokinetics

Irofulven has an elimination half-life of approximately 5 minutes. There is no accumulation of the drug over a 5-day treatment schedule.

Dose

Different regimens have been evaluated. As a daily dose for 5 days the recommended phase II dose is 11 mg/m^2/day, repeated every 28 days. Irofulven has been administered on an every other week schedule in combination with continuous infusion 5-fluorouracil. Irofulven has also been evaluated in separate studies with docetaxel, irinotecan, and gemcitabine.

Administration

Irofulven is administered IV over 5 to 60 minutes. Hydration with 500 mL of normal saline is usually given prior to each dose.

Toxicity

Hematological. Neutropenia, thrombocytopenia (40% with grade ≥ 2).
Gastrointestinal. Irofulven is highly emetogenic. Grade 3 nausea and grade 2 or worse vomiting is reported to occur in 40% to 50% of patients who do not receive aggressive antiemetic prophylaxis. Anorexia is relatively common.
Dermatological. May cause an extravasation injury if the drug leaks from the vein. Phlebitis has been reported following administration of irofulven.
Renal. Renal tubular acidosis was dose-limiting at 14 mg/m^2/day × 5 days.
Other. Fatigue (33% greater than or equal to grade 2) and visual disturbances (altered light sensitivity).

Storage and Stability

Intact vials are stored in the freezer (−10°C to −20°C). Reconstituted solutions are stable for at least 4 hours at room temperature.

Preparation

Add 0.1 mL dehydrated alcohol USP and 9.9 mL of 5% dextrose and water to the 10-mg vial to yield a concentration of 1 mg/mL.

Availability

Irofulven is an investigational agent in the United States that is available as a lyophilized powder (10 mg/vial) from the manufacturer or the National Cancer Institute.

Selected Reading

Thomas JP et al. Phase I clinical and pharmacokinetic trial of irofulven. Cancer Chemother Pharmacol 48: 467–472, 2001.

ISOTRETINOIN

Other names

Accutane®; Accutane Roche®; 13-*cis*-retinoic acid; 13-CRA; NSC-329481.

Indications

Investigational studies are evaluating the effectiveness of isotretinoin as a chemo-prevention agent for myelodysplastic syndromes, cutaneous squamous cell cancers, melanoma, head and neck cancer, cutaneous T-cell lymphoma, and other malignancies.

Classification and Mechanisms of Action

Isotretinoin is a derivative of vitamin A. The drug binds to a cellular protein that facilitates the transfer of isotretinoin from cellular cytoplasm into the nucleus. Isotretinoin is believed to increase DNA, RNA, and protein synthesis and to affect cellular mitosis. Isotretinoin affects the function of lymphocytes and monocytes, which results in a modulation of the cellular immune response. Isotretinoin possesses some anti-inflammatory activity.

Pharmacokinetics

Isotretinoin is a natural retinoic acid metabolite (basal concentrations, 3 to 4 ng/mL). After oral administration, peak plasma levels occur in approximately 3 hours. The oral bioavailability of isotretinoin is around 25%. The drug is almost totally bound to plasma albumin, is metabolized to 4-oxo-isotretinoin, and is eliminated in the urine and feces. Isotretinoin has an elimination half-life of 10 to 20 hours; 4-oxo-isotretinoin has an elimination half-life around 24 hours (range 10 to 50 hours). Because of the extensive protein binding of isotretinoin, dose adjustments are not necessary for patients undergoing dialysis.

Dose

As a chemoprevention treatment, isotretinoin has been given in doses of:
- 0.5 to 2 mg/kg/day for 3 months or longer (oral leukoplakia)
- 2.5 to 4 mg/kg/day for 8 weeks, and
- 20 to 125 mg/m²/day for up to 6 months (myelodysplastic syndromes).

Administration

Oral, as a single daily dose.

Toxicity

Hematological. Elevated sedimentation rate (40%). Thrombocytopenia, thrombo-cythemia, and anemia occur rarely.

Gastrointestinal. Nausea, vomiting, and abdominal pain (20%) xerostomia (80%), anorexia (4%), stomatitis, inflammatory bowel disease (diarrhea, rectal bleeding, and abdominal pain), cheilitis (common), glossitis (common), inflamed and/or bleeding gums (rare).

Dermatological. Almost all patients will develop cheilitis and dry skin with mild exfoliation. Pruritus (80%) and skin fragility (80%) are also common. Rash, thinning of hair, epistaxis, and nail brittleness occur infrequently (less than 10%). Photosensitivity

ISOTRETINOIN *(continued)*

(30%). Erythema nodosum, hypopigmentation or hyperpigmentation, urticaria, hirsutism, and skin infections occur in less than 5% of patients.

Hepatic. Transient elevations of hepatic enzyme levels and/or hyperbilirubinemia occur in 10% to 20% of patients and may persist for weeks after treatment is stopped. Hepatitis has been reported in some patients.

Neurological. Headache (5%), fatigue, lethargy, and mental depression occur infrequently. Pseudotumor cerebri (manifested as papilledema, headache, nausea, vomiting, and visual disturbances) has occurred in patients taking isotretinoin.

Ocular. Conjunctivitis occurs in 40% to 55% of patients. Corneal erosion, blurred vision, decreased tolerance to contact lenses, papilledema, corneal opacities, cataracts, and photophobia occur occasionally. Dry eyes and night blindness (which may occur suddenly) are infrequent toxicities but may persist after stopping therapy.

Other. Isotretinoin is teratogenic. Fetal abnormalities (e.g., thymic aplasia, craniofacial malformation, hydrocephalus, cleft palate, cerebellar malformation) are likely if in utero exposure occurs. Bone pain, myalgia, and arthralgia may occur in up to 20% of patients and in some may be dose-limiting. These symptoms may persist after treatment is stopped. Elevated serum triglyceride levels occur in approximately 25% of patients; mild to moderate decreases in high-density lipoproteins have been reported in 15% to 70% of patients taking isotretinoin. White cells in the urine (10% to 20%), proteinuria, hematuria (less than 10%), abnormal menses (less than 1%). Other uncommon toxicities that have been reported in patients taking isotretinoin include hyperglycemia, hyperuricemia, elevated creatinine phosphokinase and serum cholesterol levels (7%), and skeletal hyperostosis.

Drug Interactions

It is suggested that vitamin A-containing supplements be avoided while using oral isotretinoin, to avoid increased toxicity. Isotretinoin administered concomitantly with tetracycline or minocycline has resulted in papilledema or pseudotumor cerebri.

In patients who are receiving treatment with carbamazepine, isotretinoin may decrease serum carbamazepine concentrations.

Combined with ethanol, isotretinoin may cause disulfiram-like reactions.

Storage and Stability

Isotretinoin is stored at room temperature protected from light. Each bottle bears an expiration date.

Availability

Isotretinoin is commercially available as 10-, 20-, and 40-mg capsules.

Selected Reading

Benner SE et al. Toxicity of isotretinoin in a chemoprevention trial to prevent second primary tumors after head and neck cancer. J Natl Cancer Inst 86: 1799–1800, 1994.

KETOCONAZOLE

Other names
Nizoral®; NSC-317629.

Indications
Ketoconazole is FDA approved for oral use in the treatment of numerous fungal infections (e.g., blastomycosis, candidal infections, histoplasmosis, and others). It may also be useful as an agent in the treatment of hypercalcemia due to sarcoidosis or tuberculosis. In the oncology setting, ketoconazole may be useful in the treatment of advanced stage, metastatic prostate cancer.

Classification and Mechanisms of Action
Ketoconazole is a fungistatic agent at normal doses. The mechanism of ketoconazole activity is not fully understood; however, it is known that it alters cell membranes, which in turn increases the membrane permeability. The altered cell membrane causes secondary metabolic effects and inhibition of growth. In respect to endocrine effects exerted by ketoconazole, the drug inhibits the synthesis of both testosterone and adrenal steroids. Steroid synthesis inhibition occurs via blocking of conversion enzymes.

Pharmacokinetics
Ketoconazole is rapidly and well absorbed after oral administration. Peak plasma concentrations occur 1 to 4 hours after oral administration. Increased bioavailability of ketoconazole occurs in an acidic environment, a higher pH lowers the bioavailability of the drug. Ketoconazole is highly plasma protein-bound, up to 99%. The drug is metabolized by the liver to inactive metabolites and exhibits saturable first-pass metabolism. The drug undergoes a biphasic elimination half-life. The initial phase half-life is 2 hours and the terminal half-life is 8 hours. The majority of the drug is excreted into the bile; for patients with severe hepatic impairment, dose adjustments may be necessary. Renal excretion is minor and therefore dose adjustments for renal impairment are not necessary.

Dose
The adult dose range for ketoconazole in the treatment of fungal infections is 200 mg once a day to 400 mg twice a day. The dose varies depending on the type and severity of the infection.

The dose used for the treatment of prostate cancer is 400 mg every 8 hours (i.e., adrenocortical function may be inhibited at this dose).

Administration
Oral.

Toxicity
Hematological. Rarely leukopenia, hemolytic anemia, thrombocytopenia (less than 1%).
Gastrointestinal. Nausea and vomiting are most common. Diarrhea, constipation, abdominal pain, flatulence, and gastrointestinal bleed were rarely reported.
Dermatological. Pruritus reported in 2% of patients. Rash, dermatitis, urticaria, alopecia, purpura, and hypersensitivity reactions are all rare (less than 1%).
Hepatic. Transient increases in hepatic transaminases and alkaline phosphatase have been observed. Rare hepatocellular toxicity has been reported. Ketoconazole-induced hepatotoxicity is reversible over time, but may take several months following discontinuation of treatment.

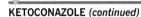

KETOCONAZOLE *(continued)*

Neurological. Headache, dizziness, insomnia, lethargy, nervousness, photophobia, asthenia, somnolence, and abnormal dreams occur rarely.

Cardiovascular. Hypertension was observed in patients treated for metastatic prostate carcinoma.

Pulmonary. Dyspnea is rare.

Other. Decreased serum cholesterol levels and hypertriglyceridemia have been reported. Gynecomastia and breast tenderness, arthralgias, chills, fever, impotence, tinnitus, and increased intracranial pressure are all rarely reported.

Drug Interactions

The oral absorption of ketoconazole will be decreased when administered with drugs that increase gastric pH. These include H_2 blockers (e.g., ranitidine, cimetidine, famotidine, nizatidine) and antacids.

Ketoconazole should not be administered concomitantly with cisapride. Ketoconazole inhibits the metabolism of cisapride, which has led to serious cardiac events.

Ketoconazole can cause hepatotoxiciy and should be used with caution in patients who may be taking other hepatotoxic drugs.

Ketoconazole administered concomitantly with rifampin has demonstrated a decrease in ketoconazole levels.

Ketoconazole administered concomitantly with cyclosporine or tacrolimus can increase circulating levels of the immunosuppressive agents. Monitor levels of these agents closely if given with ketoconazole.

Storage and Stability

Ketoconazole tablets are stored at room temperature, protected from moisture. Each bottle bears an expiration date.

Ketoconazole is also available as an antifungal shampoo and cream for treatment of fungal infections; these are not included in this monograph.

Availability

Ketoconazole is commercially available in 200-mg tablets.

Selected Reading

Small EJ et al. Simultaneous antiandrogen withdrawal and treatment with ketoconazole and hydrocortisone in patients with advanced prostate carcinoma. Cancer 80: 1755–1759, 1997.

LETROZOLE

Other names

Femara®; CGS 20267; NSC-719345.

Indications

Letrozole is FDA approved for use in the treatment of advanced breast cancer in post-menopausal women who no longer benefit from antiestrogen therapy. Letrozole is also indicated as first-line therapy for advanced breast cancer in postmenopausal women who are hormone receptor positive or whose hormone receptor status is unknown.

Classification and Mechanisms of Action

Letrozole is a competitive, nonsteroidal aromatase inhibitor. The drug produces its antitumor effects by inhibiting the peripheral tissue conversion of androstenedione to estrone and estradiol, thus significantly reducing serum estrogen levels. Letrozole does not affect the formation of adrenal corticosteroids or aldosterone. Corticosteroid replacement therapy is not necessary in patients taking letrozole.

Pharmacokinetics

Letrozole is rapidly and well absorbed after oral administration. Food does not appear to affect the absorption of letrozole. After consistent 2.5 mg daily dosing, nonlinear steady-state plasma levels occur at 2 to 6 weeks. Plasma protein binding is weak and the volume of distribution is large. The terminal half-life of letrozole is approximately 2 days. The majority of the drug is metabolized by the liver to inactive metabolites. Approximately 90% of a dose is eliminated into the urine, only 6% of which is unchanged drug.

Dose

The usual dose is 2.5 mg daily. Adjustment of dose in patients with mild to moderate renal and hepatic function impairment is not necessary; however, use with caution in patients with severe renal (i.e., creatinine clearance less than 10 mL/min) or hepatic dysfunction.

Administration

Oral.

Toxicity

Gastrointestinal. Nausea is the most commonly reported gastrointestinal toxicity observed in up to 15% of patients. Other toxicities reported in less than 10% of patients include vomiting, diarrhea, constipation, abdominal pain, anorexia, dyspepsia.
Dermatological. Rash (5%), pruritus (rare).
Neurological. Fatigue (11%), headache (9%), dizziness (8%), somnolence (3%), depression, and anxiety (rare).
Cardiovascular. Chest pain (6%), peripheral edema (5%), hypertension (5%), hot flushes (6%).
Pulmonary. Dyspnea (7%), coughing (6%).
Genitourinary. Vaginal discharge and cystitis (rare).
Other. Arthralgias (8%), decreased libido, viral infections (6%), asthenia (4%).

Storage and Stability

Letrozole tablets are stored at room temperature. Each bottle bears an expiration date.

Availability

Letrozole is commercially available in 2.5 mg tablets.

Selected Reading

Mouridsen H et al. Superior efficacy of letrozole (Femara) versus tamoxifen as first-line therapy for postmenopausal women with advanced breast cancer: results of a phase III study of the international letrozole breast cancer group. J Clin Oncol 19: 2596–2606, 2001.

LEUCOVORIN CALCIUM

Other names

Leucovorin®; Wellcovorin®; citrovorum factor; folinic acid; 5-formyltetrahydrofolate; LV; LCV; NSC-3590.

Indications

FDA approved as a rescue agent after high-dose methotrexate therapy, to counteract the effects of folic acid antagonists (e.g., trimethoprim or pyrimethamine), in combination with fluorouracil in the treatment of advanced colorectal carcinoma, and megaloblastic anemia when treatment with folic acid is not feasible. Leucovorin combined with fluorouracil may be a useful treatment for breast, head and neck, lung, stomach, and pancreatic cancers; non-Hodgkin's lymphoma; and trophoblastic neoplasms.

Classification and Mechanisms of Action

Leucovorin is a tetrahydrofolic acid derivative that acts as a biochemical cofactor for carbon transfer reactions in the synthesis of purines and pyrimidines. Leucovorin does not require the enzyme dihydrofolate reductase (DHFR) for conversion to tetrahydrofolic acid. The effects of methotrexate and other DHFR antagonists are inhibited by leucovorin.

Leucovorin can potentiate the cytotoxic effects of fluorinated pyrimidines (i.e., fluorouracil [5-FU], floxuridine, tegafur). After 5-FU is activated within the cell, it is accompanied by a folate cofactor and inhibits the enzyme thymidylate synthase, thus inhibiting pyrimidine synthesis. Leucovorin increases the folate pool, thereby increasing the binding of folate cofactor and active metabolites of 5-FU with thymidylate synthase.

Pharmacokinetics

Leucovorin is well absorbed (75% to 97%) after oral administration and is readily converted to 5-methyltetrahydrofolate after administration. Peak serum concentrations occur approximately 1.7 to 2.5 hours after an oral dose. More of the active l-isomer (versus the inactive d-isomer) is absorbed after oral dosing. Reduced accumulation of the d-isomer favors potentiation of fluorouracil-leucovorin synergy. Leucovorin is excreted into the urine as metabolites and has an elimination half-life of approximately 2 to 6 hours.

Dose

When used as a rescue agent for methotrexate, doses of 10 to 25 mg/m^2 orally or intravenously every 6 hours for 6 to 8 doses (beginning 6 to 24 hours after methotrexate) are most commonly used. Dose adjustments are made based on methotrexate serum levels and serum creatinine levels. When combined with intrathecal methotrexate, smaller doses of leucovorin may be given immediately after dosing. When used to avert trimethoprim- or pyrimethamine-induced myelosuppression, a daily leucovorin dose of 5 mg is adequate. When used to potentiate the effects of fluorinated pyrimidines, doses ranging from 20 to 500 mg/m^2 orally or intravenously have been used. High-dose (500 mg/m^2) oral leucovorin is usually given in 125 mg/m^2 increments for 4 doses.

Administration

Leucovorin has been given orally, intramuscularly, intraperitoneally, and via IV push and IV infusion in 50 mL or more of 5% dextrose or normal saline over a period of several minutes or longer.

Toxicity

Hematological. Thrombocytosis.
Gastrointestinal. Nausea, upset stomach, diarrhea.
Dermatological. Skin rash.
Allergic. Skin rash, hives, pruritus.
Pulmonary. Wheezing (possibly allergic in origin).
Other. Headache; may potentiate the toxic effects of fluoropyrimidine therapy, resulting in increased hematological and gastrointestinal (diarrhea, stomatitis) adverse effects.

Drug Interactions

As indicated above, leucovorin inhibits the activity of DHFR inhibitors, such as methotrexate, and potentiates the activity and adverse effects associated with fluorinated pyrimidines, such as fluorouracil, floxuridine, and tegafur.

Storage and Stability

All dosage forms are stored at room temperature. Each vial and bottle bears an expiration date. The reconstituted parenteral solution, 10 mg/mL, is stable for at least 7 days at room temperature. Leucovorin (0.5 to 0.9 mg/mL) is chemically stable at room temperature for at least 24 hours in normal saline, 5% dextrose, 10% dextrose, Ringer's solution, or lactated Ringer's solution.

Preparation

The 50- and 100-mg vials for injection are reconstituted with 5 and 10 mL of sterile water or bacteriostatic water, respectively, to yield a 10 mg/mL solution. The 350-mg vial is reconstituted with 17 mL of sterile water to yield a 20 mg/mL solution.

Incompatibilities

Leucovorin is incompatible with sodium bicarbonate, foscarnet, and droperidol.

Availability

Commercially available as a tablet (5, 10, 15, and 25 mg) and in parenteral formulations (5-mg ampules; 50-, 100-, 200-, and 350-mg vials).

LEUPROLIDE ACETATE

Other names

Lupron®; Lupron Depot®; Lupron Depot-3 Month; leuprorelin acetate; Viadur®.

Indications

FDA approved for the palliative treatment of advanced prostate carcinoma and management of endometriosis (including pain relief and reduction of endometriotic lesions). Leuprolide may be useful in the treatment of breast and islet cell cancers.

Classification and Mechanisms of Action

Leuprolide is a gonadotropin-releasing hormone (GnRH) analogue that binds to GnRH receptors in the pituitary, resulting in an initial increase and later a substantial decrease in secretion of luteinizing hormone (LH) and follicle-stimulating hormone (FSH). Decreases in LH and FSH result in castration levels of serum testosterone in men and postmenopausal estrogen and progesterone levels in women, which result in growth inhibition of hormone-responsive tumors. Leuprolide is usually administered in

LEUPROLIDE ACETATE *(continued)*

combination with an antiandrogen, such as flutamide or bicalutamide, for the treatment of prostate cancer.

Pharmacokinetics

Leuprolide is not absorbed by mouth. After subcutaneous administration of the acetate solution, approximately 95% is absorbed. The drug is up to 49% bound to plasma proteins. Absorption of the depot suspension is 85% to 100% after intramuscular injection. Leuprolide has an elimination half-life of 3 hours. After depot injections the initial peak plasma levels (which vary depending on the dose) are reached at approximately 4 hours, then steady-state levels are maintained over the month, 3-month, or 4-month time frame. The leuprolide implant maintains steady-state levels for up to 12 months.

Dose

For prostate carcinoma, the usual dose is 7.5 mg of the depot suspension once a month, 1 mg (0.2 mL) of the injectable solution subcutaneously once daily, 22.5 mg of the lyophilized microsphere depot once every 12 weeks, or 30 mg of the lyophilized microsphere depot once every 16 weeks. A 72-mg dose is available as an implant.

Administration

The leuprolide acetate solution is injected subcutaneously. The injectable solution is administered subcutaneously using the syringes provided by the manufacturer. Alternatively, a 0.5 mL, low-dose, disposable U-100 insulin syringe (filled to the 20-unit mark to obtain a 1-mg dose) may be used to administer the injectable solution. The leuprolide acetate depot suspension is administered intramuscularly using a 22-gauge needle.

Toxicity

Hematological. Leukopenia and anemia are rare.

Gastrointestinal. Anorexia, nausea, vomiting, constipation, taste changes, diarrhea, xerostomia.

Dermatological. Dermatitis, local skin reaction, ecchymosis, injection site reactions, hair growth or loss, itching, pigmentation, other lesions.

Hepatic. Transient, mild elevation of hepatic transaminase levels is common.

Neurological. Insomnia, depression, dizziness, and headaches are uncommon toxicities. Paresthesias, anxiety, blurred vision, lethargy, memory disorder, mood swings, insomnia, nervousness, numbness, hearing disorder, and syncope are rare.

Cardiovascular. ECG changes (20%), ischemia, high blood pressure, peripheral edema (12%); thrombosis/phlebitis, angina, cardiac arrhythmias, myocardial infarction, hypotension, pulmonary embolus, transient ischemic attack/stroke.

Endocrine. Hot flushes (50% to 60%), impotence (common), gynecomastia, breast tenderness, decrease in libido (common), decreased testicular size. In women: amenorrhea (dose-related, 98% after the second dose); hypoestrogenic symptoms, including headache, vaginitis, vaginal dryness, depression, emotional lability, decreased bone density, decreased libido, breast tenderness, myalgia, insomnia, acne, and increased serum cholesterol levels.

Other. Tumor flare, manifested as increased pain at tumor sites, sometimes causing spinal cord compression or urinary retention; myalgia, asthenia, leukopenia (rare), anemia, and urinary tract symptoms (dysuria, incontinence, bladder spasms occur infrequently). Elevated cholesterol (7%) and triglyceride concentrations (12%) occasionally occur after several months of treatment.

Storage and Stability

Leuprolide acetate injectable solution is stored in the refrigerator protected from light. However, the vial currently in use may remain at room temperature for several months. Intact vials of the depot formulation (powder for suspension) may be stored at room temperature. After reconstitution of the powder for suspension, it is stable for 24 hours.

Preparation

All strengths of leuprolide depot microspheres for injection are reconstituted with 1 mL of the provided diluent (the diluent ampule contains excess diluent). The vials should be shaken well to obtain a uniform milky suspension.

Availability

Leuprolide depot microspheres for injection are commercially available in vials containing 3.75, 7.5, 11.25, 15, 22.5, and 30 mg of lyophilized powder for suspension with a diluent ampule and syringe. Leuprolide acetate injection is commercially available as a 5 mg/mL solution in 2.8-mL multi-dose vials. Leuprolide is also available as a 72-mg single-dose implant kit.

LOMUSTINE

Other names

CeeNU®; CCNU; chloroethylcyclohexylnitrosourea; NSC-79037.

Indications

FDA approved for the treatment of brain tumors and Hodgkin's disease (secondary therapy in combination with other approved drugs). Lomustine may also be useful for the treatment of melanoma, multiple myeloma, non-Hodgkin's lymphoma, and cancers of the breast, lung, colon, rectum, and kidney.

Classification

Alkylating agent of the nitrosourea class.

Pharmacokinetics

Lomustine is thought to be well absorbed by mouth and after topical administration. Peak plasma concentrations occur 3 hours (range 1 to 6 hours) after an oral dose. The drug is widely distributed throughout the body, including breast milk. Concentrations of active metabolites in the cerebrospinal fluid may exceed those measured in the plasma. Lomustine is rapidly metabolized by the liver cytochrome P450 system to active metabolites that are eliminated by the kidneys (50% to 75%). The drug is not hemodialyzable. The elimination half-life is approximately 72 hours.

Dose

A common dose regimen is 100 to 130 mg/m^2 orally every 6 weeks. Dose reductions are recommended if renal function is impaired (e.g., a 25% reduction for creatinine clearances of 10 to 50 mL/min, a 50% reduction if the creatinine clearance is less than 10 mL/min).

LOMUSTINE *(continued)*

Administration

Oral, on an empty stomach.

Toxicity

Hematological. Lekopenia and thrombocytopenia are expected, dose-limiting, and cumulative. Nadir white blood cell and platelet counts occur approximately 4 to 6 weeks after a dose; recovery occurs 1 to 2 weeks thereafter. Anemia occurs less frequently and is also cumulative.

Gastrointestinal. Nausea, vomiting, and anorexia occur occasionally. Nausea and vomiting usually begin 45 minutes to 6 hours after administration. Antiemetic premedication is warranted. Anorexia may persist for 2 to 3 days after the nausea and vomiting have subsided. Mucositis is uncommon.

Dermatological. Alopecia is uncommon and usually mild. Skin rash, pruritus, and darkening of the skin are infrequent toxicities.

Hepatic. Elevated hepatic transaminase levels and hyperbilirubinemia are uncommon.

Neurological. Disorientation, lethargy, ataxia, confusion, slurred speech, and dysarthria are uncommon.

Pulmonary. With long-term administration, pulmonary dysfunction (shortness of breath, decreased diffusing capacity, fibrosis) can occur. Discontinue lomustine after a lifetime dose of 1,100 to 1,400 mg/m^2 has been given.

Renal. Increased serum creatinine levels and decreased creatinine clearance are uncommon and related to the cumulative dose.

Other. Fatigue, tiredness, pallor, menstrual cycle irregularities (amenorrhea), second malignancy (leukemia).

Drug Interactions

Lomustine administered concomitantly with cimetidine may increase the risk for lomustine-induced toxicity.

Alcohol use should be avoided concomitantly with lomustine therapy.

Storage and Stability

Lomustine capsules may be stored at room temperature, avoid excess heat. Containers bear expiration dates.

Availability

Lomustine is commercially available as 10-, 40-, and 100-mg capsules.

MECHLORETHAMINE

Other names

Mustargen®; nitrogen mustard; HN$_2$; NSC-762.

Indications

FDA approved for the treatment of Hodgkin's and non-Hodgkin's lymphomas, chronic myelogenous leukemia, chronic lymphocytic leukemia, polycythemia vera, cutaneous T-cell lymphoma, lung cancer, palliative treatment of metastatic carcinoma resulting in effusion (peritoneal, pericardial, or pleural).

Classification

Alkylating agent.

Pharmacokinetics
Mechlorethamine is rapidly deactivated within the blood and is undetectable within minutes of IV administration. Less than 0.01% of a dose is excreted in the urine. The drug has an elimination half-life of 15 minutes.

Dose
The usual intravenous dose for Hodgkin's disease is 6 mg/m^2 on days 1 and 8 of a monthly treatment cycle (Mustargen®-Oncovin®-procarbazine-prednisone [MOPP] regimen).

- The usual intracavitary (i.e., intrapleural) dose is 0.4 mg/kg.
- A smaller dose (0.2 mg/kg) has been used when the drug is administered intrapericardially.
- The drug has also been given as a single agent in doses up to 0.4 mg/kg monthly.
- Mechlorethamine may be used topically in the treatment of mycosis fungoides in a 10 mg/60 mL solution or a petrolatum-based ointment (10 mg/dL). Topical treatment is often administered daily (or more often if necessary) for 6 to 12 months after a complete response is attained.

Administration
Mechlorethamine is a potent vesicant and usually administered intravenously over 1 to 5 minutes using extravasation precautions. The drug may also be administered by intracavitary injection. It is recommended that ECG monitoring be conducted when mechlorethamine is administered into the pericardial cavity because the drug can cause arrhythmias when administered by this route. Intracavitary instillation is usually painful and patients should be given appropriate analgesia. Intraperitoneal administration should be avoided because intestinal adhesions and obstruction may occur. Topical application should be performed carefully in a well-ventilated area with the use of rubber gloves.

Toxicity
Hematological. Leukopenia and thrombocytopenia are expected and dose-related.
Gastrointestinal. Nausea and vomiting are common, are often severe, and usually begin within 1 hour of IV administration. Aggressive antiemetic premedication is mandatory. Diarrhea, anorexia, metallic taste, and peptic ulcers occur infrequently.
Dermatological. Discoloration of infused vein, alopecia, tissue irritation, and necrosis if extravasation occurs during IV administration. Use of the antidote sodium thiosulfate is indicated if extravasation occurs, followed by ice compresses for 6 to 12 hours. When mechlorethamine is administered topically, erythema, dermatitis, hyperpigmentation, burning, and pruritus may occur. Contact allergy occurs in approximately 50% of patients after use of mechlorethamine solution and 25% after use of the ointment formulation. Contact allergy may begin within 2 weeks or 12 months of initiating topical therapy.
Other. Amenorrhea, impaired spermatogenesis, and sterility are common. Reported toxicities include jaundice, fever, precipitation of herpes zoster, peripheral neuropathy, tinnitus, hearing loss (rare), thrombophlebitis, angioedema, and secondary malignancies.

Storage and Stability
Mechlorethamine vials are stored at room temperature. The manufacturer recommends that the reconstituted solution be used within 60 minutes because of its instability. Within 6 hours, solutions of 1 mg/mL lose 4% to 6% potency in the refrigerator and 8% to 10% potency at room temperature. The 10 mg/dL ointment has traditionally been given a 3-month expiration date.

MECHLORETHAMINE *(continued)*

Preparation

To a 10-mg vial add 10 mL of sterile water or normal saline to yield a solution of 1 mg/mL. It may be further diluted for topical administration. Mechlorethamine has also been dissolved in 95% alcohol, 1 mL/10-mg vial (5 vials), and 4.5 mL is incorporated into aquaphor (454 g) to make a 10 mg/dL ointment.

Incompatibilities

Because of its instability, mechlorethamine is incompatible with other antineoplastic agents and sodium thiosulfate.

Availability

Commercially available as a lyophilized powder in 10-mg vials.

MEDROXYPROGESTERONE ACETATE

Other names

Provera®; Depo-Provera®; Cycrin®; Amen®; Curretab®; MDA.

Indications

FDA approved for adjunctive therapy and palliative treatment of inoperable, recurrent, and metastatic endometrial or renal carcinoma. May also be used for advanced breast cancer.

Classification and Mechanisms of Action

Medroxyprogesterone is a potent progestational agent that also has androgenic activity. The drug has no estrogenic activity. The mechanism of its antineoplastic effects is unknown; it may directly inhibit tumor growth, suppress the release of gonadotropins from the pituitary and inhibit growth of hormone-sensitive tumors, or interact with other hormones. Recent evidence suggests that breast cancer tumors with high levels of androgen receptors respond to treatment more often than tumors without the receptor.

Pharmacokinetics

Medroxyprogesterone acetate (MDA) is absorbed by mouth, reaching peak plasma levels within 1 to 2 hours. Oral bioavailability is around 10% (as a result of inadequate absorption and extensive first-pass metabolism in the liver). After intramuscular injection, plasma levels of MDA remain steady from 1 to 2 hours to 7 days after injection. The elimination half-life of MDA is reported to range from 14 to 60 hours. MDA is metabolized in the liver; 20% to 40% is excreted as inactive metabolites in the urine and 5% to 15% is excreted in the feces.

Dose

Initially, 400 mg to 1,000 mg/week by intramuscular injection has been used for endometrial or renal carcinoma, with a maintenance dose of as little as 400 mg/month in responding patients. For breast and prostate cancers, up to 1,500 mg/day has been used for induction therapy, with maintenance doses of 500 mg 1 to 3 times weekly.

Administration

Oral or by intramuscular injection. The suspension for injection must be shaken well to ensure complete mixing of the drug.

Toxicity

Gastrointestinal. Nausea, cholestatic jaundice.

Dermatological. Alopecia, acne, hirsutism (all rare). Discoloration or sterile abscess at the site of injection.

Neurological. Nervousness, insomnia, somnolence, fatigue, dizziness, depression, headache.

Cardiovascular. Edema (with weight gain), thrombophlebitis, pulmonary embolism.

Endocrine. Menstrual changes (i.e., breakthrough bleeding, spotting), amenorrhea, gynecomastia, breast tenderness, galactorrhea, and hot flushes.

Hypersensitivity. Urticaria, pruritus, angioedema, generalized rash, anaphylaxis (all rare side effects).

Other. Fatigue, flare reaction at initiation of treatment for prostate cancer characterized by increased tumor (bone) pain, tremor, leg cramps, fever.

Drug Interaction

The metabolism of medroxyprogesterone to inactive metabolites may be increased two-fold by aminoglutethimide.

Storage and Stability

Medroxyprogesterone parenteral suspension and the tablets are stored at room temperature. Each container bears an expiration date.

Preparation

Shake the suspension well just before administration.

Availability

Commercially available as 2.5-, 5-, and 10-mg tablets and as a 100 mg/mL (5-mL vial), 150 mg/mL (1-mL vial), or 400 mg/mL (2.5- and 10-mL vials) suspension for injection.

MEGESTROL ACETATE

Other names

Megace®; megestrol; NSC-71423.

Indications

FDA approved for the treatment of advanced carcinoma of the breast or endometrium and for the treatment of anorexia associated with cancer or human immunodeficiency virus (HIV) infection.

Classification and Mechanisms of Action

Megestrol is a progestin that has antiestrogenic properties. Megestrol interferes with the replenishment of cytoplasmic estrogen receptors, thereby decreasing the quantity of estrogen receptors. Megestrol also inhibits the release of luteinizing hormone (a stimulus for endometrial growth).

Pharmacokinetics

Megestrol is well absorbed by mouth, reaching peak plasma levels 1 to 3 hours after dosing. The drug is metabolized by the liver and excreted in the urine as steroid metabolites and inactive compounds (57% to 80% within 10 days). Megestrol has an elimination half-life of 15 to 20 hours.

MEGESTROL ACETATE (continued)

Dose

When used for the treatment of breast cancer, 80 mg twice a day is commonly used. However, there is evidence to support once a day administration (160 mg/day). For endometrial cancer, 40 to 320 mg/day have been used. As an appetite stimulant, higher doses of 400 to 800 mg/day are indicated.

Administration

Oral.

Toxicity

Gastrointestinal. Nausea, vomiting, and abdominal pain are uncommon. Diarrhea and constipation have been reported with high doses.

Dermatological. Alopecia (uncommon), rash.

Neurological. Headache, carpal tunnel syndrome.

Cardiovascular. Hot flushes, thrombophlebitis, thromboembolism, fluid retention, edema, hypertension with high doses, congestive heart failure (rare).

Genitourinary. Vaginal bleeding or discharge, menstrual changes, amenorrhea, urinary frequency.

Metabolic. Hypercalcemia with high doses; irreversible insulin-dependent diabetes mellitus developed in a woman 6 weeks after initiation of megestrol acetate, 160 mg/day. Megestrol may cause adrenal suppression when administered in doses of 800 mg/day, necessitating the administration of corticosteroids during times of acute illness.

Other. Hyperpnea, dyspnea, weight gain and increased appetite, tumor flare (with or without hypercalcemia). Megestrol is porphyrogenic in animals and may be unsafe in patients with porphyria.

Storage and Stability

Megestrol tablets and oral suspension are stored at room temperature; bottles bear expiration dates.

Availability

Megestrol is commercially available in 20- and 40-mg tablets and as a 40 mg/mL suspension in 240-mL bottles.

MELPHALAN

Other names

Alkeran®; Alkeran IV®; L-PAM; L-phenylalanine mustard; L-sarcolysin; NSC-8806.

Indications

FDA approved for the treatment of multiple myeloma and nonresectable epithelial carcinoma of the ovary. Melphalan may also be a useful treatment for cancers of the breast, thyroid, and testes. The injectable formulation is approved for use when oral therapy is not indicated. The injectable formulation has been used in isolated limb perfusion (for melanoma) and as a part of induction regimens before bone marrow and peripheral stem cell transplantation.

Classification

Alkylating agent.

Pharmacokinetics

Melphalan is erratically absorbed (25% to 90%) from the gastrointestinal tract and reaches peak plasma levels approximately 2 hours after dosing. Approximately 30% of the drug is bound to plasma proteins. Melphalan undergoes spontaneous hydrolysis in the bloodstream and approximately 10% to 15% is eliminated in the urine as unchanged drug. Melphalan has an elimination half-life of 1.5 to 4 hours. Melphalan is not hemodialyzable.

Dose

For multiple myeloma. An oral dose of 0.25 mg/kg/day (in combination with pred-nisone 2 mg/kg/day) for 4 days repeated every 6 weeks or a dose of 6 mg/day for 2 or 3 weeks, followed by a 4-week rest, then resume melphalan at 2 mg/day. Other regimens include doses of:

- 0.1 to 0.15 mg/kg/day for 7 days every 4 weeks
- 6 to 7 mg/m^2/day for 5 days every 6 weeks
- 0.1 to 0.15 mg/kg/day for 2 to 3 weeks followed by a maintenance dose of 2 to 4 mg/day when the bone marrow has recovered.

For epithelial ovarian cancer. A dose of 0.2 mg/kg/day for 5 days repeated every 4 weeks has been administered

For isolated limb perfusion. A dose of 10 mg/L of limb volume or 0.45 mg/kg (upper extremity) and 0.9 mg/kg (lower extremity) has been given.

A 50% dose reduction of IV melphalan has been advocated for patients with a serum BUN of 30 mg/dL or higher.

Administration

Melphalan may be administered orally on an empty stomach, or intravenously as a solution of no greater than 0.45 mg/mL in normal saline over a period of 15 to 30 minutes. The duration of the infusion should not exceed 60 minutes because of drug instability. The drug has also been given intraperitoneally and via isolated limb perfusion.

Toxicity

Hematological. Leukopenia and thrombocytopenia are expected and may be cumula-tive. Recovery may be prolonged for 6 to 8 weeks. If myelosuppression is not observed after oral dosing, poor oral absorption should be suspected. Hemolytic anemia rarely occurs.

Gastrointestinal. Nausea and vomiting occur infrequently after oral dosing, but may be severe after IV administration of larger doses. Mucositis, diarrhea, and oral ulcers occur infrequently.

Dermatological. Rash, pruritus, dermatitis, alopecia (uncommon).

Hepatic. Hepatic veno-occlusive disease may occur following use of transplantation doses.

Pulmonary. Pulmonary fibrosis and interstitial pneumonitis are rare.

Hypersensitivity. Urticaria, pruritus, exanthema, rash, anaphylaxis (rare).

Other. Amenorrhea, oligospermia, and impaired fertility are relatively common toxici-ties. Cataracts, vasculitis, and second malignancies are rare. High doses may cause syndrome of inappropriate antidiuretic hormone secretion.

Drug Interactions

Administration of cyclosporine and melphalan has resulted in acute renal failure.

Cisplatin administered with melphalan may also cause renal toxicity due to decreased clearance.

MELPHALAN *(continued)*

The combination of nalidixic acid and melphalan has been associated with an increased incidence of hemorrhagic enterocolitis.

Melphalan administered concomitantly with carmustine may increase the risk of pulmonary toxicity.

Melphalan administered concomitantly with cimetidine decreases oral bioavailability and consequently plasma concentration of melphalan.

Storage and Stability

Melphalan tablets and vials are stored at room temperature and protected from light. Each container bears an expiration date. Melphalan powder diluted to a final concentration of 5 mg/mL is stable for 90 minutes. Mephalan solutions of 0.45 mg/mL are stable for 60 minutes. The reconstituted solution should not be refrigerated because the drug may precipitate.

Preparation

Reconstitute the 50-mg vial with 10 mL of the provided diluent to yield a 5 mg/mL solution. Further dilute the solution to a concentration no greater than 0.45 mg/mL in normal saline.

Availability

Melphalan is commercially available as a 2-mg tablet and a 50-mg vial provided with a 10-mL vial of diluent.

Selected Reading

Samuels BL, Bitran JD. High-dose intravenous melphalan: a review. J Clin Oncol 13: 1786–1799, 1995.

MERCAPTOPURINE

Other names

Purinethol®; 6-mercaptopurine; 6-MP; NSC-755.

Indications

The oral formulation is FDA approved for remission induction and maintenance therapy of acute lymphocytic leukemia and acute nonlymphocytic leukemia. Mercaptopurine may be a useful treatment for chronic myelogenous leukemia, non-Hodgkin's lymphoma, polycythemia vera, inflammatory bowel disease, and severe psoriatic arthritis. The injectable formulation is investigational.

Classification and Mechanisms of Action

Purine antimetabolite.

Pharmacokinetics

Mercaptopurine is well absorbed by mouth but undergoes extensive first-pass metabolism in the liver by xanthine oxidase. Thus, approximately 10% to 20% of an oral dose reaches the bloodstream. Peak concentrations occur 2 hours after dosing. Because of xanthine oxidase inhibition, the oral bioavailability of mercaptopurine increases to 60% when allopurinol is administered. Approximately 20% of a dose is bound to plasma proteins and 10% to 40% is excreted in the urine as unchanged drug. Mercaptopurine has an elimination half-life of 6 to 10 hours. Mercaptopurine is dialyzable.

Dose

A common oral dose is 70 to 100 mg/m^2/day, or 1.5 to 2.5 mg/kg/day. Doses are rounded to the nearest 25 mg. If no response is observed after 4 weeks of therapy the dose may be increased to 5 mg/kg/day. Reduce the oral dose by 75% if allopurinol is coadministered. A common IV dose is 500 to 1,000 mg/m^2/day for 2 to 3 days. Dose adjustment of mercaptopurine administered by IV is not necessary with concomitant administration of allopurinol.

Administration

Oral, administered on an empty stomach, or by IV infusion (as a 1 to 2 mg/mL solution) in normal saline or 5% dextrose over a period of 1 hour or longer.

Toxicity

Hematological. Leukopenia, thrombocytopenia, anemia. All are common, with leukopenia the most frequent dose-limiting toxicity.
Gastrointestinal. Occasionally, nausea, vomiting, anorexia, abdominal pain, diarrhea, and mucositis.
Dermatological. Hyperpigmentation, rash, and pruritus are rare. Extravasation of the IV formulation may cause tissue necrosis.
Hepatic. Jaundice, elevated hepatic transaminase levels, cholestasis, ascites, hepatic encephalopathy associated with hepatic necrosis and severe fibrosis. The onset is variable, usually occurring in 1 to 2 months. Deaths have occurred, most frequently associated with doses greater than 2.5 mg/kg/day.
Neurological. Headache.
Other. Hyperuricemia, weakness, fever, pancreatitis.

Drug Interactions

Allopurinol causes a 400% to 500% increase in the oral bioavailability of mercapto-purine because of decreased first-pass hepatic metabolism. Allopurinol inhibits xanthine oxidase, the enzyme that metabolizes mercaptopurine. The dose of oral mercaptopurine must be reduced by 75% if the patient is also taking allopurinol. Allopurinol does not significantly affect the pharmacokinetics of mercaptopurine administered by intravenous injection to patients with normal renal function. Allopurinol may increase the amount of intravenous mercaptopurine that is excreted in the urine (from 21% to 42%), and this increase could be enough to enhance the toxicity of mercaptopurine if renal function is reduced.

Co-trimoxazole (i.e., trimethoprim-sulfamethoxazole, Bactrim®, Septra®) may increase the myelosuppression of mercaptopurine.

Mercaptopurine decreases the anticoagulant effects of warfarin.

Storage and Stability

Mercaptopurine tablets and the injectable formulation are stored at room temperature. Each container bears an expiration date. Reconstituted vials are stable for 21 days at room or refrigeration temperature. Further dilution to 1 to 2 mg/mL with normal saline or 5% dextrose is stable for 3 days at room or refrigeration temperature.

Preparation

Add 49.8 mL of sterile water to the 500-mg vial to yield a concentration of 10 mg/mL. This is further diluted to 1 to 2 mg/mL in normal saline or 5% dextrose before administration.

MERCAPTOPURINE *(continued)*

Compatibilities

Mercaptopurine and methotrexate are compatible in solution.

Availability

Commercially available in 50-mg tablets. Vials containing 500-mg and 10-mg tablets are investigational and may be obtained from the NCI.

MESNA

Other names

Mesnex®; Uromitexan®; mesnum; sodium-2-mercaptoethanesulphonate; NSC-113891.

Indications

FDA approved for the prevention of ifosfamide-induced hemorrhagic cystitis. Also useful for preventing cyclophosphamide-induced hemorrhagic cystitis.

Classification and Mechanisms of Action

Uroprotectant. Mesna is a prophylactic agent used to prevent hemorrhagic cystitis induced by the oxasophosphorines (ifosfamide, cyclophosphamide). It has no intrinsic cytotoxicity and no antagonistic effects on radiotherapy or chemotherapy. Mesna binds with acrolein, the urotoxic metabolite produced by the oxasophosphorines, to produce a nontoxic thioether and slows the rate of acrolein formation by combining with the 4-hydroxy metabolites of the oxasophosphorines.

Pharmacokinetics

After IV administration, mesna is rapidly oxidized in the blood to the inactive compound dimesna, which is completely cleared from the body through the kidneys. Dimesna is reabsorbed through kidney tubules and is converted to mesna, which combines with acrolein to produce a nontoxic thioether. Approximately 50% of an oral dose of mesna is absorbed, reaching peak plasma concentrations 1 to 1.5 hours after administration (absorption half-life, 0.34 hours). Mesna and dimesna have elimination half-lives of approximately 0.5 and 1.2 hours, respectively.

Dose

The usual dose of IV mesna is 20% of the ifosfamide dose, given just before and 4 and 8 hours after ifosfamide (total IV mesna dose is 60% of the ifosfamide dose). Mesna has also been given as a continuous infusion concurrently with ifosfamide; a total dose of mesna equal to the total dose of ifosfamide is given, preceded by a loading dose of 6% to 10% of the total ifosfamide dose. Mesna may be required to infuse an additional 8 to 24 hours after a high-dose ifosfamide continuous infusion. The usual dose of IV mesna is also 20% of the cyclophosphamide dose given just before, and 4 hours and 8 hours after cyclophosphamide. An alternate schedule is 20% of the cyclophosphamide dose just before, then every 3 hours for up to 6 doses thereafter. Mesna tablets are administered at a dose that is 40% of the ifosfamide or cyclophosphamide dose (double the IV dose). Mesna tablets are administered at 2 and 6 hours after ifosfamide (or cyclophosphamide). When using mesna tablets an IV dose of mesna is given just prior to ifosfamide (or cyclophosphamide).

Administration

Oral or by IV injection in 50 mL or more of 5% dextrose or normal saline, mixed to a final concentration of 20 mg/mL over a period of 5 minutes or longer. Mesna has been given as a continuous IV infusion.

Toxicity

At the doses used for uroprotection, mesna is virtually nontoxic. However, the following adverse effects may be attributable to mesna.

Gastrointestinal. Nausea, vomiting, diarrhea, abdominal pain, and altered taste.

Dermatological. Rash, urticaria.

Other. Lethargy, headache, joint or limb pain, hypotension, fatigue, false-positive test for urinary ketones.

Storage and Stability

Mesna is stored at room temperature. The multidose vial may be stored and reused for up to 8 days. Open ampules should not be reused because mesna reacts with oxygen to form dimesna. Diluted solutions (1 to 20 mg/mL) are stable for at least 24 hours under room or refrigeration temperatures. Mesna is chemically stable in the following solutions at room temperature: 5% dextrose in water, 48 hours (20 mg/mL) or 24 hours (1 mg/mL); 5% dextrose and 0.45% NaCl, 48 hours (20 mg/mL) or 72 hours (1 mg/mL); normal saline, 24 hours (1 mg/mL); lactated Ringer's solution, 24 hours (1 mg/mL).

Preparation

The injectable solution may be further diluted in 5% dextrose, 5% dextrose and 0.2% NaCl, 5% dextrose and 0.33% NaCl, 5% dextrose and 0.45% NaCl, normal saline, or lactated Ringer's solution to a final concentration of 1 to 20 mg/mL.

Incompatibilities

Mesna is incompatible in solution with cisplatin.

Compatibilities

Ifosfamide and mesna are compatible for continuous infusion in PVC bags containing 5% dextrose or normal saline. Mesna is reported to be compatible in solution with cyclophosphamide, etoposide, lorazepam, potassium chloride, bleomycin, and dexamethasone. A pharmacist should be consulted for additional information.

Availability

Commercially available as a 400-mg tablet and in 2-mL preservative-free ampules and in 10-mL vials containing 100 mg/mL with benzyl alcohol as a preservative.

METHOTREXATE

Other names

Methotrexate LPF®; methotrexate sodium; MTX; Mexate®; Mexate-AQ®; Folex®; Folex-Pfs®; Abitrexate®; Rheumatrex®; amethopterin; NSC-740.

Indications

FDA approved for the treatment of choriocarcinoma, hydatidiform mole, acute lymphocytic leukemia; prophylaxis and treatment of meningeal lymphocytic leukemia, breast cancer, epidermal tumors of the head and neck, lung cancer, non-Hodgkin's

METHOTREXATE (continued)

lymphoma, cutaneous T-cell lymphoma, osteosarcoma, psoriasis, and rheumatoid arthritis (second- or third-line treatment). Methotrexate may be a useful treatment for acute nonlymphocytic leukemia, multiple myeloma, rhabdomyosarcoma, and cancers of the bladder, brain, cervix, esophagus, kidney, ovary, prostate, and stomach.

Classification and Mechanisms of Action
Antifolate antimetabolite.

Pharmacokinetics
Doses up to 40 mg/m^2 are well absorbed (75% to 95%) from the gastrointestinal tract. Higher oral doses are not absorbed to the same extent. Peak plasma levels occur 0.5 to 2 hours after an oral dose. Methotrexate is distributed to body water and into breast milk. Patients with significant ascites or effusions will eliminate the drug more slowly than patients without these conditions. Approximately 10% of methotrexate is metabolized to 7-hydroxymethotrexate, a less water-soluble, potentially nephrotoxic metabolite. Approximately 90% of methotrexate is eliminated from the body in the urine as unchanged drug. The patient must have relatively normal kidney function to excrete the drug adequately and avoid excessive toxicity. Renal function must be closely monitored. A 24-hour creatinine clearance before initiation of methotrexate therapy is recommended. Methotrexate has an elimination half-life of approximately 3 hours. Patients with severe renal function impairment should not receive methotrexate. Patients with lesser degrees of renal impairment should receive an attenuated dose of methotrexate with leucovorin rescue. Methotrexate is not dialyzable, but charcoal hemoperfusion may lower serum levels. Methotrexate will inhibit DNA synthesis in bone marrow at concentrations of 10 nmol per L (1×10^8 M), and will inhibit the growth of gastrointestinal epithelium at plasma concentrations as low as 5 nmol per L (5×10^9 M).

NOTE: Methotrexate 1×10^7 M is equal to 0.1 micromolar.

Dose
Parenteral doses vary from 20 to 40 mg/m^2 every 1 to 2 weeks (for the treatment of solid tumors) to 200 to 500 mg/m^2 every 2 to 4 weeks (for leukemias and lymphomas).

As adjuvant treatment for osteosarcoma, doses of 12,000 to 15,000 mg/m^2 have been given with leucovorin rescue.

The usual adult intrathecal dose is 10 to 15 mg in 7 to 15 mL of preservative-free saline (3 mL if given via an Ommaya reservoir).

Doses greater than 80 mg/week should be accompanied by leucovorin rescue. Recommended doses of leucovorin are described in the leucovorin monograph. For emergency purposes (e.g., overdose situations) carboxypeptidase may be indicated. A carboxypeptidase drug monograph is provided in this chapter. Consult the NCI if carboxypeptidase is indicated. Dose reduction is indicated for patients with renal or hepatic insufficiency.

Adminstration
"Small" doses (e.g., 100 mg) are usually administered by IV bolus (without further dilution). Larger doses are usually given by IV infusion in 50 mL or more of 5% dextrose or normal saline over a 30-minute period or longer. Methotrexate has also been given intrathecally, intramuscularly, orally, intra-arterially, intraperitoneally, and by intravesical instillation.

Toxicity

Hematological. Leukopenia and thrombocytopenia are dose-related and more common (and more severe) with prolonged drug exposure. Nadir white blood cell and platelet counts occur 7 to 10 days after dosing and recovery occurs approximately 7 days later. Anemia occurs less frequently.

Gastrointestinal. Nausea and vomiting are uncommon with conventional doses and usually mild. Stomatitis is common (more common with high doses and longer infusion durations). Diarrhea, anorexia, hematemesis, and melena are uncommon. Gastrointestinal ulceration, enteritis, and/or intestinal perforation have been reported.

Dermatological. Skin erythema and/or rash, pruritus, urticaria, alopecia (rare), photosensitivity, furunculosis, depigmentation or hyperpigmentation, acne, telangiectasia, skin desquamation (exfoliative dermatitis), bullae formation, folliculitis.

Hepatic. Mild and transient increases of hepatic transaminase levels occur occasionally. Hepatic fibrosis and cirrhosis rarely occur and are more likely to occur in patients receiving long-term continuous or daily treatment.

Neurological. Encephalopathy, more commonly with multiple intrathecal doses and in patients who have received cranial irradiation; tiredness, weakness, confusion, ataxia, tremors, irritability, seizures, and coma have also been reported. Acute side effects of intrathecal methotrexate may include dizziness, blurred vision, headache, back pain, nuchal rigidity, seizures, paralysis, and hemiparesis.

Pulmonary. Pneumonitis, pulmonary fibrosis, cough, and dyspnea are rare.

Renal. Renal dysfunction is dose-related and more likely to occur in patients with compromised renal function or dehydration, or in those receiving other nephrotoxic drugs. Renal function impairment is manifested by increased serum creatinine levels and hematuria. The patient's serum creatinine should be routinely monitored before therapy and intermittently during treatment with higher doses (e.g., greater than 200 mg). Methotrexate levels (24 hours after dosing) should also be monitored.

Ocular. Conjunctivitis, excessive lacrimation, cataracts, photophobia, cortical blindness (high doses).

Other. Malaise, osteoporosis (aseptic necrosis of the femoral head), hyperuricemia, reversible oligospermia, allergic reactions (e.g., fever, chills, rash, urticaria, anaphylaxis), vasculitis, flank pain (associated with rapid IV infusion).

Drug Interactions

Asparaginase, leucovorin, and carboxypeptidase abrogate the effects of methotrexate. Aspirin and other acetyated salicylates inhibit the renal elimination of methotrexate via competition for renal tubular secretion. The potential for methotrexate toxicity is greatly enhanced when these drugs are given simultaneously.

Enhanced methotrexate toxicity has been observed when methotrexate and nonsteroidal anti-inflammatory drugs (NSAIDs) are given simultaneously. Although the exact mechanisms are unknown, NSAIDs may reduce renal blood flow, decrease methotrexate clearance, or cause additive nephrotoxicity. These drugs should not be given to patients receiving larger doses of methotrexate. In general, NSAIDs should be discontinued 24 hours prior to methotrexate treatment and not reinitiated for at least 48 hours after the methotrexate dose.

Probenecid decreases the amount of methotrexate that is eliminated by renal tubular secretion. The combination of methotrexate and probenecid may result in a threefold to fourfold increase in methotrexate concentrations. Penicillins will interact with methotrexate in a similar manner as probenecid and toxicity may be increased. Sulfonamides may displace methotrexate from protein-binding sites, causing enhanced methotrexate toxicity.

METHOTREXATE *(continued)*

TABLE 4-1
LEUCOVORIN RESCUE DOSING GUIDELINES

MTX level at 24 hours (Molar)	Increase in serum creatinine at 24 hours	Leucovorin dose starting 24 hours after MTX (mg/m²)	Further actions
$< 5 \times 10^{-7}$ (0.5 micromolar)	$< 50\%$	10 mg every 6 hours × 6 doses	None
$< 5 \times 10^{-7}$	$> 50\%$	10 mg every 6 hours × 8 doses	Monitor 24-hour MTX level next course
$> 5 \times 10^{-7}$ but $< 1 \times 10^{-6}$	$< 50\%$	10 mg every 6 hours × 10 doses	Monitor 24-hour MTX level next course
$> 5 \times 10^{-7}$ but $< 1 \times 10^{-6}$	$> 50\%$	10 mg every 6 hours until MTX level $< 1 \times 10^{-8}$ M	Monitor 24-hour MTX and serum creatinine daily until MTX $< 1 \times 10^{-8}$ M
$> 1 \times 10^{-6}$	$< 50\%$	10 mg every 6 hours × 12 doses	Obtain 48-hour MTX; if $< 5 \times 10^{-7}$ M, do nothing further; if $> 5 \times 10^{-7}$ M, continue leucovorin until MTX $< 1 \times 10^{-8}$ M
$> 1 \times 10^{-6}$	$> 50\%$	25 mg every 6 hours until MTX $< 1 \times 10^{-8}$ M	Hydrate with 2 L NS daily until MTX level $< 1 \times 10^{-7}$ M. Monitor MTX and serum creatinine daily; hydrate and consider IV leucovorin if necessary

Trimethoprim (a component of Bactrim® and Septra®) is an inhibitor of dihydrofolate reductase. The combination of methotrexate and trimethoprim may enhance methotrexate toxicity resulting in additive bone marrow suppression.

Concomitant use of methotrexate and oral antibiotics may decrease oral absorption of methotrexate.

Methotrexate may decrease serum phenytoin concentrations.

Methotrexate may increase theophylline concentrations.

Intrathecal methotrexate given in conjunction with parenteral acyclovir therapy may cause neurological abnormalities.

Storage and Stability

Methotrexate vials and tablets are stored at room temperature and protected from light. Reconstituted solutions are stable at room temperature for at least 4 weeks. Dilute solutions (2 to 25 mg/mL) are chemically stable for at least 3 months in the refrigerator. Solutions of 50 mg/100 mL in PVC bags of 5% dextrose may be frozen at −20°C for at least 30 days when thawed in 2 minutes by microwave radiation. There is no loss of potency after 5 freeze-thaw cycles.

Preparation

Lyophilized 20-, 50-, 100-, and 250-mg vials are reconstituted with sterile water, normal saline, or 5% dextrose to a concentration no greater than 25 mg/mL. The 1,000-mg vial is reconstituted with 19.4 mL to provide a concentration of 50 mg/mL. Higher doses (greater than 100 mg) are often further diluted with 50 mL or more of 0.45% NaCl, normal saline, or 5% dextrose.

Compatibilities

Compatible with sodium bicarbonate, cytarabine, cephalothin, fluorouracil, mercaptopurine, vincristine sulfate, hydrocortisone, dacarbazine, leucovorin, furosemide, and amino acids. At the "Y-site," methotrexate is compatible with fluorouracil, cisplatin, and heparin. A pharmacist should be consulted for additional information.

Availability

Commercially available as a lyophilized powder for injection (20, 25, 50, 100, 250, and 1,000 mg/vial); as a 25 mg/mL preservative-free, isotonic solution for injection (50, 100, 200, and 250 mg/vial); as a 25 mg/mL (50- and 250-mg vials) preparation containing preservative, isotonic solution for injection, and as a 2.5-mg tablet.

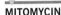

MITOMYCIN

Other names

Mutamycin®; mitomycin-C; NSC-26980.

Indications

FDA approved for the treatment of disseminated adenocarcinoma of the stomach or pancreas (in combination with other drugs). Mitomycin may be a useful treatment for cancers of the bladder, breast, cervix, colon, esophagus, gallbladder, head and neck, lung, and rectum. Mitomycin has been used as an eye drop preparation for the treatment of pterygium.

Classification

Antitumor antibiotic.

Pharmacokinetics

Mitomycin is poorly absorbed by mouth. After IV administration the drug rapidly distributes to body tissues, excluding the brain. Mitomycin is inactivated by microsomal enzymes in the liver and is also metabolized in the spleen and kidneys. The presence of ascites does not affect the elimination of mitomycin even though the drug penetrates into ascitic fluid (40% of plasma concentrations). After intra-arterial administration to the liver, approximately 25% is metabolized on first pass. Approximately 10% to 30% of the drug is eliminated unchanged in the urine. Renal dysfunction does not significantly alter mitomycin elimination. Mitomycin has an elimination half-life of 0.5 to 1 hour. The drug is not hemodialyzable.

Dose

The usual IV dose range is 10 to 20 mg/m^2 once every 6 to 8 weeks. It has been recommended that total cumulative doses not exceed 50 mg/m^2 to avoid excessive toxicity.

For instillation into the bladder, 20 to 40 mg mitomycin (mixed with 20 to 40 mL of water or saline) is given weekly for 8 weeks. Dose reduction is indicated if the creatinine clearance is less than 60 mL/minute. For intra-operative ocular instillation

MITOMYCIN *(continued)*

a 0.2 mg/mL ophthalmic solution is prepared, for pterygium a 0.02% ophthalmic solution has been used.

Administration

Using extravasation precautions (mitomycin is a potent vesicant), administer into a free-flowing IV line over 2 to 5 minutes. Mitomycin has been given intravesically, intraperitoneally, intraocularly, and intra-arterially. After intravesical instillation, patients are asked to retain the drug in the bladder for 2 to 3 hours before voiding.

Toxicity

Hematological. Leukopenia and thrombocytopenia are expected, cumulative, and dose-limiting. Nadir blood counts occur around 4 to 5 weeks after a dose with recovery 2 to 3 weeks thereafter. Anemia and hemolytic-uremic syndrome (renal failure, profound thrombocytopenia, pulmonary edema, and hypotension) are uncommon. Hemolytic-uremic syndrome is associated with a high mortality rate (approximately 50%) and may be more common with cumulative mitomycin doses in excess of 60 mg/m^2.

Gastrointestinal. Mild nausea and vomiting are common, but usually prevented by antiemetic therapy. Symptoms usually begin 1 to 2 hours after IV administration and may persist for 3 to 4 hours. Nausea occasionally persists for a few days. Anorexia is common. Stomatitis and diarrhea are uncommon.

Dermatological. Alopecia (4%), dermatitis, photosensitivity, skin rash, and pruritus (4%) are uncommon toxicities. Tissue necrosis, ulceration, and cellulitis will occur if mitomycin extravasates. Skin erythema and ulceration can occur weeks to months after administration and may appear at a site that is distant from the site of injection.

Hepatic. Veno-occlusive disease of the liver, manifested as abdominal pain, hepatomegaly, and liver failure in patients receiving mitomycin and autologous bone marrow transplantation.

Neurological. Paresthesias, lethargy, headache.

Pulmonary. Interstitial pneumonitis (with cough, dyspnea, hemoptysis, and/or pneumonia) is an infrequent toxicity and can be severe. Acute bronchospasm has been reported to occur in some patients receiving vinblastine or vindesine and mitomycin. Some advocate the administration of dexamethasone, 20 mg intravenously, before each dose of mitomycin to prevent this uncommon toxicity. Pulmonary fibrosis has been reported.

Renal. Nephrotoxicity (2% incidence overall). Frequency increases when doses exceed 50 mg/m^2.

Other. Fatigue (common), pain on injection, phlebitis, fever (rare), weakness, blurred vision (rare).

Drug Interactions

In patients who are receiving or have received mitomycin treatment, subsequent or concurrent use of vinca alkaloids (e.g., vincristine, vinblastine, vindesine) may cause bronchospasm or acute shortness of breath. Vinblastine and mitomycin may be associated with acute pneumonitis.

Storage and Stability

Mitomycin vials are stored at room temperature and protected from light. At a concentration of 0.5 mg/mL the drug is chemically stable for at least 7 days at room temperature and 14 days in the refrigerator. Further diluted to 0.2 to 0.4 mg/mL, mitomycin is stable for 3 hours in 5% dextrose, 12 hours in normal saline, and 24 hours in lactated Ringer's solution.

Preparation
Mitomycin is reconstituted with 10 (5-mg vial), 40 (20-mg vial), or 80 mL (40-mg vial) of sterile water to yield a 0.5 mg/mL solution.

Compatibilities
Mitomycin (5 to 15 mg) is compatible with heparin (1,000 to 10,000 units) in 30 mL of normal saline for 48 hours at room temperature.

Availability
Commercially available as a lyophilized powder in 5-, 20-, and 40-mg vials.

MITOTANE

Other names
Lysodren®; o,p'DDD; NSC-38721.

Indications
FDA approved for the treatment of adrenocortical cancer. Mitotane may also be useful in the treatment of Cushing's syndrome.

Classification and Mechanisms of Action
Mitotane is an adrenal cytotoxic agent; its exact mechanism of action is unknown. Mitotane may exert cytotoxic effects by damaging the mitochondria of adreno-cortical cells. Mitotane modifies extra-adrenal metabolism of exogenous and endogenous steroids and suppresses adrenocortical neoplasms by a cytotoxic effect.

Pharmacokinetics
Approximately 35% to 40% of an oral dose is absorbed and reaches peak serum concentrations 3 to 5 hours after dosing. Inhibition of adrenal function occurs after 2 to 4 weeks of continuous treatment. Serum concentrations of mitotane are not believed to correlate with antitumor effect. Mitotane is distributed to all body tissues, with adipose tissue being a primary storage site. Mitotane is metabolized by the liver and eliminated in the bile (1% to 17%) and urine (10% to 25%). The drug has an elimination half-life of 18 to 160 days.

Dose
For the treatment of adrenocortical carcinoma the usual initial adult dose is 1,000 to 6,000 mg/day in 3 to 4 divided doses. The dose is usually increased to 9,000 to 10,000 mg/day, the usual adult dose. The maximum tolerable dose is 2,000 to 16,000 mg/day. For Cushing's syndrome, initial treatment is usually 3,000 to 6,000 mg/day in divided doses followed by smaller maintenance doses administered daily or a few times each week.

Administration
Oral. Avoid administering with fatty meals, absorption may be inhibited.

Toxicity
Hematological. Thrombocytopenia and leukopenia are rare.

MITOTANE (continued)

Gastrointestinal. Anorexia, nausea, and vomiting are reported in about 80% of patients and can be dose-limiting. Diarrhea occurs in approximately 20% of patients.

Dermatological. Maculopapular rash occurs in about 15% of patients; hyperpigmentation, chloasma, urticaria, erythema multiforme, periorbital or facial swelling, and perinasal scaling rarely occur.

Hepatic. Elevation of hepatic transaminase levels and hyperbilirubinemia have been reported.

Neurological. Depression, manifested as sedation, lethargy, and dizziness or vertigo occurs in 40% of patients. Irritability, confusion, headache, weakness, fatigue, and/or tremors occur less frequently. Functional impairment and brain damage may result from prolonged use of high doses. Serum concentrations greater than 20 microg/mL are often associated with adverse central nervous system effects.

Cardiovascular. Flushing, orthostatic hypotension, and hypertension are infrequent toxicities.

Pulmonary. Shortness of breath and wheezing are infrequent toxicities.

Endocrine. Most patients develop adrenocortical insufficiency. Glucocorticoid and mineralocorticoid replacement therapy may be necessary.

Metabolic. Hypercholesterolemia and hypouricemia frequently occur.

Ocular. Visual disturbances, blurred vision, diplopia, papilledema, lens opacity, cataracts, and retinopathy are rare.

Other. Fever, hematuria, hemorrhagic cystitis, and albuminuria are rare.

Drug Interactions

Spironolactone may antagonize the effects of mitotane.

Mitotane may accelerate the metabolism of warfarin and reduce prothrombin times.

Mitotane administered concomitantly with CNS depressants (e.g., benzodiazepines, sedatives, narcotic analgesics, etc.) may cause an increase in CNS toxicity.

Chronic mitotane therapy may increase the metabolism of corticosteroids, and therefore higher doses may be necessary.

Storage and Stability

Mitotane is stored at room temperature. Containers bear expiration dates.

Availability

Commercially available as a 500-mg scored tablet.

MITOXANTRONE

Other names

Novantrone®; mitoxantrone hydrochloride; dihydroxyanthracenedione; DHAD; DHAQ; NSC-301739.

Indications

FDA approved for the treatment of acute nonlymphocytic leukemia and advanced, hormone-refractory prostate cancer. Mitoxantrone may be useful in the treatment of non-Hodgkin's lymphoma, breast cancer, hepatocellular carcinoma, and autologous bone marrow transplantation. Mitoxantrone is also FDA approved for use in multiple sclerosis.

Classification and Mechanisms of Action

Antitumor antibiotic (anthracenedione derivative).

Pharmacokinetics

Mitoxantrone is poorly absorbed after oral administration. After IV administration, it is widely distributed throughout the body, metabolized by the liver, and excreted in the bile (30% unchanged) and urine (10% unchanged). Approximately 80% of the drug is bound to plasma proteins. Elimination of the drug in patients with serum bilirubin concentrations of 1.3 to 3.4 mg/dL is similar to that observed in patients with normal bilirubin levels. Mitoxantrone has an elimination half-life of 2.3 to 13 days. Mitoxantrone is probably not removed by dialysis because of its extensive tissue binding.

Dose

A commonly used regimen for initial induction of acute nonlymphocytic leukemia is 12 mg/m^2/day for 3 days combined with cytarabine, 100 mg/m^2/day, as a 7-day continuous IV infusion. Subsequent treatments to maintain a complete remission in patients with acute leukemia utilize the same doses of mitoxantrone and cytarabine administered over 2 and 5 days, respectively. Mitoxantrone has also been administered at doses of 10 to 12 mg/m^2/day for 5 days as a treatment for patients with acute leukemia. For advanced hormone-refractory prostate cancer and for other malignancies a common dose is 12 mg/m^2 every 3 to 4 weeks.

For use in multiple sclerosis the dose range is up to 12 mg/m^2/dose administered once every 3 months.

Monitor cardiac function. The maximum recommended lifetime dose of mitoxantrone is 140 to 160 mg/m^2. For patients who have received previous anthracycline treatment the maximum recommended lifetime dose is 100 to 120 mg/m^2.

Administration

Mitoxantrone has been given as an IV bolus (over 3 minutes or longer), but it is recommended that the drug be administered by IV infusion (in 50 mL or more of 5% dextrose or normal saline) over 15 to 30 minutes or longer. The drug has also been given as a continuous IV infusion, intramuscularly, intraperitoneally, and by intravesical instillation.

Toxicity

Hematological. Leukopenia is expected and dose-limiting (nadir 10 to 14 days). Thrombocytopenia and anemia occur less frequently.

Gastrointestinal. Nausea and vomiting, diarrhea, mucositis (common), abdominal pain.

Dermatological. Alopecia is common but usually mild. Pruritus and dry skin have been reported.

Hepatic. Transient elevation of hepatic transaminase levels occur occasionally, jaundice (rare), hyperbilirubinemia is uncommon.

Neurological. Headache, seizures (rare).

Cardiovascular. Cumulative cardiomyopathy (congestive heart failure) can occur. Mitoxantrone is less cardiotoxic than doxorubicin and daunorubicin. However, monitoring left ventricular ejection fraction (LVEF) is recommended (see doxorubicin section). In patients without any risk factors for developing cardiomyopathy the risk of this toxicity appears to increase when cumulative doses exceed 140 mg/m^2. Arrhythmias, tachycardia, and chest pain occur infrequently.

Pulmonary. Cough and/or dyspnea are uncommon and may be associated with congestive heart failure.

Allergic. Hypotension, urticaria, and rash are uncommon toxicities.

MITOXANTRONE *(continued)*

Other. Blue discoloration of sclera and blue-green discoloration of the urine may persist for 24 to 48 hours after treatment. Fever, conjunctivitis, phlebitis, amenorrhea, tissue ulceration and necrosis on extravasation (rare).

Drug Interactions

Mitoxantrone may decrease the absorption of oral quinolones, such as ciprofloxacin and gatifloxacin.

Storage and Stability

Mitoxantrone vials are stored at room temperature. Storage under refrigeration may cause formation of a precipitate that redissolves upon warming to room temperature. When diluted to 0.02 to 0.5 mg/mL in normal saline or 5% dextrose, the drug is chemically stable for at least 7 days at room temperature.

Preparation

Dilute in at least 50 mL normal saline or 5% dextrose before administration.

Compatibilities

Hydrocortisone sodium succinate (0.1 to 2 mg/mL with mitoxantrone, 0.05 to 0.2 microg/mL in normal saline or 5% dextrose) is compatible for at least 24 hours at room temperature.

Incompatibilities

Heparin (1 to 10 units/mL with mitoxantrone, 50 to 200 microg/mL) causes an immediate precipitate. Hydrocortisone sodium phosphate (2 mg/mL with mitox-antrone, 50 microg/mL) causes an immediate precipitate.

Availability

Commercially available as a 2 mg/mL solution (20-, 25-, and 30-mg vials).

Selected Reading

Gisselbrecht C et al. Cyclophosphamide/mitoxantrone/melphalan (CMA) regimen prior to autologous bone marrow transplantation in metastatic breast cancer. Bone Marrow Transplantation 18: 857–863, 1996.

MOTEXAFIN GADOLINIUM

Other names

Xcytrin®; gadolinium texaphyrin; Gd-Tex; NSC-695238.

Indications

Motexafin gadolinium is an investigational agent in the United States that is undergo-ing evaluation as an enhancer of radiation treatment for patients with brain metastases.

Classification and Mechanisms of Action

Motexafin gadolinium is a porphyrin analogue. The drug is a radiation enhancer that is believed to catalyze oxidation of intracellular metabolites leading to the production of hydrogen peroxide.

Pharmacokinetics

Approximately 10% of motexafin gadolinium is detectable in the plasma 24 hours following administration. Negligible amounts of the drug are eliminated in the urine. The elimination half-life is approximately 9 hours. Concomitant administration of CYP 3A4, 5, 7 inducers has been shown to increase the clearance of motexafin gadolinium by approximately 20%.

Dose

In combination with 10 days of whole brain irradiation (30 cGy total dose), motexafin gadolinium doses have ranged from 5.0 to 6.3 mg/kg/day for 10 days. On this schedule the drug is given daily for 5 days on 2 consecutive weeks. The maximum tolerated single dose of motexafin gadolinium is 22.3 mg/kg (dose-limiting toxicities occurred at 29.6 mg/kg). The drug has also been administered 3 times weekly following the aforementioned 2-week schedule. On this schedule the maximum tolerated dose is 5 mg/kg/day.

Administration

Motexafin gadolinium is administered IV over 5 to 90 minutes. Doses are usually administered 2 to 5 hours prior to each dose of radiation therapy.

Toxicity

Motexafin gadolinium does not appear to exacerbate radiation therapy-induced toxicity to normal tissues.

Gastrointestinal. Diarrhea (25%), anorexia (25%), nausea (28%), vomiting (18%).

Dermatological. Skin rash (13%) with or without pruritus. In one study 60% of patients developed a vesiculobullous rash. Approximately 50% of patients will develop a greenish skin discoloration that resolves within 4 days following discontinuation of therapy. Some patients have experienced a burning sensation that was dose-limiting.

Hepatic. Elevation of hepatic transaminases and serum bilirubin is dose-limiting with the daily administration schedule. Significant elevations of these parameters usually occur by day 5 of a 10-day dosing regimen. Liver function tests usually resolve within a few days following the discontinuation of motexafin gadolinium.

Neurological. Cerebral edema, paralysis, and seizures have been observed in some patients. Headache occurs in approximately 10% of patients.

Pulmonary. Hypoxia, pneumonitis, and respiratory failure have been observed.

Renal. A green discoloration of the urine is common (70%). Transient elevations of BUN and creatinine have been observed with the single dose regimen. Proteinuria is uncommon.

Other. Asthenia (15% to 40%), green discoloration of the sclera (18%), photophobia, myalgia, and paresthesia of the fingertips have been reported.

Drug Interactions

Concomitant administration of CYP 3A4, 5, 7 inducers has been shown to increase the clearance of motexafin gadolinium by approximately 20%.

Storage and Stability

Motexafin gadolinium is stored at refrigeration temperatures (2° to 8°C). Do not freeze the product.

Preparation

Filter the solution through a filter with pore size of 0.45 to 0.5 micron.

MOTEXAFIN GADOLINIUM (continued)

Availability

Motexafin gadolinium is an investigational agent in the United States that is available as a 2.3 mg/mL solution from the manufacturer or the National Cancer Institute.

Selected Readings

Carde P et al. Multicenter phase Ib/II trial of the radiation enhancer motexafin gadolinium in patients with brain metastasis. J Clin Oncol 19: 2074–2083, 2001.

Sessler JL, Miller RA. Texaphyrins: new drugs with diverse clinical applications in radiation and photodynamic therapy. Biochem Pharmacol 59: 733–739, 2000.

NILUTAMIDE

Other names

Nilandron®; NSC-684588.

Indications

FDA approved for the treatment of metastatic prostate cancer (stage D2) in conjunction with surgical castration.

Classification and Mechanisms of Action

Nilutamide is a nonsteroidal selective antiandrogen that blocks the activity of testosterone at the level of the androgen receptor in prostate cancer cells.

Pharmacokinetics

Nilutamide is completely absorbed after oral administration. Moderate plasma protein binding is exhibited. The drug is almost totally metabolized by the liver to at least five metabolites. One of these metabolites is responsible for up to 50% of the pharmacological activity of the drug. After ingestion of one 150-mg dose, approximately 62% of the drug is eliminated in the urine over a period of 5 days. Nilutamide has an elimination half-life of 41 to 49 hours.

Dose

The usual dose is 300 mg/day for the first 30 days, then decreased to 150 mg/day.

Administration

Oral. Take with or without food, to begin the day after orchiectomy.

Toxicity

When nilutamide was administered in combination with an LHRH agonist, the following adverse events were observed:

Hematological. Anemia (7%) and rarely leukopenia were reported.

Gastrointestinal. Nausea (25%), constipation (20%), anorexia (10%), abdominal pain, dyspepsia, and vomiting occurred in less than 10% of patients, while diarrhea, dry mouth, melena, and gastrointestinal hemorrhage occurred in less than 2% of patients.

Dermatological. Less than 10% of patients reported rash, pruritus, sweating, alopecia, and/or dry skin.

Hepatic. Increased serum transaminases (approximately 10%).

Neurological. Insomnia and headache were most commonly reported (up to 20%). Dizziness, depression, and hypesthesia were reported in less than 10% of patients.
Cardiovascular. Hypertension reported in approximately 10% of patients.
Pulmonary. Dyspnea (10%), upper respiratory tract infections, and pneumonia. Lung disorder, increased cough, interstitial disease, and rhinitis reported in less than 5% of patients.
Genitourinary. Testicular atrophy (15%), gynecomastia (10%), urinary tract infection (10%), hematuria and nocturia (less than 10%).
Endocrine. Hot flushes (67%), loss of libido and impotence (10%).
Ocular. The most common ocular effect is an impaired adaptation to dark (57%). Also reported are chromatopsia, impaired adaptation to light, and abnormal vision. Rarely, cataracts and photophobia were reported.
Other. Pain (25%), asthenia (20%), and back pain (approximately 10%). Rarely reported were malaise, arthritis, chest pain, flu-like syndrome, bone pain, and/or fever.

When nilutamide was administered postsurgical castration, the following adverse events were observed.
Hematological. Rarely leukopenia.
Gastrointestinal. Nausea and constipation reported in less than 10% of patients.
Hepatic. Increased transaminase levels in approximately 8% of patients.
Neurological. Dizziness was reported in 7% of patients. Paresthesia and nervousness reported in less than 5% of patients.
Cardiovascular. Hypertension reported in approximately 5% of patients.
Pulmonary. Dyspnea reported in 6% of patients, lung disorder, increased cough, interstitial disease, and rhinitis reported in less than 5% of patients.
Genitourinary. Urinary tract infection reported in 8% of patients.
Endocrine. Hot flushes commonly reported in approximately 29%.
Ocular. Impaired adaptation to dark reported in 13% of patients. Rarely cataracts and photophobia were reported.

Drug Interactions
Nilutamide inhibits cytochrome P450 isoenzymes and when administered concomitantly with chronic warfarin anticoagulants may lead to prolongation of prothrombin times. Monitor PT and INR closely.

Nilutamide may also increase plasma levels of phenytoin and theophylline by inhibition of the P450 isoenzymes. Monitor levels regularly, adjust dose as necessary.

Storage and Stability
Nilutamide tablets are stored at room temperature. Containers bear expiration dates.

Availability
Nilutamide is commercially available as 50-mg and 150-mg tablets.

Selected Reading
Dijkman GA et al. Long-term efficacy and safety of nilutamide plus castration in advanced prostate cancer, and the significance of early prostate specific antigen normalization. J Urol 58: 160–163, 1997.

NITROCAMPTOTHECIN

Other names
Rubitecan; Orathecin®; 9-nitrocamptothecin; 9-NC; RFS 2000.

Indications
Nitrocamptothecin is an investigational agent in the United States. The drug appears to have activity in non-small-cell lung cancer, ovarian cancer, colorectal cancer, and other malignancies.

Classification and Mechanisms of Action
Nitrocamptothecin is, like other camptothecin antineoplastic agents, a topoisomerase I inhibitor. Topoisomerase I relaxes supercoiled DNA by incision and is necessary for DNA and RNA synthesis. Resealing of DNA is prevented by the binding of camptothecin to the DNA-enzyme complex, resulting in the accumulation of reversible enzyme-DNA cleavable complexes.

Pharmacokinetics
Nitrocamptothecin is well absorbed following oral administration. Maximum serum concentrations occur approximately 3 hours after oral administration in fasting patients. Food significantly slows oral absorption and significantly decreases the maximum concentrations and the AUC. Nitrocamptothecin is metabolized to 9-aminocamptothecin, an active metabolite.

Dose
In patients with chronic myelogenous leukemia, nitrocamptothecin has been administered at a dose of 2 mg/m^2/day for 5 days, repeated weekly (i.e., 5 days of therapy followed by 2 days of rest, repeated weekly). In patients with solid tumors the maximum tolerated dose is 2.4 mg/m^2 daily for 5 days for 2 consecutive weeks (10 days of treatment), repeated every 28 days (i.e., 2 weeks of treatment followed by 2 weeks of no treatment). Nitrocamptothecin has been administered in combination with cisplatin and other drugs. In combination with a single dose of cisplatin, 70 mg/m^2, the maximum tolerated dose of nitrocamptothecin is 1.25 mg/m^2/day for 5 days. In combination with a single dose of cisplatin, 40 mg/m^2, the maximum tolerated dose of nitrocamptothecin is 2 mg/m^2/day for 5 days.

Administration
Oral, on an empty stomach.

Toxicity
Hematological. Neutropenia is expected. Grade 3 or 4 neutropenia has been reported to occur in approximately 25% of patients. Anemia (grade 3 or 4) has been reported in approximately 15% to 33% of patients. Thrombocytopenia (grade 3 or 4) has been reported in 10% to 18% of patients.

Gastrointestinal. Nausea, vomiting, and diarrhea are dose-limiting. Nausea and vomiting (grade 3) has been reported in up to 84% of patients; diarrhea (grade 3) in approximately 40%; and significant weight loss in approximately 20% of patients.

Dermatological. Alopecia (grade 1 to 2) has been reported.

Other. Chemical cystitis and hematuria (approximately 20%, but usually grade 2), fatigue (30%), and myalgia (10%).

Storage and Stability
Nitrocamptothecin is stored at refrigeration temperature.

Availability
Nitrocamptothecin is an investigational agent in the United States that is available in an oral formulation (0.5 and 1.5 mg/capsule) from the manufacturer.

Selected Reading
Verschraegen CF et al. A phase II clinical and pharmacological study of oral 9-nitrocamptothecin in patients with refractory epithelial ovarian, tubal or peritoneal cancer. Anticancer Drugs 10: 375–383, 1999.

NOLATREXED DIHYDROCHLORIDE

Other names
Thymitaq®; AG337.

Indications
Nolatrexed dihydrochloride is an investigational agent in the United States. It is undergoing evaluation as a treatment for patients with hepatocellular cancer. It may also have activity in non-small-cell lung cancer, esophageal cancer, head and neck cancers, and other malignancies. Nolatrexed has orphan drug designation for hepatocellular carcinoma.

Classification and Mechanisms of Action
Nolatrexed is an antifolate antineoplastic agent that inhibits thymidylate synthase.

Pharmacokinetics
Nolatrexed is well absorbed (90%) by mouth. The rate of oral absorption is slowed by food; however, the AUC of the drug is not affected by food. The drug exhibits nonlinear pharmacokinetics. Approximately 20% of the drug is eliminated in the urine unchanged. The elimination half-life is approximately 2 hours.

Dose
Different doses and schedules have been evaluated. The more common regimens evaluated are 725 to 800 mg/m^2/day as a 5-day continuous infusion, repeated every 21 days. As an oral agent, 800 mg/m^2/day for 5 days, repeated every 21 days, has been evaluated. An oral regimen of 429 mg/m^2/day for 10 days, repeated every 21 days, has also been evaluated.

Administration
Nolatrexed is administered orally or intravenously as a continuous infusion over 5 days.

Toxicity
Hematological. Neutropenia (grade 3–4: 30%), febrile neutropenia (3%), thrombocytopenia.
Gastrointestinal. Stomatitis (grade 3–4: 33%), nausea, vomiting (grade 3–4: 10%).
Dermatological. Skin rash.
Other. Malaise.

Preparation
Doses for parenteral administration are usually further diluted in 500 mL or more of 5% dextrose and water.

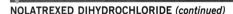

NOLATREXED DIHYDROCHLORIDE *(continued)*

Availability

Nolatrexed is an investigational agent in the United States that is available as a 16 mg/mL solution for parenteral use (80 mg/5 mL) from the manufacturer.

Selected Reading

Rafi I et al. Preclinical and phase I clinical studies with the nonclassical antifolate thymidylate synthase inhibitor nolatrexed dihydrochloride given by prolonged administration in patients with solid tumors. J Clin Oncol 16: 1131–1134, 1998.

O^6-BENZYLGUANINE

Other names

O^6-BG; 6-benzyloxyguanine; NSC-637037.

Indications

O^6-Benzylguanine is an investigational agent in the United States. It is undergoing evaluation, in combination with antineoplastic agents (such as carmustine and melphalan), for the treatment of patients with brain tumors and other malignancies.

Classification and Mechanisms of Action

O^6-BG inactivates the DNA repair enzyme O^6-alkyguanine-DNA alkyltransferase (AGT). O^6-BG may be a useful concomitant therapy with drugs whose antitumor effects are abrogated by this DNA repair enzyme. Depletion of AGT levels occurs within 1 hour of administration and approximtely 50% recovery of AGT occurs 72 hours after administration of O^6-BG.

Pharmacokinetics

O^6-BG is converted to an active metabolite that reaches peak plasma concentrations 1 to 5 hours after administration. The active metabolite has an elimination half-life of approximately 5 to 6 hours. Activation of O^6-BG is mediated by cytochrome P450 isoenzymes 1A1 and 1A2. However, in one study phenytoin did not alter the pharmacokinetics of O^6-BG and its primary metabolite 8-oxo-O^6-BG. Less than 5% of O^6-BG and its active metabolite are eliminated unchanged in the urine.

Dose

O^6-BG 100 mg/m^2/dose is administered in combination with carmustine 40 mg/m^2/dose. This treatment is repeated every 6 weeks. Dose-limiting myelosuppression occurs at a carmustine dose of 55 mg/m^2.

Administration

O^6-BG is administered IV over 1 hour. The drug has been given 1 hour prior to administration of carmustine.

Toxicity

O^6-BG will increase the toxicity of carmustine, melphalan, and other alkylating agents. The doses of the alkylating agents must be reduced when administered in combination with O^6-BG. Toxicities associated with O^6-BG alone have been negligible.

Drug Interactions

O^6-BG inhibits CYP 1A1 and CYP 1A2 activation of dacarbazine (DTIC) to its active forms.

Storage and Stability

Intact vials of O[6]-BG and its special diluent are stored in the refrigerator. Reconstituted solutions of O[6]-BG are stable for at least 24 hours at room temperature. Solutions that are diluted to approximately 0.04 mg/mL with normal saline or 5% dextrose and water are stable for at least 24 hours at room temperature.

Preparation

Add 30 mL of the special diluent to the 100-mg vial to yield a concentration of 3.3 mg/mL. Doses are usually further diluted in normal saline or 5% dextrose and water.

Availability

O[6]-BG is an investigational drug in the United States that is available as a lyophilized powder (100 mg/vial) from the National Cancer Institute. A special diluent (NSC-659805) is supplied with the drug.

Selected Readings

Dolan ME et al. O[6]-Benzylguanine in humans: metabolic, pharmacokinetic and pharmacodynamic findings. J Clin Oncol 16: 1803–1810, 1998.

Schilsky RL et al. Phase I clinical and pharmacological study of O[6]-benzylguanine followed by carmustine in patients with advanced cancer. Clin Cancer Res 6: 3025–3031, 2000.

OCTREOTIDE

Other names

Sandostatin®; L-cysteinamide; SMS 201-995. Long-acting formulations: Sandostatin LAR Depot®; octreotide pamoate (SMS 201-995 pa LAR); SMS 201-995 LAR (octreotide acetate); NSC-685403.

Indications

FDA approved for the control of symptoms in patients with carcinoid and vasoactive intestinal peptide-secreting tumors (VIPomas). Octreotide is also approved for use in acromegaly. Octreotide may be a useful treatment for pancreatic cancer, chemotherapy-induced diarrhea, graft versus host disease, and AIDS-associated diarrhea. The long-acting formulation is useful in patients who have tolerated the short-acting octreotide product.

Classification and Mechanisms of Action

Octreotide is a long-acting analogue of the natural hormone somatostatin that inhibits the secretion of serotonin, vasoactive intestinal peptide, gastrin, motilin, insulin, glucagon, secretin, and pancreatic polypeptide.

Pharmacokinetics

Octreotide solution for injection is rapidly and completely absorbed after subcutaneous injection. The drug is widely distributed throughout the body and approximately 65% is protein-bound (primarily to lipoproteins). Octreotide has an elimination half-life of 1.5 hours and its duration of action is around 12 hours. Approximately 30% of the drug is eliminated unchanged in the urine. Octreotide long-acting suspension is released via biodegradation of the microspheres that are deposited in the muscle tissue. An initial peak occurs within 1 hour after administration, followed by a slow decline over 3 to 5 days. Fourteen to 21 days after injection a plateau level is

OCTREOTIDE *(continued)*

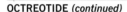

reached, which then slowly decreases. Steady-state levels occur after the second or third monthly injection, depending on the dose administered. The effect of long-acting octreotide suspension in renal or hepatically impaired patients is unknown. Renal dialysis may increase the elimination of the drug.

Dose

For the treatment of carcinoid tumors, the usual daily dose is 100 to 600 microg in two to four divided doses. For the treatment of tumors secreting vasoactive intestinal peptide, the usual daily dose is 200 to 300 microg in two to four divided doses. Doses greater than 450 microg/day are not usually necessary.

Long-acting octreotide suspension is initially administered at a dose of 20 mg every 4 weeks and doses are adjusted according to response. The subcutaneous octreotide solution should continue to be administered at the patient's maintenance dose for at least 2 weeks after initiation of treatment with the long-acting formulation.

Administration

Octreotide solution for injection is usually administered subcutaneously. Warm the solution prior to administration. Rotation of injection sites is recommended. Octreotide has also been administered as a bolus IV injection over 3 minutes and as a continuous infusion.

Octreotide long-acting suspension for injection (depot formulation) is administered intramuscularly in the gluteal muscle. Patients should begin use with octreotide long-acting suspension if they have tolerated and been maintained on octreotide solution for injection.

Toxicity

Gastrointestinal. The most frequent side effects are abdominal pain or discomfort, loose stools, anorexia, flatulence, constipation, and vomiting. These symptoms were most prominent during the first month of therapy. Fat malabsorption occurs in 1% to 3% of patients. Rarely, gastrointestinal bleeding, heartburn, swollen stomach, and cholelithiasis may occur.

Dermatological. Pain at the injection site, flushing, edema, wheal and erythema at the injection site, hair loss, thinning of skin, skin flaking, bruising, bleeding from superficial wounds, sweating, rash, and/or pruritus may occur. Pain at the injection site appears to increase with increasing doses of octreotide long-acting suspension.

Hepatic. Hepatitis, jaundice, slight elevation of liver enzyme levels. Increase in biliary tract abnormalities (e.g., cholelithiasis, gallstones, biliary obstruction, pancreatitis).

Neurological. Headache (2%), dizziness, light-headedness, fatigue, anxiety, parathesias, hypoesthesias, depression, convulsions, drowsiness, vertigo, confusion, insomnia.

Cardiovascular. Severe bradycardia, conduction abnormalities, and arrhythmias have all been reported. Hypertension, shortness of breath, thrombophlebitis, ischemia, congestive heart failure, palpitations, orthostatic hypotension, peripheral edema, and chest pain have been reported.

Metabolic. Hypoglycemia, hyperglycemia, urine hyperosmolarity, hypothyroidism (monitor thyroid function tests on chronic therapy), dehydration.

Other. Rhinorrhea, dry mouth, numbness, oliguria, prostatitis, hyperhidrosis, visual disturbance, flu-like symptoms, chills, fever, throat discomfort, cough, elevated creatine phosphokinase levels.

Drug Interactions

Octreotide administered concurrently with oral cyclosporine may alter cyclosporine absorption.

Octreotide may alter blood glucose levels; monitor glucose closesly when octreotide is administered with antidiabetic agents such as insulin, oral hypoglycemic agents, sulfonylureas, glucagon, diazoxide, or any other agent known to affect blood glucose.

Storage and Stability

Ampules and vials of octreotide solution for injection are stored in the refrigerator. Octreotide solution can be stored at room temperature for at least 14 days if protected from light. At concentrations of 5, 50, or 100 microg/mL in normal saline, octreotide is stable for at least 96 hours at room temperature. Vials of octreotide long-acting powder for suspension (depot formulation) are stored in the refrigerator and should be brought to room temperature when ready to mix. Do not leave the sterile powder at room temperature until ready to mix.

Preparation

Octreotide injection may be further diluted in normal saline or 5% dextrose to concentrations of 5 to 100 microg/mL. Vials of octreotide powder for suspension (depot formulation) and diluent should be brought to room temperature (do not heat) for 30 to 60 minutes prior to mixing. Tap the vial gently on a countertop, using the provided diluent draw up 2 mL into a syringe and inject the 2 mL into the sidewall of the vial that is to be mixed. Allow the vial to remain idle for approximately 2 minutes, this allows the wetting process to occur. After 2 minutes have elapsed, lift the vial and observe it for any unsaturated powder. If unsaturated powder exists, place the vial down, without agitation, and reobserve after 30 seconds. Continue this observation until complete saturation is observed, it may take as long as 5 minutes. Once the powder is saturated, gently swirl the vial for 30 to 60 seconds, do not shake the mixture. A white cloudy suspension is formed. This is drawn up into a syringe and immediately administered to the patient. Use the needle provided with the drug for administration.

Compatibilities

Octreotide is compatible with heparin and certain total parenteral nutrition (TPN) solutions. However, the manufacturer does not recommend mixing of octreotide with TPN solutions. A pharmacist should be consulted for additional information.

Incompatibilities

Octreotide is incompatible with 10% fat emulsion.

Availability

Octreotide solution for injection is commercially available in 1-mL ampules containing 0.05, 0.1, and 0.5 mg/mL. Octreotide is also available in a 5-mL multidose vial containing 0.2 and 1 mg/mL.

Octreotide powder for suspension (depot formulation) is commercially available in kits of 10-, 20- and 30-mg vials. All vials contain mannitol and a 2-mL diluent that also contains mannitol.

Selected Reading

Rubin J et al: Octreotide acetate long-acting formulation versus open-label subcutaneous octreotide acetate in malignant carcinoid syndrome, J Clin Oncol 17: 600–606, 1999.

OXALIPLATIN

Other names

Eloxatin®; Eloxatine®; L-OHP; NSC-266046.

Indications

Oxaliplatin is FDA approved for the treatment of patients with advanced colorectal cancer when administered in combination with 5-fluorouracil and leucovorin. Oxaliplatin also has activity in non-small-cell lung cancer, esophageal cancer, head and neck cancers, ovarian cancer, and other malignancies.

Classification and Mechanisms of Action

Oxaliplatin is a platinum-containing antineoplastic agent. Metabolites of oxaliplatin interact with DNA to form inter- and intra-strand cross-links.

Pharmacokinetics

Oxaliplatin is metabolized by nonenzymatic degradation to active metabolites. Oxaliplatin metabolites are eliminated via the urine within 5 days of administration. The terminal elimination half-life of platinum is approximately 9 days. Elimination of platinum in the feces is negligible. Although moderate to severe renal dysfunction reduces clearance of inactive platinum species by 40%, the NCI Organ Dysfunction Working Group does not recommend dose reductions for patients with moderate to severe renal dysfunction (defined as creatinine clearance 20 to 59 mL/minute). However, the manufacturer does not recommend the use of oxaliplatin when the creatinine clearance is less than 30 mL/minute.

Dose

The FDA-approved dose is 85 mg/m^2 on day 1 every 2 weeks in combination with leucovorin and 5-fluorouracil given on days 1 and 2. Leucovorin, 200 mg/m^2, is given after oxaliplatin on day 1 as a 2-hour infusion followed by a 400 mg/m^2 bolus of 5-fluorouracil which is followed by a 22-hour infusion of 5-fluorouracil, 600 mg/m^2. These doses of leucovorin and 5-fluorouracil are repeated on day 2. Oxaliplatin has also been given at a dose of 130 mg/m^2 every 3 weeks, in combination with 5-fluorouracil and leucovorin. Other doses and schedules of oxaliplatin have been used. Oxaliplatin has been used in combination with other drugs. Some of these regimens are:

- Oxaliplatin 130 mg/m^2 on day 1; vinorelbine 26 mg/m^2 on days 1 and 8; repeated every 3 weeks.
- Paclitaxel 175 mg/m^2 over 3 hours followed by oxaliplatin 130 mg/m^2; repeated every 3 weeks.
- Pemetrexed 500 mg/m^2 over 30 minutes followed by oxaliplatin 120 mg/m^2; repeated every 3 weeks.
- Oxaliplatin 100 mg/m^2 on day 1; gemcitabine 1,000 mg/m^2 on day 1; repeated every 2 weeks.
- Oxaliplatin 85 mg/m^2 on day 1; irinotecan 200 mg/m^2 on day 1; repeated every 3 weeks.
- Oxaliplatin 85 mg/m^2 and irinotecan 175 mg/m^2 on day 1, 5-fluorouracil 240 mg/m^2/day and leucovorin 20 mg/m^2/day on days 2 through 5; repeated every 3 weeks.
- Oxaliplatin 130 mg/m^2 on day 1; capecitabine 1,000 or 1,250 mg/m^2 twice daily on days 1 through 14; repeated every 3 weeks. The lower dose of capecitabine was administered to previously treated patients.

Administration

Oxaliplatin is administered IV in 250 to 500 mL of 5% dextrose and water over 2 to 6 hours. Oxaliplatin should be administered prior to 5-fluorouracil. Oxaliplatin is not a vesicant.

Toxicity

Hematological. Following oxaliplatin 130 mg/m^2 as a single agent the incidence of grade 3 and 4 neutropenia and thrombocytopenia is less than 3% and grade 3 and 4 anemia is less than 4%. Combined with 5-fluorouracil the incidence of grade 3 or 4 neutropenia is approximately 40% and grade 3 and 4 thrombocytopenia and anemia is approximately 4%. Febrile neutropenia is uncommon (less than 2%).

Gastrointestinal. Nausea and vomiting will occur and prophylactic antiemetics are recommended. Diarrhea, dehydration hypokalemia, and metabolic acidosis may occur, especially when oxaliplatin is administered in combination with 5-fluorouracil. Anorexia and abdominal pain have been reported.

Dermatological. Alopecia is not common (2%) and usually moderate. Hand-foot syndrome and skin rash have been reported.

Hepatic. Elevation of transaminase enzymes (usually grade 1 or 2) is common. Hyperbilirubinemia has been reported.

Cardiovascular. Tachycardia supraventricular arrhythmia, hypertension, phlebitis, and thromboembolism have been reported in patients receiving oxaliplatin.

Renal. Renal dysfunction is uncommon (approximately 3%).

Neurological. Two forms of neurological toxicity have been reported.

Acute neurological symptoms include: paresthesias of the hands, feet, and perioral area, jaw tightness, and laryngopharyngeal dysesthesia (sensations of dysphagia, dyspnea, but no evidence of hypoxia, laryngospasm, or bronchospasm). The acute symptoms may occur during the infusion or within hours after administration. These symptoms often occur upon exposure to cold and may increase in severity and/or duration with repeated treatment. Prolonging the rate of oxaliplatin infusion (i.e., from 2 hours to 6 hours) is recommended for patients who develop laryngopharyngeal dysesthesia. Other, less common, neurological adverse events include loss of deep tendon reflexes and Lhermittes's sign. Rarely, deafness and loss of visual acuity have been reported.

Chronic neurologic symptoms may include peripheral sensory neuropathy, which is common and may be dose-limiting. It is aggravated by exposure to cold. Some degree of sensory neuropathy occurs in almost all of patients treated with oxaliplatin, and grade 3 and 4 neuropathy is reported in approximately 45% of patients. In approximately 15% of patients, paresthesias and function impairment lasted longer than 2 weeks and occurred after a median cumulative dose of 874 mg/m^2. In the majority of patients this adverse event improves slowly after oxaliplatin is discontinued. In some studies, 40% of patients had resolution of peripheral sensory neuropathies 6 to 8 months after discontinuation of oxaliplatin.

Other. Anaphylactic reactions and ototoxicity (mild hearing loss) are uncommon (< 1%). Hypersensitivity reactions, defined as dyspnea, chills, wheezing, rigors, rash, decreased oxygen saturation or hypotension during or within hours of administration, is reported to occur in 8% of patients.

Despite receiving dexamethasone prophylaxis, approximately two-thirds of reactive patients will continue to develop a hypersentivity reaction. A prophylactic regimen including dexamethasone, cimetidine, diphenhydramine, and acetaminophen in combination with a 6-hour infusion of oxaliplatin, may be effective at minimizing and/or preventing these reactions. Other adverse events may include fatigue; back pain and arthralgia are common.

OXALIPLATIN *(continued)*

Storage and Stability

Intact vials are stored at room temperature. Reconstituted solutions are chemically stable for at least 48 hours at room and refrigeration temperatures.

Preparation

Add 10 mL of sterile water or 5% dextrose to the 50-mg vial or add 20 mL of sterile water or 5% dextrose to the 100-mg vial to yield a concentration of 5 mg/mL. Doses of oxaliplatin are further diluted in 250 to 500 mL of 5% dextrose and water.

Compatibilities

In vitro, no significant displacement of oxaliplatin binding to plasma proteins has been observed with erythromycin, salicylates, granisetron, paclitaxel, or valproic acid.

Incompatibilities

Oxaliplatin is not compatible with aluminum- or chloride-containing and basic solutions (including 5-fluorouracil).

Availability

Oxaliplatin is available as a lyophilized powder (50 mg/vial and 100 mg/vial) from the manufacturer.

Selected Reading

Raymond E et al. Oxaliplatin: a review of preclinical and clinical studies. Ann Oncol 9: 1053–1071, 1998.

PACLITAXEL

Other names

Taxol®; Onxol®; NSC-125973.
Investigational agent: polyglutamate paclitaxel; Xyotax®.

Indications

FDA approved for the treatment of advanced ovarian cancer, breast cancers, non-small-cell lung cancer, and AIDS-related Kaposi's sarcoma. Paclitaxel may be useful for the treatment of cancers of the head and neck, esophagus, prostate, and stomach.

Classification

Plant alkaloid (antimicrotubule agent).

Pharmacokinetics

Paclitaxel is 95% to 98% protein-bound and is metabolized to 7-epitaxol. Only 1.3% to 12% is excreted unchanged in the urine, indicating clearance is primarily nonrenal. The drug is metabolized by the cytochrome P450 system isoenzymes CYP 2C8 and CYP 3A4. The elimination half-life of paclitaxel depends on the dose and infusion duration, the half-lives range from 13 hours (at 135 mg/m^2 dose over 3 hours) to 53 hours (at 135 mg/m^2 dose over 24 hours). Paclitaxel distributes to ascitic fluid, achieving concentrations approximately 40% of plasma levels. Elimination of paclitaxel is reduced by one-third when the drug is administered immediately after administration of cisplatin.

Dose

A variety of doses and schedules have been used including the following:

For ovarian cancer. 135 to 175 mg/m^2 over 3 hours, repeated every 3 weeks, or 135 mg/m^2 as a continuous infusion over 24 hours, repeated every 3 weeks.

For breast cancer. 175 mg/m^2 over 3 hours, every 3 weeks, doses up to 200 to 250 mg/m^2 have been administered every 3 weeks. Doses of 70 to 100 mg/m^2/week, as a 1-hour infusion, have been evaluated.

For non-small-cell lung cancer. 135 mg/m^2 every 3 weeks as a continuous infusion over 24 hours. Higher doses of paclitaxel (e.g., 175 mg/m^2 to 200 mg/m^2) have been given in combination with carboplatin doses targeted at AUC of 6.

For Kaposi's sarcoma. 135 mg/m^2 every 3 weeks over 3 hours.

Administration

Paclitaxel is further diluted as an IV infusion (as a 0.3 to 1.2 mg/mL solution in 5% dextrose or normal saline) over 1, 3, or 24 hours. Use of an in-line 0.2-micron filter is recommended when administering paclitaxel. Premedication is recommended to reduce the incidence of hypersensitivity reactions: dexamethasone 20 mg orally, 6 and 12 hours before paclitaxel, plus diphenhydramine 50 mg intravenously, and ranitidine 50 mg intravenously (or cimetidine 300 mg intravenously, or famotidine 20 mg intravenously) 30 to 60 minutes before administration of paclitaxel. If patients forget to take the oral doses of dexamethasone before paclitaxel, then an IV dose of dexamethasone 20 mg is administered 30 minutes before administration of paclitaxel. Some clinicians give this IV dexamethasone dose 30 minutes before paclitaxel, regardless of whether the two oral doses were taken, just to be cautious. Paclitaxel has also been given as a 96-hour continuous IV infusion and intraperitoneally (maximum tolerated dose, 175 mg/m^2).

Toxicity

Hematological. Neutropenia is dose-limiting and does not appear to be cumulative; it occurs more often when a 24-hour (versus 3-hour) infusion of paclitaxel is administered. Nadir counts occur by day 8 to 11 with recovery occurring by day 21. Thrombocytopenia is usually not severe. Myelosuppression is most severe in patients who have received extensive prior treatment and in patients who receive cisplatin just before paclitaxel. Mild anemia is seen in approximately 20% of patients.

Gastrointestinal. Mucositis is dose-related and cumulative (3% have greater than grade I mucositis), occurs within 3 to 7 days, and resolves 5 to 7 days thereafter. Nausea and vomiting are infrequent (4% incidence), as are diarrhea, taste changes, typhlitis (neutropenic enterocolitis), ischemic colitis, and pancreatitis.

Dermatological. Alopecia is universal, complete, and often sudden. Hair loss usually occurs 14 to 21 days after treatment and often affects all body hair (i.e., eyebrows, pubic hair). Many patients experience regrowth of hair after five to seven cycles of treatment. Infrequent dermatological toxicities include: injection site reactions (erythema, induration, tenderness, skin discoloration), infiltration (phlebitis, cellulitis, ulceration, and necrosis), nail changes (e.g., discoloration, separation from the nail bed), radiation recall reactions, and rashes.

Hepatic. Minor elevation of hepatic transaminase levels, hyperbilirubinemia, hepatic failure, and hepatic necrosis have been reported.

Neurological. Peripheral neuropathy, more frequent with longer infusions, with doses over 170 mg/m^2, and in patients with a history of substantial alcohol use, diabetes, or diabetic neuropathy. Grade 2 peripheral neuropathies have been seen after 9 of 281 courses and appear to be cumulative. Transient myalgias and arthralgias begin within

PACLITAXEL (continued)

2 to 3 days after treatment, occasionally resolve within 2 to 4 days, are amenable to treatment with nonsteroidal anti-inflammatory drugs, and occur more often after higher doses. Mood alterations, light-headedness, neuroencephalopathy, hepatic encephalopathy, motor neuropathy, autonomic neuropathy, paralytic ileus, generalized weakness, and seizures are rare.

Cardiovascular. Bradycardia (40 to 60 bpm) is common, usually transient, and usually asymptomatic. Ventricular tachycardia (usually asymptomatic but potentially serious) and atypical chest pain occur less frequently. In patients with no prior history of cardiac problems and taking no cardiac medications, routine cardiac monitoring is not recommended. Syncope, hypotension, ventricular tachycardia, bigeminy, complete heart block requiring a pacemaker, and myocardial infarction have been reported rarely. Hypertension, possibly related to concomitant administration of dexamethasone, has been reported.

Pulmonary. Interstitial pneumonitis has been reported in some patients.

Hypersensitivity. Anaphylactic reactions (2% to 4%) manifested as cutaneous flushing, hypotension, dyspnea with bronchospasm, and bradycardia (40 to 60 bpm). Urticaria, abdominal and extremity pain, angioedema, and diaphoresis have also occurred. Half of the reported reactions occurred within 2 to 3 minutes of initiation of treatment (78% within 20 minutes), 50% occur after the first dose, and 40% after the second dose. Hypersensitivity reactions are of the same frequency for 24- and 3-hour infusions. Premedication is recommended. Patients who experience hypersensitivity reactions can be desensitized using a desensitization regimen in order to receive further paclitaxel doses.

Other. Fatigue, headache, minor elevations in serum creatinine and triglyceride levels, light-headedness, myopathy, sensation of flashing lights, and blurred vision.

Drug Interactions

The clearance of paclitaxel is significantly reduced when administered after cisplatin or carboplatin; this leads to an increase in toxicity, (e.g., myelosuppression). When combination therapy is used, always administer paclitaxel prior to platinum compounds.

The plasma clearance of doxorubicin is decreased when administered concomitantly with paclitaxel, resulting in an increase in doxorubicin toxicity.

Potential drug interactions may occur when paclitaxel is administered with any medication that either induces or inhibits the cytochrome P450 isoenzyes CYP 2C8 or CYP 3A4.

Storage and Stability

Paclitaxel vials may be stored at room temperature and protected from light. Refrigeration and freezing do not affect the potency of paclitaxel. Solutions diluted to a concentration of 0.3 to 1.2 mg/mL in normal saline or 5% dextrose are stable for at least 27 hours at room temperature.

Preparation

The concentrated solution must be diluted before use in normal saline, 5% dextrose, or 5% dextrose in Ringer's solution to a concentration of 0.3 to 1.2 mg/mL. Solutions exhibit a slight haze, common to all products containing nonionic surfactants. Glass, polypropylene, or polyolefin containers and non-PVC-containing (nitroglycerin) infusion sets should be used.

Incompatibilities

Avoid the use of PVC bags and infusion sets because of leaching of di-(2-ethylhexyl)phthalate (DEHP) (plasticizer).

Availability

Paclitaxel is commercially available as a 6 mg/mL solution in 30-, 100-, 150-, and 300-mg vials.

PAMIDRONATE

Other names

Aredia®; pamidronate disodium; aminohydroxypropylidene biphosphonate; APD; NSC-720699.

Indications

FDA approved for the treatment of hypercalcemia of malignancy, and for treatment of patients with osteolytic bone metastases due to breast cancer, multiple myeloma, and Paget's disease. It may also be useful for other bone-resorptive diseases.

Classification and Mechanisms of Action

Pamidronate is a biphosphonate that inhibits bone resorption. The drug exerts its actions through its effects on osteoclast precursors, possibly by adsorption of the drug to hydroxyapatite crystals in bone. The drug also inhibits parathyroid hormone-induced bone resorption.

Pharmacokinetics

Pamidronate is poorly absorbed (1% to 5%) after oral administration. In animals the drug is widely distributed throughout the body, primarily to bone, spleen, and liver. Pamidronate has an elimination half-life of 27 hours, and approximately 50% is eliminated unchanged in the urine.

Dose

For hypercalcemia of malignancy. In conjunction with vigorous saline hydration for the treatment of hypercalcemia, pamidronate is given at a dose of 60 to 90 mg. The drug should be administered by IV infusion, in 1,000 mL of 5% dextrose, normal saline, or 0.45% NaCl over a 4- (60-mg dose) to 24-hour (90-mg dose) period. Others have recommended that pamidronate (90 mg/500 mL maximum concentration) be administered at a rate no greater than 15 mg/hour. The drug has been given over a 1- to 4-hour period (60 mg/hour maximum). If retreatment is necessary, it is recommended that at least 7 days elapse from the time of the initial dose. The manufacturer recommends a dose of 60 to 90 mg for moderate hypercalcemia (serum calcium corrected for albumin, 12 to 13.5 mg/dL) and a starting dose of 90 mg for severe hypercalcemia (serum calcium corrected for albumin, greater than 13.5 mg/dL). (Corrected serum calcium (mg/dL) = measured serum calcium in mg/dL + 0.8 × [4.0 − serum albumin in g/dL].)

For osteolytic bone metastases. Multiple myeloma: 90 mg/month administered in 500 mL of 5% dextrose, normal saline, or 0.45% NaCl over 4 hours.

Breast cancer. 90 mg in 250 mL of 5% dextrose, normal saline, or 0.45% NaCl over 2 hours; repeated every 3 to 4 weeks.

For Paget's disease. The recommended dose is 30 mg/day in 500 mL of 5% dextrose, normal saline, or 0.45% NaCl for 3 days. Monitor renal function regularly.

PAMIDRONATE *(continued)*

Administration

Pamidronate is administered as an IV infusion in 1,000, 500, or 250 mL of 5% dextrose, normal saline, or 0.45% NaCl over 2 to 24 hours depending upon the indication for use.

Toxicity

Hematological. Anemia, leukopenia, and thrombocytopenia (rare).

Gastrointestinal. Nausea, vomiting, abdominal pain (2%), anorexia (1% to 12%), constipation (up to 6%), gastrointestinal hemorrhage (up to 6%).

Neurological. Insomnia (1% to 2%), somnolence (1% to 6%), abnormal vision (2%), psychosis (0% to 4%), headache, seizures.

Cardiovascular. Atrial fibrillation, hypertension, syncope, and tachycardia have been reported in up to 6% of patients treated with pamidronate, 90 mg.

Pulmonary. Upper respiratory infection (2%), rales (up to 6%).

Electrolyte. Hypocalcemia (2% to 12%), hypokalemia (4% to 18%), hypomagnesemia (4% to 12%), hypophosphatemia (9% to 18%).

Other. Fatigue (12% with 90-mg dose), fever (18% to 50%), infusion site reaction (4% to 18%), hypothyroidism (6% with 90-mg dose), generalized pain (15%), bone pain (15%), uveitis, scleritis, iritis.

Drug Interactions

Concomitant use of vitamin D may antagonize the effects of pamidronate and should be avoided.

Storage and Stability

Pamidronate is stored at room temperature. Vials bear expiration dates. Reconstituted solutions (30 mg/10 mL) are stable for at least 24 hours in the refrigerator. Further diluted (30 to 90 mg in 1,000 mL of 5% dextrose, normal saline, or 0.45% NaCl), pamidronate is stable for at least 24 hours at room or refrigeration temperatures.

Preparation

Add 10 mL of sterile water to the 30- or 90-mg vial to yield concentrations of 3 or 9 mg/mL, respectively.

Incompatibilities

Pamidronate is incompatible with calcium-containing solutions, such as Ringer's solution.

Availability

Pamidronate is commercially available as a lyophilized powder in 30- and 90-mg vials. Vials contain mannitol.

PEMETREXED DISODIUM

Other names

Alimta®; MTA; LY231514; NSC-698037.

Indications

Pemetrexed is an investigational agent undergoing evaluation for the treatment of malignant mesothelioma, non-small-cell lung cancer, breast cancer, and other malignancies. The drug has been evaluated in combination with cisplatin, gemcitabine, carboplatin, and other drugs.

Classification and Mechanisms of Action
Pemetrexed is a multitargeted antifolate drug. Pemetrexed inhibits several folate-dependent enzymes, including thymidylate synthase, dihydrofolate reductase, and glycinamide ribonucleotide formyltransferase.

Pharmacokinetics
Pemetrexed clearance occurs primarily (80% to 90%) via the urine. Creatinine clearance has been shown to correlate with the clearance of pemetrexed. However, doses of 500 mg/m^2 have been safely administered to patients with mild renal dysfunction (i.e., GFR ≥ 40 mL/minute). The elimination half-life is approximately 20 hours.

Dose
The maximum tolerated doses of pemetrexed are 500 to 600 mg/m^2 every 3 weeks; 4 mg/m^2/day × 5 days repeated every 3 weeks; and 40 mg/m^2/week × 4 weeks. Pemetrexed has been used in combination with other drugs. Some of these regimens are:

- Pemetrexed 500 mg/m^2 and cisplatin 75 mg/m^2, repeated every 3 weeks.
- Pemetrexed 500 mg/m^2 and carboplatin, AUC = 5, repeated every 3 weeks.
- Gemcitabine 1,250 mg/m^2 on days 1 and 8, pemetrexed 500 mg/m^2 on day 8, repeated every 3 weeks.
- Pemetrexed 500 mg/m^2 over 30 minutes followed by oxaliplatin 120 mg/m^2, repeated every 3 weeks.

Administration
Pemetrexed is administered IV over 10 to 30 minutes.

Toxicity
Hematological. Neutropenia (grade 3–4) is dose-limiting and occurs in approximately 40% of patients administered a dose of 500 mg/m^2 every 3 weeks. Thrombocytopenia (grade 3–4) and anemia (grade 3) occur in approximately 5% of patients who received 500 mg/m^2 every 3 weeks. Anemia (grade 2) occurs in approximately 30% of patients.
Gastrointestinal. Stomatitis (up to 17% grade 3), diarrhea (3% grade 2), anorexia (6%), nausea (30% grade 1), vomiting (less than 10% grade 1).
Dermatological. A diffuse erythematous maculopapular skin rash is occasionally severe. The rash has a primarily truncal distribution. Prophylactic administration of dexamethasone, 4 mg twice daily, for 3 days prior to subsequent doses of pemetrexed may prevent or lead to improvement. With dexamethasone prophylaxis, skin rash (grade 1–2) is reported to occur in approximately 20% of patients.
Hepatic. Transient, grade 1 to 2 elevations of transaminase levels occur in up to 70% of patients. Recovery to baseline transaminase levels usually occurs between treatment cycles. Hyperbilirubinemia (grade 2–3) has been reported in approximately 5% of patients.
Other. Grade 3 fatigue has been reported in approximately 8% of patients receiving pemetrexed.

Nutritional status has been correlated with life-threatening hematological and nonhematological (e.g., mucositis, diarrhea) toxicity. Vitamin supplementation with folic acid 350 to 1,000 microg/day and vitamin B12, 1,000 microg every 9 weeks, has been shown to decrease the incidence of grade 4 hematological and grade 3 to 4 nonhematological toxicities from 37% to approximately 6%.

PEMETREXED DISODIUM *(continued)*

Storage and Stability

Reconstituted solutions are chemically stable for at least 72 hours at room and refrigeration temperatures.

Preparation

Add 10 mL normal saline to the 100-mg vial to yield a concentration of 10 mg/mL.

Availability

Pemetrexed is an investigational agent in the United States that is available as a lyophilized powder (100 mg/vial) from the manufacturer or the National Cancer Institute.

Selected Readings

Curtin NJ, Hughes AN. Pemetrexed disodium, a novel antifolate with multiple targets. Lancet May 2: 298–306, 2001.

Fizazi K, John WJ, Vogelzang NJ. The emerging role of antifolates in the treatment of malignant pleural mesothelioma. Semin Oncol 29: 77–81, 2002.

PENTOSTATIN

Other names

Nipent®; 2′-deoxycoformycin; dCF; co-vidarabine; NSC-218321.

Indications

FDA approved for the treatment of hairy-cell leukemia in patients whose disease is no longer controlled by interferon alfa. Pentostatin may also be useful in the treatment of non-Hodgkin's lymphoma and cutaneous T-cell lymphoma.

Classification and Mechanisms of Action

Antimetabolite (adenosine deaminase inhibitor).

Pharmacokinetics

Approximately 4% of pentostatin is bound to plasma proteins. The majority of pentostatin is excreted unchanged in the urine. The plasma elimination half-life of pentostatin in patients with normal renal function (i.e., creatinine clearance of 60 mL/minute or better) is 5 to 6 hours. In patients with impaired renal function (i.e., creatinine clearance less than 50 mL/minute) the elimination half-life may exceed 18 hours. High levels of deoxyadenosine can accumulate in the blood and brain. Urinary deoxyadenosine may exceed solubility in patients with sensitive neoplasms, such as acute lymphoblastic leukemia, unless a forced diuresis is arranged.

Dose

A common regimen is 4 mg/m^2 every 2 weeks. Dose modification may be necessary for renal dysfunction exhibited by a creatinine clearance less than 60 mL/minute.

Administration

Pentostatin is usually administered by IV bolus over 5 minutes or further diluted in 25 to 50 mL of 5% dextrose or normal saline and administered as an IV infusion over a 20-minute or longer period. The final diluted concentration should be 0.18 to 0.33 mg/mL. It is recommended that a total of 1,000 to 2,000 mL of 5% dextrose/0.45% NaCl hydration be given prior to and following each treatment.

Toxicity

Hematological. Severe leukopenia and lymphopenia occur commonly and can lead to serious infection. Thrombocytopenia and anemia are common (32% to 35%).

Gastrointestinal. Nausea (up to 63%) and vomiting are not usually severe. Stomatitis (3% to 10%), diarrhea (15%), anorexia (16%), and altered taste are infrequent toxicities.

Dermatological. Skin rashes occur in up to 26% of patients, may be severe, and worsen with continued therapy. Other dermatological toxicities include dry skin (3% to 17%), diaphoresis (3% to 10%), pruritus, skin discoloration, seborrhea, and eczema.

Hepatic. Elevated hepatic transaminase levels (19%), hepatitis (rare), hyper-bilirubinemia.

Neurological. In phase I studies, neurological toxicities were often dose-limiting. Neurological toxicities observed in these studies included lassitude, confusion, headache, fatigue, insomnia, expressive aphasia, slurred speech, depression, hallucinations, agitation, cerebral edema, seizures, and coma. The more severe toxicities rarely occur with conventional doses (i.e., 4 mg/m^2 every 2 weeks).

Pulmonary. Cough (17%). Shortness of breath, respiratory insufficiency, and/or pulmonary infiltrates on chest radiographs are all rare.

Renal. Elevated serum creatinine, acute tubular necrosis, hematuria, dysuria, and renal failure are uncommon.

Other. Keratoconjunctivitis, photophobia, fever (42%), chills (11%), arthralgia, myalgia (11%).

Drug Interactions

Allopurinol may increase pentostatin toxicity.

Combined treatment with pentostatin and fludarabine is contraindicated because of the increased risk of fatal pulmonary toxicity.

Pentostatin enhances the effects of vidarabine and is not recommended because of the increased risk of toxicity of both agents.

Storage and Stability

Pentostatin vials are stored in the refrigerator. Each vial bears an expiration date. Reconstituted solutions (2 mg/mL) are chemically stable for 72 and 96 hours at room and refrigeration temperatures, respectively. The manufacturer recommends discarding unused reconstituted solutions after 8 hours, due to lack of preservative. Dilute solutions (10 mg/500 mL) are chemically stable at room temperature for 24 hours in 5% dextrose and 48 hours in normal saline or lactated Ringer's solution.

Preparation

The 10-mg vial is reconstituted with 5 mL of sterile water or normal saline to yield a 2 mg/mL solution. The desired dose is further diluted to concentrations of 1 mg/mL or less in normal saline, lactated Ringer's solution, or 5% dextrose.

Availability

Pentostatin, 10 mg/vial, is commercially available as a lyophilized powder.

Selected Reading

Flinn IW et al. Long-term follow-up of remission duration, mortality, and second malignancies in hairy cell leukemia patients treated with pentostatin. Blood 96: 2981–2985, 2001.

PLICAMYCIN

Other names
Mithracin®; mithramycin; NSC-24559.

Indications
FDA approved for the treatment of malignant tumors of the testis and hypercalcemia and hypercalcuria associated with a variety of advanced neoplasms. Plicamycin may be useful in the treatment of chronic myelogenous leukemia in blast crisis.

Classification
Antitumor antibiotic.

Pharmacokinetics
Plicamycin is not well absorbed by mouth. After IV administration the drug predominately distributes to the liver, kidney, bone, and cerebrospinal fluid. Plicamycin is liver metabolized, and approximately 25% to 40% is eliminated unchanged in the urine. Plicamycin has an elimination half-life of approximately 2 hours.

Dose
For the treatment of testicular cancer, doses of 25 to 30 microg/kg/day for 8 to 10 days have been given. For the treatment of hypercalcemia of malignancy, doses of 25 to 30 microg/kg may be administered 1 to 3 times a week. Dose must be adjusted for creatinine clearance less than 60 mL/minute. In hypercalcemic patients with hepatic dysfunction the recommended dose is 12 microg/kg. Use ideal body weight in the presence of edema.

Administration
Plicamycin is administered by slow IV infusion (in 100 to 500 mL of normal saline or 5% dextrose) over a 30- to 60-minute or longer period (usually over 4 to 6 hours).

Toxicity
Hematological. Leukopenia and anemia occur infrequently. Thrombocytopenia (nadir 5 to 10 days) and hemorrhage occur more frequently and are dose-related. Bleeding episodes occur approximately 12% of the time and are fatal in up to 6% of patients who receive doses greater than 30 microg/kg/day and/or receive more than 10 doses. Facial flushing, epistaxis, and prolonged prothrombin time are frequent signs of this toxicity. Treatment should be withheld if any of these signs are present. An alternate-day schedule instead of daily dosing reduces the incidence of bleeding problems.
Gastrointestinal. Nausea and vomiting (more common with rapid IV infusion), anorexia, stomatitis, diarrhea.
Dermatological. Skin and soft-tissue damage (cellulitis, phlebitis) if extravasated, hyperpigmentation, toxic epidermal necrolysis, acneiform skin rash.
Hepatic. Elevated hepatic transaminase levels, hyperbilirubinemia.
Neurological. Headache, depression, dizziness, nervousness, drowsiness.
Renal. Proteinuria, azotemia, elevated serum creatinine levels.
Electrolyte. Hypocalcemia, hypophosphatemia, hypokalemia, hypomagnesemia, rebound hypercalcemia on discontinuation of treatment.
Other. Fever, weakness, fatigue, lethargy, periorbital pallor.

Drug Interactions
Plicamycin, administered concomitantly with calcitonin, may cause clinically significant hypocalcemia.

Storage and Stability

Unreconstituted drug should be stored in the refrigerator. Unreconstituted plicamycin is stable for 3 months at room temperature. At a concentration of 500 microg/mL, the drug is chemically stable for at least 24 and 48 hours at room and refrigeration temperatures, respectively. After dilution in 5% dextrose or normal saline to a concentration of 24 microg/mL, plicamycin is stable for at least 24 hours at room temperature.

Preparation

The 2,500-microg (2.5-mg) vial is reconstituted with 4.9 mL of sterile water to yield a 500 microg/mL (0.5 mg/mL) solution. The desired dose of plicamycin is usually further diluted in 100 to 500 mL of normal saline or 5% dextrose.

Incompatibilities

Cellulose ester filters, iron, trace element solutions.

Availability

Plicamycin is commercially available as a lyophilized powder in 2,500-microg (2.5-mg) vials.

PREDNISONE

Other names

Deltasone®; Orasone®; Meticorten®; Panasol-S®; Liquid Pred; deltacortisone; and others; NSC-10023.

Indications

FDA approved indications include the treatment of endocrine disorders (adrenocortical insufficiency, hypercalcemia of malignancy, nonsuppurative thyroiditis), rheumatic disorders (rheumatoid arthritis, psoriatic arthritis, ankylosing spondylitis, bursitis, gouty arthritis, osteoarthritis, epicondylitis), collagen diseases (lupus, polymyositis), dermatological diseases (pemphigus, erythema multiforme, mycosis fungoides, psoriasis, seborrheic dermatitis), ophthalmic diseases (severe acute and chronic allergic and inflammatory processes), respiratory diseases (sarcoidosis, Löeffler's syndrome, berylliosis, aspiration pneumonitis), hematological disorders (idiopathic thrombocytopenic purpura [ITP] in adults, secondary thrombocytopenia in adults, hemolytic anemia, erythroblastopenia, congenital hypoplastic anemia), neoplastic diseases (leukemias and lymphomas in adults, acute leukemia of childhood), edematous states, gastrointestinal disorders (ulcerative colitis, regional enteritis), acute exacerbations of multiple sclerosis, tuberculous meningitis, and trichinosis with neurological or myocardial involvement.

Classification and Mechanisms of Action

Prednisone is a potent synthetic glucocorticoid. It has anti-inflammatory, immuno-suppressant, minimal mineralocorticoid activity and antineoplastic properties. As an antineoplastic agent, prednisone may bind to specific proteins (receptors) within the cell, forming a steroid-receptor complex. Binding of the receptor-steroid complex with nuclear chromatin alters mRNA and protein synthesis within the cell.

Pharmacokinetics

Approximately 80% of a dose is absorbed by mouth and 75% of the drug is bound to plasma proteins. Prednisone is metabolized by the liver and has an elimination half-life of 3.5 hours.

PREDNISONE *(continued)*

Dose

Common regimens include:

- 40 mg/m^2/day for 14 days, repeated every 28 days
- 20 mg/m^2/day for 7 days
- 100 mg/m^2/day for 5 days, repeated every 3 to 4 weeks.

Dosing is specific to the disease and combination of antineoplastic drugs being used. A dose taper is required if patients have been on chronic therapy.

Administration

Orally, in the morning with food.

Toxicity

Hematological. Leukocytosis, thrombocytosis.

Gastrointestinal. Nausea, vomiting, anorexia, increased appetite, weight gain, pancreatitis, aggravation of peptic ulcers, peptic ulceration.

Dermatological. Rash, skin atrophy, hirsutism, acne, facial erythema, ecchymoses, poor wound healing.

Neurological. Insomnia, muscle weakness, euphoria, psychosis, depression, headache, vertigo, seizures.

Cardiovascular. Fluid retention and edema, hypertension, thromboembolism.

Genitourinary. Menstrual changes (amenorrhea, menstrual irregularities).

Ocular. Cataracts, increased intraocular pressure, exophthalmos.

Metabolic. Hyperglycemia, decreased glucose tolerance, aggravation or precipitation of diabetes mellitus, adrenal suppression (with Cushingoid features), hypokalemia, sodium retention, hypokalemia.

Other. Osteoporosis (and resulting back pain), serious infections (including herpes zoster, varicella zoster, fungal infections, *Pneumocystis carinii* pneumonia, tuberculosis), muscle wasting, aseptic necrosis of femoral head, suppression of reactions to skin tests.

Drug Interactions

The metabolism of prednisone may be reduced by agents that inhibit the cytochrome P450 enzymes. These agents include, but are not limited to, itraconazole, calcium channer blockers, cimetidine, and macrolides. Dose adjustments may be necessary or the toxicity of prednisone may increase if this inhibition occurs.

The metabolism of prednisone may be increased by agents that induce the cytochrome P450 enzymes. These agents include, but are not limited to, phenytoin, rifampin, and phenobarbital. The concentrations and efficacy of prednisone may decrease if this inhibition occurs and dose adjustments may be necessary.

Prednisone administered concomitantly with nonsteroidal anti-inflammatory agents may increase the risk of gastrointestinal toxicity.

Storage and Stability

Prednisone is stored at room temperature. Each bottle bears an expiration date.

Availability

Commercially available in 1-, 2.5-, 5-, 10-, 20-, 25-, and 50-mg tablets. Also available as a 1 mg/mL oral solution or 1 mg/mL oral syrup and as a 5 mg/mL oral solution.

PROCARBAZINE

Other names
Matulane®; Natulan®; ibenzmethyzin; *N*-methylhydrazine; NSC-77213.

Indications
FDA approved for the treatment of Hodgkin's disease (stages III and IV) as
a part of the Mustargen®-Oncovin®-procarbazine-prednisone (MOPP) regimen.
Procarbazine may also be useful in the treatment of non-Hodgkin's lymphoma,
multiple myeloma, melanoma, brain tumors, lung cancer, and polycythemia vera.

Classification
Alkylating agent.

Pharmacokinetics
Procarbazine is almost completely absorbed after oral administration and reaches peak
plasma concentrations in 1 hour. Procarbazine penetrates into the cerebrospinal fluid,
is metabolized by the liver, and less than 5% is eliminated in the urine as unchanged
drug. Procarbazine has an elimination half-life of approximately 1 hour.

Dose
As a part of the MOPP and C-MOPP (cyclophosphamide-Oncovin®-procarbazine-
prednisone) regimens, procarbazine is given in a dose of 100 mg/m^2/day for 14 days
and repeated every 4 weeks.

As a part of the PCV (procarbazine, lomustine, and vincristine) regimen,
procarbazine is given in a dose of 60 mg/m^2/day for 14 days, days 8 through 21.

Administration
Oral. Administer with food or after a meal.

Toxicity
Hematological. Leukopenia and thrombocytopenia occur frequently, with the nadir up
to 4 weeks after cessation of therapy. Anemia occurs less frequently.
Gastrointestinal. Nausea and vomiting occur commonly and may be dose-limiting.
Antiemetic drugs may be necessary. Anorexia, diarrhea (uncommon), stomatitis
(uncommon), xerostomia, dysphagia, and constipation have been reported.
Dermatological. Skin rash, photosensitivity, urticaria, dermatitis, flushing, alopecia.
Neurological. Paresthesias, lethargy, weakness, dizziness, somnolence, nightmares,
depression, insomnia, headache, visual disturbances, hallucinations, ataxia, nystag-
mus, seizures. Concomitant use with tricyclic antidepressants, opiate analgesics, or
benzodiazepines may lead to enhanced central nervous system toxicities.
Cardiovascular. Hypotension, tachycardia, syncope. Concomitant use with sympathomimetics or foods with high tyramine content may lead to a sudden increase in blood
pressure and hypertensive crisis.
Ocular. Photophobia, diplopia, papilledema, and retinal hemorrhage have been reported.
Other. Urinary frequency, hematuria, nocturia, gynecomastia, sterility, menstrual
irregularities, fever, myalgia, arthralgia, second malignancy, allergic pneumonitis.

Drug/Food Interactions
Concurrent use of drugs and/or foods listed below may result in adverse effects such
as headache, tremor, excitation, cardiac arrhythmia, nausea, vomiting, and visual
disturbances. Procarbazine is a weak monoamine oxidase inhibitor, and this is the
basis for some of the drug interactions listed.

PROCARBAZINE *(continued)*

Drugs. Ethanol, sympathomimetics (e.g., ephedrine, pseudoephedrine, isoproterenol, epinephrine), tricyclic antidepressants (e.g., imipramine, nortriptyline, amitriptyline, desipramine), monoamine oxidase inhibitors (e.g., pargyline), seratonin reuptake inhibitors, opiate analgesics (especially meperidine), antihistamines, phenothiazines, antihypertensive agents, and barbiturates.

Foods. Alcohol and procarbazine may cause a disulfuram-like reaction. Tyramine-rich foods (imported beer, fermented cheese, smoked meats or salami, some wines, yogurt, bananas), chocolate, and fava beans should be avoided.

Storage and Stability

Procarbazine is stored at room temperature; containers bear expiration dates.

Availability

Procarbazine is commercially available in 50-mg capsules.

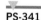

PS-341

Other names

Bortezomib; Velcade®; MLN341; NSC-681239.

Indications

PS-341 is an investigational agent in the United States. The drug may be effective in patients with multiple myeloma, renal cell cancer, prostate cancer, and other malignancies.

Classification and Mechanisms of Action

PS-341 is a proteasome inhibitor. The drug induces apoptosis in cells that overexpress Bcl-2. PS-341 also has antiangiogenesis properties, inhibits interleukin-6-mediated cell growth, and inhibits cellular adhesion molecules.

Pharmacokinetics

PS-341 has linear pharmacokinetics. The drug is rapidly distributed following IV injection. The elimination half-life is approximately 8 hours. The inhibition of proteasomes lasts approximately 72 hours following administration.

Dose

PS-341 is administered at a dose of 1.3 mg/m^2 on days 1, 4, 8, and 11 (i.e., twice weekly × 2 weeks) followed by 10 days of no treatment. A 72-hour interval between doses is required. PS-341 has also been administered at a dose of 1.04 mg/m^2/dose twice weekly for 4 weeks followed by 2 weeks of no treatment. The manufacturer recommends that doses be calculated using actual body weight (i.e., no modifications for obese patients).

PS-341 1 mg/m^2/dose twice weekly for 4 weeks has been evaluated in combination with 5-fluorouracil 500 mg/m^2 and leucovorin 20 mg/m^2 administered weekly for 4 consecutive weeks of a 6-week cycle.

PS-341 1 mg/m^2/dose twice weekly for 2 consecutive weeks and gemcitabine 1,000 mg/m^2/dose weekly for 2 consecutive weeks has been evaluated.

Administration

PS-341 is administered by rapid IV push (usually into a running IV over 3 to 5 seconds).

Toxicity

Hematological. Neutropenia (5% grade 3), thrombocytopenia (15% to 40% grade 3), anemia.

Gastrointestinal. Diarrhea was a dose-limiting toxicity in phase I studies of PS-341. Nausea, vomiting, anorexia, and abdominal cramps have been reported. Reversible ileus has been reported (i.e., resolution occurred within 24 hours without the need for surgery).

Neurological. Peripheral neuropathy was a dose-limiting toxicity in phase I studies of PS-341 (3% grade 3). Peripheral neuropathy, which may be painful, usually appeared during the first or second course of therapy. Dizziness and headache have been reported.

Cardiovascular. Orthostatic hypotension, atrial flutter, hypertension.

Pulmonary. Dyspnea has been reported.

Other. Fatigue, fever (5% grade 3), arthralgia, myalgia, conjunctivitis.

Storage and Stability

Intact vials of PS-341 are stored at refrigeration temperatures. Although reconstituted solutions are stable at room temperature for at least 43 hours, the National Cancer Institute recommends that the dose be administered within 8 hours of preparation.

Preparation

Reconstitute the 3.5-mg vial with 3.5 mL of normal saline to yield a concentration of 1 mg/mL.

Availability

PS-341 is an investigational agent in the United States that is available as an injectable solution (3.5 mg/vial) from the manufacturer or the National Cancer Institute.

Selected Readings

Adams J. Proteasome inhibition in cancer: development of PS-341. Semin Oncol 28: 613–619, 2001.

Teicher BA et al. The proteasome inhibitor PS-341 in cancer therapy. Clin Cancer Res 5: 2683–2685, 1999.

RALTITREXED

Other names

Tomudex®; ZD1694; NSC-639186.

Indications

Raltitrexed is an investigational agent in the United States. In Canada, Europe, and Australia it is approved for the treatment of patients with metastatic or advanced colorectal cancer. Raltitrexed also has activity in non-small-cell lung cancer, esophageal cancer, head and neck cancers, and other malignancies.

Classification and Mechanisms of Action

Raltitrexed is a thymidylate synthase inhibitor. Thymidylate synthase is a key enzyme in the synthesis of thymidine triphosphate, a nucleotide required for DNA synthesis.

Pharmacokinetics

Raltitrexed exhibits a triexponential pattern of elimination after IV administration. The beta half-life ranges from approximately 1 to 3 hours; the elimination half-life varies

RALTITREXED (continued)

widely, from 8 to 105 hours. The drug does not appear to accumulate with repeated administration. Approximately 40% to 50% of the drug is eliminated unchanged in the urine.

Dose

Raltitrexed has been administered as a single agent at a dose of 3 mg/m^2 every 3 weeks. The combination of irinotecan and raltitrexed has been evaluated. Irinotecan, 350 mg/m^2, is administered on day 1 followed by raltitrexed, 3 mg/m^2, on day 2; both drugs are repeated every 3 weeks.

The combination of raltitrexed and oxaliplatin has been evaluated. Raltitrexed, 3 mg/m^2, is administered 1 hour prior to oxaliplatin, 130 mg/m^2, repeated every 3 weeks.

The combination of raltitrexed and gemcitabine has been evaluated. Raltitrexed, 3 mg/m^2, is administered on day 1, gemcitabine 1,000 mg/m^2 is administered on days 1 and 8, repeated every 3 weeks.

Administration

IV infusion over a 15-minute period or longer, in 50 to 250 mL of normal saline or 5% dextrose and water.

Toxicity

Hematological. Leukopenia is dose-limiting and has occurred in approximately 60% of patients receiving a dose of 3 mg/m^2 every 3 weeks. Approximately one-third of the patients will develop grade 3 to grade 4 nadir leukocyte counts. The nadir leukocyte count occurs around day 8 (range, days 7 to 21) with recovery occurring approximately 10 days later. Thrombocytopenia has been reported to occur in 25% of patients and to be clinically significant in a small percentage of these patients. Thrombocytopenia leading to fatal pulmonary hemorrhage has been reported. Anemia occurs but is rarely clinically significant.

Gastrointestinal. Diarrhea has been dose-limiting in some patients. At a dose of 3 mg/m^2, diarrhea has been reported to occur in 60% of patients, with 26% of patients experiencing severe or life-threatening diarrhea. Severe diarrhea generally occurs 1 week after the second dose but may begin a few days after the dose. Nausea, vomiting, and anorexia have been observed in 35% to 50% of patients who have received doses of 1.6 mg/m^2 or greater. Grade 2 mucositis is observed in approximately 50% of patients who receive raltitrexed at a dose of 3 mg/m^2.

Dermatological. Rash (35%) with pruritus, hair thinning.

Hepatic. Reversible elevations of hepatic transaminase levels occur in approximately 15% of patients. Hyperbilirubinemia has also been observed. In combination with irinotecan 350 mg/m^2 every 3 weeks, doses of raltitrexed in excess of 3 mg/m^2 are associated with dose-limiting elevations of hepatic transaminase levels.

Neurological. Dizziness is uncommon.

Pulmonary. Dyspnea is uncommon.

Other. Dose-limiting malaise may occur in up to 40% of patients receiving raltitrexed at a dose of 3.5 mg/m^2 every 3 weeks. This adverse effect is prolonged in some patients. Fever and flu-like symptoms occur occasionally. Arthralgia and myalgia have been reported.

Storage and Stability

Intact vials are stored at room temperature. Following reconstitution or further dilution in 50 to 250 mL of normal saline or 5% dextrose and water, raltitrexed is stable for at least 24 hours at room temperature. Solutions do not require protection from light.

Preparation
Reconstitute the 2-mg vial with 4 mL of sterile water for injection to yield a concentration of 0.5 mg/mL. The drug may be diluted with 5% dextrose or normal saline.

Availability
Raltitrexed is an investigational agent in the United States that is available from the manufacturer or the National Cancer Institute in 2-mg vials of lyophilized powder.

Selected Reading
Cocconi G et al. Open, randomized, multicenter trial of raltitrexed versus fluorouracil plus high-dose leucovorin in patients with advanced colorectal cancer. Tomudex Colorectal Cancer Study Group. J Clin Oncol 16: 2943–2952, 1998.

RANPIRNASE

Other names
Onconase®; P-30 Protein.

Indications
Ranpirnase is an investigational agent in the United States. It appears to have activity in malignant mesothelioma.

Classification and Mechanisms of Action
Ranpirnase is a ribonuclease protein that is derived from the eggs and embryos of the leopard frog. The drug binds to cell surfaces and degrades tRNA.

Dose
Ranpirnase has been administered at a dose of 480 microg/m^2 weekly. Doses of 960 microg/m^2 weekly are dose-limiting.

Administration
Ranpirnase is administered IV over 30 minutes.

Toxicity
Hematological. Ranpirnase does not appear to have significant hematological effects.
Gastrointestinal. Nausea (grade 3 in 2% of patients), vomiting (infrequent and usually grade 1), and anorexia.
Cardiovascular. Transient hypotension usually preceded by flushing has been observed in a few patients. In each patient volume expansion ameliorated the event. Anaphylactoid reactions with hypotension, flushing, and/or a vasovagal reaction have occurred in a few patients. Administration of a test dose followed by 15 minutes of observation does not appear to be predictive.
Neurological. Paresthesias, dizziness.
Renal. Proteinuria with or without azotemia and peripheral edema is dose-limiting.
Other. Myalgia and arthralgia (grade 3 in 2% to 3% of patients), fatigue, asthenia.

Storage and Stability
Ranpirnase is stored in the freezer.

Preparation
Doses are usually further diluted in 50 to 100 mL of normal saline.

RANPIRNASE (continued)

Availability

Ranpirnase is an investigational agent in the United States that is available in vials (1 mg/2-mL vial) from the manufacturer.

Selected Reading

Mikulski SM et al. Phase II trial of single weekly intravenous dose of ranpirnase in patients with unresectable malignant mesothelioma. J Clin Oncol 20: 274–281, 2002.

STREPTOZOCIN

Other names

Zanosar®; streptozotocin; NSC-85998.

Indications

FDA approved for the treatment of metastatic islet cell carcinoma of the pancreas. Streptozocin may be a useful treatment for carcinoid tumors, Hodgkin's disease, colorectal, liver, and pancreatic carcinoma.

Classification

Alkylating agent.

Pharmacokinetics

Streptozocin is poorly absorbed by mouth. After IV administration, the drug is primarily distributed in the kidneys, pancreas, and liver. Metabolites of streptozocin penetrate the cerebrospinal fluid (CSF), and drug levels in the plasma and CSF are equivalent 2 hours after administration. Streptozocin is extensively metabolized, and 10% to 20% is eliminated in the urine as unchanged drug. Streptozocin has an elimination half-life of 35 to 40 minutes; metabolites of the drug have half-lives of around 40 hours.

Dose

Streptozocin is commonly given every 4 to 6 weeks at a dose of 500 to 1,000 mg/m^2/day for 5 days. Doses of 1,000 to 1,500 mg/m^2/week have also been used. A single daily dose of 1,500 mg/m^2 should not be exceeded because this may increase the likelihood of severe nephrotoxicity. Doses should be reduced if the creatinine clearance is less than 50 mL/minute.

Administration

Streptozocin has been given by IV bolus, but is usually administered by slow IV infusion (in 100 mL or more of normal saline or 5% dextrose), usually over a period of 30 to 60 minutes. The drug has been given as a 5-day continuous IV infusion.

Toxicity

Hematological. Leukopenia and thrombocytopenia are rarely dose-limiting. However, cumulative myelosuppression has been reported. Anemia and eosinophilia occur infrequently.

Gastrointestinal. Nausea and vomiting are common, often severe, and require antiemetic pretreatment. Symptoms begin 1 to 4 hours after administration of the drug. Anorexia, diarrhea, and abdominal cramps occur less frequently.

Hepatic. Mild, transient increases in hepatic enzyme levels occur in approximately 25% of patients. Hypoalbuminemia has also been reported.

Neurological. Confusion, depression, and lethargy are rare and tend to occur most often in patients receiving streptozocin as a continuous 5-day IV infusion.

Renal. Nephrotoxicity in the form of renal tubular damage is common, dose-related, and sometimes irreversible. Early signs include hypophosphatemia, aminoaciduria, and/or proteinuria. Other manifestations may include renal tubular acidosis, Fanconi syndrome, azotemia, acetonuria, acute tubular necrosis, hyperchloremia, decreased creatinine clearance, and nephrogenic diabetes insipidus (rare).

Metabolic. Mild to moderate hyperglycemia, severe hypoglycemia, and insulin shock have been rarely reported in patients with insulinoma.

Other. Fever (rare), vein irritation during administration, second malignancy.

Drug Interactions

Streptozocin used concomitantly with other nephrotoxic drugs can increase the risk of renal toxicity.

Increased glucose levels may occur in patients receiving streptozocin and cortico-steroids concomitantly.

Storage and Stability

Streptozocin is stored in the refrigerator (2° to 8°C) and protected from light. Each vial bears an expiration date. Streptozocin is stable at room temperature for at least 1 year after the date of manufacture. After reconstitution to a concentration of 100 mg/mL and after dilution to a concentration of 2 mg/mL in 5% dextrose or normal saline, the drug is chemically stable for at least 48 hours at room temperature and 96 hours under refrigeration. However, it is recommended that reconstituted solutions be used within 24 hours.

Preparation

The 1,000-mg vial is reconstituted with 9.5 mL of 5% dextrose or normal saline to yield a 100 mg/mL solution. The desired dose may be further diluted in 5% dextrose, normal saline, or 5% dextrose and normal saline.

Availability

Streptozocin, 1,000 mg/vial, is commercially available as a lyophilized powder.

SURAMIN

Other names

Suramin sodium; Antrypol; Metaret®; Bayer 205; Germanin; Moranyl; Naganin; Naphuride; Naganol; Fourneau 309; NSC-34936.

Indications

Suramin is an investigational drug that has been shown to have activity against prostate cancer. Suramin may be a useful treatment for patients with adrenal carcinoma.

Classification and Mechanisms of Action

Suramin is a glycosaminoglycan (GAG) agonist-antagonist and a potent antitrypanoso-mal agent that may inhibit malignant cell growth by binding to growth factors, such as platelet-derived growth factor (PDGF), epidermal growth factor (EGF), transforming growth factor beta (TGF beta), and basic fibroblast growth factor (bFGF). Suramin may also exert antitumor activity by other mechanisms, including inhibition of growth-regulatory proteins (such as transferrin), inhibition of glycosaminoglycan catabolism, and inhibition of DNA polymerases.

SURAMIN *(continued)*

Pharmacokinetics

After IV administration, suramin is almost completely (i.e., 99%) and tightly bound to plasma proteins, primarily albumin. Suramin distributes primarily to the kidneys; 2% is eliminated unchanged in the bile, and the remainder is eliminated in the urine by renal excretion. Suramin has an elimination half-life of 40 to 50 days. Anticonvulsant medications do not affect suramin pharmacokinetics.

Dose

Many different regimens have been evaluated. For prostate cancer the following regimen has been used:

Cycle 1. 1,100 mg/m^2 on day 1, 400 mg/m^2 on day 2, 300 mg/m^2 on day 3, 250 mg/m^2 on day 4, 200 mg/m^2 on day 5, then 275 mg/m^2 on days 8, 11, 15, 19, 22, 29, 36, 43, 50, 57, 64, 71, and 78.

Cycle 2. Begins approximately 12 weeks later and is given as: 750 mg/m^2 on day 1, 400 mg/m^2 on day 2, 300 mg/m^2 on day 3, 250 mg/m^2 on day 4, 200 mg/m^2 on day 5 followed by 275 mg/m^2 on days 8, 11, 15, 19, and 22.

Administration

Suramin has been given by IV bolus and by IV infusion over a period of 1 hour or longer. The drug has also been administered as a continuous IV infusion until the plasma suramin level reaches 250 to 300 microg/mL.

Toxicity

The most significant toxicities (e.g., neurotoxicity) are dose-dependent.

Hematological. Leukopenia (usually mild); thrombocytopenia (may be dose-limiting); elevated thrombin, prothrombin, and partial thromboplastin times; hemorrhage; anemia.

Gastrointestinal. Nausea, vomiting, metallic or salty taste in the mouth, constipation.

Dermatological. Erythematous rash (usually transient), urticaria, pruritus.

Hepatic. Elevated hepatic enzyme levels and hyperbilirubinemia.

Neurological. Paresthesias (distal end of the extremity and perioral); polyradiculo-neuropathy (muscle weakness progressing to generalized flaccid paralysis), with maximum plasma level 386 microg/mL or more.

Renal. Proteinuria, decreased creatinine clearance, elevated serum creatinine levels, hypophosphatemia, hypomagnesemia, hematuria.

Adrenal. Adrenocortical insufficiency (increased adrenocorticotropin [ACTH] and plasma renin concentrations, decreased serum cortisol level, lack of response to ACTH stimulation).

Ocular. Vortex keratopathy, with lacrimation, photophobia, and blurred vision.

Other. Fever, malaise, and lethargy (often severe); hypocalcemia, pericardial effusion (rare).

Storage and Stability

Intact vials are stored at room temperature. At concentrations of 2, 10, and 20 mg/mL in normal saline (PVC containers), the drug is chemically stable for at least 21 days at room temperature. At a concentration of 8 mg/mL in 5% dextrose in Deltec cassette reservoirs, suramin is stable for 3 weeks at 4°C and 20°C.

Preparation

The 1,000-mg vial is reconstituted with 10 mL of sterile water to yield a 100 mg/mL solution. The desired dose is further diluted to concentrations of 2 to 10 mg/mL in normal saline or 5% dextrose.

Availability

Suramin is an investigational drug that is available as a lyophilized powder from the National Cancer Institute in 1,000-mg vials.

Selected Reading

Stein CA, LaRocca R, Myers C. Suramin: an old compound with new biology. In DeVita VT Jr, Hellman S, Rosenberg SA, eds. Principles and Practice of Oncology. PPO Updates 4: 1–12, 1990.

TAMOXIFEN

Other names

Nolvadex®; tamoxifen citrate; Alpha-Tamoxifen®; Med Tamoxifen®; Nolvadex-D®; Novo-Tamoxifen®; Tamofen®; Tamone®; Tamoplex®; NSC-180973.

Indications

FDA approved for the treatment of breast cancer in an adjuvant setting after initial surgical and/or radiation treatment. Tamoxifen is also approved for the treatment of metastatic breast cancer, and the prevention of breast cancer in the high-risk female population. The drug may be a useful treatment for mastalgia, gynecomastia, malignant melanoma, and cancers of the pancreas, endometrium, and liver.

Classification and Mechanisms of Action

Tamoxifen is a hormone antagonist (antiestrogen). Tamoxifen and its metabolites possess antiestrogenic activity as a result of their ability to compete with estradiol for binding to receptors in the cells of tumors that contain high amounts of estrogen receptors (such as breast cancer). The tamoxifen-estrogen receptor complex is translocated from the cytoplasm of cancer cells to the nucleus, where it reduces DNA synthesis and cellular responses to estrogen. Tamoxifen also has weak estrogenic properties.

Pharmacokinetics

Tamoxifen is well absorbed following oral administration, reaching peak serum concentrations in 3 to 6 hours. Tamoxifen is metabolized by the liver to several metabolites; the major one is *N*-desmethyltamoxifen. With continued dosing, serum concentrations of *N*-desmethyltamoxifen often exceed those of tamoxifen by twofold. Negligible amounts of *N*-desmethyltamoxifen and unchanged tamoxifen are excreted in the bile or urine. Tamoxifen and *N*-desmethyltamoxifen have elimination half-lives of approximately 7 and 14 days, respectively.

Dose

The usual dose is 10 mg twice daily. Once-daily doses (20 mg) may also be used. For breast cancer prevention and as adjuvant therapy, the dose is 20 mg per day for 5 years. There is no data to support use for a period of time exceeding 5 years.

Administration

Oral.

TAMOXIFEN *(continued)*

Toxicity

Hematological. Thrombocytopenia is usually mild and transient. Leukopenia and anemia are infrequent (5% to 10%).

Gastrointestinal. Nausea (5% to 25%), vomiting, and anorexia occur occasionally and are rarely dose-limiting. Diarrhea or constipation occurs infrequently.

Dermatological. Rash and erythema are uncommon. Mild hair loss has been reported.

Hepatic. Increased hepatic enzyme levels and cholestasis are rare. A few cases of severe hepatotoxicity (fatty liver, hepatitis, cholestasis, hepatic necrosis) have been reported.

Neurological. Depression, dizziness, light-headedness, headache, confusion, lassitude, and/or syncope are uncommon.

Cardiovascular. Hot flushes are the most common side effect (25% to 32% incidence). Thrombophlebitis, thromboembolism, pulmonary embolism, fluid retention, and edema are infrequent toxicities.

Genitourinary. Vaginal bleeding or discharge, amenorrhea (16%), menstrual irregularities (12%), pruritus vulvae, and endometriosis are infrequent toxicities.

Secondary malignancy. The long-term use (> 2 years) of tamoxifen increases the risk of developing endometrial cancer. Yearly gynecological pelvic examinations are recommended for patients on tamoxifen therapy.

Ocular. Retinopathy, decreased visual acuity, cataracts, optic neuritis, and/or corneal opacity are rare with conventional doses.

Other. Tumor "flare" may occur in the first month of therapy, manifested as an increase in tumor-related symptoms, such as bone pain (sometimes accompanied with hypercalcemia), increase in tumor size, and/or erythema. This reaction subsides quickly. Increased thyroxine concentrations occur rarely.

Drug Interactions

Phenobarbital may decrease and bromocriptine may increase serum concentrations of tamoxifen.

Tamoxifen may potentiate the anticoagulant effects of warfarin, through a potential liver enzyme inhibition. Case reports have demonstrated a significant increase in PT (1.5–2×) in patients who have been stabilized on warfarin and begin tamoxifen therapy. In one patient taking warfarin 3 days after beginning tamoxifen, 10 mg twice daily, the prothrombin time (PT) was 39 seconds (baseline is 34 seconds). Three weeks later the PT was 206 seconds. A 40% decrease in the dose of warfarin was required to maintain the baseline PT.

Aminoglutethimide may decrease serum concentrations of tamoxifen and potentially reduce its effectiveness.

Storage and Stability

Tamoxifen is stored at room temperature; containers bear expiration dates.

Availability

Tamoxifen is commercially available in 10- and 20-mg tablets.

Selected Readings

Fisher B et al. A randomized clinical trial evaluating tamoxifen in the treatment of patients with node-negative breast cancer who have estrogen-receptor-positive tumors. N Engl J Med 320: 479–484, 1989.

Fisher B et al. Endometrial cancer in tamoxifen-treated breast cancer patients: findings from the National Surgical Adjuvant Breast and Bowel Project (NSABP) B-14. J Natl Cancer Inst 86: 527–537, 1994.

Nayfield SG et al. Potential role of tamoxifen in prevention of breast cancer. J Natl Cancer Inst 83: 1450–1459, 1991.

TEGAFUR

Other names
Ftorafur (Ftegafur alone); UFT; Uftoral® and Orzel® (uracil combined with tegafur).

Indications
UFT (uracil and tegafur) is an investigational agent in the United States. UFT combined with leucovorin is approved in Canada, the United Kingdom, Japan, and other countries, primarily for the treatment of patients with advanced colorectal cancer. UFT plus leucovorin has activity in other cancers for which fluorinated pyrimidines are a useful treatment.

Classification
Pyrimidine antimetabolite.

Pharmacokinetics
Tegafur is metabolized to 5-fluorouracil after administration. Peak serum levels of 5-fluorouracil occur approximately one hour after oral administration of tegafur.

Dose
Doses are calculated based upon the tegafur component of UFT. UFT has been administered at a dose of 300 mg/m^2/day for 28 days followed by 7 days of rest. This 5-week cycle is repeated until the patient no longer benefits from the therapy. Daily doses are calculated, rounded up or down to the nearest 100 mg, and each daily dose is divided into three equal parts taken approximately every 8 hours. UFT is most often administered with oral leucovorin, 90 mg/day, in three divided doses.

Administration
Oral.

Toxicity
Hematological. Leukopenia and thrombocytopenia are uncommon (less than 3% incidence of severe myelosuppression). Anemia has been reported to occur rarely in studies conducted in Japan.
Gastrointestinal. Diarrhea (10%) and abdominal cramps (3%) are dose-related and are the most common adverse effects. Nausea, vomiting (5%), and anorexia occasionally occur. Hemorrhagic enteritis, mucositis, and pancreatitis have been reported.
Dermatological. Rash or itching occur infrequently; urticaria (rare).
Hepatic. With prolonged use, elevations of liver enzyme levels may occur and be dose-limiting. Fulminant hepatitis has rarely been reported.
Neurological. Headache, malaise, or vertigo (rare). Leukoencephalopathy has been reported in patients receiving UFT in Japan.
Pulmonary. Interstitial pneumonia has been rarely observed in patients receiving UFT in Japan.
Renal. Proteinuria or hematuria (rare).
Other. Fatigue (5%); fever, arthralgia, or glycosuria (rare).

Drug Interactions
Tegafur and other fluorinated pyrimidines adversely interact with halogenated antiviral agents (e.g., sorivudine, netivudine). The catabolism of the fluorinated pyrimidine is inhibited, and life-threatening myelosuppression may occur. Deaths have been

reported when tegafur or 5-fluorouracil has been administered to patients receiving sorivudine or netivudine.

TEGAFUR *(continued)*

Storage and Stability

Capsules are stored at room temperature; containers bear expiration dates.

Availability

UFT is an investigational drug in the United States. In the United States and in countries where the drug is approved it is available from the manufacturer in capsules for oral administration. Each capsule contains 100 mg of tegafur and 224 mg of uracil.

Selected Reading

Pazdur R et al. Phase II trial of uracil and tegafur plus oral leucovorin: an effective oral regimen in the treatment of metastatic colorectal carcinoma. J Clin Oncol 12: 2296–2300, 1994.

TEMOZOLOMIDE

Other names

Temodar®; methozolastone; CCRG 81045; SCH 52365; NSC-362856.

Indications

Temozolomide is FDA approved for refractory anaplastic astrocytomas. It may also be useful for patients with types of brain tumors, melanoma, and other malignancies.

Classification and Mechanisms of Action

An imidazotetrazine derivative of mitozolomide, also related to dacarbazine (DTIC). Temozolomide is an alkylating agent. It is a prodrug whose active metabolite – monomethyl triazenoimidazole carboxamide (MTIC) – is formed by chemical degradation at physiological pH.

Dose

The initial dose is 150 mg/m^2/day for 5 consecutive days (total dose of 750 mg/m^2) with the intent to titrate up to 200 mg/m^2/day for 5 consecutive days (total dose of 1,000 mg/m^2). Doses need to be rounded to the nearest 5 mg to accommodate for capsule strength. Treatment cycles have been repeated every 28 days, and continued until disease progression is evident.

Administration

Oral. Temozolomide may be taken with or without food; however, it should be taken the same time each day with regard to meals. It is known that food minimally decreases the rate and extent of absorption. To lessen nausea associated with this drug take the capsules at bedtime or on an empty stomach. The capsules should not be crushed, chewed, opened, or dissolved.

Toxicity

Hematological. Leukopenia, lymphopenia, thrombocytopenia, and anemia usually occur 2 to 8 weeks after the start of treatment, and are dose-limiting.
Gastrointestinal. Nausea; vomiting is usually preventable and limited to the first day of treatment. Constipation, anorexia, diarrhea, and stomatitis have been reported.
Dermatological. Alopecia (usually mild to moderate), skin rash, and pruritus have been reported.
...tic. Elevation of hepatic enzyme levels is uncommon and usually mild.

Neurological. Headache, fatigue, and seizures are most common. Lethargy, insomnia, dizziness, parathesias, and weakness are less common.

Other. Hyperglycemia, impaired renal function, fever, back pain, peripheral edema.

Drug Interactions

Temozolomide administered concomitantly with valproic acid may reduce the clearance of temozolomide by approximately 5%.

Storage and Stability

Temozolomide capsules should be stored at room temperature in the original packaging and should be protected from moisture. Medication should be dispensed to patients in amber plastic containers. Each bottle bears an expiration date.

Availability

Temozolomide is commercially available in 5-, 20-, 100-, and 250-mg capsules.

Selected Reading

Yung WKA et al. A phase II study of temozolomide vs procarbazine in patients with glioblastoma multiforme at first relapse. Br J Cancer 83: 588–593, 2000.

TENIPOSIDE

Other names

Vumon®; VM-26; PTG; thenylidene-lignan-P; NSC-122819.

Indications

FDA approved for the treatment of children with relapsed or refractory acute lymphoblastic leukemia (in combination with cytarabine). Teniposide has been found to have activity in other neoplasms, including adult leukemias, non-Hodgkin's lymphoma, and small-cell lung cancer.

Classification

Plant alkaloid (topoisomerase II inhibitor).

Pharmacokinetics

After IV administration, teniposide is extensively (99%) bound to plasma albumin. The drug is metabolized by the liver, and 4% to 14% is eliminated unchanged in the urine. Teniposide has a terminal half-life of approximately 5 hours.

Dose

Treatment of acute lymphocytic leukemia: teniposide is administered in a dose of 165 mg/m^2 in combination with cytarabine 300 mg/m^2 intravenously, twice weekly for 8 to 9 doses. Occasionally, maintenance doses of teniposide, 250 mg/m^2/week, are given for a period of 4 to 8 weeks.

   Several other regimens have been used, including:
- 100 mg/m^2 once or twice weekly
- 20 to 60 mg/m^2/day for 5 days, and
- 250 mg/m^2/week for a period of 4 to 8 weeks.

   As a single agent in the treatment of small-cell lung cancer, a dose of 80 to 90 mg/m^2/day for 5 days has been used.

Administration

Teniposide for injection is administered by slow IV infusion, as a 0.1 to 0.4 mg/mL solution in 5% dextrose or normal saline, over at least 30 to 60 minutes. The drug has also been given as a continuous IV infusion and intraperitoneally.

TENIPOSIDE (continued)

Toxicity

Hematological. Leukopenia is expected and dose-limiting (nadir 10 to 14 days). Thrombocytopenia and anemia occur less frequently.

Gastrointestinal. Nausea and vomiting occur occasionally (29%) and are usually preventable with antiemetic drugs. Anorexia, diarrhea (33%), stomatitis (76%), and abdominal pain (with intraperitoneal administration) may also occur. Abdominal pain may be dose-limiting when teniposide is administered intraperitoneally.

Dermatological. Alopecia occurs in 10% to 30% of patients and is generally mild. Skin rashes have been reported in 3% of patients.

Hepatic. Elevated hepatic transaminase levels, hyperbilirubinemia.

Neurological. Fatigue, seizures, paresthesias (all rare). Somnolence and hypotension have been reported in children receiving sedative antiemetics (e.g., promazine and diphenhydramine) in combination with teniposide and cytarabine.

Cardiovascular. Hypotension is associated with rapid IV administration.

Hypersensitivity. Anaphylaxis (rare); reactions may include blood pressure changes, bronchospasm, tachycardia, urticaria, facial flushing, diaphoresis, periorbital edema, vomiting, and/or fever. Hypersensitivity reactions are secondary to the vehicle diluent Cremaphor®-EL, pretreatment with a corticosteroid and antihistamine may be necessary.

Other. Fever (rare); elevated levels of BUN and serum creatinine (rare); local IV site phlebitis, secondary malignancy (acute nonlymphocytic leukemia).

Drug Interactions

The clearance of teniposide is increased two- to threefold in patients receiving anticonvulsant enzyme-inducing medications (e.g., phenobarbital, phenytoin, carbamazepine).

Storage and Stability

Teniposide should be stored at refrigeration temperature and protected from light. Freezing does not adversely affect the stability of teniposide. After dilution in normal saline or 5% dextrose to concentrations of 0.1 to 0.4 mg/mL, the drug is chemically stable for at least 24 hours at room or refrigeration temperatures in glass containers. In plastic containers, 0.1 mg/mL of teniposide in normal saline is stable for 8 hours at room and refrigeration temperatures. Teniposide exhibits poor stability in plastic containers when mixed with 5% dextrose and precipitation may occur within 4 hours.

Preparation

Teniposide is often diluted in glass containers to a concentration of 0.4 mg/mL or less in normal saline or 5% dextrose. Teniposide has also been diluted to a concentration 1.0 mg/mL in normal saline or 5% dextrose. Use of non-DEHP PVC containers such as polyolefin, polypropylene, or glass is recommended.

Incompatibilities

Teniposide and heparin are incompatible; precipitation of teniposide may occur.

Availability

Teniposide is commercially available in 50-mg (10 mg/mL) ampules.

THALIDOMIDE

Other names

Thalomid®; K-17; NSC-66847.

Indications

FDA approved for the acute treatment of erythema nodosum leprosum (ENL), cutaneous manifestations, and for maintenance therapy of these lesions to prevent further lesions and suppress reoccurrence. Thalidomide has has activity against multiple myeloma, myelodysplatic syndrome, and other malignancies. Thalidomide has also been used as a potential treatment for graft versus host disease and aphthous ulcers.

Classification and Mechanisms of Action

Thalidomide is classified as an immunomodulatory drug that also possesses antiangiogenic properties. The mechanisms of action are not completely characterized; however, it is thought that thalidomide may suppress excess tumor necrosis factor-alfa and down-modulate selected sites on the cell surface. As an anticancer agent, thalidomide is thought to prevent or stunt microvessel formation through inhibition of vascular endothelial growth factor or basic fibroblast growth factor.

Pharmacokinetics

Thalidomide is slowly absorbed from the gastrointestinal tract, due to the drug's poor aqueous solubility. The time to peak plasma levels ranges from 2.9 to 5.7 hours. Thalidomide is plasma protein-bound, 55% for the (R) isomer to 66% of the (S) isomer. Thalidomide does appear to distribute to semen. Thalidomide undergoes a nonenzymatic hydrolysis in the plasma resulting in the formation of numerous metabolites. It does not appear to be extensively metabolized by the liver. The elimination half-life of thalidomide is 5 to 7 hours, with less than 1% of the drug excreted unchanged in the urine. Characterization of thalidomide elimination is not well known.

Dose

For ENL, the standard dose is 100 mg to 300 mg per day.

For oncology indications, the dose is not a standard and often a titration schedule is used (commonly increasing the dose by 200 mg every 2 weeks). The dose for single agent thalidomide has a range of 100 mg to 1,200 mg.

The median daily dose of single agent thalidomide in multiple myeloma is 400 mg (with a range of 50 mg to 800 mg).

Administration

Thalidomide must only be prescribed and dispensed by S.T.E.P.S. (System for Thalidomide Education and Prescribing Safety) registered physicians and pharmacies and administered to patients in compliance with all of the terms set forth by the manufacturer in their S.T.E.P.S. program. Consult the manufacturer for specific details.

Oral. Administer at bedtime with a full glass of water or one hour after the evening meal.

Toxicity

Teratogenicity. Thalidomide will cause severe birth defects and possibly death to the unborn child. When used in women of child-bearing potential or in sexually active men (due to levels of thalidomide in semen), adherence to strict guidelines adopted by the FDA is required. The specific guidelines fall under the term "S.T.E.P.S program" or "System for Thalidomide Education and Prescribing Safety." All prescribers, distributors, and patients must adhere to these guidelines.

THALIDOMIDE *(continued)*

Hematological. Neutropenia occurs in approximately 25% of patients. Anemia and lymphadenopathy have been reported in HIV-positive patients.

Gastrointestinal. Constipation is reported in up to 9% of patients. Nausea, vomiting, diarrhea, oral moniliasis, and tooth pain have been reported in ENL patients. Anorexia, dry mouth, and flatulence were reported in less than 10% of HIV-positive patients.

Dermatological. Rash is reported in up to 20% of ENL patients, and more frequently in the HIV-positive patient population. Fungal dermatitis, urticaria, maculopapular rash, and nail disorders have been reported. Stevens-Johnson syndrome and toxic epidermal necrolysis are rare; however, if the rash presents as purpuric, exfoliative, or bullous, therapy must be discontinued.

Genitourinary. Impotence is reported in approximately 10% of ENL patients. Albuminuria and hematuria in HIV-positive patients have been reported.

Hepatic. Hyperlipidemia and increased transaminase levels have been reported.

Neurological. Neurological toxicities, particularly somnolence and sedation, are common. Other toxicities may include dizziness, weakness, fatigue, confusion, mood changes, tremor, incoordination, and peripheral neuropathy. Peripheral neuropathy may be irreversible and dose-limiting. The presentation may include sensory symptoms such as paresthesias of the hands and feet, pain, hyperesthesia, extremity coldness, sensory loss, muscle cramps or weakness, decreased muscle stretch reflexes, brittle nails, and redness.

Pulmonary. Sinusitis, rhinitis, and pharyngitis are reported in approximately 5% of patients.

Cardiovascular. Orthostatic hypotension was observed in up to 19% of patients. Less commonly reported were peripheral edema and bradycardia.

Other. Abdominal pain, asthenia, back pain, chills, facial edema, malaise, neck pain or rigidity. Fever and infection were reported in the HIV-positive patient population.

Drug Interactions

Thalidomide administered concurrently with barbiturates, chlorpromazine, reserpine, alcohol, or other sedatives may cause an increase in sedation.

Thalidomide should be used with caution when administered with any other agent known to cause peripheral neuropathy. Frequent clinical assessments are recommended.

Storage and Stability

Thalidomide capsules are stored at room temperature and protected from light. Each container bears an expiration date.

Availability

Thalidomide is commercially available as a 50-mg, 100-mg, and 200-mg hard gelatin capsules. It is supplied in cardboard prescription packs that contain either 14 or 28 capsules each.

Selected Readings

Alexanian R, Weber D. Thalidomide for resistant and relapsing myeloma. Sem Hematol 37(1;suppl. 3): 22–25, 2000.

Barlogie B et al. In DeVita VT, Hellman S, Rosenberg SA, eds. Progress in Oncology 2001. Boston, Jones and Bartlett, 2001: p117.

THIOGUANINE

Other names
6-Thioguanine; 6-TG; Lanvis; Thioguanine Tabloid®; aminopurine-6-thiol-hemihydrate; NSC-752.

Indications
Oral thioguanine is FDA approved for remission induction, consolidation, and maintenance therapy of acute nonlymphocytic leukemia. Thioguanine may be a useful treatment for acute lymphocytic leukemia and chronic myelogenous leukemia. The injectable formulation of thioguanine is investigational.

Classification
Purine antimetabolite.

Pharmacokinetics
Thioguanine is incompletely (14% to 46%) and slowly absorbed by mouth and reaches maximum plasma concentrations approximately 8 hours after dosing. Thioguanine is extensively liver metabolized forming several metabolites. Negligible amounts of thioguanine are eliminated unchanged in the urine. The elimination half-life of the drug is reported to range from 1.5 to 11 hours.

Dose
As a single agent or as maintenance therapy the dose range is 2 to 3 mg/kg/day orally for both adults and children greater than 3 years of age. In each course of remission induction combination therapy a dose range of 75 to 200 mg/m^2/day orally for 5 to 7 days has been used. Combined with daunorubicin and cytarabine in the treatment of acute nonlymphocytic leukemia, thioguanine has been given at a dose of 100 mg/m^2 every 12 hours for a 14-day period. The IV formulation of thioguanine has been evaluated in patients with solid tumors at a dose of 55 mg/m^2/day for 5 days, repeated every 4 weeks. The dose should be attenuated in patients with hepatic or renal dysfunction.

Administration
Thioguanine is taken orally on an empty stomach, if possible. The drug may also be given by IV infusion in 250 to 500 mL of 5% dextrose or normal saline over a period of at least 30 minutes or longer. Rapid IV infusion may induce bronchospasm and cardiovascular collapse.

Toxicity
Hematological. Leukopenia and thrombocytopenia, with nadirs occurring 10 to 14 days after administration. Anemia occurs occasionally.
Gastrointestinal. Nausea (infrequent), vomiting (infrequent), anorexia, stomatitis, diarrhea.
Dermatological. Rash and dermatitis have been reported.
Hepatic. Elevated hepatic transaminase levels, hyperbilirubinemia, jaundice, veno-occlusive disease.
Neurological. Loss of vibratory sensation, unsteady gait.
Cardiovascular. Bronchospasm and cardiovascular collapse may be associated with rapid IV infusion (i.e., infusion over a period of less than 30 minutes).
Renal. Elevated BUN and serum creatinine concentrations, hyperuricemia (caused by tumor cell lysis).

THIOGUANINE *(continued)*

Drug Interactions

The risk of hepatotoxicity may be increased when thioguanine is administered with busulfan.

Storage and Stability

Tablets are stored at room temperature; containers bear expiration dates. Intact vials are stable for at least 4 years under refrigeration and 3 years at room temperature. At a concentration of 15 mg/mL the drug is chemically stable for at least 24 hours at refrigeration temperatures. After further dilution in 500 mL of 5% dextrose or normal saline, thioguanine is chemically stable for at least 24 hours at room and refrigeration temperatures.

Preparation

The 75-mg vial is reconstituted with 5 mL of normal saline to yield a 15 mg/mL solution. The desired dose may be further diluted with 500 mL of 5% dextrose or normal saline. An oral suspension of thioguanine can be made from the tablets. A pharmacist should be consulted for additional information.

Compatibilities

A 1 mg/mL solution containing 0.5 mEq of sodium bicarbonate for every 75 mg of thioguanine is stable for 8 hours in 5% dextrose or normal saline.

Availability

Thioguanine 40-mg tablets are commercially available. The injectable formulation, 75 mg/vial, is investigational and is available as a lyophilized powder from the National Cancer Institute.

THIOTEPA

Other names

Thioplex®; triethylenephosphoramide; *N,N',N''*-triethylene-thiophosphoramide; tris(1-aziridinyl)phosphine sulfide; TESPA; TSPA; NSC-6396.

Indications

FDA approved for the treatment of adenocarcinoma of the breast, adenocarcinoma of the ovary, intracavitary effusions, superficial papillary bladder cancer, and Hodgkin's and non-Hodgkin's lymphomas. Thiotepa is also used for the treatment of carcinomatous meningitis. Thiotepa may be useful in bone marrow transplantation treatment programs and as a treatment for lung cancer.

Classification

Alkylating agent.

Pharmacokinetics

Thiotepa administered orally is poorly absorbed from the gastrointestinal tract. Between 10% and 100% is absorbed through bladder mucosa after intravesical instillation. Thiotepa is extensively liver metabolized, its major metabolite (TEPA) has cytotoxic activity, and only trace amounts of thiotepa and TEPA appear in the urine. Thiotepa has an elimination half-life of 2 to 3 hours (from plasma) and 8 hours (from cerebrospinal fluid after intrathecal administration). TEPA has an elimination half-life of 15 to 18 hours.

Dose

Nontransplant doses: 12 to 16 mg/m^2 every 1 to 4 weeks.
  Intravesical instillation: 30 to 60 mg every week for 4 weeks.
  Intrathecal doses: 1 to 10 mg/m^2 once or twice weekly.

Administration

Thiotepa has been given by IV push, but it may be administered by IV infusion in 50 mL or more of 5% dextrose or normal saline, over a 10-minute period or longer. Thiotepa has also been administered as an ophthalmic instillation, intrathecally, as an intravesical instillation, intra-arterially (i.e., regional perfusion), intratumorally, intrapleurally, intraperitoneally, intrapericardially, and intramuscularly.

Toxicity

Systemic effects may occur after intravesical instillation or intracavitary administration.

Hematological. Leukopenia is expected and often dose-limiting (nadir, 10 to 14 days after administration). Thrombocytopenia and anemia occur less frequently. Myelosuppression may be cumulative.

Gastrointestinal. Nausea and vomiting are uncommon with nontransplantation doses. Anorexia, diarrhea, and abdominal pain are uncommon. Stomatitis may be severe with bone marrow transplantation doses.

Dermatological. Alopecia (rare with conventional doses), hives, rash, pruritus, contact dermatitis, fingernail changes; bronzing, erythema, and desquamation of the skin in patients receiving greater than 900 mg/m^2 before bone marrow transplantation.

Hepatic. Elevated hepatic transaminase levels occur and are usually mild and transient.

Neurological. Headache, dizziness, weakness of lower extremities, paresthesias (with intrathecal injection). Cognitive impairment (e.g., stupor, coma) is the dose-limiting toxicity of high-dose thiotepa (first observed at 1125 mg/m^2 and increasing in severity at higher doses).

Pulmonary. Apnea (in patients receiving succinylcholine).

Urinary (in patients receiving thiotepa by intravesical instillation). Abdominal pain, hematuria, hemorrhagic cystitis (rare), dysuria, frequency, urgency, ureteral obstruction, and impairment of renal function (rare).

Ocular (after ophthalmic instillation). Irritation, skin pigmentation in the periorbital region, blurred vision, conjunctivitis.

Other. Second malignancy (i.e., leukemia), pain at site of injection (rare), impaired fertility (i.e., azoospermia, amenorrhea), fever (rare), angioedema (rare), hypersensitivity reactions (e.g., rash, urticaria, laryngeal edema, wheezing).

Drug Interactions

Intraperitoneal thiotepa given 90 minutes after pancuronium caused one patient to experience increased neuromuscular blockade, prolonged respiratory depression, and periods of apnea.

Storage and Stability

Thiotepa is stored in the refrigerator. At a concentration of 10 mg/mL the drug is stable for at least 24 hours at room temperature and 5 days in the refrigerator. After dilution in normal saline to concentrations of 1 or 3 mg/mL in polyvinylchloride containers, thiotepa is stable for at least 48 hours in the refrigerator and 24 hours at room temperature. At a concentration of 5 mg/mL the drug is stable for at least 24 hours at room and refrigeration temperatures. Solutions of thiotepa, 0.5 mg/mL, are unstable at 24 hours and should be used immediately.

218

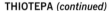

THIOTEPA *(continued)*

Preparation
The 15-mg vial is reconstituted with 1.5 mL of sterile water to result in a 10 mg/mL solution. The desired dose is further diluted with normal saline. The reconstituted solution should be filtered using a 0.22-micron filter. Solutions that remain opaque or that have particulate matter after filtration should not be used.

Compatibilities
Thiotepa is compatible with 2% procaine hydrochloride and/or epinephrine 1:1000.

Availability
Thiotepa, 15 mg/vial, is commercially available as a lyophilized powder.

TIPIFARNIB

Other names
R115777; Zarnestra®; NSC-702818.

Indications
Tipifarnib is being evaluated as a targeted therapy for hematological and nonhematological malignancies. Tipifarnib appears to have activity in breast cancer, gliomas, myelodysplastic syndromes, and other malignancies. The drug does not appear to have activity against prostate cancer or pancreatic cancer.

Classification and Mechanisms of Action
Tipifarnib is an inhibitor of Ras oncogene farnesylation (activation).

Pharmacokinetics
Peak plasma levels occur 0.5 to 5 hours after administration. The drug does not affect the pharmacokinetics of irinotecan or capecitabine. The drug has a terminal half-life of approximately 16 hours. Less than 0.1% of a dose is eliminated in the urine as unchanged drug. Approximately 16% of the drug is eliminated in the urine as a glucuronide conjugate.

Dose
Tipifarnib has been administered at a dose of 300 to 400 mg twice daily for 21 days followed by a 1-week rest period. This 3 weeks on, 1 week off regimen is repeated every 28 days. The 400 mg twice a day dose has been used in patients with hematological malignancies. Higher doses (600 mg twice daily) have been evaluated in patients with leukemia and myelodysplastic syndromes and in patients who are also taking hepatic enzyme-inducing antiepileptic drugs (EIAIDs), such as phenytoin or phenobarbital. In phase I studies dose-limiting toxicities occurred at the 900 mg twice daily dose level. Tipifarnib 200 to 300 mg twice daily for 21 days has been administered in combination with several drugs, including:

Topotecan, 1 mg/m^2/day for 5 consecutive days.
Irinotecan, 350 mg/m^2 every 3 weeks.
Trastuzumab (Herceptin®), 4 mg/kg followed one week later by 2 mg/kg per week.
Capecitabine, 2,000 mg/day for 14 days followed by one week of no treatment.
Gemcitabine, 1,000 mg/m^2/ week for 7 consecutive weeks, then weekly for 3 out of every 4 weeks.

Administration
Oral. The drug should be administered with a meal.

Toxicity
Hematological. Neutopenia (grade 3 to grade 4 in 14% at 300 mg twice daily), febrile neutropenia in a few patients, thrombocytopenia, anemia (grade 3 to grade 4 in 16% at 300 mg twice daily).
Gastrointestinal. Nausea (all grades: 49%), anorexia (all grades: 50%), diarrhea (all grades: 35%, grade 3–4: 8%), vomiting (uncommon).
Dermatological. Skin rash, occasionally grade 3. The rash occurs within two weeks of treatment and can be dose-limiting with the doses that have been used in patients with leukemia and myelodysplastic syndromes.
Hepatic. Grade 3 elevations of transaminases and bilirubin have been reported.
Neurological. Confusion was dose-limiting in phase I studies. Peripheral neuropathies (grade 3) have been observed in approximately 8% of patients. Neuropathy is more common with a continuous dosing regimen compared to dosing for 21 out of every 28 days. Cerebellar symptoms have been observed in patients receiving 700 mg twice a day.
Other. Fatigue is relatively common and often dose-limiting. Grade 3 to grade 4 fatigue has been observed in up to 25% of patients in some studies. Uncommon adverse events include: arthralgia, myalgia, headache, hypokalemia, hypomagnesemia, hypotension, photophobia, and acute renal failure. Bone pain has been observed in patients with myelodysplastic syndromes at doses of 700 mg twice a day.

Storage and Stability
Room temperature.

Availability
Tipifarnib is an investigational agent in the United States that is available as an oral formulation (50-mg and 100-mg tablets) from the manufacturer or the National Cancer Institute.

Selected Readings
Harousseau J-L et al. Interim results from a phase II study of R115777 (Zarnestra) in patients with relapsed and refractory acute myelogenous leukemia. Proc Am Soc Clin Oncol 21: 265a, 2002.
Zujewski J et al. Phase I and pharmacokinetic study of farnesyl protein transferase inhibitor R115777 in advanced cancer. J Clin Oncol 18: 927–941, 2000.

TIRAPAZAMINE

Other names
Tirazone®; TPZ; SR259075; SR4233; Win 59075; NSC-130181.

Indications
Tirapazamine is an investigational agent in the United States that is being evaluated in a number of malignancies. The drug has activity in non-small-cell lung cancer, esophageal cancer, head and neck cancers, and other malignancies.

Classification and Mechanisms of Action
Tirapazamine is a benzotriazine antineoplastic agent that has been shown to be more toxic to certain hypoxic tumor cells compared to aerobic cells. It is believed that tirapazamine produces radical anions that cause strand breaks in DNA.

Pharmacokinetics
The terminal half-life is approximately 20 to 60 minutes.

TIRAPAZAMINE *(continued)*

Dose

As a single agent, administered intravenously, tirapazamine, 390 mg/m^2, repeated every 21 to 28 days is the maximum tolerated dose. This dose of tirapazamine has been administered in combination with cisplatin, 75 mg/m^2.

The combination of tirapazamine 330 mg/m^2 on day 1, cisplatin 75 mg/m^2 on day 1, and gemcitabine 1,250 mg/m^2 on days 1 and 8 has been evaluated on a 21-day schedule. Other regimens have been evaluated. Tirapazamine has also been administered with radiation therapy for patients with glioblastoma multiforme. In this setting, tirapazamine has been administered at a dose of 260 mg/m^2/dose 3 times each week for 4 consecutive weeks.

Administration

Tirapazamine is administered IV in 250 mL of normal saline over 2 hours.
Tirapazamine is administered before cisplatin when the drugs are administered on the same day.

Toxicity

Hematological. Leukopenia and thrombocytopenia (uncommon and not usually clinically significant).
Gastrointestinal. Nausea and vomiting occur but rarely exceed grade 2. In combination with cisplatin 75 mg/m^2 the incidence of grade 3 nausea and vomiting is approximately 15%. Diarrhea is rarely severe; approximately 5% of patients have developed grade 3 diarrhea. Esophagitis has been reported when tirapazamine is administered in combination with radiation therapy.
Dermatological. An erythematous skin rash has been reported in approximately 15% of patients.
Cardiovascular. Cardiac ischemia has been reported.
Other. Visual disturbances, loss of consciousness, muscle cramping (less than 5% is grade 3), tinnitus has been reported. Grade 3 fatigue has been reported in up to 8% of patients receiving tirapazamine.

Storage and Stability

Intact vials and capsules are stored at room temperature. Do not refrigerate tirapazamine. After further dilution, the parenteral formulation may be stored at room temperature for up to 48 hours. It is recommended that the drug be protected from light during storage and during administration.

Preparation

Doses are usually further diluted in 250 mL of normal saline.

Availability

Tirapazamine is an investigational agent in the United States that is available in parenteral and oral formulations. The parenteral product is available as a 0.7 mg/mL solution (175-mg/vial) and the oral formulation is available in 50-mg capsules from the manufacturer or the National Cancer Institute.

Selected Readings

Gandara DR et al. Tirapazamine: prototype for a novel class of therapeutic agents targeting tumor hypoxia. Semin Oncol 29: 102–109, 2002.
Von Pawel J et al. Tirapazamine plus cisplatin versus cisplatin in advanced non-small-cell lung cancer: a report of the international CATAPULT I study group. J Clin Oncol 18: 1351–1359, 2000.

TOPOTECAN

Other names

Hycamptin®; topotecan hydrochloride; topotecan AC/AF; hycamptamine; SKF 104864-A; NSC-609699.

Indications

FDA approved for the treatment of patients with metastatic ovarian carcinoma after failure of initial or second-line therapy. Also approved for small-cell lung cancer sensitive disease after failure of first time chemotherapy. Topotecan has activity in non-small-cell lung cancer, non-Hodgkin's lymphoma, acute myelogenous leukemia, and other malignancies.

Classification

Topoisomerase I inhibitor.

Pharmacokinetics

Approximately 22% to 48% of a dose of topotecan is eliminated unchanged in the urine. Topotecan has an elimination half-life of approximately 2 to 3 hours. There does not appear to be a strong correlation with AUC (area under the plasma concentration time curve) and ANC (absolute neutrophil count). Approximately 35% of topotecan is bound to plasma proteins. Elimination of topotecan is delayed in patients with compromised renal function. Patients with hyperbilirubinemia appear to eliminate the drug more slowly than patients with normal serum bilirubin levels, but clinically significant differences in toxicity between the two groups have not been observed.

Dose

The approved dose of topotecan is 1.5 mg/m^2/day for 5 days by IV infusion over a 30-minute period for the first four courses of treatment. Subsequent treatments should be administered at a dose of 1.25 mg/m^2/day for 5 days. It is recommended that the daily dose be reduced to 0.75 mg/m^2 for patients with moderate renal impairment (i.e., creatinine clearance 20 to 40 mL/min). Dose adjustments are not necessary for patients with hyperbilirubinemia (i.e., bilirubin 1.7 to 15 mg/dL). Other doses and regimens of topotecan have been evaluated, including:

- Single dose of 1.3 to 1.6 mg/m^2/dose by IV infusion over a 0.5-, 2-, and 24-hour period; repeated every 3 to 4 weeks.
- Weekly dose of 1.5 to 1.75 mg/m^2/dose by IV infusion over a 24-hour period.
- Weekly doses of up to 3 mg/m^2/dose by intravenous intermittent infusion.
- Continuous infusion over a 72-, 96-, or 120-hour period at a dose of 0.65 to 2 mg/m^2/day, repeated every 3 to 4 weeks.

Administration

Topotecan is administered intravenously usually in 100 mL or more of normal saline or 5% dextrose over a 30-minute period or longer.

Toxicity

Hematological. Dose-limiting leukopenia is the major toxicity of topotecan (nadir, days 10 to 12; recovery by days 15 to 21 after the consecutive day 1 through 5 regimen). With the doses recommended for the treatment of women with ovarian cancer, neutropenia (500 cells/mm^3 or less) is reported to occur in 81% of patients. Thrombocytopenia occurs frequently but is rarely dose-limiting. Anemia is common (i.e., 2% decline in hematocrit in 80%, 4% decline in 30% to 50%) and occasionally (14%) precipitous.

TOPOTECAN *(continued)*

Approximately 50% of patients have required red blood cell transfusions during treatment with topotecan. Myelosuppression induced by topotecan (1.25 mg/m^2/day for 5 days) is more severe if combined with cisplatin (50 mg/m^2 on day 1).

Gastrointestinal. Severe (grades 3 and 4) nausea and vomiting are reported to occur in approximately 10% of patients. Diarrhea is common (25% to 42%) but is severe in approximately 5% of patients. Diarrhea usually begins during or shortly after infusion of topotecan and lasts 2 to 3 days. Anorexia, constipation, abdominal pain, mucositis, and xerostomia are rarely dose-limiting.

Dermatological. Total alopecia is common (42%). Skin rash (mild) occurs infrequently and on occasion may be accompanied by pruritus and/or urticaria. Acne and fever blisters have been reported.

Hepatic. Elevated hepatic enzyme levels and hyperbilirubinemia are uncommon toxicities.

Neurological. Headache occurs frequently. Dizziness, light-headedness, peripheral neuropathy, and Horner's syndrome have been reported.

Cardiovascular. Hypertension and tachycardia have been reported infrequently.

Pulmonary. Dyspnea has been reported to occur in 20% of patients, severe (grades 3 and 4) in 4% to 6%.

Renal. Elevated serum creatinine concentrations and hematuria rarely occur.

Other. Fever, fatigue (severe in 8%), malaise (severe in 2%), arthralgia (severe in 1%), asthenia (severe in 5%), myalgia, and weight loss have been reported.

Drug Interactions

Cisplatin administered concomitantly with topotecan increases the degree of myelo-suppression.

Storage and Stability

Topotecan is stored at room temperature and protected from light. After reconstitution to concentrations from 10 microg/mL to 500 microg/mL, the solution is chemically stable for 21 days at room and refrigeration temperatures. Dilution to concentrations of 20 microg/mL and 100 microg/mL in plastic containers with 5% dextrose or normal saline are stable for at least 48 hours at room temperature.

Preparation

Add 4 mL of sterile water to the 4-mg vial to yield a concentration of 1 mg/mL.

Availability

Topotecan is commercially available as a single use 4-mg vial.

Selected Reading

Homesley HD et al. A dose escalation study of weekly bolus topotecan in previously treated ovarian cancer patients. Gyn Oncol 83: 394–399, 2001.

TOREMIFENE

Other names

Fareston®; toremifene citrate; toremifenum; FC-1157a.

Indications

FDA approved for the treatment of advanced breast cancer in postmenopausal women.

Classification and Mechanisms of Action

Toremifene has a high affinity for estrogen receptors. Thus part of its mechanism of action may involve binding to estrogenic receptors that become translocated in the nucleus where DNA synthesis is inhibited. However, toremifene has also been shown to have cytostatic effects in estrogen receptor-negative cells.

Pharmacokinetics

Toremifene is rapidly absorbed after oral administration and reaches peak serum concentrations within 3 to 4 hours of dosing. Toremifene is almost totally bound to serum proteins (92% to albumin). Toremifene exhibits a biphasic elimination pattern with a distribution half-life of approximately 4 to 4.5 hours and an elimination half-life of approximately 5 to 6 days. Toremifene is metabolized in the liver to at least two metabolites (i.e., *N*-desmethyl-toremifene, 4-hydroxy-toremifene) that have equivalent antiestrogenic activity.

Dose

The standard dose is 60 mg/day. Phase I studies evaluated doses ranging from 20 to 400 mg/day for 8 weeks. Phase II studies have employed doses of 60 and 200 mg/day. Toremifene 60 mg/day has equivalent antiestrogenic activity to tamoxifen 60 mg/day.

Administration

Oral, once daily, with or without food.

Toxicity

Hematological. Marked decline in erythrocyte sedimentation rate (common), rarely leukopenia or thrombocytopenia.
Gastrointestinal. Nausea (6% to 31%), upper abdominal pain (4% to 10%), vomiting (0% to 12%), anorexia (0% to 9%), diarrhea (4%), constipation (3%), increased appetite (2%).
Cardiovascular. Thrombophlebitis, thrombosis, edema, transient ischemic attacks (rare).
Dermatological. Urticaria (rare).
Neurological. Dizziness or vertigo (10%), lethargy/fatigue (10%), headache (9%), insomnia, tremulousness.
Pulmonary. Pulmonary embolism (rare).
Ocular. Dryness and cataracts have been reported in a few patients.
Other. Hot flushes (10% to 30%), sweating (13%), tumor or bone pain on intiation of therapy, hypercalcemia (rare), vaginal discharge (8%), vaginal bleeding (3%), mildly reduced levels of antithrombin III (58%), elevated liver function tests.

Drug Interactions

Toremifene may inhibit the metabolism of warfarin and increase its anticoagulant effect.

Toremifene elimination may be reduced by agents that inhibit the cytochrome P450 enzymes. These agents include, but are not limited to, itraconazole, ketoconazole, calcium channer blockers, cimetidine, and macrolides.

Toremifene elimination may be increased by agents that induce the cytochrome P450 enzymes. These agents include, but are not limited to, phenytoin, rifampin, and phenobarbital. The concentrations and efficacy of toremifene may decrease if this inhibition occurs.

Storage and Stability

Store at room temperature. Each bottle bears an expiration date.

Availability

Toremifene is commercially available as 60-mg tablets.

TREOSULFAN

Other names
Ovastat®.

Indications
Treosulfan is an investigational agent in the United States. In the United Kingdom (and other countries) it is approved as a second-line treatment of ovarian cancer. Treosulfan also has activity in non-small-cell lung cancer, esophageal cancer, head and neck cancers, and other malignancies.

Classification and Mechanisms of Action
Treosulfan is a bifunctional alkylating agent similar to busulfan.

Pharmacokinetics
Treosulfan is well absorbed (97%) after oral administration. The maximum concentration occurs approximately 1.5 hours after oral administration. The drug is converted to active metabolites and is primarily eliminated by the kidneys. Approximately 15% is eliminated unchanged in the urine. The elimination half-life is approximately 2 hours.

Dose
Several oral treatment regimens have been used, including:
- 250 mg four times daily × 4 weeks followed by 4 weeks of no treatment
- 250 mg four times daily × 2 weeks followed by 2 weeks of no treatment
- 500 mg three times daily × 2 weeks followed by 2 weeks of no treatment
- 500 mg three times daily × 1 week followed by 3 weeks of no treatment.

Intravenous treatment regimens, 3 to 10 g/m^2 every 3 to 4 weeks, have also been used.

Treosulfan has been administered via intraperitoneal instillation at a dose of 1,500 mg/m^2.

High-dose treosulfan, 47 g/m^2, has been used in combination with bone marrow rescue. A dose of 56 g/m^2 was dose-limiting.

Administration
Treosulfan is administered by mouth or by IV infusion. Doses less than 3,000 mg/m^2 have been administered over 5 to 10 minutes. Larger doses are usually administered over at least 30 minutes. Treosulfan has also been administered by intraperitoneal instillation. Because of the risk of hemorrhagic cystitis it is recommended that patients remain well hydrated for up to 24 hours after the IV infusion.

Toxicity
Hematological. Leukopenia is dose-limiting and cumulative. Nadir leukocyte and platelet counts usually occur 4 weeks after initiation of treatment.
Gastrointestinal. Nausea and vomiting are usually preventable. Grade 3 and grade 4 diarrhea and grade 3 stomatitis were dose-limiting toxicities with high-dose treosulfan.
Dermatological. Skin rash, with pruritus, may occur. Hyperpigmentation (bronze discoloration) may occur in up to 30% of patients. This side effect usually resolves a few months after treatment has been discontinued. Alopecia is usually mild and observed in approximately 15% of patients. Toxic epidermal necrolysis was observed in one patient who received high-dose treosulfan.
Local effects. Vesicant if extravasated.

Pulmonary. Allergic alveolitis, pneumonia, and pulmonary fibrosis have been reported.
Other. The manufacturer indicates that after long-term treatment with treosulfan the incidence of developing acute leukemia is approximately 1.4%. Rare side effects include: flu-like symptoms, hemorrhagic cystitis, Addison's disease, hypoglycemia, paresthesias, and acidosis.

Storage and Stability
Room temperature.

Preparation
Add 20 mL of sterile water to the 1,000-mg vial or add 100 mL of sterile water to the 5,000-mg vial to yield a concentration of 50 mg/mL.

Availability
Treosulfan is an investigational agent in the United States. Treosulfan is available in other countries as a 250-mg capsule and as a lyophilized powder (1,000 mg and 5,000 mg/vial) for parenteral use.

Selected Reading
Scheulen ME et al. Clinical phase I dose escalation and pharmacokinetic study of high-dose chemotherapy with treosulfan and autologous peripheral blood stem cell transplantation in patients with advanced malignancies. Clin Cancer Res 6: 4209–4216, 2000.

TRETINOIN

Other names
Vesanoid®; all-trans-retinoic acid; TRA; ATRA; vitamin A acid; NSC-122758.

Indications
FDA approved for the treatment of acute promyelocytic leukemia.

Classification and Mechanisms of Action
Tretinoin is a derivative of vitamin A. The drug binds to a cellular protein that facilitates the transfer of tretinoin from cellular cytoplasm into the nucleus. Within the nucleus, tretinoin binds to a chromosomal receptor that is near the chromosomal lesion that is associated with acute promyelocytic leukemia (APL). Differentiation of APL cells occurs after administration of tretinoin.

Pharmacokinetics
Tretinoin is a natural retinoic acid metabolite (basal concentrations, 3 to 4 ng/mL). After oral administration, peak plasma levels (e.g., 1 microM after an 80-mg dose) occur in 1 to 4 hours. The drug is highly plasma protein-bound. The drug rapidly disappears from the systemic circulation (elimination half-life, 40 minutes), does not penetrate into the cerebrospinal fluid, and is almost totally metabolized (i.e., 1% eliminated unchanged in the urine). Patients on low-fat diets may not absorb retinoic acid adequately. With continued treatment, plasma levels decline and increased urinary excretion of metabolites occurs, indicating increased metabolism of the drug, which often coincides with relapse of acute promyelocytic leukemia (APL).

Dose
For the treatment of APL: 45 mg/m^2/day (rounded up to the nearest 10 mg) for 30 days. If a partial response is obtained, treatment is continued until a complete response is achieved or there is progression of disease. If a complete response is

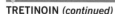

TRETINOIN *(continued)*

attained, treatment is continued for another 60 days (maximum, 90 total days of treatment). Doses of 175 mg/m^2/day have been evaluated in the treatment of other malignancies. In a study evaluating tretinoin in patients with brain tumors, each 8-week course of tretinoin consisted of daily administration for 6 weeks followed by a 2-week period of no treatment.

Administration

Oral, once daily in the morning with food. The daily dose has also been administered in two divided fractions.

Toxicity

Hematological. Leukocytosis (40%). A rapid increase in white blood cell count has resulted in leukostasis and hemorrhage in a few patients. Leukocyte counts tend to reach peak levels within 6 to 16 days after initiation of treatment. Less common toxicities include anemia, increased erythrocyte sedimentation rate, and thrombocytosis.

Gastrointestinal. Nausea, vomiting, and anorexia are uncommon. Xerostomia occurs occasionally, and pancreatitis is rare.

Dermatological. Dry skin and mild exfoliation occur in most patients. Rash, cheilitis, cracked lips, inflamed lips, pruritus, and photosensitivity are also common side effects. Alopecia (mild thinning) is an infrequent toxicity.

Hepatic. Transient elevation of hepatic enzyme levels (50% to 60%) and hyperbilirubinemia occur occasionally but may persist for weeks after treatment is discontinued.

Neurological. Headache is common, occurs several hours after dosing, and is managed with mild analgesics. Lethargy, fatigue, pseudotumor cerebri (dose-limiting in children), and mental depression occur infrequently.

Cardiovascular. Fluid retention, including generalized, facial, and peripheral edema. Flushing, hypotension, hypertension, chest discomfort, rarely MI or cardiac failure.

Cardiopulmonary. "Retinoic acid syndrome" occurs in up to 25% of patients, occurs within 2 days to 3 weeks after initiation of treatment, and can be fatal. High fever, respiratory distress, pulmonary infiltrates, and pericardial and/or pleural effusion may be accompanied by heart failure and hypotension. Some patients have required intubation and mechanical ventilation. Initiation of treatment with corticosteroids at the first sign of dyspnea has been recommended (generally intravenous dexamethasone for 3 days or more until symptoms resolve).

Ocular. Dryness, corneal erosion, blurred vision, papilledema, corneal opacities, night blindness, conjunctivitis, xerophthalmia.

Other. Tretinoin is teratogenic. Fetal abnormalities (e.g., thymic aplasia, craniofacial malformation) are likely if in utero exposure to tretinoin occurs. Nasal congestion, bone pain (10% to 25%), myalgia and arthralgia (common), muscle weakness, osteophyte formation, elevated cholesterol and triglyceride levels (common), fever, and xanthomas (rare) have been reported in patients receiving tretinoin.

Hyperhistaminemia (100 times normal) resulting in shock and severe gastric and duodenal ulceration have been reported.

Drug Interactions

Tretinoin elimination may be reduced by agents that inhibit the cytochrome P450 enzymes. These agents include, but are not limited to, itraconazole, calcium channel blockers, cimetidine, and macrolides. The toxicity of tretinoin may be increased. A 72% increase in the area under the plasma concentration curve was demonstrated when ketoconazole was administered with tretinoin.

Tretinoin elimination may be increased by agents that induce the cytochrome P450 enzymes. These agents include, but are not limited to, phenytoin, rifampin, and phenobarbital. The concentrations and efficacy of tretinoin may be decreased.

It is suggested that topical tretinoin (Retin-A®) and other vitamin A-containing supplements be avoided while using oral tretinoin.

Storage and Stability
Tretinoin capsules are stored at room temperature and protected from light. Each bottle bears an expiration date.

Incompatibilities
Tretinoin is contraindicated in patients allergic to parabens or vitamin A.

Availability
Tretinoin is commercially available as a 10-mg capsule.

Selected Reading
Levien TL, Baker DE. Reviews of tramadol and tretinoin, Hosp Pharm 31: 54–73, 1996.

TRIMETREXATE

Other names
Neutrexin®; TMQ; TMTX; NSC-352122.

Indications
FDA approved for the treatment of patients with *Pneumocystis carinii* infection who are intolerant of or refractory to trimethoprim-sulfamethoxazole therapy. Trimetrexate may be a useful treatment for cancers of the lung, head and neck, prostate, and colon.

Classification
Antimetabolite.

Pharmacokinetics
Trimetrexate is rapidly absorbed (19% to 67%) after oral administration, reaching peak plasma concentrations in 1 hour. After IV administration the drug distributes throughout the body but does not appear to accumulate in pleural or ascitic fluid. Trimetrexate is metabolized by the liver, with 6% to 25% appearing in the urine as unchanged drug. Trimetrexate has an elimination half-life of 11 to 16 hours. However, trimetrexate clearance is decreased and toxicity is increased in patients with hypoalbuminemia (i.e., serum albumin less than 3.5 g/dL).

Dose
The recommended dose for the treatment of *Pneumocystis carinii* infection is 45 mg/m^2/day for 21 days with concomitant leucovorin. Leucovorin must be administered for 3 days after cessation of treatment with trimetrexate. Leucovorin may be administered orally or by IV infusion at a dose of 20 mg/m^2 every 6 hours for 24 days. For the treatment of patients with cancer, doses of 8 to 12 mg/m^2/day for a 5-day period repeated every 3 to 4 weeks have been evaluated. When followed by leucovorin rescue, trimetrexate (110 mg/m^2) has been administered in combination with fluorouracil (500 mg/m^2) on a weekly basis for a 6-week period followed by 2 weeks of no treatment.

TRIMETREXATE *(continued)*

Administration

Trimetrexate has been given by IV push, but it is usually administered by IV infusion, in 50 mL or more of 5% dextrose only over a 60- to 90-minute period. Trimetrexate has also been given by shorter IV infusions and as a continuous IV infusion.

Toxicity

Patients with hypoalbuminemia (i.e., serum albumin less than 3.5 g/dL) are more likely to experience severe or life-threatening anemia, mucositis, and thrombocytopenia.

Hematological. Myelosuppression (leukopenia, thrombocytopenia, anemia) is dose-related and occasionally dose-limiting. Concomitant leucovorin significantly reduces the incidence of these toxicities.

Gastrointestinal. Mucositis can be dose-limiting and severe. Nausea, vomiting, anorexia, and diarrhea occur infrequently.

Dermatological. Maculopapular skin rash (occasionally with erythroderma), pruritus, hyperpigmentation, partial alopecia, radiation recall reactions (rare).

Hepatic. Transient elevations of liver enzyme levels (17%).

Renal. Transient elevation of serum creatinine level (4% to 8%).

Other. Fever (40%), shaking chills, malaise (12%).

Drug Interactions

Trimetrexate administered concomitantly with other hepatotoxic agents, such as ethanol, methotrexate, asparaginase, and nonsteroidal anti-inflammatory agents, may increase the risk of hepatotoxicity.

The elimination of trimetrexate may be reduced by agents that inhibit cytochrome P450 enzymes. These agents include, but are not limited to, itraconazole, calcium channer blockers, cimetidine, and macrolides. The toxicity of trimetrexate may be increased.

The elimination of trimetrexate may be increased by agents that induce the cytochrome P450 enzymes. These agents include, but are not limited to, phenytoin, rifampin, and phenobarbital. The concentrations and efficacy of trimetrexate may be decreased.

Trimetrexate's antitumor activity may be decreased when administered concomitantly with rescue agents leucovorin and thymidine.

Storage and Stability

Unreconstituted vials are stored at room temperature and protected from light. At a concentration of 12.5 mg/mL, trimetrexate is stable for 2 days at room temperature and 5 days refrigerated. Trimetrexate can also be frozen for up to 8 days. After dilution in 5% dextrose to a concentration of 0.25 to 2 mg/mL, the drug is chemically stable for at least 24 hours at room and refrigeration temperatures.

Preparation

The 25-mg vial is reconstituted with 2 mL of sterile water to yield a 12.5 mg/mL solution. The 200-mg vial is reconstituted with 16 mL of sterile water to yield a 12.5 mg/mL solution. The desired dose may be further diluted in 5% dextrose to achieve a final concentration of 0.25 to 2 mg/mL. Do not use chloride-containing solutions to reconstitute or dilute trimetrexate, or a black precipitate will form.

Incompatibilities

Trimetrexate is incompatible with leucovorin and chloride- or anion-containing (i.e., chloride) solutions, precipitation will occur.

Availability

Trimetrexate is commercially available as a lyophilized powder in 25- and 200-mg vials.

TRIPTORELIN PAMOATE

Other names

Trelstar Depot®; Trelstar LA®; AY-25650; triptoreline; d-Trp(6)-LHRH; CL-118532; tryptoreline.

Indications

FDA approved for the palliative treatment of advanced carcinoma of the prostate.

Classification and Mechanisms of Action

Triptorelin is a luteinizing hormone-releasing hormone (LHRH) analogue. In men, administration of pharmacological doses inhibits gonadotropin release, resulting in decreased serum concentrations of luteinizing hormone (LH), follicle-stimulating hormone (FSH), and testosterone. After an initial surge of levels, 2 to 4 weeks later triptorelin causes down-regulation of LHRH receptors with reduced LH and FSH secretion and castration levels of testosterone (by week 4) or estradiol.

Pharmacokinetics

Triptorelin is not absorbed after oral administration. Triptorelin microsphere formulation is slowly released following intramuscular injection with concentrations maintained for up to 4 weeks. Peak serum concentrations occur within 7 days after administration. There is no clinically relevant plasma protein binding. The metabolic fate of triptorelin is uncertain; potential mechanisms may include rapid tissue or plasma degradation, or renal clearance. Triptorelin undergoes a three-compartment model of elimination, involving both the liver and kidneys. The initial half-life is approximately 6 minutes, followed by 45 minutes, then a terminal half-life of 3 hours. Patients with renal or hepatic insufficiency demonstrate decreased elimination of the triptorelin and increased exposure to the drug. The clinical relevance of this is unknown and dose adjustment recommendations have not been established.

Dose

Recommended doses are 3.75 mg every 28 days, or once a month.

Administration

Intramuscular injection, in rotating sites.

Toxicity

Gastrointestinal. Infrequent vomiting and diarrhea.
Dermatological. Pain at injection site (4%) and pruritus (less than 2%).
Neurological. Headache (5%), dizziness (less than 2%), insomnia (2%), and emotional lability.
Endocrine. Hot flushes (58%) and impotence (7%).
Tumor flare. Patients with carcinoma of the prostate may experience tumor flare within the first weeks of therapy. This consists of increased bone pain, urethral or bladder obstruction, hematuria, spinal cord compression, and other symptoms.

TRIPTORELIN PAMOATE *(continued)*

Other. Skeletal pain (12%), hypertension (3%), muscle weakness (rare), leg pain (2%), fatigue (2%), anemia (2%), urinary retention and urinary tract infections (less than 2%)

Storage and Stability

Store at room temperature. The reconstituted suspension should be used immediately after dilution.

Preparation

Add 2 mL of sterile water and shake well. A milky white suspension will be formed. Withdraw the suspension from the vial immediately prior to injection.

Availability

Commercially available in 3.75-mg vials of lyophilized microgranules for reconstitution with mannitol.

Selected Reading

Hellstrom M et al. A 3-year follow-up of patients with localized prostate cancer operated on with or without pre-treatment with the GnRH-agonist triptorelin. Br J Urol 78: 432–436, 1996.

TROXACITABINE

Other names

Troxatyl®; BCH-4556; troxicitabine.

Indications

Troxacitabine is an investigational agent in the United States. In phase I and phase II studies, troxacitabine has shown some activity in non-small-cell lung cancer, melanoma, acute myelogenous leukemia, and other malignancies.

Classification and Mechanisms of Action

Troxacitabine is a nucleoside analogue. The drug is phosphorylated and incorporated into DNA, inducing degradation of DNA.

Pharmacokinetics

Elimination of troxacitabine occurs primarily by renal excretion (approximately 70% unchanged). The elimination half-life is approximately 39 hours with measurable levels 15 to 21 days after initiation of treatment.

Dose

Various dose regimens are under evaluation. As a daily × 5 regimen, repeated every 3 weeks, the phase II recommended dose is 1.5 mg/m^2/dose for "lightly pretreated" patients and 1.2 mg/m^2/dose for heavily pretreated patients. As a weekly × 3 regimen, repeated every 4 weeks, the phase II recommended dose is 3.2 mg/m^2/week. As a once every 3 weeks regimen the phase II recommended dose is 10 mg/m^2. For the treatment of acute leukemia 8 mg/m^2/day × 5 days was the maximum tolerated dose.

Administration

Troxacitabine is administered IV in 50 mL of normal saline over 30 minutes.

Toxicity

Hematological. Neutropenia is dose-limiting with nadir counts occurring around day 15 and recovery 7 days thereafter. There is evidence that neutropenia may be cumulative. Severe thrombocytopenia and anemia occur less commonly.

Gastrointestinal. Mild nausea and vomiting. Routine prophylaxis with antiemetic drugs is not necessary. Mild stomatitis has been reported; however, in the treatment of patients with leukemia, stomatitis occurs in approximately 30% of patients with grade 4 stomatitis occurring in approximately 5% of patients. Anorexia and diarrhea have also been reported, but these effects have not been dose-limiting.

Dermatological. Skin rash (local and patchy erythematous maculopapular) with pruritus occurs in approximately 50% of patients. A more generalized rash, with bullous eruptions, has been observed in some patients. The rash usually begins within 5 to 8 days of treatment, peaks within 15 days of treatment, and often resolves 7 days thereafter. Asymptomatic hyperpigmentation (face, extremities, tongue, and buccal mucosa) has been observed. Alopecia is uncommon.

Other. Hand-foot syndrome with blistering and pain, which may worsen with continued treatment, has been observed and may be dose-limiting (24% grade 3 at 8 mg/m^2/day × 5 days). Mild to moderate malaise, which does not appear to be dose-related, has been observed in some patients.

Storage and Stability

Unreconstituted vials are stored in the refrigerator.

Preparation

Add 5 mL normal saline to the 10-mg vial to yield a concentration of 2 mg/mL. Doses are usually further diluted in 50 mL of normal saline.

Availability

Troxacitabine is an investigational agent in the United States that is available as a lyophilized powder (10 mg/vial) from the manufacturer.

Selected Readings

De Bono JS et al. Troxacitabine, a L-stereoisomeric nucleoside analog, on a five-times-daily schedule: a phase I and pharmacokinetic study in patients with advanced solid malignancies. J Clin Oncol 20: 96–109, 2002.

Giles FJ et al. Phase II study of troxacitabine, a novel dioxolane nucleoside analog, in patients with refractory leukemia. J Clin Oncol 20: 656–664, 2002.

VALRUBICIN

Other names

Valstar®; *N*-trifluoroacetyladriamycin-14-valerate; AD 32.

Indications

FDA approved for use in BCG-refractory urinary bladder cancer in situ, in patients who are unable to undergo an immediate cystectomy.

Classification and Mechanisms of Action

Anthracycline antitumor antibiotic.

Pharmacokinetics

Upon intravesical administration, valrubicin is well absorbed into the tissue of the bladder wall. During retention of the drug in the bladder, negligible amounts are

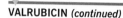

VALRUBICIN (continued)

absorbed systemically. The drug is excreted almost completely upon voiding. Systemic exposure to valrubicin is minimal; however, plasma concentrations are dependent upon the condition of the bladder. Patients who have a perforated bladder are more likely to have systemic exposure.

Dose

The usual dose of valrubicin in 800 mg administered intravesically into the bladder once a week for 6 weeks. Patients who have undergone transurethral resection or fulguration should wait 14 days before beginning valrubicin therapy.

Administration

Intravesical through a urethral catheter.

Toxicity

Gastrointestinal. Observed in less than 5% of patients are: nausea, vomiting, diarrhea, abdominal pain, and flatulence.
Genitourinary. Urinary frequency and urgency, dysuria, bladder spasms, hematuria, bladder pain, cystitis, urinary incontinence, nocturia, urethral pain, pelvic pain, and burning.
Neurological. Observed in less than 5% of patients: headache, dizziness.
Other. Observed in less than 5% of patients: pneumonia, myalgia, vasodilation, fever, rash, chest pain, malaise, back pain, and anemia.

Storage and Stability

Valrubicin vials are stored in the refrigerator. Each vial bears an expiration date. Do not freeze the vials.

Availability

Valrubicin is commercially available as a 40 mg/mL solution in 5-mL vials.

Selected Reading

Patterson AL et al. Pilot study of the tolerability and toxicity of intravesical valrubicin immediately after transurethral resection of superficial bladder cancer. Urology 56: 232–235, 2000.

VINBLASTINE

Other names

Velban®; Velsar®; Alkaban AQ®; Velbe; vinblastine sulfate; vincaleukoblastine; VLB; NSC-49842.

Indications

FDA approved for the treatment of Hodgkin's disease, non-Hodgkin's lymphoma, cutaneous T-cell lymphoma (advanced stages), carcinoma of the testis, Kaposi's sarcoma, histiocytosis X, choriocarcinoma, and breast cancer. Vinblastine may be useful in the treatment of chronic myelogenous leukemia, melanoma, neuroblastoma, and cancers of the kidney, bladder, cervix, head and neck, ovary, and lung.

Classification and Mechanisms of Action

Plant alkaloid (tubulin inhibitor). The drug binds to microtubular proteins of the mitotic spindle leading to mitotic arrest.

Pharmacokinetics

Vinblastine is poorly absorbed by mouth. After IV administration the drug is quickly and widely distributed throughout the body (excluding the cerebrospinal fluid). The drug is liver metabolized to the active metabolite, desacetylvinblastine, and nonactive metabolites. Approximately 14% of vinblastine is eliminated in the urine. Vinblastine is not hemodialyzable and has an elimination half-life of approximately 20 hours.

Dose

Commonly used doses range from 6 to 10 mg/m^2 every 2 to 4 weeks in combination with other drugs.

Vinblastine has also been given weekly and as a continuous infusion in a dose of 1.7 to 2 mg/m^2/day over a 96-hour period.

Administration

Vinblastine is most commonly given by IV push over 1 to 5 minutes using extravasation precautions. The drug has been administered by continuous IV infusion in 50 mL or more of 5% dextrose or normal saline over a 96-hour period.

Toxicity

Hematological. Leukopenia is dose-limiting. Thrombocytopenia and anemia occur less frequently.

Gastrointestinal. Nausea and vomiting are infrequent toxicities, and constipation occurs occasionally (see neurological side effects). Abdominal pain (cramps), anorexia, diarrhea, mucositis, and gastrointestinal hemorrhage are rare.

Dermatological. Alopecia (uncommon), epilation, skin and soft-tissue damage if extravasated (the manufacturer recommends subcutaneous injection of hyaluronidase and application of heat to help disperse the drug), rash, photosensitivity.

Neurological. Neurological adverse effects are dose-related and occur infrequently with conventional doses. Toxicities may include peripheral neuropathy (loss of deep tendon reflexes, paresthesias, paralysis), autonomic neuropathy (constipation, paralytic ileus, urinary retention, orthostasis), vocal cord paralysis, myalgias, Raynaud's phenomenon, headache, seizures, depression, dizziness, and malaise.

Pulmonary. Bronchospasm and acute dyspnea are uncommon and more commonly occur when vinblastine and mitomycin are administered in combination. Pulmonary edema has been rarely reported.

Other. Severe pain in the jaw, pharynx, bones, back, or limbs after injection; syndrome of inappropriate antidiuretic hormone (SIADH), fever, and ischemic cardiotoxicity.

Drug Interactions

Vinblastine administered with paclitaxel or cisplatin may increase the risk of neurotoxicity.

The elimination of vinblastine may be reduced by agents that inhibit cytochrome P450 enzymes. These agents include, but are not limited to, itraconazole, calcium channer blockers, cimetidine, erythromycin, and macrolides. The toxicity of vinblastine may be increased.

Vinblastine may decrease phenytoin levels and increase the risk for seizure activity.

Vinblastine administered concomitantly with mitomycin can result in acute increased pulmonary toxicity (e.g., severe bronchospasm). Avoid this combination of chemotherapy drugs.

VINBLASTINE *(continued)*

Storage and Stability

Vials are stored in the refrigerator. Vinblastine, reconstituted to a concentration of 1 mg/mL, is stable for 14 and 30 days at room and refrigeration temperatures, respectively. Further diluted to a concentration of 0.01 mg/mL in normal saline or 5% dextrose, vinblastine is stable for at least 5 days at room temperature.

Preparation

The 10-mg vial of lyophilized powder is reconstituted with 10 mL of bacteriostatic normal saline to yield a concentration of 1 mg/mL. Doses for continuous infusion may be further diluted with 50 mL or more of normal saline or 5% dextrose in water.

Incompatibilities

Furosemide, heparin, Infusaid® pumps.

Compatibilities

Vinblastine is physically stable in normal saline solutions for at least 5 days, alone or mixed with doxorubicin, at room or refrigeration temperatures. Vinblastine is also compatible in solution with metoclopramide, dacarbazine, or bleomycin. A pharmacist should be consulted for additional information.

Availability

Vinblastine is commercially available in 10-mg vials, as a lyophilized powder, and as a 1 mg/mL solution.

VINCRISTINE

Other names

Oncovin®; Vincasar PFS®; Vincrex®; vincristine sulfate; VCR; leucocristine; NSC-67574.

Indications

FDA approved for the treatment of acute leukemia, Hodgkin's disease, non-Hodgkin's lymphoma, rhabdomyosarcoma, neuroblastoma, Ewing's sarcoma, and Wilm's tumor. Vincristine may be useful in the treatment of chronic leukemias, Kaposi's sarcoma, soft-tissue sarcomas, osteosarcoma, multiple myeloma, trophoblastic neoplasms, malignant melanoma, and cancers of the colon, rectum, brain, breast, cervix, head and neck, ovary, lung, and thyroid.

Classification and Mechanisms of Action

Plant alkaloid (tubulin inhibitor). The drug binds to microtubular proteins of the mitotic spindle leading to mitotic arrest.

Pharmacokinetics

Vincristine is poorly absorbed by mouth. After IV dosing the drug is quickly and widely distributed throughout the body (excluding the cerebrospinal fluid). Vincristine is metabolized by the liver with 40% to 80% of the drug excreted in the bile and feces; 10% to 20% is excreted unchanged in the urine. Vincristine is not hemodialyzable and has an elimination half-life of approximately 85 hours.

Dose

Commonly used doses range from 0.5 to 1.4 mg/m^2 per dose every 1 to 4 weeks. Limiting a total individual dose to 2 mg is advocated by many but may not be necessary. Continuous infusion regimens of 0.5 mg/day to 0.5 mg/m^2/day for 4 days have also been used.

Administration

Usually given through a free-flowing IV line over 1 to 5 minutes using extravasation precautions. Occasionally it is administered by continuous IV infusion in 50 mL or more of 5% dextrose or normal saline over a 96-hour period.

Toxicity

Hematological. Leukopenia (mild and rare), thrombocytopenia (rare), anemia.
Gastrointestinal. Nausea and vomiting are rare, constipation (see neurological side effects), abdominal pain (cramps), anorexia, diarrhea.
Dermatological. Alopecia (12% to 45%), skin and soft-tissue damage if extravasated (the manufacturer recommends subcutaneous injection of hyaluronidase and application of heat to help disperse the drug), rash (uncommon).
Hepatic. Elevations of hepatic transaminase levels are usually mild and transient.
Neurological. Peripheral neuropathy (loss of deep tendon reflexes, paresthesias, paralysis), autonomic neuropathy (constipation, paralytic ileus, urinary retention, orthostasis), ataxia, hoarseness, myalgia, cortical blindness, headache, seizures. Fatal ascending paralysis follows intrathecal administration. Foot pain with severe motor weakness has been observed after treatment with vincristine and filgrastim (granulocyte colony-stimulating factor [G-CSF]).
Pulmonary. Bronchospasm and acute dyspnea have been reported and appear to occur more frequently when vincristine is administered with mitomycin.
Ocular. Diplopia, ptosis, photophobia, cortical blindness (see neurological toxicity), optic atrophy, ophthalmoplegia, corneal hypesthesia.
Other. Severe pain in the jaw, pharynx, bones, back, and limbs after injection, syndrome of inappropriate antidiuretic hormone (SIADH), fever, pancreatitis (rare).

Drug Interactions

Vincristine administered to patients on chronic digoxin or phenytoin therapy has decreased the serum levels of these medications.

Asparaginase administered prior to or with vincristine may cause increased vincristine toxicity, due to decreased hepatic clearance of vincristine. Administer vincristine 12 to 24 hours prior to asparaginase.

Vincristine administered in combination with filgrastim (granulocyte colony-stimulating factor [G-CSF], Neupogen®) may cause severe atypical neuropathy.

Vincristine may decrease the oral absorption of quinolone antibiotics (e.g., ciprofloxacin, gatifloxacin).

Vincristine administered with paclitaxel or cisplatin may increase the risk and severity of neurotoxicity.

The elimination of vincristine may be reduced by agents that inhibit cytochrome P450 enzymes. These agents include, but are not limited to, itraconazole and macrolides. The toxicity of vincristine may be increased.

Storage and Stability

Vincristine is stored in the refrigerator. The drug is stable for at least 30 days at room temperature. Vincristine is chemically stable when further diluted in normal saline or 5% dextrose for at least 4 days at room temperature (7 days in the refrigerator), alone or mixed with doxorubicin in glass or PVC containers.

VINCRISTINE (continued)

Preparation

Doses for continuous infusion are further diluted with 50 mL or more of normal saline or 5% dextrose, and should be administered through a central line.

Incompatibilities

Furosemide, idarubicin, some in-line filters, polysiloxane containers used in portable delivery devices.

Compatibilities

Vincristine is compatible with doxorubicin, bleomycin, cytarabine, fluorouracil, methotrexate, and metoclopramide. A pharmacist should be consulted for additional information.

Availability

Vincristine is commercially available as a solution in a concentration of 1 mg/mL in 1-, 2-, and 5-mL vials and 1- and 2-mg syringes (Hyporet).

Selected Reading

Weintraub M et al. Severe atypical neuropathy associated with colony-stimulating factors and vincristine, J Clin Oncol 14: 935–940, 1996.

VINDESINE

Other names

Eldisine®; deacetylvinblastine amide sulfate; DAVA; VDS; NSC-245467.

Indications

Vindesine is an investigational agent in the United States that has activity against Hodgkin's and non-Hodgkin's lymphomas, non-small-cell lung cancer, breast cancer, and other malignancies. In Canada and other countries vindesine is approved as a single agent or in combination with other drugs. Vindesine is approved in these countries as a single agent for acute lymphoblastic leukemia of childhood, resistant to other drugs; blast crisis of chronic myeloid leukemia; malignant melanoma unresponsive to other forms of therapy; and advanced carcinoma of the breast unresponsive to appropriate endocrine surgery and/or hormonal therapy.

Classification and Mechanisms of Action

Vindesine is a vinca alkaloid derivative that is similar to vinblastine. The drug binds to microtubular proteins of the mitotic spindle leading to mitotic arrest.

Pharmacokinetics

Vindesine is metabolized by the liver and primarily excreted into the bile. Approximately 15% of the drug is eliminated unchanged in the urine. The elimination half-life is approximately 20 hours.

Dose

Several regimens have been evaluated, including 2 to 4 mg/m² every 1 to 2 weeks, 1 to 1.5 mg/m²/day for 5 to 7 days repeated every 3 weeks, and 1.5 to 2 mg/m² twice weekly. The manufacturer recommends a 50% dose reduction if the patient's total bilirubin is 25 to 50 micromol/L (1.5 to 2.9 mg/dL) and to omit the dose if the bilirubin exceeds 50 micromol/L (2.9 mg/dL).

Administration
Vindesine is administered by IV push, using extravasation precautions.

Toxicity
Hematological. Leukopenia is common and often dose-limiting with nadir counts occurring 4 to 10 days after administration. Recovery occurs within 7 to 10 days. Thrombocytopenia and anemia occur less often.
Gastrointestinal. Nausea, vomiting, anorexia, diarrhea, and stomatitis are uncommon.
Dermatological. Alopecia is common but usually mild. If the drug extravasates, tissue damage (blistering, ulceration, necrosis) is likely to occur.
Neurological. Peripheral neuropathy is common, cumulative, and dose-limiting in some patients.
Other. Fatigue, malaise, photophobia, and fever are uncommon side effects.

Drug Interactions
The elimination of vindesine may be reduced by agents that inhibit cytochrome P450 3A4 enzymes. These agents include, but are not limited to, itraconazole and macrolides. The toxicity of vindesine may be increased.

Vinca alkaloids when administered in combination with mitomycin resulted in an increase in acute pulmonary reactions.

Storage and Stability
Intact vials are stored in the refrigerator. Reconstituted solutions (1 mg/mL) are chemically stable for at least 14 days at room or refrigeration temperatures. Solutions that are further diluted in 5% dextrose or normal saline are stable for at least 24 hours at room temperature.

Preparation
Add 5 mL of sterile water to the 5-mg vial to yield a concentration of 1 mg/mL.

Compatibilities
Dilution of vindesine in electrolyte-containing solutions such as lactated Ringer's may cause precipitation.

Availability
Vindesine is an investigational agent in the United States that is available as a lyophilized powder (5 mg/vial) from the manufacturer.

Selected Reading
Vats T et al. A study of toxicity and comparative therapeutic efficacy of vindesine-prednisone vs. vincristine-prednisone in children with acute lymphoblastic leukemia in relapse. Invest New Drugs 10: 231–234, 1992.

VINORELBINE

Other names
Navelbine®; vinorelbine tartrate; 5′-noranhydrovinblastine; NVB.

Indications
FDA approved for the treatment of non-small-cell lung cancer as a single agent or in combination with cisplatin. Vinorelbine may also be useful in the treatment of breast cancer, uterine-cervical cancer, platinum-resistant ovarian cancer, Hodgkin's disease, and advanced Kaposi's sarcoma.

VINORELBINE (continued)

Classification

Vinca alkaloid (tubulin inhibitor).

Pharmacokinetics

Approximately 26% of vinorelbine is bioavailable after oral administration. The drug is metabolized in the liver and has an elimination half-life of approximately 23 hours.

Dose

The usual IV dose, as a single agent or in combination with cisplatin, is 30 mg/m^2/week. Adjust dose based on absolute neutrophil count and bilirubin.

Vinorelbine has been evaluated in oral doses of 50 to 80 mg/m^2/week.

Administration

Vinorelbine is a moderate vesicant and can produce phlebitis. The drug is most often administered intravenously (using extravasation precautions) over 6 to 10 minutes. Adequate flushing of the vein with 100 to 200 mL of 5% dextrose or normal saline after administration is recommended to decrease the risk of phlebitis. The orally administered drug is generally taken on an empty stomach as a single dose.

Toxicity

Hematological. Leukopenia and neutropenia are the most frequent dose-limiting toxicities. Leukopenia generally begins 1 week after administration with recovery 8 to 10 days thereafter. Mild to moderate anemia is infrequent. Thrombocytopenia rarely occurs. Hematological toxicity does not appear to be cumulative.

Gastrointestinal. Nausea and vomiting after IV administration are generally mild and controllable with standard anti-emetic drugs. Severe nausea and vomiting have been reported more frequently after oral administration. Mild to moderate constipation, anorexia, stomatitis, diarrhea, and abdominal pain have been reported in approximately 18% to 38% of patients.

Dermatological. Significant alopecia is uncommon and appears to be related to the duration of the treatment. Phlebitis, characterized by erythema, vein discoloration, and tenderness extending over the length of the infused vein, is an occasional toxicity. Chemical phlebitis occurs in up to 10% of patients and manifests along the vein proximal to the site of injection; this can be an immediate or delayed reaction. Vinorelbine is a moderate vesicant, similar to vincristine and vinblastine. Radiation recall reactions may occur with the administration of vinorelbine in patients who have received prior or concommitant radiation therapy.

Hepatic. Transient and mild elevations of hepatic enzyme levels have been reported.

Neurological. Fatigue has been reported in 27% of patients treated with vinorelbine and tended to worsen with continued treatment. Severe peripheral neuropathy is rare (less than 1%) and may appear as decreased deep tendon reflexes, constipation, paresthesias, and/or hypesthesia. Loss of deep tendon reflexes (less than 5%) may be cumulative. Tumor pain and jaw pain are infrequent, but may be severe.

Cardiovascular. Chest pain, with or without ECG changes, has been reported in several patients treated with vinorelbine. Many of the patients experiencing chest pain had either a history of cardiovascular disease or a tumor within the chest. The precise cause of the chest pain has not been determined. Myocardial infarction has also been reported in a few patients; all of these patients had a prior history of severe cardiovascular disease.

Pulmonary. Acute reversible dyspnea after IV administration has been reported and may be an allergic phenomenon, as with other vinca alkaloids. Hypoxemia and interstitial pneumonitis have been reported infrequently. Treatment with corticosteroids may be beneficial in patients who develop pulmonary toxicities.

Other. Mild to moderate asthenia is common. Syndrome of inappropriate secretion of antidiuretic hormone (SIADH), fatigue, and hemorrhagic cystitis have been rarely reported after administration of vinorelbine.

Drug Interactions

The elimination of vinorelbine may be reduced by agents that inhibit cytochrome P450 3A4 enzymes. These agents include, but are not limited to, itraconazole and macrolides. The toxicity of vinorelbine may be increased.

Vinorelbine administered with paclitaxel may increase the risk of neurotoxicity.

Vinca alkaloids when administered in combination with mitomycin resulted in an increase in acute pulmonary reactions.

Storage and Stability

Intact vials are stored in the refrigerator (2° to 8°C) and protected from light. The parenteral formulation is stable at room temperature for at least 72 hours. Vials should not be frozen. Vinorelbine, diluted in 50 to 100 mL of 5% dextrose or normal saline, is stable for at least 24 hours at room and refrigeration temperatures.

Preparation

Vinorelbine must be diluted before administration. Concentrations of 1.5 or 3 mg/mL have been diluted with 5% dextrose or normal saline and administered with a syringe. For administration in an IV container, vinorelbine may be diluted in 5% dextrose, normal saline, 0.45% NaCl, 5% dextrose and 0.45% NaCl, Ringer's solution, or lactated Ringer's solution to a concentration of 0.5 to 2 mg/mL.

Availability

Commercially available as a 10 mg/mL solution in 1-mL and 5-mL vials. Oral capsules, 10 and 40 mg, are investigational.

ZOLEDRONIC ACID

Other names

Zometa®; Zoledronic acid for injection; CGP-42446; CGP-42446A; ZOL 446; NSC-721517.

Indications

FDA approved for the treatment of hypercalcemia of malignancy. Zoledronic acid may also be useful for treatment of patients with osteolytic lesions or osteolytic bone metastases (e.g., breast cancer, multiple myeloma, and prostate cancer), Paget's disease, and other bone-resorptive diseases.

Classification and Mechanisms of Action

Zoledronic acid is a biphosphonate that prevents bone resorption. The drug exerts its actions by inhibiting osteoblast proliferation and osteoclast formation. It also causes apoptosis of osteoclasts, and inhibits osteoclast mineralized bone resorption. The drug also inhibits stimulatory factors that induce osteoclast activity and skeletal release of calcium.

ZOLEDRONIC ACID *(continued)*

Pharmacokinetics

Zoledronic acid exhibits triphasic elimination with a terminal half-life of 167 hours. Low plasma concentrations are detected up to 28 days after a 4-mg dose. Zoledronic acid is minimally plasma protein-bound (22%) and rapidly taken up by the bone. The majority of drug is eliminated in the urine as parent compound with up to 60% recovered in the urine 24 hours following administration. The remainder of zoledronic acid is slowly released from the bone. Clearance does not depend on dose, patient weight, gender, race, or body mass index, but it does correlate closely with creatinine clearance.

Dose

Treatment of hypercalcemia. The maximum dose of zoledronic acid is 4 mg, given in conjunction with vigorous saline hydration. If retreatment is necessary, it is recommended that at least 7 days elapse from the time of the initial dose.
Treatment of osteolytic bone lesions. The maximum dose of zoledronic acid is 4 mg.

Administration

Zoledronic acid is administered by IV infusion in 100 mL of 5% dextrose or normal saline over at least a 15-minute period.

Toxicity

Hematological. Anemia (22%).
Gastrointestinal. Nausea (29%), vomiting (14%), abdominal pain (16%), anorexia (9%), constipation (26%), diarrhea (17%).
Neurological. Insomnia (15%), anxiety (14%), agitation (12%), confusion (12%).
Cardiovascular. Hypotension.
Pulmonary. Dyspnea (22%).
Renal. Renal dysfunction, renal failure manifested by an increase in serum creatinine. Monitor renal function frequently.
Electrolyte. Hypocalcemia, hypokalemia (11%), hypomagnesemia (10%), hypophosphatemia (12%).
Other. Fever (44%), chills, bone pain.

Storage and Stability

Zoledronic acid is stored at room temperature. Vials bear expiration dates. The drug must be administered within 24 hours after reconstitution. Immediate use of the reconstituted solution is recommended; if not used immediately, store reconstituted solution in the refrigerator.

Preparation

Add 5 mL of sterile water to the 4-mg vial. Withdraw the entire vial contents (4 mg) and further dilute in 100 mL 0.9% sodium chloride or 5% dextrose and water.

Incompatibilities

Zoledronic acid is incompatible with calcium-containing solutions, such as Ringer's solution. Use a dedicated intravenous line for administration of this drug.

Availability

Zoledronic acid is commercially available as a 4-mg vial of sterile powder for reconstitution.

Selected Readings

Berenson JR et al. Zoledronic acid reduces skeletal-related events in patients with osteolytic metastases. A double-blind, randomized dose-response study. Cancer 91: 144–154, 2001.

Major P et al. Zoledronic acid is superior to pamidronate in the treatment of hypercalcemia of malignancy: a pooled analysis of two randomized, controlled clinical trials. J Clin Oncol; 19: 558–567, 2001.

Rosen LS et al. Zoledronic acid versus pamidronate in the treatment of skeletal metastases in patients with breast cancer or osteolytic lesions of multiple myeloma: a phase III, double-blind, comparative trial. The Cancer J 7: 337–387, 2001.

GENERAL REFERENCES

American Medical Association. AMA Drug Evaluations. Chicago, 1996.

Beckwith MC, Tyler LS, eds. Facts and Comparisons: Cancer Chemotherapy Manual. St. Louis, Facts and Comparisons, 2001.

Chabner BA, Longo DL. Cancer Chemotherapy and Biotherapy: Principles and Practice, 3rd ed. Philadelphia, Lippincott, Williams and Wilkins, 2001.

DeVita VT Jr, Hellman S, Rosenberg SA, eds. Cancer: Principles and Practice of Oncology, 6th ed. Philadelphia, Lippincott, Williams and Wilkins, 2001.

Durivage HJ, Burnham NL. Prevention and management of toxicities associated with antineoplastic drugs. J Pharm Pract 4: 27–48, 1991.

Gelman RS et al. Actual versus ideal weight in the calculation of surface area effects on dose of 11 chemotherapy agents. Cancer Treat Rep 71: 907–911, 1987.

Georgiadis MS et al. Obesity and therapy-related toxicity in patients treated for small-cell lung cancer. J Natl Cancer Inst 87: 361–366, 1995.

Gisselbrecht C et al. Cyclophosphamide/mitoxantrone/melphalan (CMA) regimen prior to autologous bone marrow transplantation in metastatic breast cancer. Bone Marrow Transplantation 18: 857–863, 1996.

Goss PE et al. Aromatase inhibitors in the treatment and prevention of breast cancer. J Clin Oncol 19: 881–894, 2001.

Grochow LB, Baraldi C, Noe D. Is dose normalization to weight or body surface area useful in adults? J Natl Cancer Inst 82: 323–325, 1990.

Gurney H. Dose calculation of anticancer drugs: a review of the current practice and introduction of an alternative. J Clin Oncol 14: 2590–2611, 1996.

Gurney H. How to calculate the dose of chemotherapy. Br J Cancer 86: 1207–1208, 2002.

Gurney HP et al. Factors affecting epirubicin pharmacokinetics and toxicity: evidence against using body-surface area for dose calculation. J Clin Oncol 16: 2299–2304, 1998.

Hebel SK et al, eds. Antineoplastic agents. In Facts and Comparisons: Drug Information. St. Louis, Facts and Comparisons, 2001, pp642–689.

Hensley ML et al. American Society of Clinical Oncology clinical practice guidelines for the use of chemotherapy and radiotherapy protectants. J Clin Oncol 17: 3333–3335, 1999.

McEvoy JK, ed. AHFS Drug Information. Washington, DC, American Society of Health-System Pharmacists, 2002.

Physician's Desk Reference. Montvale, NJ, Medical Economics, 2002.

Rosner GL et al. Relationship between toxicity and obesity in women receiving adjuvant chemotherapy for breast cancer: results from cancer and leukemia group B study 8541. J Clin Oncol 14: 3000–3008, 1996.

Southwest Oncology Group. Dosing Principles for Patients on Clinical Trials. Policy Memorandum No. 38, October 2001. Available at SWOG website, www.SWOG.org.

United States Pharmacopeial Convention. USP Drug Information. Rockville, MD, The Convention, 1996.

BIOTHERAPY

The immune system is responsible for protecting the body from harmful substances such as bacteria, viruses, and cancer. External defenses, such as the skin, mucous membranes, and gastric acid, prevent the absorption of harmful substances. Internal defenses, such as the lymphoid organs, tissues, and cells, rid the body of substances that have penetrated our external defenses. Internal defenses can be either nonspecific (e.g., neutrophils, macrophages) or specific (e.g., T-lymphocytes). The immune system is responsible for recognizing foreign substances (antigens), eliminating them, and remembering that they were once present. Re-exposure to the antigen produces an immune response. Many investigators believe the immune system is responsible for the elimination of malignant cells. In a patient with a rapidly progressive malignancy, the immune system has failed to function properly.

Early work with nonspecific stimulators of the immune system, such as bacillus Calmette-Guérin (BCG), methanol-extracted residue of BCG, *Corynebacterium parvum* (*C. parvum*), and levamisole, yielded few successes. Most studies failed to demonstrate any benefit when these agents were used alone as systemic therapy for advanced disease or as an adjuvant to surgery for "localized" malignancies.

More recent investigations of immunological responses and approaches for the treatment of cancer followed these early disappointments. These studies have increased our knowledge of tumor immunology and, coupled with recombinant DNA technology, have led to the development of many of the biological response modifiers and monoclonal antibody targeting agents that are viable cancer treatment options.

This chapter contains a brief discussion of tumor immunology, general classes of available biological response modifiers, and monoclonal antibodies. Some targeted therapy agents that can be classified as biotherapy or monoclonal antibody therapy will be located in this chapter, all others have been listed in Chapter 4. For an extensive review of tumor immunology, see the general references provided at the end of this chapter.

ANTITUMOR IMMUNITY

When the immune system responds to the presence of a foreign substance, or antigen, it does so in two possible ways. In the humoral response, B-lymphocytes recognize and attach to the antigen. Plasma cells are then formed that produce antibodies against the antigen. In the cell-mediated response, T-lymphocytes (T-helper cells or cytotoxic T-lymphocytes) recognize the foreign substance and either directly kill the invader or elicit the production of antibody from plasma cells. Regulation of T-lymphocyte proliferation and activity is largely mediated by cytokines such as interleukin-1 (IL-1), interleukin-2 (IL-2), and tumor necrosis factor (TNF).

The concept known as natural immunity or immune surveillance implies that the immune system is capable of recognizing all tumor cells as foreign. Natural killer (NK) cells (another type of lymphocyte) and macrophages confer this type of immunity. However, views are divided on the concept of immune surveillance because not all human tumors elicit an immune response or they are not particularly sensitive to the effects of NK cells. Although it is not precisely known how NK cells, macrophages, and certain lymphocytes recognize and kill tumor cells, studies with these cell types have resulted in antitumor therapies. These cells can be removed from the body, can be induced by cytokines (such as IL-2), and later can be reinfused to the patient as a form of treatment. As will be discussed in this chapter, many of the cytokines that are a natural part of the immune system are presently available for the treatment of cancer or will be in the future.

CLINICAL DEVELOPMENT OF THE BIOLOGICAL RESPONSE MODIFIERS

The target cells of the biological response modifiers are the host effector cells, such as the T-helper lymphocytes, not the cancer cells. As a result, classical dose-response relationships that exist for antineoplastic drugs may not exist for agents that are intended to augment the immune system. Administration of a biological response modifier at its maximally tolerated dose may not be the optimal dose for modulation of the immune system. In some cases, the maximally tolerated dose may be inferior to a lower dose. Alternatively, the higher dose may increase the severity of adverse effects without a concomitant increase in the desired biological effect. The clinical development and early human testing of biological response modifiers are designed to determine the optimal biological dose (OBD), the relationship between the OBD and the optimal therapeutic effect and, if necessary, the maximally tolerated dose (MTD). Unfortunately, it is often unclear which of the many effector cell functions are directly related to tumor response.

HEMATOPOIETIC GROWTH FACTORS

Hematopoietic growth factors are glycoproteins that bind to specific cell surface receptors and stimulate the proliferation, differentiation, and activation of blood cells from different lineages. They were discovered and are defined by their ability to support colony formation in vitro, hence the name colony-stimulating factor. Blood cell formation involves a complex network of cytokines. The goal of therapy with hematopoietic growth factors is to increase the number of functional white blood cells so that host defense mechanisms can be maintained, to increase the number of platelets so that bleeding problems can be avoided, and/or to increase the number of red blood cells so that red blood cell transfusions can be avoided. In addition, white blood cell colony-stimulating factors are used to mobilize stem cells into the pool of peripheral blood. The stem cells can then be collected through a pheresis process and later reinfused into patients undergoing stem cell transplants. Success of treatment with growth factors will be measured in terms of decreased neutropenia, infection, use of antibiotics, transfusion requirements, hospital admissions for fever, decreased length of stay, and reduced treatment costs. Other applications will be to examine the efficacy of increasing dose intensity of chemotherapy using growth factors to minimize myelosuppression. The success of these studies will be measured by increases in tumor response, disease-free interval, and survival.

INTERFERONS

The phenomenon known as viral interference (i.e., prevention of viral infection after initial exposure) has been known for many years. While studying viral interference in vitro, Isaacs and Lindemann (1957) reported the discovery of a substance that was able to induce cellular resistance to viral challenge. They called this substance interferon. In 1969, the interferons were shown to have antitumor effects. In 1973, methods were developed that permitted the isolation of interferons from human blood. Interferons are a family of species-specific proteins that, among other functions, induce antiviral resistance in cells. After viral challenge, human cells naturally secrete them. The interferons were originally described according to their cell of origin, later according to physical-chemical properties, and now according to their antigenic type. Experimental studies in man in the 1970s and early 1980s were performed with interferon prepared from human leukocytes exposed to the Sendai virus. Interferon was isolated from leukocytes that were collected primarily by the Finnish Red Cross. These preparations contained approximately 0.5% pure interferon and at least 16 other species of interferon alfa. Since then, recombinant DNA technology has provided a way to produce massive amounts of pure interferon of a single species. Interferons are available for use in the treatment of patients with cancer and other disease as a mixture of alfa interferons (interferon alfa-n3, Alferon®; interferon alfa-n1, Wellferon®) or as single recombinant proteins (interferon alfa-2a, Roferon®; interferon alfa-2b, Intron® A; or interferon gamma-1b, Actimmune®).

Although the interferons are described in the following sections as single agents for the treatment of malignant and other conditions, some studies suggest that they may be useful when combined with antineoplastic drugs or other biological agents.

INTERLEUKINS

The interleukins are cytokines, substances secreted by T-cells, monocytes, macrophages, and other cells, and are important mediators of many immune responses. The recent advances in genetic engineering have enabled researchers to identify and evaluate the biological activities of several different interleukins. As of July 2000, there have been 18 identified interleukins (Rieger, 2001); not all of the interleukins that have been identified have been evaluated in humans and some are in preclinical testing. Others have undergone extensive study and are no longer being pursued as potential treatments for patients with cancer. The interleukins included in this chapter are those that have been approved for the treatment of cancer (IL-2, aldesleukin), and a few others currently undergoing clinical evaluation.

CLINICAL DEVELOPMENT OF TARGETED THERAPY

The concept of drug-specific targeting agents has evolved over the past 20 years. In 1986, large-scale testing of monoclonal antibodies was made possible by Kohler and Milstein through the publication of the hybridoma methodology (Dillman, 2001). This opened the door for increased clinical testing of monoclonal antibodies.

Monoclonal antibodies are classified and named based on their derivation. Murine monoclonal antibodies have the suffix ending "momab", are cleared quickly from the body, and have a greater chance of inducing a HAMA reaction (human anti-mouse antibody). Chimeric antibodies are a human-mouse antibody mixture; they possess the suffix ending "imab" and are more efficient and effective at destroying cells via CDC (complement-dependent cytotoxicity) and ADCC (antibody-dependent cell-mediated cytotoxicity) (Maloney & McLaughlin, 2001). Chimeric antibodies circulate longer in the human body and are less likely to invoke a HAMA reaction. Humanized monoclonal antibodies posses the suffix ending "umab" and are not likely to invoke a HAMA reaction.

Monoclonal antibody therapy is based on the ability to target markers and bind to cell membrane antigens with great specificity (Weiner, 1999). Many times the enhanced specificity demonstrated toward the tumor antigens allows normal cells to be protected against harmful effects, unlike conventional chemotherapy. There are several mechanisms by which monoclonal antibodies destroy or prevent further replication of malignant cells. Some monoclonal antibodies utilize tumor immunology and components of the host natural defense mechanism to exert their desired effect. For example,

PREVENTION AND MANAGEMENT OF TOXICITIES

monoclonal antibodies can utilize tumor effector cells to promote tumor cell lysis or they have the ability to directly modulate tumor function (Weiner, 1999). Conjugated monoclonal antibodies can be used as carriers of toxic therapy, such as radionuclides (e.g., Zevalin®), cytotoxic drugs, or cell toxins, to specific cell targets. They are also being employed to create tumor vaccines, by stimulating a host antibody reaction causing the production of anti-idiotype antibodies (Weiner, 1999).

In the last two to five years, selected monoclonal antibodies have become a standard of care for certain malignancies. Rituximab, a chimeric monoclonal antibody used against CD20-positive B-cell non-Hodgkin's lymphoma, is now utilized in combination with the standard of care chemotherapy regimen CHOP. Trastuzumab, a humanized monoclonal antibody, is a weekly maintenance therapy for HER2neu-positive metastatic breast cancer patients. Despite the many obstacles that continue to challenge this therapeutic modality, monoclonal antibody therapy provides a new venue in the realm of oncology therapy that has only just begun.

PREVENTION AND MANAGEMENT OF TOXICITIES

Most biological response modifiers (BRMs) produce similar side effects, although a few unique toxicities have been observed. As outlined for interferon, treatment with a BRM produces predictable acute and chronic constitutional symptoms. The flu-like syndrome of fevers, chills, rigors, and myalgias is the most common acute side effect for most of the BRMs. Exceptions include granulocyte colony-stimulating factor (G-CSF) and BCG. Common acute and chronic side effects include fatigue, confusion, depression, and neurological side effects. Less predictable, except for high-dose IL-2 therapy, is the broad range of potential organ system toxicities. Most side effects that are observed, however, are dependent on dose, duration of treatment, schedule, route of administration, or a combination of these variables.

A common toxicity of monoclonal antibodies that react with antigen is the potential to produce a side effect referred to as an infusion-related symptom complex. The probability of this reaction occurring increases in patients with a large tumor burden. This reaction is generally observed with the first or second dose of the monoclonal antibody; however, it is important to note that mild to severe latent reactions have occurred. The symptom complex is characterized by one or more of the following: fever, chills, rigors, dyspnea, bronchospasm, headache, hypotension, rash, nausea, throat tightness, flushing, and urticaria. This reaction can range from very mild symptoms to a severe and/or fatal reaction. It is vital to assess each patient on an individual basis due to the variability of reactions. The management of infusion-related reactions begins with stopping the infusion, assessing the patient, and administering hypersensitivity medications as needed (e.g., diphenhydramine, meperidine, H2 blockers, corticosteroids, epinephrine). Once patient symptoms have resolved, many patients can have the infusion restarted at a slower rate, under clinical observation.

Patients need to be aware of the side effects that are likely to occur, and they must be informed about what they can do to prevent or minimize the severity of these side effects. They also need to know that virtually all of the side effects are reversible, most subsiding within a few days after stopping treatment. The severity of symptoms varies from patient to patient. The lack of acute side effects is not usually predictive of adverse effects that may occur after weeks to months of treatment. Many of the side effects are subjective (i.e., fatigue, bone pain) and accurate documentation requires frequent communication and the cooperation of the patient and healthcare provider. Neurological side effects, such as mood or behavior changes, may be subtle. Family members and friends are a valuable source of information regarding these types of side effects. Healthcare providers must be aware of the full range of possible toxicities associated with BRM and monoclonal antibody treatments. Factors that may intensify a particular toxicity or mask its detection must be eliminated before treatment is begun and avoided during therapy. Premedication and other preventative measures must be instituted at the onset of treatment and adjusted accordingly as therapy continues.

Several biological agents are discussed in this revision along with the addition of monoclonal antibodies that were not included in the previous edition. The format and general guidelines for the listing of biological and monoclonal agents is alphabetical.

ALDESLEUKIN

Other Names
Proleukin®; interleukin-2; IL-2; rIL-2; T-cell growth factor; T-cell replacing factor; TRF; NSC-373364.

Indications
FDA approved for the treatment of metastatic renal cell carcinoma in adults. Aldesleukin may be useful as a single agent, or combined with other drugs as treatment for patients with malignant melanoma, Kaposi's sarcoma (combined with zidovudine [AZT]), and non-Hodgkin's lymphoma.

Classification and Mechanisms of Action
Aldesleukin is a glycoprotein produced and released during an immune response by stimulated T-helper cells. Aldesleukin has been called T-cell growth factor because of its role in regulating the maturation and replication of T-lymphocytes. Aldesleukin mediates the expansion of reactive T-lymphocytes (cells that possess IL-2 receptors) after they contact an antigen. Four subsets of T-lymphocytes (i.e., T-helper cells, cytolytic T-cells, suppressor T-cells, and memory T-cells) as well as monocytes and B-lymphocytes are influenced by aldesleukin.

Pharmacokinetics
Aldesleukin is not absorbed after oral administration. After IV administration, aldesleukin rapidly distributes throughout the body, including the cerebrospinal fluid. Aldesleukin is metabolized in the kidneys and has an elimination half-life of 30 to 90 minutes. Elimination occurs via glomerular filtration and tubular secretion. The elimination of aldesleukin is not dramatically affected in patients with reduced creatinine clearance because of tubular secretion.

Dose
For the treatment of renal cell carcinoma, the recommended dose is 600,000 IU/kg every 8 hours for a total of 14 doses over 5 consecutive days. After a 9-day period of no treatment, the same dose and schedule is repeated. Of the 28 doses intended, an average of eight doses are withheld because of toxicity. In patients who appear to be obtaining benefit from the first course of treatment, a second course may be administered. It is recommended that the second course be initiated 7 weeks after the date the patient was discharged from the hospital. Similar dosing has been used for metastatic melanoma.

It is recommended that therapy be permanently discontinued if any of the following toxicities are observed: sustained ventricular tachycardia, unresponsive or uncontrolled cardiac arrhythmia, recurrent chest pain with ECG changes, documented angina or myocardial infarction, pericardial tamponade, intubation required for more than 72 hours, renal dysfunction requiring greater than 72 hours of dialysis, coma or toxic psychosis lasting more than 48 hours, uncontrolled seizures, bowel ischemia, bowel perforation, or gastrointestinal bleeding requiring surgery.

Administration

Aldesleukin is administered intravenously, usually in 50 mL or more of 5% dextrose and water over a period of 20 to 30 minutes. Aldesleukin has also been administered by continuous IV (more toxic by this route), subcutaneously, intramuscularly, intraperitoneally, via intrahepatic intra-arterial infusion, and by isolated limb perfusion.

Toxicity

High-dose aldesleukin also causes capillary leak and suppression of hematopoiesis, leading to anemia, thrombocytopenia, and neutropenia. High-dose aldesleukin is an intensive therapy that causes many adverse effects. Aldesleukin affects the endothelium, causing increased capillary permeability and emigration of lymphoid cells and proteinaceous fluids from the peripheral blood into the interstitium of many organs. Most of the serious toxicities are a result of capillary leak syndrome.

Hematological. Eosinophilia greater than $40,000/mm^3$ (21% to 30%), thrombocytopenia less than $25,000/mm^3$ (16%), platelet transfusion required in 36%, anemia requiring transfusion (62% required 4 units of packed red blood cells, 43% required 8 units), lymphocytosis (75%), leukopenia, transient neutropenia less than $500/mm^3$ (0% to 3%), lymphocytopenia, mildly elevated prothrombin time.

Gastrointestinal. Nausea or vomiting (81%), dyspepsia, diarrhea (67% to 84%), abdominal distention, mucositis (32%), xerostomia, anorexia (27%), gastrointestinal necrosis and perforation (1% to 2%), gastrointestinal bleeding requiring surgery (13%), pancreatitis (rare).

Dermatological. Erythema (41%), rash (26%), pruritus (20% to 48%), dry skin (15%), exfoliative dermatitis (14%), bullous dermatitis, alopecia, vitiligo, injection site reactions after subcutaneous administration. Skin rash (cutaneous macular erythema) usually begins 2 to 3 days after the onset of treatment and is most prominent on the head and neck but may involve the entire body. Within 72 hours after treatment is discontinued the erythema resolves and desquamation follows. Although pruritus may persist for 3 to 6 weeks, normal-appearing skin is usually present within 2 to 3 weeks.

Hepatic. Reversible cholestasis. Hyperbilirubinemia occurs commonly and generally returns to baseline 5 to 6 days after stopping therapy. Transient elevation of hepatic enzyme levels (56%). Jaundice has been reported in 11% of patients receiving aldesleukin.

Neurological. Changes in mental status (73%), impaired memory, irritability, aphasia, headache (12%), somnolence (5% to 13%), disorientation (13% to 35%), stupor, coma (2% to 8%), dizziness (17%), sleep disorders, vivid dreams, paranoia, emotional lability, light-headedness, motor neurological disorders, abnormalities of special senses. Rare neurological toxicities include transient ischemic attack, leukoencephalopathy, peripheral neuropathy, carpal tunnel syndrome, brachial plexopathy, and seizure.

Cardiovascular. Arrhythmias (6% to 17%), hypotension requiring vasopressors (50% to 70%), tachycardia (70%), severe peripheral edema (3%), weight gain greater than 10% of body weight (32%), angina/ischemic attacks (1% to 3%), myocardial injury (0.5% to 2%). Rare reports of thrombosis, pericardial effusion, stroke, myocarditis, and congestive heart failure. Hypotension begins within a few hours of beginning treatment and returns to baseline within 24 to 48 hours of discontinuing therapy.

Pulmonary. Dyspnea (52%), respiratory distress (3% to 23%), intubation required (1% to 6%), pulmonary edema (10%), pleural effusion (3% to 7%), wheezing (6%), tachypnea (8%). Rare reports of apnea, pneumothorax, and hemoptysis.

ALDESLEUKIN *(continued)*

Renal. Transient increase in serum creatinine levels (61% to 83%) and oliguria begin within 24 to 48 hours after starting treatment (29% to 44%). Renal function returns to normal in 7 days (64%), 14 days (84%), and 30 days (95%). In earlier studies, approximately 2% of patients have required dialysis. With current treatment guidelines the need for dialysis is rare.

Metabolic. Hypomagnesemia (16%), acidosis (16%), hypocalcemia (15%), hypophosphatemia (11%), hypokalemia (9%), hyperuricemia (9%), hypoalbuminemia (8%), hyponatremia (7%), adrenal insufficiency (rare), hypothyroidism (may persist for months).

Other. Fatigue and malaise (53%), fever and chills (41% to 89%), myalgia (6%), 10% or greater increase in weight (32%), nasal congestion, central line sepsis malignant hyperthermia (rare).

Drug Interactions

Aldesleukin administered with any drug that may be hepatotoxic, cardiotoxic, myelotoxic, or nephrotoxic may increase the risk of these organ system toxicities.

Corticosteroids, administered concomitantly, may decrease the antitumor effects of the aldesleukin.

Aldesleukin-associated hypotension may be exacerbated by administration of antihypertensive agents.

Aldesleukin administered concomitantly with interferon alfa may cause an increase in autoimmune disease and inflammatory reactions.

Nonsteroidal anti-inflammatory agents administered concomitantly with aldesleukin may increase the capillary leak syndrome.

Aldesleukin administered concomitantly with central nervous system agents potentiates the risk for additional alteration of CNS function.

Storage and Stability

Intact vials are stored in the refrigerator. Once reconstituted, aldesleukin is stable for 48 hours at refrigerated and room temperatures when further diluted in 5% dextrose.

Preparation

Aldesleukin is provided as a lyophilized powder containing 22 million IU/vial. Vials are reconstituted with 1.1 mL sterile water to yield an 18 million IU/mL solution. Direct the diluent down the side of the vial to avoid foaming. The diluted solution is to be added to 50 mL of 5% dextrose in a polyvinylchloride container.

Incompatibilities

Aldesleukin is incompatible with normal saline (results in a precipitate) and bacteriostatic solutions. The manufacturer has indicated that dilution of aldesleukin with albumin should be avoided. Do not use an in-line filter.

Availability

Aldesleukin is commercially available as a lyophilized powder in vials containing 22 million IU (1.3 mg).

Selected Readings

Mier JW, Atkins MB. Pharmacology of cancer biotherapeutics: interleukin-2. In DeVita VT Jr, Hellman S, Rosenberg SA, eds. Principles and Practice of Oncology, 6th ed. Philadelphia, Lippincott Williams and Wilkins, 2001.

Schwartzentruber DJ. Biologic therapy with interleukin-2: clinical applications: principles of administration and management of side effects. In DeVita VT Jr, Hellman S, Rosenberg SA, eds. Biologic Therapy of Cancer, 2nd ed. Philadelphia, JB Lippincott, 1995, pp235–249.

Sznol M. Biologic therapy with interleukin-2: clinical applications, other cancers. In DeVita VT Jr, Hellman S, Rosenberg SA, eds. Biologic Therapy of Cancer, 2nd ed. Philadelphia, JB Lippincott, 1995, pp269–278.

ALEMTUZUMAB

Other Names
Campath® monoclonal antilymphocyte antibody; anti-human lymphocyte antibody; NSC-715969.

Indications
FDA approved for the treatment of B-cell chronic lymphocytic leukemia. Approved in patients who have received alkylating agent therapy and who no longer benefit from treatment with fludarabine. Alemtuzumab also has activity against T-cell prolymphocytic leukemia.

Classification and Mechanisms of Action
Alemtuzumab is a recombinant DNA-derived humanized monoclonal antibody. It has affinity for cells that express the 21–28 kDa cell surface glycoprotein CD52. This CD52 glycoprotein is located on normal and malignant B and T lymphocytes. It also resides on natural killer cells, macrophages, monocytes, and male reproductive tissues. Alemtuzumab binds the antigen CD52 on the cell surface causing the leukemic cells to lyse via antibody-dependent cell-mediated cytotoxicity (ADCC).

Pharmacokinetics
Significant interpatient variability has been observed. The half-life of alemtuzumab is approximately 12 days. Increased serum levels have been observed after several weeks of treatment. Steady-state levels occur approximately 6 weeks after initiation of treatment.

Dose
The standard dose of alemtuzumab is as follows:
Initially, a 3-mg dose is administered daily until infusion-related toxicities are ≤ grade 2. Once this dose is tolerated, the dose is increased to 10 mg until infusion-related toxicities are ≤ grade 2. Once the 10-mg dose is tolerated, the maintenance dose of alemtuzumab is 30 mg per day three times per week for a maximum of 12 weeks. The maintenance dose of 30 mg should be reached in 3 to 7 days. Modify dose for severe hematological toxicity.

Administration
It is recommended that patients be premedicated with acetaminophen and diphenhydramine prior to the initial dose of alemtuzumab, with each dose increase, and per physician clinical judgment.
It is also recommended that prophylactic *Pneumocystis carinii* anti-infective therapy and antiviral therapy be used due to expected decreases in CD4 counts.
The alemtuzumab dose is administered intravenously, diluted in 100 mL of 0.9% sodium chloride or 5% dextrose in water as a 2-hour infusion. Alemtuzumab has also been administered subcutaneously in recent studies.

ALEMTUZUMAB *(continued)*

Toxicity

Hematological. The most commonly observed hematological grade 3 or 4 toxicities include: anemia (47%), neutropenia (70%), and thrombocytopenia (52%). Lymphopenia is also common. Pancytopenia and marrow hypoplasia are rare. Coagulation disorders, hematoma, thrombocythemia, agranulocytosis, aplasia, marrow depression are rare.

Gastrointestinal. Nausea was reported in 54% of patients, with vomiting in 41%. Diarrhea (22%), stomatitis (14%), abdominal pain, dyspepsia, and constipation are reported less commonly. Rarely reported are duodenal ulcer, hematemesis, paralytic ileus, esophagitis, gastroenteritis, intestinal obstruction, colitis, peritonitis, and pancreatitis.

Dermatological. Most commonly observed are rash, maculopapular or erythematous. Pruritus (24%), urticaria (30%), and increased sweating (19%) have all been reported. Rarely observed are bullous eruptions and cellulitis.

Infusion reactions. Most commonly observed with the first week of therapy. Symptoms include rigors (86%), fever (85%), nausea (47%), vomiting (33%), and hypotension (15%). Also observed are rash (30%), fatigue (22%), urticaria (22%), dyspnea (17%), pruritus (14%), headache (13%), and diarrhea.

Hepatic. Rare reports exist of hyperbilirubinemia, hepatocellular damage or hepatic failure, hypoalbuminemia, and biliary pain.

Neurological. Most commonly reported are headache, insomnia, depression, dysesthesia, somnolence, and dizziness. Rarely reported: coma, convulsions, aphasia, meningitis, abnormal gait, confusion, nervousness.

Cardiovascular. Hypotension (32%), hypertension (11%), and tachycardia. Rarely reported: cardiac arrest, ventricular tachycardia, ventricular arrhythmias, myocardial infarction, atrial fibrillation, cardiac failure.

Pulmonary. Most commonly reported are cough (25%), dyspnea (26%), bronchitis and pneumonitis (21%). Also observed: pneumonia, pharyngitis, bronchospasm, and rhinitis. Rarely observed: hypoxia, asthma, pulmonary edema, respiratory depression, throat irritation, pleurisy, pneumothorax, pleural effusion, chronic obstructive pulmonary disease.

Renal. Rare renal toxicity has been reported, including abnormal renal function, acute renal failure, hematuria, toxic nephropathy, urinary retention, and urinary tract infection.

Metabolic. Hyperglycemia, hypoglycemia, hyperkalemia, hyponatremia, hypokalemia, hyperthyroidism, and respiratory alkalosis.

Other. Opportunistic infections, myalgias, rare reactions, vascular disorders resulting in cerebral hemorrhage, deep vein thrombosis, phlebitis, subarachnoid hemorrhage, arthritis, endophthalmis, ascites, anaphylactoid reactions, syncope, and taste loss.

Drug Interactions

Avoid live viral vaccinations.

Storage and Stability

Alemtuzumab intact ampules are stored in the refrigerator at a temperature of 2°–8°C. Do not freeze. Once reconstituted, alemtuzumab is stable for 8 hours at room or refrigerated temperatures. Protect from direct sunlight and do not shake ampules.

Preparation
The desired dose should be withdrawn from the ampule and passed through a 5-micron, low protein-binding filter before further dilution in 100 mL 0.9% sodium chloride or dextrose 5% in water.

Availability
Alemtuzumab is commercially available as a preservative-free 10 mg/mL solution in vials containing 30 mg per 3 mL.

Selected Readings
Dearden CE et al. High remission rate in T-cell prolymphocytic leukemia with CAMPATH-1H. Blood 98: 1721–1726, 2001.

Osterborg A et al. Phase II multicenter study of human CD52 antibody in previously treated chronic lymphocytic leukemia. J Clin Oncol 15: 1567–1574, 1997.

Lundin J et al. CAMPATH-1H monoclonal antibody therapy for previously treated low-grade non-Hodgkin's lymphomas: a phase II multicenter study. J Clin Oncol 16: 3257–3263, 1998.

BACILLUS CALMETTE-GUÉRIN

Other Names
TheraCys®; Pacis®; Tice BCG; BCG; NSC-614388.

Indications
FDA approved for the treatment of primary and relapsed carcinoma in situ of the urinary bladder. Theracys® is approved to eliminate residual tumor cells and reduce the frequency of recurrence. Tice BCG is approved as first- or second-line treatment for patients who cannot undergo radical surgery. BCG is not approved for the treatment of papillary tumors occurring in the absence of carcinoma in situ. Other forms of BCG are approved for immunization against tuberculosis and are not discussed.

Classification and Mechanisms of Action
It is unclear whether the effects of BCG are the result of an immune reaction to the bacillus that extends to tumor antigens on the surface of the neoplastic cell or to a nonspecific inflammatory reaction. It has been proposed that the antitumor effects of BCG are mediated by release of tumor necrosis factor (TNF) from activated macrophages.

Dose
When administered by intravesical instillation, BCG is administered in 50 to 53 mL of normal saline. Patients should avoid urinating for 2 hours after BCG has been given. Treatment is usually repeated weekly for 6 weeks. The usual dose of Tice BCG is one ampule (i.e., 50 mg). The usual weekly dose of BCG live (TheraCys®) is one vial of 81 mg. Six-week courses of treatment with TheraCys® may be repeated at 3, 6, 12, 18, and 24 months after the initial treatment, and 6-week courses of Tice BCG may be repeated monthly for 6 to 12 months. Pacis® is administered at a dose of 120 mg as a bladder instillation once a week for 6 weeks, repeated if clinically necessary.

Administration
BCG is administered intravesically for the treatment of in situ bladder cancer. Treatment is usually initiated within 1 to 2 weeks after biopsy or resection. Other routes of administration (i.e., intradermal, intralesional, intrapleural) have been evaluated in the treatment of other malignancies. It is not recommended that BCG be

BACILLUS CALMETTE-GUÉRIN *(continued)*

administered if the patient has hematuria or an active urinary tract infection because these conditions increase the risk of developing post-treatment systemic tuberculosis. Do NOT administer subcutaneously or intravenously.

Toxicity

Hematological. Anemia and leukopenia, rarely severe, have been reported. Aplastic anemia has been reported.

Gastrointestinal. Nausea and vomiting have been reported in 3% to 16% of patients, anorexia in 2% to 10%, diarrhea in 1% to 6%, and mild abdominal pain in 1.5% to 3%.

Dermatological. Skin rash (erythema nodosum). When administered intradermally, the expected reaction is a small red papule that scales, ulcerates, and dries, leaving a small pink or bluish scar after about 3 months. More severe ulceration, abscesses, and granulomas may occur and are worse with larger doses. Generalized rashes, lymphadenitis, or lymphangitis can also occur.

Genitourinary. Intravesical administration is frequently associated with dysuria (62%, severe in 3% to 10%), hematuria (40%, severe in 7% to 17%), urinary frequency (40%, severe in 2% to 7%), and cystitis (6% to 30%, severe in 2%), which may require interruption or discontinuation of therapy. Bladder irritation usually occurs 2 to 4 hours after instillation and may last 1 to 2 days. Other genitourinary toxicities are rarely severe and may include urinary urgency (6% to 18%), urinary incontinence (2% to 6%), pain (4% to 6%), nocturia (0% to 4%), and urethritis (0% to 1%).

Other. Almost all patients will develop positive conversion of the tuberculin skin test. This usually occurs after 3 to 12 weeks of intravesical therapy and is not permanent. Flu-like symptoms including fever, chills, lethargy, and malaise are common (41%). Osteomyelitis, tuberculous meningitis, anaphylaxis, and Guillain-Barré syndrome have occurred rarely. The presence of cough may be a sign of a systemic BCG infection. Disseminated BCG infection occasionally occurs and may be fatal. The likelihood of developing a systemic BCG infection may be increased if treatment is administered when the patient has a urinary tract infection.

Drug Interactions

The therapeutic effectiveness of BCG live may be altered by antimicrobial agents.

BCG live administered concomitantly with immunosuppressant agents may decrease the therapeutic effectiveness of BCG, increase the potential for BCG disseminated infection, and/or increase the risk of developing osteomyelitis.

Storage and Stability

The intact ampules and vials are stored in the refrigerator. After reconstitution, BCG preparations are to be used within 2 hours. It is recommended that BCG preparations be protected from light (i.e., sunlight and artificial light).

Preparation

Care should be taken by those handling BCG to avoid contact with the product. Contact with live BCG (TheraCys®) may cause conversion to tuberculin reactivity.

TheraCys® is reconstituted with the provided diluent, 3 mL/vial. The vial is further diluted with 50 mL of normal saline (53 mL total/dose). Gently shake until an even suspension is formed. Tice BCG is reconstituted with 1 mL of sterile water per ampule. One ampule is further diluted with 49 mL of normal saline, gently swirl until an even suspension is obtained. Pacis® is reconstituted by adding 1 mL of sterile preservative-free normal saline to the ampule, allow for 60-second contact time, then mix by removing the contents from the ampule with a syringe, then gently squirt the mixture back into the ampule. Repeat this procedure several times to obtain a uniform suspension. This 1 mL of suspension is further diluted with 49 mL of normal saline.

Disposal

Containers that have come in contact with BCG preparations are to be considered as biohazardous material. It is recommended that containers, syringes, and other equipment used for handling the vaccine be sterilized before disposal.

Availability

Tice BCG contains 100 to 800 million colony-forming units (approximately 50 mg) of BCG bacillus as a freeze-dried suspension for reconstitution, in 2-mL ampules. Each 3-mL vial of BCG live (TheraCys®) contains $10.5 \pm 8.7 \times 10^8$ colony-forming units (approximately 81 mg) of BCG bacillus as a freeze-dried suspension for reconstitution. Pacis® contains 240 to 1,200 million colony-forming units (approximately 120 mg) of BCG bacillus as a freeze-dried suspension.

Selected Reading

Batts CN. Adjuvant intravesical therapy for superficial bladder cancer. DICP Ann Pharmacother 26: 1270–1276, 1992.

Bcl-2 ANTISENSE OLIGONUCLEOTIDE

Other Names

Genasense®; Oblimersen; G3139; phosphorothioate antisense oligonucleotide; NSC-683428.

Indications

G3139 is undergoing evaluation as a treatment for patients with multiple myeloma, acute myelogenous leukemia, chronic lymphocytic leukemia, malignant melanoma, and other malignancies.

Classification and Mechanisms of Action

G3139 is an antisense compound that blocks Bcl-2 production by cancer cells by binding to a portion of mRNA that is responsible for Bcl-2 production. The Bcl-2 protein is believed to prevent or slow the rate of apoptosis by malignant cells. The Bcl-2 protein is overexpressed in many different types of malignancies. G3139 may be more effective when given in combination with other drugs, such as taxanes, irinotecan, gemtuzumab ozogamicin, fludarabine, dexamethasone, or cyclophosphamide.

Pharmacokinetics

Steady-state plasma concentrations are attained within 24 hours after initiation of a continuous IV infusion. The drug is primarily eliminated in the urine. The elimination half-life is approximately 2 hours.

Dose

Dose-limiting toxicity has been observed at a dose of 7 mg/kg/day for 21 days. In combination with dacarbazine, 1,000 mg/m² on day 5, G3139 has been administered as a 5-day continuous infusion (5 to 9 mg/kg/day) and a 14-day continuous infusion (up to 6.5 mg/kg/day). As a 14-day continuous subcutaneous infusion, the maximum tolerated dose was 147 mg/m²/day (i.e., approximately 4 mg/kg/day).

Bcl-2 ANTISENSE OLIGONUCLEOTIDE *(continued)*

G3139, 5 mg/kg/day as an 8-day continuous infusion, combined with irinotecan 280 mg/m^2 on day 6 has been administered as an every-3-weeks regimen. Dose-limiting neutropenia (grade 4) and diarrhea (grade 3 and 4) were observed when the dose of irinotecan was escalated to 350 mg/m^2. Combinations of G3139 with docetaxel, mitoxantrone, and fludarabine have also been evaluated.

Administration

G3139 is administered IV as a continuous infusion over 4 to 14 days. G3139 has also been administered as a continuous subcutaneous infusion over 7 to 14 days.

Toxicity

Hematological. Anemia, leukopenia, thrombocytopenia, elevations of prothrombin and partial thromboplastin times.
Gastrointestinal. Anorexia, nausea, vomiting.
Dermatological. Rash, urticaria.
Hepatic. Elevations of alkaline phosphatase, hepatic transaminases, and bilirubin may be dose-limiting with the 14-day continuous infusion schedule. These abnormalities have not been dose-limiting with the 5-day continuous infusion schedule.
Cardiovascular. Edema, fluid retention, hypotension, tachycardia.
Renal. Elevations of serum creatinine have been observed in some patients.
Other. Hypersensitivity, fatigue, fever, hot flushes, hyperglycemia, and hypophosphatemia have been reported.

Storage and Stability

Stable for at least 24 hours at room temperature.

Compatibility

Compatible with ambulatory infusion pumps.

Availability

G3139 is an investigational agent in the United States that is available from the manufacturer.

Selected Reading

Walters JS et al. Phase I clinical and pharmacokinetic study of Bcl-2 antisense nucleotide therapy in patients with non-Hodgkin's lymphoma. J Clin Oncol 18: 1812–1823, 2000.

BEVACIZUMAB

Other Names

Avastin®; rhuMAb VEGF; anti-VEGF humanized Mab; NSC-704865.

Indications

Bevacizumab is an investigational agent in the United States. Bevacizumab is undergoing evaluation and appears to have activity in renal cell cancer, acute myelogenous leukemia, non-small-cell lung cancer, and other malignancies.

Classification and Mechanisms of Action

Bevacizumab is a recombinant human IgG monoclonal antibody against vascular endothelial growth factor (VEGF). Vascular endothelial growth factor (VEGF) is required for blood vessel formation and is produced by the majority of malignant cells.

Pharmacokinetics

Linear pharmacokinetic pattern for doses greater than 1 mg/kg. The terminal half-life is approximately 15 days.

Dose

Phase I doses have ranged from 0.1 mg/kg to 10 mg/kg on days 0, 28, 35, and 42. Doses of 5 mg/kg to 15 mg/kg have been administered every 2 to 3 weeks. Bevacizumab, 3 mg/kg, has been used in combination with doxorubicin, carboplatin/paclitaxel, or 5-FU/leucovorin.

Administration

Bevacizumab is administered IV in 250 to 500 mL of 5% dextrose and water over 90 minutes.

Toxicity

Hematological. Mild neutropenia, hemorrhagic events (without thrombocytopenia) including CNS hemorrhage, epistaxis, hematemesis, and hemoptysis.

Gastrointestinal. Grade 1 and 2 nausea. Vomiting is uncommon. Constipation has been reported.

Dermatological. Skin rash

Cardiovascular. Hypertension, occasionally grade 2 or 3. Deep venous thrombosis has been observed infrequently.

Renal. Proteinuria is usually grade 1.

Pulmonary. Pulmonary hemorrhage occurred in 10% of patients with non-small-cell lung cancer in one study. Cavitation and/or necrosis of squamous cell lung cancer lesions appeared to be a risk factor for the development of pulmonary hemorrhage. The NCI prohibits enrollment of patients to clinical trials if they have "gross or frank hemoptysis at baseline."

Other. Tumor-related bleeding has been observed in a few patients. Grade 1 and 2 asthenia and headache have been observed. Arthralgia, dyspnea, and hyponatremia have been reported.

Storage and Stability

Intact vials are stored in the refrigerator. Vials must not be frozen. The National Cancer Institute recommends administration of the agent within 8 hours of preparation.

Preparation

Doses may be further diluted with normal saline. Doses greater than 1,000 mg may be administered without further dilution.

Availability

Bevacizumab is an investigational agent in the United States that is available as sterile liquid (10 mg/mL, 100 mg/vial) from the manufacturer or the National Cancer Institute.

Selected Reading

Novotny WF et al. Identification of squamous cell histology and central, cavitary tumors as possible risk factors for pulmonary hemorrhage in patients with advanced NSCLC receiving bevacizumab. Proc Am Soc Clin Oncol 20: 330a, 2001.

CEA VACCINE

Other Names
CeaVAC™; NSC-720063.

Indications
CEA vaccine is an investigational agent in the United States that is under evaluation as a treatment for colon and rectal carcinoma.

Classification and Mechanisms of Action
CEA vaccine is an anti-idiotope monoclonal antibody.

Dose
For patients with advanced colorectal cancer CEA vaccine has been administered at a dose of 2 mg every other week for 4 doses followed by 2 mg every month until disease progression.

Administration
CEA vaccine is administered by subcutaneous injection.

Toxicity
Dermatological. Mild erythema, induration, and, occasionally, swelling at the site of the injection are the most common toxicities.
Other. Mild fever and chills.

Storage and Stability
Vials are stored upright at refrigeration temperatures (4°–8°C).

Preparation
Do not freeze or shake the suspension.

Compatibilities
CEA vaccine has been administered concurrently with 5-fluorouracil in colorectal cancer patients. Immune response was not affected by 5-fluorouracil. CEA vaccine has been admixed with the adjuvants QS-21 and aluminum hydroxide.

Availability
CEA vaccine is an investigational agent in the United States that is available as a 2 mg/mL suspension (1.2 mL/vial) from the manufacturer.

Selected Reading
Foon KA et al. Clinical and immune responses in resected colon cancer patients treated with anti-idiotype monoclonal antibody vaccine that mimics the carcino-embryonic antigen. J Clin Oncol 17: 2889–2895, 1999.

CETUXIMAB

Other Names
Erbitux®; IMC-225; C225; NSC-632307.

Indications
Cetuximab is an investigational agent that is undergoing evaluation in the treatment of colorectal cancer and other malignancies. The drug has been evaluated as a single agent and combined with irinotecan for patients with colorectal cancer. Cetuximab has

orphan drug designation for squamous cell carcinoma of the head and neck that expresses epidermal growth factor receptor.

Classification and Mechanisms of Action

Cetuximab is a mouse-human chimeric anti-epidermal growth factor receptor (EGFR) monoclonal antibody. Cetuximab binds to its receptor blocking activation of tyrosine kinase and down-regulation of EGFR.

Pharmacokinetics

The pharmacokinetics of cetuximab have been described as nonlinear. It appears that doses of 200 to 400 mg/m^2 may saturate clearance mechanisms. Cetuximab has a terminal half-life of approximately 8 days.

Dose

As a single-agent, cetuximab has been given as a 20 mg/m^2 test dose followed by a 400 mg/m^2 loading dose followed in one week by 250 mg/m^2/week. In combination with conventional radiation therapy (7,000 cGy, 200 cGy/day), cetuximab has been administered as a 400 to 500 mg/m^2 loading dose followed by 250 mg/m^2/week for 7 to 8 weeks.

The single-agent regimen of cetuximab has been combined with the following regimens:

Paclitaxel 225 mg/m^2 and carboplatin AUC 6 every 3 weeks.

Gemcitabine 1,000 mg/m^2 days 1 and 8 and carboplatin AUC 5.5 every 3 weeks.

Cisplatin 60 mg/m^2 every 3 weeks or 100 mg/m^2 every 4 weeks.

Docetaxel 75 mg/m^2 every 3 weeks.

Irinotecan 100 mg/m^2, 5-fluorouracil 400 mg/m^2, and leucovorin 20 mg/m^2 every week for 4 weeks; cycles repeated every 6 weeks.

Administration

Cetuximab is administered over 1 to 2 hours. The infusion line is primed with cetuximab and when the infusion is completed the infusion line is flushed with normal saline.

Toxicity

Hematological. Leukopenia, thrombocytopenia, and anemia (all grade 1) have been reported.

Gastrointestinal. Anorexia, diarrhea, nausea (common but primarily grade 1), vomiting (uncommon).

Dermatological. Acneiform follicular rash, primarily of the face, scalp, and trunk, is the most common toxicity. The rash occurs in up to 80% of patients (grade 3 in 16%) and usually appears within the first 2 to 3 weeks of weekly treatment. The rash resolves without scarring following discontinuation of treatment. Occasionally, a generalized maculopapular rash may occur.

Constitutional. Asthenia is reported to occur in approximately 50% of patients (grade 3 in 5%). Fever and chills have been observed in approximately 15% of patients. Other flu-like symptoms have been observed.

Hepatic. Grade 1 elevations of transaminase enzymes have been reported.

Other. Allergic reactions during the infusion have occurred, including anaphylaxis (2% grade 4). Prophylactic antihistamines have allowed continuation of treatment in some patients who experienced a hypersensitivity reaction.

Storage and Stability

Cetuximab is stored at refrigeration temperatures (2°C to 8°C).

CETUXIMAB *(continued)*

Preparation
Cetuximab is administered undiluted. Before infusion, cetuximab is filtered with a 0.22-micron protein-sparing filter.

Availability
Cetuximab is an investigational agent in the United States that is available as a 2 mg/mL solution (40 mg/20-mL vial and 100 mg/50-mL vial) from the manufacturer.

Selected Readings
Baselga J et al. Phase I studies of anti-epidermal growth factor receptor chimeric antibody C225 alone and in combination with cisplatin. J Clin Oncol 18: 904–914, 2000.

Herbst RS, Langer CJ. Epidermal growth factor receptors as a target for cancer treatment: the emerging role of IMC-C225 in the treatment of lung and head and neck cancers. Semin Oncol 29 (suppl 4): 27–36, 2002.

Robert F et al. Phase I study of anti-epidermal growth factor receptor antibody cetuximab in combination with radiation therapy in patients with advanced head and neck cancer. J Clin Oncol 19: 3234–3243, 2001.

DENILEUKIN DIFTITOX

Other Names
Ontak®; interleukin-2 fusion protein; LY-335348; DAB-389 interleukin-2; DAB389-IL2; NSC-714744.

Indications
Denileukin diftitox is FDA approved for use in cutaneous T-cell lymphoma, in patients whose disease expresses the CD25 component of the IL-2 receptor.

Classification and Mechanisms of Action
Denileukin diftitox targets the IL-2 receptor of the malignant cells. The drug interacts at the receptor and utilizes the diphtheria toxin to destroy cells via inhibition of protein synthesis.

Pharmacokinetics
Lymphoma patients were treated with a range of doses to determine the pharmacokinetics. After an intravenous infusion, a two-compartment model was observed. The distribution half-life was 2 to 5 minutes, while the terminal half-life was 60 to 80 minutes. Clearance is increased with the formation of antibodies to the drug. Multiple doses do not cause accumulation of the drug.

Dose
The recommended adult dose of denileukin diftitox is 9 microg/kg/day or 18 microg/kg/day administered once a day for 5 consecutive days. This 5-day treatment is repeated every 21 days.

Administration
Denileukin diftitox is administered intravenously over at least 15 minutes.
    Do not administer unless serum albumin is >3 gm/dL.

Toxicity
Hematological. Anemia (18%) was most common, followed by thrombocytopenia (8%) and leukopenia (6%).

Gastrointestinal. Nausea/vomiting (64%), anorexia (36%), diarrhea (29%) were common. Less than 10% of patients experienced constipation, dyspepsia, and dysphagia.

Dermatological. Rashes in the form of maculopapular, vesicular bullous, eczematous, petechial, and urticarial have all been observed. Pruritus and sweating also reported.

Infusion reactions. Classified either as acute hypersensitivity (69%) or a flu-like (91%) symptom complex. Acute hypersensitivity reactions occur within 24 hours of infusion and are manifested as hypotension (50%), back pain (30%), vasodilation (28%), shortness of breath (28%), rash (25%), chest pain or tightness (24%), tachycardia (12%), dysphagia or laryngismus (5%), syncope (3%), and/or anaphylaxis (1%). Treat these reactions as clinically indicated with IV corticosteroids, antihistamines, and epinephrine. Results from a small study indicate that steroid premedication significantly reduced these reactions without compromising clinical response.

The flu-like symptom complex can be experienced hours to days after the infusion. The signs and symptoms reported include chills and fever (81%), asthenia (66%), nausea and vomiting (64%), myalgias (18%), arthralgias (8%). Treatment of these symptoms can include acetaminophen and antiemetic therapy.

Vascular leak syndrome. Occurs in approximately 27% of patients, and occurs within 2 weeks of infusion. Symptoms include hypotension, edema, and hypoalbuminemia.

Hepatic. Elevated transaminase levels, generally observed with course 1 and resolve within 2 weeks.

Neurological. Dizziness, nervousness, and paresthesias are most common. Confusion and insomnia have been reported in less than 10% of patients.

Cardiovascular. Hypotension (36%), tachycardia (22%), vasodilation (12%), and thrombotic events (7%) are the most common cardiovascular toxicities. Hypertension and arrhythmias have been reported.

Pulmonary. Dyspnea (29%), cough (26%), pharyngitis (17%), rhinitis (13%), and lung disorders (8%).

Storage and Stability

Denileukin diftitox is stored frozen at a temperature of $-10°C$. The vials can thaw in refrigerated temperatures for a maximum of 24 hours or at room temperature for up to 2 hours. Do not refreeze.

Preparation

Allow vials to come to room temperature, the solution will appear clear and colorless at room temperature. Gently swirl the drug, do not shake or agitate vigorously. Observe the product for discoloration or particulate matter. Using aseptic technique, withdraw the desired dose from the vials using plastic syringes and inject it into an empty intravenous infusion bag. Further dilute the drug with preservative-free normal saline to maintain a concentration of 15 microg/mL. (For every 1 mL of drug, dilute with no more than 9 mL of normal saline.) The final product should be administered within 6 hours of preparation.

Availability

Denileukin diftitox is commercially available in 2-mL vials that contain 300 microg of drug.

Selected Readings

Foss FM et al. Biological correlates of acute hypersensitivity events with DAB (389)IL-2 (denileukin diftitox, ONTAK) in cutaneous T-cell lymphoma: decreased frequency and severity with steroid premedication. Clin Lymphoma 1: 298–302, 2001.

Olsen ED et al. Pivotal phase III trial of two dose levels of denileukin diftitox for the treatment of cutaneous T-cell lymphoma. J Clin Oncol 19: 376–388, 2001.

EDRECOLOMAB

Other Names
Mab 17-1A; Panorex®; Adjuqual®; NSC-377963.

Indications
Edrecolomab is an investigational agent in the United States. In Germany it is approved as an adjuvant treatment for patients with Duke's C colorectal cancer, following surgery.

Classification and Mechanisms of Action
Edrecolomab is a murine monoclonal IgG2a antibody that is directed to the 17-1A cell surface antigen. This antigen has been found on epithelial cells.

Dose
Edrecolomab 500 mg is administered within 4 weeks following surgery followed by 100 mg every 4 weeks for 4 months (4 additional doses are given). The total dose of edrecolomab administered is 900 mg.

Administration
Edrecolomab is administered IV in 250 mL of normal saline over 2 hours.

Toxicity
Hematological. Neutropenia and thrombocytopenia are rare.
Gastrointestinal. Diarrhea has been reported to occur in 19% of patients, nausea in 10%, vomiting in 5%, and stomatitis in approximately 2%. Anorexia is also reported.
Dermatological. Skin rash, pruritus, and alopecia are rare.
Hepatic. Elevations of transaminase levels have been reported.
Cardiovascular. Hypotension has been reported in approximately 3% of patients.
Other. Flu-like symptoms (i.e., fever, chills, malaise, arthralgia, headache) are common and generally last for one week following administration. Abdominal pain has been reported in approximately 7% of patients, hot flushes in 5%, and musculoskeletal pain in 3%. Hypersensitivity reactions have occurred, including anaphylaxis on rare occasions.

Storage and Stability
Diluted solutions of edrecolomab are stable for at least 6 hours at room temperature.

Preparation
Edrecolomab is further diluted in 250 mL of normal saline.

Availability
Edrecolomab is an investigational agent in the United States that is available as an injectable 10 mg/mL solution (100-mg vials) from the manufacturer.

Selected Readings
Atkins JC, Spencer CM. Edrecolomab (monoclonal antibody 17-1A). Drugs 56: 619–626, 1998.
Riethmuller G et al. Monoclonal antibody therapy for resected Duke's C colorectal cancer: seven year outcome of a multicenter randomized trial. J Clin Oncol 16: 1788–1794, 1998.

ENDOSTATIN

Other Names
Rh-Endostatin; NSC-704805.

Indications
Endostatin is an investigational agent in the United States. It is undergoing evaluation in pancreatic cancer, carcinoid tumor, malignant melanoma, and other malignancies.

Classification and Mechanisms of Action
Endostatin is an angiogenesis inhibitor.

Pharmacokinetics
Endostatin has a linear pharmacokinetic profile. Bioavailability of endostatin administered by subcutaneous injection is equivalent to intravenous administration. The elimination half-life is approximately 10 hours.

Dose
Intravenous doses up to 600 mg/m^2/day have been administered. A continuous IV infusion for 4 weeks followed by subcutaneous injections, 15 mg/m^2/day, is under evaluation.

Administration
Endostatin has been administered as a 20- to 60-minute IV infusion, by continuous IV infusion, and by subcutaneous injection. Subcutaneous doses have been divided into two equal daily doses.

Toxicity
Dermatological. Grade 1 skin rashes have been observed.

Storage and Stability
Endostatin is stored at a temperature of −70°C.

Preparation
Thaw at room temperature. Do not shake or use a microwave to thaw. Endostatin is further diluted to a total volume of 75 mL in the buffered solution provided with the product. It is recommended that endostatin be added to the buffered solution, which has already been added to an empty container.

Compatibilities
Endostatin is compatible with normal saline.

Availability
Endostatin is an investigational agent in the United States that is available as a frozen liquid (8 mg/mL, 40 mg/vial) from the manufacturer or the National Cancer Institute.

Selected Reading
Thomas JP et al. A phase I pharmacokinetic and pharmacodynamic study of recombinant human endostatin. Proc Am Soc Clin Oncol 20: 70a, 2001.

EPOETIN ALFA/DARBOPOETIN ALFA

Other Names

Epogen®; Procrit®; Neo-Recormon®; erythropoietin; EPO; erythropoietin alfa; NSC-628281; Aranesp®; darbopoetin alfa; NESP.

Indications

Epoetin alfa is FDA approved for the treatment of anemia associated with chronic renal failure, zidovudine (AZT) therapy in patients with HIV infection, and cancer chemotherapy for nonmyeloid malignancies. Also administered to patients undergoing elective surgery for noncardiac or nonvascular conditions.

Darbopoetin alfa is FDA approved for the treatment of anemia associated with chronic renal failure and for the treatment of anemia secondary to cancer chemotherapy for nonmyeloid malignancies.

Classification and Mechanisms of Action

Epoetin alfa (EPO) is a lineage-specific inducer of erythrocyte production. EPO stimulates the division and differentiation of erythrocyte progenitor cells within the bone marrow. EPO does not have any effects on leukocytes, platelets, or their progenitors. Reticulocyte counts begin to rise within 10 days of initiating treatment. Elevation of hematocrit, hemoglobin, and red blood cell levels usually occurs within 2 to 6 weeks of treatment onset. The rate of the elevation of red blood cell levels, hemoglobin, and hematocrit is dose-dependent.

Darbopoetin alfa is similar to epoetin alfa, the chemical difference being that darbopoetin alfa has 2 additional N-linked oligosaccharide chains, totaling 5 versus 3 on EPO. The mechanism of action and response time of darbopoetin is comparable to EPO.

Pharmacokinetics

Epoetin alfa demonstrates peak serum levels of EPO within 5 to 24 hours, after subcutaneous administration. EPO has an elimination half-life of 4 to 13 hours. The elimination half-life does not appear to be affected by renal function, although the half-life of EPO is approximately 20% shorter in normal volunteers.

Darbopoetin alfa administered intravenously exhibits a 1.4-hour distribution half-life with a terminal half-life of 21 hours (approximately). Darbopoetin alfa administered subcutaneously exhibits a slower absorption; this translates into a 49-hour terminal half-life and a peak serum concentration at approximately 34 hours. Darbopoetin alfa is distributed mainly into the vascular space, and utilizing the once a week schedule, steady-state levels are reached within 4 weeks of dosing.

Dose

Prior to treating anemia secondary to chemotherapy treatment, a full assessment of hemoglobin levels, TSAT/ferritin levels, epoetin level, and evaluation of other potential causes of anemia (e.g., bleeding, iron deficiency, etc.) should be completed. The manufacturer's recommended starting dose for patients with anemia caused by cancer chemotherapy is 150 units/kg, 3 times each week. The dose of 40,000 units once a week is common practice. The manufacturer recommends that if anemia is not corrected after 8 weeks of treatment, the dose may be increased to 300 units/kg 3 times weekly. Doses are adjusted to maintain the desired hematocrit and hemoglobin levels.

Darbopoetin alfa for treatment of anemia in chronic renal failure patients is 0.45 microg/kg administered once weekly. A hemoglobin concentration of 12 g/dL should not be exceeded. For the treatment of cancer-related anemia, a starting dose of 2.25 microg/kg of darbopoetin alfa is administered weekly with a dosing range up to 4.5 microg/kg/week.

Administration
Epoetin alfa is administered by subcutaneous injection.
Darbopoetin alfa is administered by subcutaneous injection or intravenously.

Toxicity
The adverse events described are those reported after the use of EPO in patients receiving cancer chemotherapy:
Gastrointestinal. Diarrhea (21%), nausea (17%), vomiting (17%).
Dermatological. Pain at site of injection, rash.
Cardiovascular. Edema, hypertension, thrombotic events, tachycardia, myocardial infarction, transient ischemic attacks.
Neurological. Paresthesia (11%), dizziness (5%).
Other. Fever (29%), asthenia (13%), fatigue (13%), shortness of breath (13%).
   The adverse events reported after the use of darbopoetin alfa in patients with chronic renal failure:
Gastrointestinal. Diarrhea (16%), nausea (14%), vomiting (15%), abdominal pain (12%), and constipation (5%).
Dermatological. Pruritus (8%), pain at injection site (7%).
Cardiovascular. The reports of cardiovascular events were higher in patients with higher hemoglobin levels, upwards toward 14 g/dL. Hypertension (23%), darbopoetin alfa should not be used to treat patients with uncontrolled hypertension. Hypotension (22%), arrhythmias and cardiac arrest (10%), chest pain (8%), thrombosis vascular access (8%), peripheral edema and congestive heart failure (6%). Myocardial infarction occurred in less than 1% of patients.
Neurological. Headache (16%), dizziness (8%), transient ischemic attacks and stroke occurred in less than 1% of patients.
Respiratory. Upper respiratory infection (14%), shortness of breath (12%), cough (10%), bronchitis (6%).
Other. Myalgia (21%), arthralgia (11%), limb pain (10%), back pain (8%), fever (9%), asthenia (5%), fatigue (9%), flu-like symptoms (6%), infection (6%), fluid overload (6%), death (7%).

Storage and Stability
Epoetin alfa is stored in the refrigerator. The 1-mL vials do not contain a preservative and it is recommended that one vial be used per dose. The 2-mL (20,000-unit) vial contains a preservative and may be stored in the refrigerator for at least 21 days. Epoetin alfa should not be frozen.
Darbopoetin alfa is stored in the refrigerator. Darbopoetin alfa should not be frozen, and it should be protected from light. Discard excess drug due to lack of preservative.

Preparation
Epoetin alfa and darbopoetin alfa are administered without further dilution. Do not shake the vial because this may adversely affect potency.

Compatibilities
Epoetin alfa is compatible with bacteriostatic normal saline.

EPOETIN ALFA/DARBOPOETIN ALFA *(continued)*

Availability

Epoetin alfa is commercially available as an injectable solution in 1-mL vials containing 2,000, 3,000, 4,000, 10,000, 20,000 and 40,000 units and a 2-mL vial containing 20,000 units (10,000 units/mL).

Darbopoetin is formulated in two separate solutions. The albumin solution is available in 25 microg, 40 microg, 60 microg, and 100 microg/mL vials. The polysorbate solution is available in 25 microg, 40 microg, 60 microg, and 100 microg/mL vials.

Selected Reading

Glaspy J et al. A dose-finding and safety study of novel erythropoiesis stimulatin protein (NESP) for the treatment of anaemia in patients receiving multicycle chemotherapy. Br J Cancer 84 (suppl 1): 17–23, 2001.

FILGRASTIM AND PEGFILGRASTIM

Other Names

Neupogen® (filgrastim); granulocyte colony-stimulating factor; G-CSF; rG-CSF recombinant-methionyl human granulocyte colony-stimulating factor; r-met HuG-CSF; NSC-614629. Neulasta® (pegfilgrastim).

Indications

Filgrastim (G-CSF) is FDA approved to decrease the incidence of infection in patients with nonmyeloid tumors receiving myelosuppressive chemotherapy and to reduce the duration of neutropenia in patients receiving bone marrow transplantation. Filgrastim may also be useful as a rescue treatment for febrile neutropenic patients; as a treatment for aplastic anemia, cyclic neutropenia, congenital neutropenia, and myelodysplastic disorders; and to augment peripheral stem cell collection.

Pegfilgrastim is FDA approved to decrease the incidence of infection in patients with nonmyeloid tumors receiving myelosuppressive chemotherapy. There is no data to date to support the use of pegfilgrastim for radiation-induced neutropenia or mobilization of peripheral blood stem cells. Until clinical trials demonstrate safety and efficacy, it should not be used for these purposes.

Mechanisms of Action

Filgrastim and pegfilgrastim are both colony-stimulating factors that possess the same mechanism of action. Filgrastim is produced by monocytes, fibroblasts, and endothelial cells of the bone marrow. Filgrastim supports the proliferation, differentiation, and activation of committed progenitor cells of the granulocyte series. Filgrastim also enhances neutrophil chemotaxis and phagocytosis. After a single subcutaneous dose of filgrastim the absolute neutrophil count (ANC) decreases 50% to 75% for the first 30 minutes before rising to a maximum 8 to 10 hours later. If filgrastim is not administered again, the ANC will normalize within 24 to 48 hours. The level of neutrophilia observed is dose-related.

Pharmacokinetics

Filgrastim is not absorbed by mouth. Filgrastim can be detected in the serum within 5 minutes of a subcutaneous injection; peak serum concentrations occur within 2 to 8 hours. Filgrastim is metabolized in the liver and kidneys. It has an elimination half-life of 3 to 5 hours.

Pegfilgrastim exhibits nonlinear pharmacokinetics. As the dose is increased, the clearance is decreased. The half-life of pegfilgrastim, after it is administered subcutaneously, lasted as short as 15 hours and as long as 80 hours.

Dose

The recommended starting adult dose of filgrastim is 5 microg/kg/day for up to 14 days beginning 24 hours after completion of chemotherapy. Higher doses of filgrastim may be administered in subsequent cycles according to the duration and severity of myelosuppression. In general, filgrastim may be discontinued when the ANC is greater than 10,000/mm^3 after the expected chemotherapy-induced nadir. Filgrastim has also been administered as a 5-day course of treatment at a dose of 5 microg/kg/day on days 15 through 19 of a 3-week chemotherapy regimen. For the bone marrow transplant population, filgrastim is administered at a dose of 10 microg/kg/day as a 4- or 24-hour intravenous infusion, or a 24-hour subcutaneous infusion; adjust dose based on neutrophil counts. To reduce wastage and cost, daily doses are often rounded off to the nearest vial size (300 or 480 microg). Doses of 100 microg/kg/day or greater have been administered without the occurrence of dose-limiting toxicities.

Pegfilgrastim is given as a single 6-mg dose, administered once during a chemotherapy cycle. The dose should not be given within 14 days prior to chemotherapy and not within 24 hours after a dose of chemotherapy.

Administration

Subcutaneous injection is the preferred route of administration for both filgrastim and pegfilgrastim. Filgrastim may also be administered intravenously, usually as an infusion over at least 30 minutes. Continuous infusions, by either the intravenous or subcutaneous route, have also been used.

Toxicity

The toxicity profile represents patients who had received chemotherapy prior to filgrastim or pegfilgrastim therapy. Therefore many toxicities listed can be attributed to patient disease or chemotherapy.

Hypersensitivity reactions. Allergic-type reactions, anaphylaxis, urticaria, and skin rash have all been reported with filgrastim therapy. These reactions were not noted in the clinical trials with pegfilgrastim.

Hematological. Filgrastim causes an initial decrease in ANC (within 5 minutes, may last up to 1 hour). Transient decreases in platelet counts have been reported in patients receiving "high doses." Progression of myelodysplastic syndromes (especially in patients with "excess blasts") may occur. Filgrastim has caused exacerbation of severe sickle cell crisis (a fatality has been documented) when administered to patients with sickle cell disease. Use filgrastim or pegfilgrastim in the sickle cell population with great caution and clinical oversight. Avoid use in this population if possible.

Pegfilgrastim rarely (< 1%) caused a significant leukocytosis (WBC greater than 100×10^9/L), this was not associated with any adverse outcomes.

Gastrointestinal. Nausea, vomiting, diarrhea, anorexia, dyspepsia, constipation, stomatitis, mucositis.

Dermatological. Local inflammation at the injection site, skin rash (rare), cutaneous vasculitis (rare), flare in psoriasis, mild alopecia with long-term administration (rare), Sweet's syndrome (acute febrile neutrophilic dermatosis).

Hepatic. Filgrastim exhibited mild elevation of lactic dehydrogenase (29%), alkaline phosphatase (16%), and uric acid levels (9%); pegfilgrastim exhibited mild elevation of lactic dehydrogenase (19%), alkaline phosphatase (9%), and uric acid levels (8%).

FILGRASTIM AND PEGFILGRASTIM *(continued)*

Cardiovascular. Fluid retention; pericardial effusion (rare).

Neurological. Severe motor weakness and foot pain have been observed after the use of G-CSF in combination with chemotherapy regimens containing vincristine. Headache, dizziness.

Pulmonary. Neutropenic septic patients have demonstrated adult respiratory distress syndrome (ARDS) secondary to filgrastim therapy and risk exists with pegfilgrastim therapy also. Presentation consists of lung infiltrates, fever, and respiratory distress.

Musculoskeletal. Transient bone pain (15% to 39% incidence), usually mild to moderate in severity, occurs with both filgrastim and pegfilgrastim. The pain has been described as a pulsating deep pain in the lower back, pelvis, or sternum. The pain usually begins after initiation of treatment and just before the onset of neutrophil recovery. Nonnarcotic analgesics are useful in controlling this adverse reaction. Resolution usually occurs without stopping treatment and always resolves within a few hours after discontinuation.

Other. Fatigue, flushing (rare), generalized weakness, sore throat, and chest tightness. Splenomegaly is relatively common in patients receiving chronic therapy with filgrastim; splenic rupture has occurred with filgrastim when used as a mobilizing agent in both donors and recipients.

Drug Interactions

Concomitant use of filgrastim or pegfilgrastim with lithium may potentiate the release of neutrophils and monitoring may be required.

Storage and Stability

Filgrastim should be refrigerated and not allowed to freeze. It is stable for at least 10 months when refrigerated. There is significant loss of activity when the product is stored above or below 2°C to 8°C. Filgrastim is stable in plastic syringes for at least 24 hours or 7 days at room and refrigeration temperatures, respectively. At a concentration of 5 microg/mL or greater in 5% dextrose, filgrastim is stable for 7 days at room or refrigerator temperatures. At dilutions from 2 to 15 microg/mL, albumin in a final concentration of 2 mg/mL should be added to protect against adsorption. Addition of albumin is unnecessary when the drug is diluted to a concentration greater than or equal to 15 microg/mL in 5% dextrose. Concentrations of less than 2 microg/mL should not be used. Dilutions of filgrastim in 5% dextrose are stable in glass bottles, polyvinylchloride, polyolefin, or polypropylene bags and IV sets, and Travenol infusors.

Pegfilgrastim should be refrigerated and protected from light. Do not shake. In the original carton, pegfilgrastim can be allowed to reach room temperature for up to 48 hours. Discard syringe if left at room temperature longer than 48 hours. Pegfilgrastim should not be frozen; however, if this does occur the syringe can be thawed in the refrigerator and used. Do not allow refreezing.

Preparation

If utilizing vials, draw appropriate dose into a syringe for subcutaneous injection. If filgrastim is further diluted for IV administration, use only 5% dextrose.

Incompatibilities

Normal saline.

Availability
Filgrastim is commercially available as a 300 microg/mL solution in vials containing 1 mL (300 microg/vial) and 1.6 mL (480 microg/vial), and prefilled syringes in 300 microg/0.5 mL and 480 microg/0.8 mL. Pegfilgrastim is commercially available as a 6 mg in 0.6 ml prefilled syringe.

Selected Readings
American Society of Clinical Oncology. Update of recommendations for the use of hematopoietic colony-stimulating factors: evidence-based clinical practice guidelines. J Clin Oncol 18: 3558–3585, 2000.

ASCO Ad Hoc Colony-Stimulating Factor Guidelines Expert Panel. American Society of Clinical Oncology recommendations for the use of hematopoietic colony-stimulating factors: evidence-based, clinical practice guidelines. J Clin Oncol 12: 2471–2508, 1994.

GEMTUZUMAB OZOGAMICIN

Other Names
Mylotarg®; anti-CD33 antibody; NSC-720568.

Indications
FDA approved for the treatment of CD33-positive patients who are 60 years or older who have relapsed acute myelocytic leukemia, and who are not considered candidates for other cytotoxic chemotherapy.

Mechanisms of Action
Gemtuzumab ozogamicin is a recombinant humanized monoclonal antibody that is combined with the cytotoxic antibiotic calicheamicin. This targeted antibody/ chemotherapy combination is directed against the CD33 antigen which is found on specific hematopoietic cells, including the myeloid stem cell, erythrocytes, thrombocytes, monocytes, macrophages, and neutrophils. The pluripotent hematopoietic stem cell does not express CD33 positivity. Once binding of the antigenic site occurs, the drug complex is internalized into the cell and the cytotoxic calicheamicin component is released. Calicheamicin causes DNA double-strand breaks and ultimately cell death.

Pharmacokinetics
After the initial dose of gemtuzumab ozogamicin, the serum half-life of the total compound is approximately 45 hours and the half-life of the unconjugated calicheamicin is 100 hours. Following the second dose of the total compound, the serum half-life of the total compound increases to approximately 60 hours. The half-life of unconjugated calicheamicin does not change with the second dose of gemtuzumab ozogamicin. The area under the curve increases to twice that of the initial dose. The metabolic pathways and isoenzymes involved in the metabolism of these drug components have not yet been completely identified. It appears that the calicheamicin is released from the gemtuzumab ozogamicin via a hydrolytic reaction.

Dose
The dose of gemtuzumab ozogamicin is 9 mg/m^2. Two doses are given, 14 days apart. Prior to administering gemtuzumab ozogamicin, patients should have a peripheral white blood count less than 30,000/microL. Dose with caution in patients with bilirubin > 2 mg/dL.

GEMTUZUMAB OZOGAMICIN *(continued)*

Administration

It is recommended that acetaminophen 650 to 1,000 mg and diphenhydramine 50 mg be administered 1 hour prior to each dose of gemtuzumab ozogamicin. Acetaminophen should be given every 4 hours for two additional doses. Monitor vital signs during and up to 4 hours after the infusion.

Gemtuzumab ozogamicin is administered intravenously in 100 mL of normal saline over 2 hours. The intravenous tubing must contain a 1.2-micron low protein-binding filter.

Toxicity

Hematological. Almost all patients will experience grade 3 or 4 neutropenia and thrombocytopenia. Approximately 20% of patients developed neutropenic fever following treatment. Approximately 50% of patients will develop grade 3 or 4 anemia and 15% will develop bleeding (e.g., disseminated intravascular coagulation, epistaxis, cerebral hemorrhage, and hematuria). The median time to obtain an ANC greater than 500/microL and platelets greater than 25,000/microL is around 40 days.

Gastrointestinal. Commonly reported with gemtuzumab ozogamicin therapy are nausea in 70% of patients, vomiting (63%), diarrhea (38%), stomatitis (32%), anorexia (29%), constipation (25%), and dyspepsia (11%).

Dermatological. Most commonly observed are local reactions (25%), rash (22%), and petechia (20%). Herpes simplex was reported in 22% of patients.

Hepatic. Transient elevations of liver transaminases have been observed. Hyperbilirubinemia (grade 3 or 4) has been reported in 23% of patients. Veno-occlusive disease (VOD) has occurred in the transplant setting, up to 3 weeks post gemtuzumab ozogamicin therapy, and can be fatal. The symptoms of VOD included right upper quadrant pain, rapid weight gain, ascites, and hepatomegaly.

Neurological. Dizziness and insomnia were reported in 15% of patients. Depression has been reported less frequently.

Cardiovascular. Hypotension and hypertension were equally reported in 20% of patients. Tachycardia was reported in 11% of patients.

Pulmonary. Most commonly reported are dyspnea, cough, and epistaxis. Less than 15% of patients developed pharyngitis, pneumonia, rhinitis, and abnormal pulmonary findings upon clinical examination.

Renal. Hematuria is reported in 10% of patients. Tumor lysis syndrome leading to renal failure has been reported.

Metabolic. Hypokalemia (31%), hypomagnesemia (10%), hyperuricemia, and hyperglycemia.

Infusion reactions. A post-infusion symptom complex is most commonly observed following the first infusion and less commonly following subsequent infusions. The recommended premedication may prevent this reaction. The reaction usually occurs at the end of the 2-hour intravenous infusion, but can occur within 24 hours of infusion. The most common symptoms are chills and fever; less common are nausea, vomiting, shortness of breath, and hypotension. Resolution of symptoms is aided by administration of acetaminophen, diphenhydramine, and fluid replacement. Other symptoms less commonly observed with these infusion reactions are hypertension, hyperglycemia, hypoxia, and dyspnea.

Hypersensitivity reactions. Anaphylaxis and other severe hypersensitivity reactions, which may include pulmonary complications, have been reported.

Other. Fever (85%), chills (73%), headache (35%), sepsis (25%), asthenia (44%), abdominal pain (37%), enlarged abdomen (9%), back pain (15%), generalized pain (21%), and arthralgias (8%).

Storage and Stability

Intact vials are stored at refrigeration temperatures (i.e., $2°$ to $8°C$). The drug should be protected from light, prior to mixing and while being administered. Once reconstituted, gemtuzumab ozogamicin is stable for 8 hours protected from light, at refrigerated temperatures and in the original vial. Diluted solutions should be administered immediately.

Preparation

Vials of gemtuzumab ozogamicin should be equilibrated to room temperature prior to mixing. Each 5-mg vial is reconstituted with 5 mL of sterile water for injection, to yield a concentration of 1 mg/mL. Do not shake the final product, swirl gently. While preparing this drug the fluorescent light in the biological safety cabinet should be turned off. The desired dose of gemtuzumab ozogamicin is added to 100 mL of normal saline. This final product should be protected from UV light and administered immediately.

Availability

Gemtuzumab ozogamicin, 5 mg/vial, is commercially available as a sterile lyophilized powder in amber vials.

Selected Reading

Sievers EL et al. Efficacy and safety of gemtuzumab ozogamicin in patients with CD33-positive acute myeloid leukemia in first relapse. J Clin Oncol 19: 3244–3254, 2001.

HSPPC-96

Other Names

Oncophage™; heat shock protein peptide complex-96; gp-96.

Indications

Oncophage™ is an investigational agent in the United States that is being evaluated as a treatment for patients with renal cell cancer, colon cancer, malignant melanoma, and other malignancies.

Classification and Mechanisms of Action

Oncophage™ is an autologous vaccine that is derived from heat shock proteins. Heat shock proteins are transport peptides that may activate CD8+ and CD4+ lymphocytes and induce maturation of dendritic cells.

Dose

Doses between 2.5 microg and 100 microg have been administered. Treatment is usually given every week for 4 consecutive weeks, then every other week until all of the vaccine that was prepared has been used. Two 4-weekly vaccination regimens, separated by a 4-week interval of no treatment, have also been evaluated. The vaccine has been administered in combination with interleukin-2.

Administration

Oncophage™ is administered by intradermal injection.

Toxicity

Gastrointestinal. Anorexia, nausea.

HSPPC-96 (continued)

Dermatological. Rash.
Other. Injection site reactions, flu-like symptoms (fever, headache, weakness), myalgia, and hyponatremia have been reported.

Storage and Stability

Oncophage™ is stored in the freezer.

Preparation

The vaccine is prepared from the patient's tumor by the manufacturer.

Availability

Oncophage™ is an investigational agent in the United States that is prepared by the manufacturer using the patient's tumor.

Selected Reading

Hertkorn C et al. Phase I trial of vaccination with tumor-derived gp96 (oncophage) in patients after surgery for gastric cancer. Proc Am Soc Clin Oncol 21: 30a, 2002.

IBRITUMOMAB TIUXETAN

Other Names

Zevalin®; IDEC-2B8; IDEC-Y2B8 (yttrium[90]-ibritumomab tiuxetan); IDEC-In2B8 (indium[111]-ibritumomab tiuxetan); NSC-710085.

Indications

FDA approved for the treatment of CD20-positive, relapsed or refractory, B-cell low grade or follicular non-Hodgkin's lymphoma. Ibritumomab tiuxetan is approved for use in conjunction with rituximab.

Classification and Mechanisms of Action

Ibritumomab is a murine-derived monoclonal antibody directed against CD20-positive cells. Rituximab is the chimeric (murine/human monoclonal antibody) derivative of ibritumomab; it is also directed against CD20-positive cells. The tiuxetan portion of this compound acts as a linker-chelate that allows the beta emitter yttrium[90] to be covalently bound to ibritumomab. Once the radioimmunotherapy is attached, the compound is administered and selectively targets B-cells that possess the CD20 antigen. High levels of expression are found on B-cell malignancies such as non-Hodgkin's lymphomas. Similar to rituximab, ibritumomab binds the antigen CD20 on the cell surface, the effector cells are recruited, and cell lysis occurs via complement-dependent cytotoxicity (CDC), antibody-dependent cell-mediated cytotoxicity (ADCC), and apoptosis.

Pharmacokinetics

Yttrium[90], a beta emitter, is not detectable by external scanning, but is extensively taken up by tumor cells, does not appear to be metabolized, and is removed from circulation by tumor binding and limited (6% to 11%) renal excretion. The blood and plasma yttrium[90] mean elimination half-life is approximately 28 hours, while the biological half-life is 48 hours. The indium[111]-labeled antibody, which is a gamma ray emitter and can be detected by external scans, is used for dosimetry purposes. Dosimetry dosing provides information regarding distribution of radiation absorbed following administration of a radiolabeled isotope. Since yttrium[90] and indium[111] have similar biodistribution patterns, indium^{111} acts as a surrogate isotope used to determine the sites of radiation uptake expected from administering the dose of yttrium^{90}.

Dose

The standard treatment with ibritumomab tiuxetan is a series of therapy and scans over several days.

Day 1 – Rituximab 250 mg/m^2 is administered. This is followed by a 5 mCi imaging dose of indium^{111}-labeled ibritumomab tiuxetan (Zevalin®) and a whole body scan completed between hour 2 and hour 24.

Day 3 or Day 4 – Whole body scan between hour 48 and hour 72.

Day 4 or Day 5 – Whole body scan between hour 90 and hour 120. This is an optional scan.

Day 8 – A second dose of rituximab 250 mg/m^2 is administered. This is followed by yttrium^{90} Zevalin®, 0.4 mCi/kg of yttrium^{90} (or 0.3 mCi/kg for a platelet count of 100,000–149,000/microL). The total dose should not exceed 32 mCi. Do not treat if the platelet count is less than 100,000 cells/microL, the ANC is less than 1,500 cells/microL, or if the patient exhibits abnormal indium^{111} biodistribution scans.

Administration

It is recommended that patients receive acetaminophen and diphenhydramine prior to each dose of rituximab.

Rituximab is administered intravenously, diluted to a concentration of 1 to 4 mg/mL in normal saline or 5% dextrose in water. Rituximab infusions are rate-dependent. The initial infusion rate is 50 mg/hour, the rate is then increased by 50 mg/hour every 30 minutes, as the patient tolerates the drug, to a maximum rate of 400 mg/hour. As long as the patient has tolerated the initial infusion, subsequent doses can be administered at an initial rate of 100 mg/hour, increased by 100 mg/hour to the maximum of 400 mg/hour.

Indium^{111}-labeled ibritumomab tiuxetan is administered intravenously over 10 minutes and yttrium^{90}-labeled ibritumomab tiuxetan is administered over 10 minutes.

Toxicity

For additional rituximab-associated toxicities refer to the rituximab monograph.

Infusion reactions. Rituximab – most common with the first infusion (usually within 30–120 minutes after initiation), incidence decreases with subsequent infusions. For mild to moderate reactions the most common symptoms are chills, fever, rigors. Also observed are nausea, vomiting, headache, bronchospasm, throat irritation, pruritus, asthenia, hypotension or hypertension, dizziness, myalgia, and angioedema.

Severe/fatal infusion reactions have occurred within 24 hours of rituximab administration. The severe symptoms associated with these were hypoxia, pulmonary infiltrates, myocardial infarction, ventricular fibrillation or cardiogenic shock, and acute respiratory distress.

Hematological. Neutropenia (57% of patients exhibited ANC less than 1,000/microL), thrombocytopenia (approximately 60% of patients developed a platelet count less than 50,000/microL). Hemorrhage, some of which was fatal, has occurred. Anemia is common and reversible. The median time to nadir ANC and platelet counts was 7 to 9 weeks, with recovery occurring 22 to 35 days later.

Gastrointestinal. Nausea, anorexia, abdominal pain, diarrhea, or constipation.

Dermatological. Most commonly observed are rash, pruritus, and urticaria. Rituximab has been associated with severe and potentially fatal mucotaneous reactions, including Stevens-Johnson syndrome, paraneoplastic pemphigus, lichenoid dermatitis, vesiculobullous dermatitis, and toxic epidermal necrolysis.

IBRITUMOMAB TIUXETAN *(continued)*

Hepatic. Hyperbilirubinemia and increased LDH levels have been reported.

Neurological. Dizziness and headache.

Cardiovascular. Angioedema. Rituximab induced hypotension or hypertension. Cardiac failure has been observed weeks after administration of rituximab. It is recommended that patients with a history of arrhythmias and angina be carefully monitored.

Pulmonary. Rituximab induced cough and rhinitis, dyspnea, bronchospasm. Rarely reported but severe are acute bronchospasm, acute pneumonitis with a delayed presentation, and bronchiolitis obliterans.

Renal. Rituximab has been associated with acute renal failure due to tumor lysis syndrome in patients with a large tumor burden or with concurrent cisplatin therapy.

Metabolic. Rituximab-associated hyperglycemia and less commonly hypoglycemia. Hyperkalemia, hyperuricemia, hypocalcemia, and hyperphosphatemia have been observed 12 to 24 hours after an infusion due to an association with a reduction in tumor burden.

Other. Fever, chills, infection, asthenia, flushing, back pain, secondary malignancies.

Storage and Stability

Ibritumomab tiuxetan kits are stored at refrigeration temperatures, (i.e., 2° to 8°C). Following reconstitution the indium^{111}-ibritumomab tiuxetan is stable for 12 hours and the yttrium^{90}-labeled ibritumomab tiuxetan is stable for 8 hours.

Preparation

The desired dose of rituximab is added to either a polyvinylchloride or polyethylene infusion container with normal saline or 5% dextrose in water. The final concentration should be 1 to 4 mg/mL. Ibritumomab tiuxetan kits are to be processed by nuclear medicine facilities in accordance with local, state, and federal regulations for handling of radioactive material and biohazardous waste. Specific preparation and handling guidelines are provided to personnel responsible for radiolabeling these products.

Availability

Ibritumomab tiuxetan is commercially available as two separate kits. Each of the kits contain four vials; one vial contains 3.2 mg of ibritumomab tiuxetan in 2 mL of normal saline, one vial contains a formulation buffer, one vial contains 50 mM of sodium acetate, and one vial is an empty "reaction vial."

Rituximab is commercially available as a sterile, preservative-free 10 mg/mL solution in vials containing 100 mg/10 mL and 500 mg/50 mL.

Selected Readings

Wiseman GA et al. Radiation dosimetry results for Zevalin radioimmunotherapy of rituximab-refractory non-Hodgkin's lymphoma. Cancer 94(suppl 4): 1349–1357, 2002.

Wiseman GA et al. Radioimmunotherapy of relapsed non-Hodgkin's lymphoma with Zevalin, a 90Y-labeled anti-CD20 monoclonal antibody. Clin Cancer Res 5(suppl 10): 3281s–3286s, 1999.

INTERFERONS

Interferon is a glycoprotein with a molecular weight of 20,000 composed of approximately 150 amino acids. It consists of multiple species. Interferons are available as a mixture of alfa interferons (interferon alfa-n3: Alferon®, interferon alfa-n1: Wellferon®) or as single recombinant proteins (interferon alfa-2a: Roferon®, interferon alfa-2b: Intron-A®, or interferon gamma-1b: Actimmune®).

ALFA INTERFERONS

Other Names

Interferon alfa-2a; IFN alfa-2a; Roferon®; NSC-367982.
Interferon alfa-2b; IFN alfa-2b; Intron-A®; NSC-377523.
Interferon alfa-n1; IFN alfa-n1; Wellferon®.
Interferon alfa-n3; IFN alfa-n3; Alferon®.
Peginterferon alfa-2a; Pegasys®.
Peginterferon alfa-2b; PEG-Intron®.
Interferon alfacon-1; Infergen®.

Indications

Interferon alfa-n1. Investigational orphan drug status for Kaposi's sarcoma of AIDS, human papillomavirus. Approved in Canada for hairy-cell leukemia and condylomata acuminata.

Interferon alfa-n3. Condylomata acuminata.

Interferon alfa-2a. Hairy-cell leukemia, Kaposi's sarcoma of AIDS, chronic myelogenous leukemia. Also useful for adjuvant treatment of malignant melanoma, chronic hepatitis B, chronic hepatitis non-A non-B/C, condylomata acuminata, multiple myeloma, bladder carcinoma (intravesical instillation), low-grade non-Hodgkin's lymphoma, cutaneous T-cell lymphoma, essential thrombocythemia, and renal cell carcinoma.

Interferon alfa-2b. Hairy-cell leukemia, adjuvant treatment of malignant melanoma, Kaposi's sarcoma of AIDS, chronic hepatitis B, chronic hepatitis non-A non-B/C, condylomata acuminata. Also useful for multiple myeloma, chronic myelogenous leukemia, bladder carcinoma (intravesical instillation), low-grade non-Hodgkin's lymphoma, cutaneous T-cell lymphoma, essential thrombocythemia, renal cell carcinoma.

Peginterferon alfa-2a. Chronic hepatitis C. Also useful in renal cell carcinoma and chronic myelogenous leukemia (designated orphan drug status).

Interferon alfacon-1. Chronic hepatitis C. May also be useful for the treatment of hairy-cell leukemia. In addition to these indications, the alfa interferons may be useful in the treatment of multiple myeloma, chronic myelogenous leukemia, bladder carcinoma (intravesical instillation), low-grade non-Hodgkin's lymphoma, cutaneous T-cell lymphoma, essential thrombocythemia, and renal cell carcinoma. In patients with chronic myelogenous leukemia, cytogenetic conversion to Ph1 chromosome negativity occurs in approximately 40% of patients after a median of 9 months of treatment, and 90% of responding patients maintain their remission with continued therapy.

Classification and Mechanisms of Action

The interferons induce antiviral proteins in cells without directly influencing the virus. Interferons also inhibit tumor growth via an interaction with 2',5'-oligoadenylate synthetase and other means, namely by increasing tumor antigenicity, down-regulation of

ALFA INTERFERONS *(continued)*

oncogenes (e.g., c-myc, c-fos), inducing differentiation, affecting antibody production, negative regulation of angiogenesis, and regulating cytotoxic effector cells. Its direct antiproliferative properties (e.g., inhibition of cell growth) may explain its activity in certain malignancies. Interferons also inhibit P450 enzymes. This phenomenon may result in reduced hepatic metabolism of aminophylline, barbiturates, carmustine, and other drugs.

Pharmacokinetics

Interferons are not absorbed by mouth; they must be administered parenterally. Interferons are metabolized almost totally by renal tubules. Very little interferon is reabsorbed into the circulation from the kidneys. There is no need to reduce the dose of interferon in patients with reduced creatinine clearance. Although the interferons have a short elimination half-life, their antiviral and other effects persist for up to 72 hours after a single dose.

Interferon alfa-n1. Well absorbed after intramuscular or subcutaneous injection with a peak concentration at 6–9 hours for both administration routes, and a half-life of 7–10 hours. Elimination occurs via glomerular filtration and is completely cleared through the renal tubules.

Interferon alfa-2a. Well absorbed after IM injection, up to 80%. In a healthy population the elimination half-life is approximately 5 hours (range 3.7 to 8.5 hours). Significant variability is demonstrated with serum concentration of interferon alfa-2a. Renal catabolism and glomerular filtration are the primary excretion pathways, with minimal excretion via the liver and biliary tract.

Interferon alfa-2b. Maximum serum levels occur approximately 3 to 12 hours after intramuscular administration. By hour 16 they are no longer detectable. The half-life is approximately 2 to 3 hours for IFN alfa-2b, and it is thought to undergo catabolism in the kidney.

Peginterferon alfa-2a. Peak plasma concentrations are demonstrated at 15 to 44 hours after a dose and last for 48 to 72 hours. The drug is approximately 60% bioavailable and bioavailability increases with multiple doses. Peginterferon exhibits an absorption half-life of 4.6 hours and an elimination half-life of approximately 40 hours. Peginterferon is 30% renally cleared, less than the nonpegylated interferon. Dose adjustment may be required in patients with a creatinine clearance less than 50 mL/min.

Interferon alfacon-1. Plasma levels remain undetectable after dosing in healthy subjects, but 24 to 36 hours after dosing peak levels of gene products were detected.

Dose

Hairy-cell leukemia.

IFN alfa-2b. A dose of 2 million IU/m^2 SC or IM 3 times weekly.

IFN alfa-2a. A dose of 3 million IU SC or IM daily for a period of 16 to 24 weeks, then 3 times weekly. Administration of the dose at bedtime may reduce the severity of some side effects. Treatment is usually administered for 1 year.

IFN alfacon-1. A dose of 10 microg/m^2 SC 3 times weekly (combined with filgrastim daily therapy).

Kaposi's sarcoma of AIDS.

IFN alfa-2b. A dose of 30 million IU/m^2 SC or IM 3 times weekly.

IFN alfa-2a. A dose of 36 million IU SC or IM daily for a period of 10 to 12 weeks, then 36 million IU 3 times weekly. The dose needs to be reduced in patients also receiving zidovudine (AZT). Dose-limiting toxicity is seen in most of the patients taking AZT, 100 to 200 mg every 4 hours with IFN alfa-2a, 9 million IU/day.

Condylomata acuminata.

IFN alfa-2b. A dose of 1 million IU, injected into each lesion 3 times weekly for 3 weeks (repeat the 3-week treatment in 12 to 16 weeks if necessary).

IFN alfa-n3. A dose of 250,000 IU injected into each lesion twice weekly for a period up to 8 weeks.

Chronic hepatitis non-A, non-B/C.

IFN alfa-2b. A dose of 3 million IU subcutaneously 3 times weekly for a 16-week period.

Chronic hepatitis B.

IFN alfa-2b. A dose of 5 million IU/day SC or 10 million IU 3 times weekly (30 to 35 million IU/week) for a 16-week period.

Chronic hepatitis C.

IFN alfa-2b. A dose of 3 million IU SC or IM 3 times per week for a 16-week period, for an improved response therapy can be extended to 18 to 24 months.

IFN alfacon-1. A dose of 9 microg administered SC 3 times per week for a 24-week period.

PegIFN alfa-2b. Weight-based dosing is utilized; see Table 5-1 for single agent dosing. The desired dose is administered SC once a week for 12 months. (When peginterferon is used in combination with rebetol the dose of peginterferon is 1.5 microg/kg/week.)

Adjuvant treatment for malignant melanoma.

IFN alfa-2b. A dose of 20 million IU/m^2/day intravenously for 5 days, repeated weekly for 4 weeks, followed by 10 million IU/m^2 SC 3 times each week for 48 weeks.

Chronic myelogenous leukemia.

IFN alfa-2a. An induction dose of 9 million IU SC or IM daily. (Use titration to this dose; 3 million IU/day x 3 days, then 6 million IU/day x 3 days to desired dose of 9 million IU/day.) Maintenance dose is variable.

Multiple myeloma.

IFN alfa-2a. 2 million IU/m^2 3 times weekly as maintenance therapy in patients who attain a response to induction chemotherapy.

Other malignancies.

Various doses (i.e., 3 to 20 million IU/m^2) and schedules (i.e., daily, daily for 5 days repeated every 3 to 4 weeks, or every other day) have been used.

Administration

The preferred route of administration is subcutaneous, preferably in the evening. Interferons (excluding peginterferon) have also been given intramuscularly,

TABLE 5-1

SINGLE AGENT DOSING FOR PegIFN ALFA-2B

Vial size	Weight in kilograms	Amount of PegIFN to administer (microg/ml)
100 microg/ml	37–45	40 microg in 0.4 ml
	46–56	50 microg in 0.5 ml
160 microg/ml	57–72	64 microg in 0.4 ml
	73–88	80 microg in 0.5 ml
240 microg/ml	89–106	96 microg in 0.4 ml
	107–136	120 microg in 0.5 ml
300 microg/ml	137–160	150 microg in 0.5 ml

Adapted from pharmaceutical company product information.

ALFA INTERFERONS (continued)

intravenously, intralesionally, intravesically, intraperitoneally, and topically. When interferon is administered intravenously, it is often mixed in 50 to 100 mL of normal saline and given over a period of 10 to 15 minutes. Alfa interferons have also been administered as a continuous IV or subcutaneous infusion.

Toxicity

The toxicity listed below is for alfa interferon therapy in general; each specific agent may have more or less toxicity reported based on its individual toxicity profile in each patient population studied. Consult product information for details.

Hematological. Mild leukopenia (50%), thrombocytopenia (35%), and anemia (27%) are not usually dose-limiting.

Peginterferon exhibited 7% thrombocytopenia and 6% neutropenia. IFN alfacon-1 exhibited granulocytopenia (23%), thrombocytopenia (19%), and leukopenia (15%). Less common are bruising, lymphadenopathy, and lymphocytosis.

Gastrointestinal. Mild nausea (30% to 50%), vomiting (10% to 17%), diarrhea (30% to 40%), anorexia (45% to 65%), aberrant taste, flatulence, constipation, and gastric distress have been reported. These side effects occasionally occur and are rarely severe. Ulcerative and hemorrhagic colitis has been reported, maybe severe or fatal.

Peginterferon compared to interferon 2b demonstrated a slight increase in nausea (26% vs. 20%), anorexia, diarrhea, and abdominal pain.

IFN alfacon-1 patients reported nausea (40%), abdominal pain, anorexia (20%), diarrhea and dyspepsia. Less common are vomiting, constipation, flatulence, toothache, hemorrhoids, and dry mouth.

Dermatological. Mild alopecia is observed in some patients after 4 months of therapy. Skin rash and injection site reactions occur in 21% to 25% of patients. Other uncommon side effects include dry skin, flushing, increased eyelash growth, and urticaria.

Peginterferon compared to interferon 2b demonstrated a slight increase in pruritus, dry skin, and flushing.

IFN alfacon-1 toxicity includes alopecia (14%), pruritus, rash, erythema, and dry skin.

Hepatic. Mild elevations of hepatic transaminase levels occur in approximately 25% to 46% of patients with hairy-cell leukemia. Hyperbilirubinemia, hepatomegaly, and hepatitis rarely occur. Severe and fatal pancreatitis has been reported.

Liver tenderness was reported with IFN alfacon-1.

Neurological. Depression, suicide, suicidal ideation, homicidal ideation, aggressiveness, and relapsed drug addiction/overdose are severe side effects of interferon therapy. Patients and/or family members should be aware of this side effect toxicity and report any abnormalities immediately to their physician.

Somnolence and mild paresthesias occur in about 25% of patients. Dizziness has been reported in 21% to 41% of patients. Depression, visual and sleep disturbances, tremor, seizures, acute paranoid reactions, aphasia, agitation, anxiety, and dizziness have occurred with high doses (i.e., 20 million units/m^2).

Peginterferon compared to interferon 2b demonstrated a slight increase in headache, depression, and dizziness, and less associated anxiety, irritability, and emotional instability.

IFN alfacon-1 most commonly causes headache (82%) nervousness, depression (as above), anxiety, emotional lability, insomnia, dizziness, paresthesias, amnesia, and hypoesthesia. Less common are abnormal thinking, agitation, decreased libido.

Cardiovascular. Cough (27%), dyspnea (11%), hypotension (5%), edema (3% to 9%), chest pain (4%), hypertension. Arrhythmias (atrial or ventricular), tachycardia, and myocardial infarction have been rarely reported.

Hypertension and palpitations were reported rarely with IFN alfacon-1.

Peginterferon caused less than 1% of reported cardiac events.

Renal. Proteinuria and elevations of serum creatinine levels occur in less than 2% of patients; elevation of BUN levels have been reported to occur in 4% of patients.

Respiratory. Rhinorrhea (4%), sinusitis (0% to 3%), coughing (6%), and pharyngitis (7% to 10%). Monitor patients with pulmonary infiltrates or dysfunction; dyspnea, pneumonitis, and pneumonia have been reported.

IFN alfacon-1 exhibited pharyngitis (34%), upper respiratory infections (31%), cough (22%), sinusitis (17%), rhinitis (13%), and, less commonly, upper respiratory congestion, epistaxis, dyspnea, and bronchitis.

Flu-like symptoms. Fever, chills, diaphoresis, and rigors occur universally regardless of dose, route, or schedule. The usual onset occurs 1 to 2 hours after a dose, peaks within 4 to 8 hours, and may persist for 18 hours. These effects tend to lessen with continued dosing. Prophylactic treatment with acetaminophen blunts the severity of these side effects.

Approximately 50% of peginterferon patients will experience flu-like symptoms, these may improve with increased duration of therapy.

Approximately 15% of IFN alfacon-1 patients will experience flu-like symptoms.

Constitutional symptoms. Most common with all interferon therapy is fatigue (up to 90%), myalgias, arthralgias, and headaches (up to 70%), which may be dose-limiting. These symptoms usually occur during the first or second week of treatment. Chronic fatigue is dose-limiting when doses are greater than 3 to 4 million units 3 times weekly. In patients' with Kaposi's sarcoma of AIDS, an 84% incidence of chronic fatigue has been reported.

Other. Weight loss (14% to 25%), impotence (6%), night sweats (8%). Rarely reported toxicities include hypothyroidism, conjunctivitis, injection site inflammation, bronchospasm, tachypnea, cyanosis, earache, eye irritation, hypersensitivity reactions. Injection site reactions (irritation, inflammation, bruising, itching) are very common (47%) with administration of peginterferon. Peginterferon can exacerbate autoimmune disorders and should be used cautiously in this population.

Conjunctivitis, earache, eye pain, and tinnitus were reported in less than 10% of patients receiving IFN alfacon-1.

Drug Interactions

Theophylline clearance has been reduced by 33% to 88% and theophylline half-life increased by 70% within 24 hours of an intramuscular injection of interferon alfa-2b. The effect was greatest in fast metabolizers of theophylline (i.e., smokers). Theophylline serum concentrations should be monitored closely during and after discontinuation of interferon treatment. Aminophylline clearance will also be significantly reduced by interferon alfa-2b and alfa-2a.

Interferon has been shown to inhibit the metabolism of aminophylline by as much as 33% to 81%.

Interferon alfa-2b may cause serum levels of melphalan to decrease.

Interferon alfa-2b administered concurrently with vidarabine may cause an increase in neurotoxicity.

Antiviral effects may be potentiated by administering interferon alfa-2b with other antiviral agents, i.e., zidovudine and acyclovir.

Interferon alfa-2a administered concomitantly with interleukin-2 (aldesleukin) may increase the risk of renal failure.

Alfa interferons can potentially decrease hepatic cytochrome P450 enzyme activity, thus altering metabolism of other drugs that utilize these enzymes.

ALFA INTERFERONS (continued)

Storage and Stability

The intact vials of IFN alfa-2a, IFN alfa-2b, IFN alfa-n3, and IFN alfacon-1 are stored in the refrigerator. PegIFN is to be stored at controlled room temperature, and can be kept in the refrigerator for 24 hours after dilution. Do not shake vigorously. All containers bear expiration dates.

Preparation

IFN alfa-2a powder for injection: add 3 mL of accompanying diluent to the vial containing 18 million IU to yield 6 million IU/mL (Table 5-2).

For IV injection, it is recommended that IFN alfa-2b be administered as a 100,000 IU/mL solution to minimize adsorption of the drug to glass and plastic containers. The manufacturer does not recommend use of the 10, 18, or 25 million IU vials for IV administration.

Peginterferon is prepared by adding **only** 0.7 ml of provided diluent (sterile water for injection) to the desired vial size, then administer immediately.

Incompatibilities

IFN alfa-2b is incompatible with 5% dextrose solution and with a component of the Travenol infusor.

Compatibilities

IFN alfa-2b is compatible in normal saline, Ringer's injection, lactated Ringer's solution, and 5% sodium bicarbonate injection.

Availability

IFN alfa-2a is commercially available as a vial of injectable solution (3, 6, and 36 million IU/mL, 9 million IU/0.9 mL, and 6 or 9 million IU/0.5 mL prefilled syringes), also as a vial of powder for injection of 6 IU/mL, total of 18 million IU with diluent.

IFN alfa-2b is commercially available as a lyophilized powder in vials containing 3, 5, 10, 18, 25, and 50 million IU and as an injectable solution in vials containing 3 million IU/0.5 mL, 5 million IU/0.5 mL, 10 million IU/1 mL, 22.8 million IU/3.8 mL (6 million IU/mL), and 32 million IU/3.2 mL (10 million IU/mL).

IFN alfa-2b multidose injectable pens available as an 18 million IU pen (6 doses of 3 million IU), 30 million IU pen (6 doses of 5 million IU), and 60 million IU pen (6 doses of 10 million IU).

TABLE 5-2

IFN ALFA-2B POWDER FOR INJECTION

Vial strength (million IU)	Diluent (mL)	Final concentration (million IU/mL)
3	1	3
5	5	5
10*	1	10
18	1	18
25	5	5
50†	1	50

*For condylomata acuminata.
†For Kaposi's sarcoma of AIDS.

IFN alfa-n3 is commercially available as an injectable solution in 1-mL vials containing 5 million IU/mL.

Peginterferon is commercially available as lyophilized powder for injection in vial sizes of 100 microg/mL, 160 microg/mL, 240 microg/mL, and 300 microg/mL; a 5-mL sterile vial of diluent is provided.

Interferon alfacon-1 is commercially available as a 9 microg/0.3 mL and a 15 microg/0.5 mL single dose preservative-free solution.

Selected Readings

Browman GP et al. Randomized trial of interferon maintenance in multiple myeloma: a study of the National Cancer Institute of Canada Clinical Trials Group. J Clin Oncol 13: 2354–2360, 1995.

Heathcote EJ et al. Peginterferon alfa 2a in patients with chronic hepatitis C and cirrhosis. N Engl J Med 343: 1673–1680, 2000.

Manns MP et al. Peginterferon alfa-2b plus ribavirin compared with interferon alfa-2b plus ribavirin for initial treatment of chronic hepatitis C: a randomized trial. Lancet 358: 958–965, 2001.

INTERFERON BETA-1A AND 1B

Other Names

1A – Avonex®; 1B – Betaseron®; interferon beta; IFN-beta; recombinant beta interferon; rIFN-B; IFN-Bser; NSC-373361.

Indications

Interferon beta-1a is FDA approved for use in the treatment of relapsing forms of multiple sclerosis, and interferon beta-1b is FDA approved for ambulatory patients with relapsing-remitting multiple sclerosis. IFN-beta may also be useful in the treatment of AIDS-related Kaposi's sarcoma, renal cell carcinoma, melanoma, cutaneous T-cell lymphoma, non-small-cell cancer of the lung, and acute non-A, non-B hepatitis.

Classification and Mechanisms of Action

Interferon-beta binds to the same cellular receptor sites as the alfa interferons. Interferon-beta has antiviral, antiproliferative (cytostatic), and immunomodulatory properties. Its direct antiproliferative properties (e.g., inhibition of cell growth and differentiation) may account for its activity in certain malignancies. The mechanisms by which interferon-beta exerts its effects on multiple sclerosis are not known.

Pharmacokinetics

After intravenous administration of interferon beta-1a, peak serum biological response marker levels increase within 12 hours of dosing and peak 48 hours after dosing. The elimination half-life after IM or SC dosing is 10 and 8.6 hours, respectively.

Peak serum concentrations of interferon beta-1b occur within 1 to 8 hours after subcutaneous injection. The apparent bioavailability of interferon beta after subcutaneous administration is 50%. The elimination half-life has been calculated as 8 minutes to 4.3 hours.

Dose

Interferon beta-1a. For the treatment of multiple sclerosis the recommended dose is 30 microg per dose, intramuscularly once a week.

Interferon beta-1b. For the treatment of multiple sclerosis, the recommended dose is 0.25 mg subcutaneously every other day. Various doses have been evaluated in the treatment of malignancies, including 90 million IU/day for 10 days, repeated every 21 days, and 180 million IU 3 times a week.

INTERFERON BETA-1A AND 1B *(continued)*

Administration

IFN-beta has been administered subcutaneously, intramuscularly, intranasally, intravesically, intraperitoneally, intrathecally, topically, and intravenously, usually as an infusion over a 10- to 15-minute period.

Toxicity

Hematological.
Interferon beta-1a. Anemia, eosinophilia (>10%) decreased hematocrit, and bruising at injection site.
Interferon beta-1b. Neutropenia (18% may have an absolute neutrophil count less than 1,500/mm^3), lymphopenia (84% will have a lymphocyte count less than 1,500/mm^3), thrombocytopenia (uncommon), anemia (rare).
Gastrointestinal.
Interferon beta-1a. Nausea (33%), diarrhea (16%), dyspepsia (11%), and anorexia (7%).
Interferon beta-1b. Mild nausea, vomiting (21%), mild diarrhea (35%), constipation (24%).
Dermatological.
Interferon beta-1a. Urticaria, alopecia, nevus, and herpes infections (zoster and simplex), injection site reactions (4%).
Interferon beta-1b. Rash, alopecia (4%), injection site reaction (85%), diaphoresis (23%), photosensitivity (rare).
Hepatic.
Interferon beta-1a. 3% of patients experienced an AST greater then three times the upper limit of normal.
Interferon beta-1b. Significant elevation of hepatic transaminase levels has been reported to occur in 5% to 19% of patients.
Neurological. Depression and suicidal ideation are not uncommon with interferon beta therapy. Patients and/or family members should be aware of these side effects and report any abnormalities immediately to their physician.
Interferon beta 1a. Insomnia (19%), dizziness (15%), muscle spasm (7%), less than 5% of patients experienced speech disorder, convulsions, ataxia.
Interferon beta-1b. Hypertonia (26%), Somnolence (6%), confusion (at high doses), paresthesia, tremor, seizures (rare), paranoia (rare), aphasia (3%), agitation (2%), anxiety, dizziness (35%), transient visual disturbances (7%).
Cardiovascular.
Interferon beta-1a. Syncope and vasodilation reported in less than 5% of patients.
Interferon beta-1b. Tachycardia (6%), migraine (12%), palpitations (8%), generalized edema (8%), hypertension (7%), arrhythmias, myocardial infarction (rare).
Flu-like symptoms. Flu-like symptoms occur in up to 76% of patients receiving interferon beta-1b and up to 61% of patients receiving interferon beta-1a. Fever, chills, diaphoresis, and rigors occur regardless of dose, route, or schedule. The usual onset occurs 1 to 2 hours after a dose, peaks within 4 to 8 hours, and may persist for 18 hours. These effects tend to lessen with continued dosing. Prophylactic treatment with acetaminophen blunts the severity of these side effects.
Constitutional symptoms. Fatigue (common), myalgias, arthralgias, and headaches may be dose-limiting. These symptoms usually occur during the first or second week of treatment. Chronic fatigue is dose-limiting with higher doses.

BIOTHERAPY DRUGS

Other.

Interferon beta-1a. Infection (11%), abdominal pain (9%), chest pain (6%), ovarian cyst (3%), hypersensitivity reactions (3%), vaginitis (4%), upper respiratory tract infection (31%), sinusitis (18%), dyspnea (6%).

Interferon beta-1b. Asthenia (49%), abdominal pain (32%), sinusitis (36%), dyspnea (8%), laryngitis (6%), hypoglycemia (15%), proteinuria (6%), weight gain (4%), weight loss (4%), conjunctivitis (12%), menstrual abnormalities (17%), cystitis (15%).

Storage and Stability

Interferon beta-1a. Unreconstituted vials are preferably stored at refrigeration temperatures, avoid freezing. The unreconstituted vials may be kept at room temperature for no more than 30 days. Once reconstituted, use solution within 6 hours, keep at refrigerated temperature.

Interferon beta-1b. Unreconstituted vials are stored at refrigeration temperatures, avoid freezing. The manufacturer recommends that reconstituted solutions be used within 3 hours.

Preparation

Interferon beta-1a. The lyophilized product is reconstituted by adding 1.1 mL of the provided diluent to the 33-microg vial. Completely dissolve powder by swirling the vial gently.

Interferon beta-1b. The lyophilized product is reconstituted by adding 1.2 mL of the provided diluent to the 0.3-mg vial (9.6 million IU) to result in a concentration of 0.25 mg/mL (8 million IU/mL). For intravenous injection interferon beta-1b may be further diluted with 5% dextrose or normal saline.

Availability

Interferon beta-1a is commercially available as a lyophilized powder in 33-microg (6.6 million IU) vials.

Interferon beta-1b is commercially available as a lyophilized powder in 0.3-mg (9.6 million IU) vials.

INTERFERON GAMMA

Other Names

Actimmune®; interferon gamma-1b; IFN-gamma; lymphocyte interferon; T-interferon.

Indications

FDA approved to decrease the severity and frequency of serious infections associated with chronic granulomatous disease. Also approved for use in malignant osteopetrosis, to delay time to disease progression. Interferon gamma may be a useful treatment for patients with ovarian carcinoma or combined with melphalan and tumor necrosis factor (TNF) given by isolated limb perfusion for patients with melanoma of the extremity.

Pharmacokinetics

Interferon gamma is not absorbed by mouth. Approximately 90% of the drug is absorbed after subcutaneous administration. Peak plasma concentrations occur 4 and 7 hours after administration by intramuscular and subcutaneous routes, respectively. The elimination half-life is approximately 6 hours after subcutaneous administration, 40 minutes after intravenous administration, and 3 hours after intramuscular dosing. The maximum serum concentration occurs 7 hours after subcutaneous injection.

INTERFERON GAMMA *(continued)*

Dose

For patients with a body surface area greater than 0.5 m^2: 50 microg/m^2/dose (1 million IU/m^2/dose).

For patients with a body surface area less than or equal to 0.5 m^2: 1.5 microg/kg/dose.

One dose is administered 3 times each week (usually on a Monday, Wednesday, and Friday). For patients with ovarian carcinoma, interferon gamma has been administered intraperitoneally at a dose of 20 million IU/m^2 twice weekly for a period of 3 to 4 months. Combined with melphalan and tumor necrosis factor (TNF) administered by isolated limb perfusion (ILP), interferon gamma has been administered subcutaneously at a dose of 200 microg/day on the 2 days preceding ILP. Interferon gamma, 200 microg, was also added to the perfusate containing TNF and melphalan. For metastatic renal cell carcinoma a dose of 100 microg once a week has produced some clinical responses.

Administration

Subcutaneous injection is the preferred route of administration. Interferon gamma has also been given intramuscularly, intravenously over a 1-minute or longer period, intraperitoneally, and by isolated limb perfusion. When administered into the peritoneal cavity, interferon gamma has been diluted in 250 mL of normal saline and infused over a 2-hour period.

The administration of acetaminophen, beginning 4 hours prior to dosing interferon gamma and continuing up to 24 hours after administration, can aid in reducing the expected flu-like symptoms.

Toxicity

Hematological. Leukopenia occurs frequently but is rarely of clinical significance. Decreased hemoglobin and hematocrit (uncommon), thrombocytopenia, prolonged PT and PTT, and hemolysis (rare). Deep venous thrombosis and pulmonary embolism have been reported. After intraperitoneal administration, grade 3 neutropenia and anemia were observed in 4% and 3% of patients, respectively.

Gastrointestinal. Diarrhea (14%), nausea (10%), vomiting (13%), abdominal pain (8% after SC use, 13% after intraperitoneal use), anorexia (3%), weight loss, stomatitis, pancreatitis, gastrointestinal bleeding in patients with a prior history (rare).

Dermatological. Rash, injection site reactions, exacerbated dermatomyositis.

Hepatic. Increased hepatic transaminase levels and serum bilirubin occur frequently.

Neurological. Headache (33%) decreased alertness, confusion, dizziness, Parkinson-like symptoms, disorientation, hallucinations, transient ischemic attack, depression, and seizures. Paresthesias have been reported in 6% of patients receiving interferon gamma via the intraperitoneal route.

Cardiovascular. Hypotension, primary atrioventricular block, peripheral vasoconstriction, syncope, tachyarrhythmia, myocardial infarction.

Pulmonary. Tachypnea, interstitial pneumonitis, bronchospasm.

Renal. Elevated BUN or creatinine levels, proteinuria, and acute renal failure.

Constitutional symptoms. Flu-like symptoms including fever which commonly occurs after all routes of administration; chills (14%), myalgias (6%), fatigue (14%), night sweats, rigors, diaphoresis, malaise.

Other. Psoriatic arthritis, hyponatremia, hyperglycemia, increased triglyceride levels.

Preparation

Available as a sterile liquid.

Drug Interactions

A potential decrease in hepatic cytochrome P450 enzymes has been observed in pre-clinical rodent studies. This in turn can lead to decreased metabolism of hepatically metabolized drugs. Interferon gamma-1b administered concomitantly with other myelosuppressive agents may cause an increase in myelosuppressive effects.

Storage and Stability

Interferon gamma-1b is stored in the refrigerator. Do not freeze. It is stable for 12 hours at room temperature. The manufacturer recommends discarding any unused portion of a vial after withdrawing the desired dose.

Availability

Commercially available as 100 microg (2 million units) per 0.5-mL vial.

ISIS 3521

Other Names

Affinitac®; ISI641A; LY900003; CGP64128A; NSC-719337.

Indications

ISIS 3521 is an investigational agent in the United States that is undergoing evalua-tion in non-small-cell lung cancer, ovarian cancer, non-Hodgkin's lymphoma, and other malignancies.

Classification and Mechanisms of Action

ISIS 3521 is an antisense inhibitor of protein kinase C-alfa (PKC-alfa). The drug binds to a messenger RNA sequence that is specific to PKC-alfa.

Pharmacokinetics

ISIS 3521 exhibits a nonlinear pharmacokinetic profile. With increasing doses the total body clearance decreases and the half-life increases. The elimination half-life following a single 2-hour IV infusion of 6 mg/kg is approximately 90 minutes. Twenty-four hours after administration less than 1% of the product is eliminated in the urine.

Dose

As a 21-day continuous infusion followed by 7 days of no treatment, the maximum tolerated dose is 2 mg/kg/day. Dose-limiting thrombocytopenia and fatigue occurred at a dose of 3 mg/kg/day on this schedule. ISIS 3521 has also been administered at doses up to 6 mg/kg/day by continuous infusion for 14 days, repeated every 21 days (i.e., 14 days of treatment followed by 7 days of rest).

ISIS 3521, 2 mg/kg/day by continuous infusion for 14 days, has been adminis-tered with docetaxel 75 mg/m^2 on day 3.

The same dose and schedule of ISIS 3521 has been administered with cisplatin 80 mg/m^2 on day 1 and gemcitabine 1,000 mg/m^2 on days 1 and 8.

Administration

ISIS 3521 has been administered by continuous IV infusion. It has also been administered as a 2-hour IV infusion.

Toxicity

Hematological. Thrombocytopenia is dose-limiting with a dose of 3 mg/kg/day for 21 days. Transient increases in activated PTT have been observed.

ISIS 3521 *(continued)*

Gastrointestinal. Mild to moderate nausea and vomiting is an uncommon adverse event.
Other. Fatigue may be dose-limiting in some patients. Fever and chills have been
reported.

Storage and Stability

Intact vials are stored at refrigeration temperatures (2°C to 8°C).

Preparation

Doses are usually further diluted in 50 mL or more of normal saline.

Availability

ISIS 3521 is an investigational agent in the United States that is available as an
injectable solution 10 mg/mL (10 mg/1-mL vial and 100 mg/10-mL vial) from the
manufacturer.

Selected Readings

Nemunaitis J et al. Phase I evaluation of ISIS 3521, an antisense oligodeoxynucleotide to
    protein kinase C-alfa, in patients with advanced cancer. J Clin Oncol 17: 3586–3595, 1999.
Yuen AR et al. Phase I study of an antisense oligonucleotide to protein kinase C-alfa (ISIS 3521/CGP
    64128A) in patients with cancer. Clin Cancer Res 5: 3357–3363, 1999.

KEYHOLE LIMPET HEMOCYANIN (MODIFIED)

Other Names

KLH; BCI Immune Activator™; NSC 713762.

Indications

Modified KLH is an investigational agent in the United States that is undergoing evaluation as a treatment for patients with superficial bladder cancer or cancer in situ (CIS)
with disease that is refractory to BCG treatment.

Classification and Mechanisms of Action

Keyhole limpet hemocyanin is derived from a variety of the giant mollusk. Modified
KLH is an antigenic protein that elicits humoral and cellular immune responses.

Dose

1 mg intradermally, followed by 50 mg every week for 12 consecutive weeks.

Administration

Instillation into the bladder in 50 mL of normal saline.

Toxicity

Dermatological (following intradermal injection). Erythema, induration, and ulceration
have been reported.
Urinary (following intravesicular administration). Incontinence, urinary retention,
dysuria, bladder pain, hematuria, increased urgency, and increased frequency have
been reported following administration.
Other. Malaise, asthenia, low-grade fever, and chills have been reported following
intradermal and intravesicular administration. These effects are usually mild. A few
patients have experienced hypersensitivity reactions, including bronchospasm,
hypotension, and serum sickness.

Storage and Stability
The product is stable for at least 15 months at 2° to 8°C. The manufacturer recommends that the product not be frozen.

Preparation
The product is filtered through a 0.22 micron filter prior to administration.

Availability
Modified KLH is an investigational agent in the United States that is available as a 5 mg/mL solution (1.2 mL in a 3-mL vial) from the manufacturer.

Selected Reading
Jennemann R et al. Specific immunization using keyhole limpet hemocyanin-ganglioside conjugates. J Biochem 115: 1047–1052, 1994.

MELANOMA THERACCINE

Other Names
Melacine®; NSC-653041.

Indications
Melacine® is an investigational agent in the United States. In Canada it is approved for the treatment of patients with stage IV metastatic melanoma. The vaccine appears to be effective as an adjuvant treatment for a subset of patients with melanoma.

Classification and Mechanisms of Action
Melacine® is an allogeneic vaccine. It consists of lysed cells from two melanoma cell lines combined with Detox TM® adjuvant. Detox TM® adjuvant is a mixture of monophosphoryl lipid A and mycobacterial cell wall skeleton.

Dose
Melacine®, for the treatment of metastatic melanoma, is administered once a week for 5 consecutive weeks. This 5-week course is repeated after a 2-week break. Responding patients receive one dose each month and a single 5-week course every 6 months. As an adjuvant treatment for melanoma Melacine® has been administered over 2 years, in 6-month cycles. Each 6-month cycle is separated by 3 weeks of no treatment. During each 6-month cycle 10 doses are administered as weekly injections for 4 consecutive weeks followed by every other week injections for 4 weeks followed by monthly injections for 4 months. Each dose is administered as two 0.625-mL injections (i.e., 0.5 mL Melacine® and 0.125 mL Detox® per injection).

Administration
Intramuscular injection.

Toxicity
Approximately 23% of patients will experience adverse events no greater than grade 1, 65% grade 2 as the maximum toxicity, and 9% will experience grade 3 adverse event(s). Injection site reactions and flu-like symptoms are the most common adverse events associated with Melacine®.
Hematological. Leukopenia (2% grade 1), thrombocytopenia (3% grade 1).
Gastrointestinal. Diarrhea (4% grade 1), nausea (16%).
Dermatological. Erythema (15%), skin rash, urticaria.

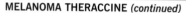

MELANOMA THERACCINE *(continued)*

Local reactions. Injection site reactions are the most common adverse events associated with Melacine®. In one study involving approximately 300 patients, 11% discontinued treatment due to toxicity. Local toxicities included granulomas (55% grade 2), sterile abscesses (38% grade 2), and other local reactions (60% grade 1, 24% grade 2, 3% grade 3).

Hepatic. Hyperbilirubinemia (3% grade 2), elevations of transaminase levels (5% grade 1).

Other. Chills (15% grade 1, 7% grade 2), fever without infection (12% grade 1 or 2), asthenia (35%), myalgia (30%), visual changes, sweats, headache (16%), and dizziness.

Storage and Stability

Melacine® is to be prepared just prior to injection.

Availability

Melacine® is an investigational agent in the United States. In Canada it is commercially available.

Selected Reading

Sandak VK et al. Adjuvant immunotherapy of resected, intermediate-thickness, node-negative melanoma with an allogeneic tumor vaccine: overall results of a randomized trial of the Southwest Oncology Group. J Clin Oncol 20: 2058–2066, 2002.

ONYX-015

Other Names

CI-1042; d11520; NSC-688653.

Indications

ONYX-015 is an investigational agent in the United States. The compound is undergoing evaluation in glioblastoma, colon cancer, head and neck cancers, ovarian cancer, and other malignancies.

Classification and Mechanisms of Action

ONYX-15 is a modified human adenovirus that is believed to be active against cancer cells that are deficient in p53 suppressor gene activity. ONYX-015 has been shown to replicate and lyse tumor cells that are deficient in p53 suppressor gene activity. It has been postulated that many drug-resistant tumor cells do not have functional p53.

Pharmacokinetics

The presence of viral activity has been noted 10 days following the last dose of ONYX-015.

Dose

By direct injection into the tumor, in head and neck cancer patients, doses up to 5×10^{10} plaque-forming units (pfu)/day for 5 days. This 5-day course is repeated every 3 weeks. In combination with cisplatin, on day 1, and 5-fluorouracil, as a continuous infusion for 5 days, ONYX-015 has been administered at a dose of 1×10^{10} pfu/day for 5 days. For intraperitoneal use doses up to 10^{11} plaque-forming units (pfu)/day for 5 days have been administered. This treatment was repeated every 3 weeks. ONYX-015 has been administered by hepatic artery infusion: 2×10^{12} pfu/week for 2 consecutive weeks. ONYX-015 has been evaluated as a mouthwash for oral dysplasia: 10^{10} pfu/week for 12 consecutive weeks.

Administration
ONYX-015 is administered directly into the tumor (e.g., head and neck cancer). The appropriate volume of ONYX-015 solution is a percentage (i.e., 30%) of the estimated tumor volume. ONYX-015 has also been administered via intraperitoneal instillation, in 500 mL of normal saline, in patients with ovarian cancer. ONYX-015 has also been administered as a mouthwash for oral dysplasia.

Toxicity
Gastrointestinal. Nausea, vomiting, heartburn, anorexia, and diarrhea have been observed following intraperitoneal administration. Diarrhea (grade 3) was dose-limiting in one of 16 ovarian cancer patients.
Constitutional. Flu-like symptoms are the most common toxicity associated with ONYX-015. Symptoms included fever, headache, myalgia and malaise. These symptoms occur following direct tumor and peritoneal administration. In one series of 16 ovarian cancer patients who received intraperitoneal ONYX-015, the incidence of grade 2 and grade 3 flu-like symptoms was: asthenia 47%, fever 33% to 50%, chills 25%, headache 25%, myalgia 6%, and malaise 6%.
Cardiovascular. Atrial flutter (rare), facial edema (rare).
Neurological. Confusion (rare).
Other. Pain (grade 1 to 2) at the site of the intratumoral injection is common ($>50\%$) and usually resolves within 24 hours following the injection. A few patients have developed hemorrhage at the site of intratumoral injection. Abdominal pain is common following intraperitoneal administration.

Storage and Stability
ONYX-015 is stored in the freezer ($-20°C$).

Preparation
Doses are usually further diluted in 500 mL of normal saline for intraperitoneal administration or the appropriate volume of 5% dextrose and water for intratumoral injection.

Availability
ONYX-015 is an investigational agent in the United States that is available in vials containing 0.5 mL of virus solution from the manufacturer or the National Cancer Institute.

Selected Reading
Nemunaitis J et al. Phase II trial of intratumoral administration of ONYX-015, a replication-selective adenovirus, in patients with refractory head and neck cancer. J Clin Oncol 19: 289–298, 2001.

OPRELVEKIN

Other Names
Neumega®; recombinant human interleukin-11; IL-11; rhIL-11.

Indications
Oprelvekin is FDA approved for use as an adjunctive treatment to myelosuppressive chemotherapy in patients with nonmyeloid cancers. Oprelvekin is useful because of its ability to stimulate the production of platelets, prevent severe thrombocytopenia, and decrease the number of platelet transfusions a patient requires.

OPRELVEKIN (continued)

Classification and Mechanisms of Action

Oprelvekin is an inducer of platelet production via stimulation of megakaryocytopoiesis and thrombopoiesis. Platelet increases are observed 5 to 9 days after initiation of treatment.

Pharmacokinetics

Following administration of one 50 microg/kg subcutaneous dose, peak plasma concentrations of oprelvekin occur at approximately 3.2 hours. The terminal half-life is approximately 7 hours. Oprelvekin is greater than 80% bioavailable and multiple doses do not cause accumulation of the drug. Clearance of oprelvekin decreases with age and with severe renal function.

Dose

The recommended adult dose of oprelvekin is 50 microg/kg administered once a day for 10 to 21 days. Treatment should begin 6 to 24 hours after chemotherapy has been completed and should continue through the platelet nadir until the platelet count rises above 50,000 cells/mm^3. Oprelvekin therapy should be discontinued at least 2 days prior to the next chemotherapy cycle.

Administration

Oprelvekin is administered subcutaneously. The recommended sites include the hip, abdomen, thigh, or upper arm.

Toxicity

Many reported side effects can be related to chemotherapy treatments and were reported in both the placebo and oprelvekin-treated patients.

Gastrointestinal. Oral moniliasis was reported in 14% of patients. Nausea, vomiting, and diarrhea were reported in a slightly higher percentage of oprelvekin patients than placebo.

Dermatological. Most commonly observed in 1% of patients is a transient rash at the injection site.

Neurological. Dizziness and insomnia, reported slightly higher than the placebo group.

Cardiovascular. Tachycardia, atrial fibrillation, atrial flutter, and palpitations were significantly higher in the oprelvekin-treated patients. Fluid retention manifested as peripheral edema and increased shortness of breath on exertion are commonly reported in oprelvekin patients. This is reversible upon discontinuing the oprelvekin. Monitor patients who may have pre-existing fluid conditions (e.g., pleural effusions).

Pulmonary. Most commonly observed in oprelvekin patients was dyspnea (48%) and pleural effusions (10%). Rhinitis, cough, and pharyngitis were reported in a slightly higher percentage of oprelvekin patients than placebo-treated patients.

Other. Blurred vision and papilledema.

Storage and Stability

Oprelvekin vials are stored in the refrigerator at a temperatures of 2° to 8°C. Do not freeze. Once reconstituted, oprelvekin is stable for 3 hours at room or refrigerated temperatures. Protect from light.

Preparation

Reconstitute the 5-mg vial with 1 mL of preservative-free sterile water (provided). Inject the diluent at the sidewall of the vial, do not shake or agitate vigorously.

Observe the product for discoloration or particulate matter. Withdraw dose from the vial and administer subcutaneously.

Availability
Oprelvekin is commercially available in 5-mg vials of sterile, white lyophilized powder. A vial of diluent is provided with the drug.

Selected Readings
Reynolds CH. Clinical efficacy of rhIL-11. Oncology 14(suppl 8): 32–40, 2000.
Rust DM et al. Oprelvekin: an alternative treatment for thrombocytopenia. Clin J Oncol Nurs 3: 57–62, 1999.

RITUXIMAB

Other Names
Rituxan®; anti-CD20 antibody; NSC-687451.

Indications
FDA approved for the treatment of CD20-positive, relapsed or refractory, B-cell low-grade or follicular non-Hodgkin's lymphoma. Rituximab has also demonstrated activity in other CD20-positive malignancies such as chronic lymphocytic leukemia, lympho-plasmacytic tumors, and small subsets of multiple myeloma.

Classification and Mechanisms of Action
Rituximab is a chimeric murine/human monoclonal antibody directed against CD20-positive cells. Normal mature B-cells possess the CD20 antigen and high levels of expression are found on B-cell malignancies such as non-Hodgkin's lymphomas. Rituximab binds the antigen CD20 on the cell surface, the effector cells are recruited, and cell lysis occurs. Rituximab can induce cell lysis via complement-dependent cytotoxicity (CDC) or antibody-dependent cell-mediated cytotoxicity (ADCC). It is also thought that rituximab binding may directly prevent cell replication.

Pharmacokinetics
Rituximab rapidly saturates CD20-positive sites on the B-cells in the blood, then spleen, marrow, and lymph nodes. The serum half-life of rituximab increases with each dose due to variability in tumor burden and the number of saturable sites that remain after each week of treatment. After the initial infusion the half-life is 76 hours, after the fourth infusion the half-life is often greater than 200 hours. Detectable levels of rituximab have been demonstrated at 3 and 6 months post-infusion.

Dose
The standard dose of rituximab is 375 mg/m^2/week for 4 doses. Doses are calculated using the patient's actual body weight. Alternative dosing schedules have included additional weekly cycles of rituximab beyond the initial 4 doses, three times per week dosing, and rituximab in combination with chemotherapy for non-Hodgkin's lymphoma (e.g., rituximab plus CHOP).

Administration
It is recommended that patients be premedicated with acetaminophen and diphenhydramine prior to each dose of rituximab.

Rituximab is administered intravenously, diluted to a concentration of 1 to 4 mg/mL in 0.9% sodium chloride or 5% dextrose in water. Rituximab infusions are rate-dependent.

RITUXIMAB *(continued)*

The initial infusion rate is 50 mg/hour, the rate is then increased by 50 mg/hour every 30 minutes, as the patient tolerates the drug, to a maximum rate of 400 mg/hour. As long as the patient has tolerated the initial infusion, subsequent doses can be administered at an initial rate of 100 mg/hour and increased by 100 mg/hour to the maximum of 400 mg/hour.

Toxicity

Hematological. Lymphopenia is most common and observed in up to 48% of patients, with a median duration of 14 days. Observed in less than 15% of patients are: leukopenia, anemia, neutropenia (median duration 13 days), and thrombocytopenia. The incidence of grade 3 or 4 hematological toxicity was approximately 12%. The incidence of anemia and neutropenia is higher in patients with bulky disease (i.e., greater than 10 cm).

Gastrointestinal. Nausea was reported in 23% of patients, with vomiting and diarrhea less commonly reported. Rarely, anorexia and dyspepsia have been reported.

Dermatological. Most commonly observed are rash, pruritus, and urticaria. Severe and potentially fatal mucotaneous reactions have been reported. These reactions included: Stevens-Johnson syndrome, paraneoplastic pemphigus, lichenoid dermatitis, vesiculobullous dermatitis, and toxic epidermal necrolysis.

Hepatic. Increase in LDH was observed in 7% of patients.

Neurological. Dizziness and anxiety most common. Rarely, insomnia, depression, nervousness, neuritis, neuropathy, paresthesia, somnolence, and vertigo.

Cardiovascular. Hypotension (10%) and hypertension (6%). Rare cardiac failure has been observed with the onset observed weeks after rituximab infusion. It is recommended to monitor carefully patients with a history of arrhythmias and angina during rituximab infusions.

Pulmonary. Most commonly reported are cough and rhinitis. Dyspnea and bronchospasm were reported in less than 10% of patients. Rarely reported, but severe, are acute bronchospasm, acute pneumonitis with a delayed presentation, and bronchiolitis obliterans.

Renal. Acute renal failure, associated with tumor lysis syndrome in patients with a high number of circulating cells or large tumor burden, and with concurrent cisplatin therapy.

Metabolic. Hyperglycemia, and less commonly hypoglycemia. Observed 12–24 hours after an infusion due to an association with a reduction in tumor burden, hyperkalemia, hyperuricemia, hypocalcemia, and hyperphosphatemia have been observed.

Infusion reactions. Most common with the first infusion (usually within 30 to 120 minutes after initiation), incidence decreases with subsequent infusions. For mild to moderate reactions the most common symptoms are chills, fever, and rigors. Also observed are nausea, vomiting, headache, bronchospasm, throat irritation, pruritus, asthenia, hypotension or hypertension, dizziness, myalgia, and angioedema.

Severe/fatal infusion reactions have occurred within 24 hours of rituximab administration. The severe symptoms associated with these were hypoxia, pulmonary infiltrates, myocardial infarction, ventricular fibrillation or cardiogenic shock, and acute respiratory distress.

Other. Fever (55%) and chills (33%), infection (31%, only 2% of which were grade 3 or 4), asthenia (25%), abdominal pain (14%), throat irritation (9%), back pain (10%), flushing (5%), sinusitis (6%), angio- (11%) or peripheral (8%) edema, and night sweats (15%). Rare reactions: agitation, arthritis, conjunctivitis, hyperkinesia, hypertonia, pain at injection site, weight loss, uveitis, pleuritis, serum sickness, and vasculitis with rash.

Drug Interactions

Rituximab administered concomitantly with cisplatin in clinical trials resulted in renal toxicity.

Storage and Stability

Intact vials are stored in the refrigerator at temperatures of 2° to 8°C. Reconstituted solutions are stable for 24 hours at refrigerated temperatures and an additional 24 hours at room temperature.

Preparation

The desired dose is rituximab is drawn into a syringe and added to either polyvinylchloride or polyethylene bags of 0.9% sodium chloride or 5% dextrose in water to a final concentration of 1 to 4 mg/mL. Discard any remaining drug.

Availability

Rituximab is commercially available as a sterile, preservative-free 10 mg/mL solution in vials containing 100 mg and 500 mg.

Selected Readings

Byrd JC et al. Rituximab using a thrice weekly dosing schedule in B-cell chronic lymphocytic leukemia and small lymphocytic lymphoma demonstrated clinical activity and acceptable toxicity. J Clin Oncol 19: 2153–2164, 2001.

Czuczman MS et al. Treatment of patients with low-grade B-cell lymphoma with the combination of chimeric anti-CD20 monoclonal antibody and CHOP chemotherapy. J Clin Oncol 17: 268–276, 1999.

Hainsworth JD et al. Rituximab monoclonal antibody as initial systemic therapy for patients with low-grade non-Hodgkin's lymphoma. Blood 95: 3052–3056, 2000.

Maloney DG, McLaughlin P. Rituximab for the treatment of patients with B-cell non-Hodgkin's lymphoma. In DeVita VT Jr, Hellman S, Rosenberg SA, eds. Progress in Oncology. Boston, Jones and Bartlett, 2001: pp204–227.

SARGRAMOSTIM

Other Names

Leukine®; Prokine®; granulocyte-macrophage colony-stimulating factor; GM-CSF; rGM-CSF; NSC-617589.

Sargramostim is derived from yeast.

Indications

Sargramostim (GM-CSF) is FDA approved for myeloid reconstitution after autologous bone marrow transplantation (ABMT) and to abrogate myelosuppression associated with chemotherapy, including patients with acute leukemia, non-Hodgkin's lymphoma, and Hodgkin's disease. Use of GM-CSF is contraindicated in patients whose bone marrow or peripheral leukemic myeloid blast cell counts are greater than or equal to 10%. GM-CSF may also be useful as a rescue treatment for febrile, neutropenic, elderly AML patients; as a recovery agent for allogeneic or autologous bone marrow transplant patients with engraftment delay or failure; as a treatment for aplastic anemia, cyclic neutropenia, congenital neutropenia, or myelodysplastic disorders; to augment autologous peripheral stem cell collection; and to reduce the severity of mucositis after chemotherapy.

SARGRAMOSTIM *(continued)*

Mechanisms of Action

GM-CSF supports the production of granulocyte and monocyte precursors. GM-CSF is produced by T-cells, fibroblasts, and endothelial cells of the bone marrow. GM-CSF supports the production, differentiation, and activation of granulocyte and monocyte precursors. In "high" doses, GM-CSF may increase the production of red blood cell and platelet precursors.

Pharmacokinetics

GM-CSF is not absorbed by mouth and is degraded by the liver and kidneys. GM-CSF can be detected in the serum within 5 minutes of a subcutaneous injection; peak serum concentrations occur within 2 hours. GM-CSF is metabolized in the liver and kidneys. GM-CSF has an elimination half-life of approximately 2 to 3 hours and remains detectable in the serum for up to 6 hours after subcutaneous injection.

Dose

Phase I studies have demonstrated that the maximum tolerated dose of GM-CSF is approximately 30 microg/kg/day. In addition, the dose and peak serum levels have been shown to correlate with adverse side effects.

In the treatment of neutropenia after ABMT, sargramostim is given at a dose of 250 microg/m^2/day for 21 consecutive days. Treatment with GM-CSF is begun 2 to 4 hours after infusion of the bone marrow. The manufacturer recommends stopping GM-CSF if the absolute neutrophil count (ANC) exceeds 20,000/mm^3. GM-CSF has been given at a dose of 5 microg/kg/day for 10 to 14 days beginning 24 hours after completion of chemotherapy. Higher doses of GM-CSF have been administered in subsequent cycles according to the duration and severity of myelosuppression.

In the elderly AML population for neutrophil recovery the dose is 250 microg/m^2/day intravenously over 4 hours. This therapy begins on day 11 or 4 days after the end of induction chemotherapy.

For PBSC collection, administer 250 microg/m^2/day intravenously over 24 hours or subcutaneously, the duration will vary with marrow response.

Post PBSC transplant for engraftment, the same dose of 250 microg/m^2/day is used until the ANC >1,500/mm^3 for 3 consecutive days.

For delayed engraftment or failure of engraftment post BMT, dose 250 microg/m^2/day for an initial 14 days as a 2-hour intravenous infusion. This dose can be repeated after a 7-day hiatus, for another 14 days. If engraftment has still not occurred, a third 14-day cycle can be administered after an additional 7 days off, but at an increased dose of 500 microg/m^2/day.

To reduce wastage and cost, doses are often rounded off to the nearest vial size.

Administration

GM-CSF is usually mixed in 50 mL of normal saline and administered to bone marrow transplant patients as a 2- to 4-hour intravenous infusion. GM-CSF has also been given by subcutaneous injection and as a continuous IV infusion.

Toxicity

The adverse effects of GM-CSF are dose-related. Doses of 30 microg/kg/day or greater may induce capillary leak and a host of related adverse effects. Lower doses (e.g., 5 microg/kg/day or 250 microg/m²/day) produce side effects that are similar to those caused by G-CSF.

First-dose effect. Flushing sensation, hypotension (58%), hypertension (21%), tachycardia, dyspnea, hypoxia, nausea, vomiting, fever, rigor, syncope, and leg spasms. The symptoms usually begin 1 to 2 hours after injection, and are more common when GM-CSF is administered intravenously.

Hematological. Initial decrease in ANC for 4 to 24 hours. Transient but sometimes significant decrease in platelet counts with high doses. Thrombosis at the catheter tip has occurred in patients receiving doses above 30 microg/kg/day. Progression of myelodysplastic syndromes (especially in patients with "excess blasts") may occur.

Gastrointestinal. Anorexia, nausea, vomiting, abnormal taste, dysphagia, hematemesis, constipation, abdominal distinction.

Dermatological. Local erythema, skin rash, injection site reactions, alopecia, pruritus.

Hepatic. Mild elevation of hepatic enzyme levels, abnormal clotting times, and hypoalbuminemia have been reported.

Neurological. Headache, confusion, neuropathies, paresthesia, insomnia, anxiety.

Cardiovascular. Dose-related. Fluid retention, pericardial effusion, thrombophlebitis, chest pain, pericarditis, cardiac arrhythmias, atrial fibrillation.

Pulmonary. At high doses: dyspnea (caused by fluid retention and capillary leak syndrome), pleuritis, lung disorder, epistaxis, rhinitis.

Musculoskeletal. Transient bone pain, usually mild to moderate in severity. The pain has been described as a pulsating deep pain in the lower back, pelvis, or sternum. The pain usually resolves without stopping treatment and always resolves within a few hours after discontinuation.

Other. Fever, infections, weight loss, metabolic disorder, sepsis, eye hemorrhage, back pain, sweats, flu-like syndrome (chills, rigors, myalgias), fatigue, arthralgias, hypersensitivity reactions.

Drug Interactions

Concomitant use of sargramostim with lithium or corticosteroids may potentiate the release of neutrophils and monitoring is recommended.

Storage and Stability

Intact vials should be kept refrigerated. Solutions of GM-CSF that have been reconstituted with 1 mL sterile water or 1 mL bacteriostatic sterile water are stable in the vial or in a polypropylene syringe for at least 30 days at room or refrigeration temperatures. Dilute solutions (2.5, 8, or 12 microg/mL) are stable in PVC containers for at least 48 hours at room or refrigeration temperatures. Solutions diluted to a concentration less than 10 microg/mL require the addition of albumin at a concentration of 1 mg/mL to minimize adsorption of GM-CSF to the container and IV tubing.

Preparation

When mixing GM-CSF, care must be taken to keep the product from foaming and to avoid excess agitation. The diluent should be injected against the side of the vial. Do not shake the vial. Add 1 mL of sterile water for injection to the 250- or 500-microg vial to achieve final concentrations of 250 or 500 microg/mL. GM-CSF may be further diluted with normal saline to a concentration of no less than 10 microg/mL. Solutions containing less than 10 microg/mL may require the addition of albumin (at a final concentration of 0.1%) to prevent GM-CSF from adhering to glass or plastic containers.

SARGRAMOSTIM *(continued)*

Availability

Sargramostim is commercially available as a lyophilized powder in vials containing 250 and 500 microg, and as a 500 microg/mL solution in a 1-mL vial.

Selected Reading

Rowe JM et al. A randomized placebo-controlled phase III study of granulocyte macrophage colony-stimulating factor in adult patients (55 to 70 years of age) with acute myelogenous leukemia: a study of the Eastern Cooperative Oncology Group (E1490). Blood 86: 457–462, 1995.

TOSITUMOMAB

Other Names

Bexxar®; iodine[131] tositumomab; NSC-715818.

Indications

Tositumomab is an investigational agent that has been used in the treatment of patients with CD20-positive, follicular low-grade non-Hodgkin's lymphomas (NHL), including patients with transformed low-grade NHL, and patients who have relapsed after or are refractory to chemotherapy.

Classification and Mechanisms of Action

Tositumomab is a murine IgG2a monoclonal antibody directed against CD20-positive cells.

Pharmacokinetics

Tositumomab is extensively taken up by tumor cells, does not appear to be metabolized, and is removed from circulation by tumor binding and renal excretion. The radioisotope half-life is 8 days.

Dose

Unlabeled tositumomab, 450 mg, is administered prior to 5 mCi (35 mg) of iodine I[131] tositumomab (for dosimetry purposes). Total body gamma counts are obtained three times over the ensuing week. Using standard dosimetry methods, a patient-specific dose is calculated to deliver 75 cGy to patients with a prestudy platelet count greater than 150,000/mm^3 or to deliver 65 cGy to patients with a prestudy platelet count less than 150,000/mm^3. Premedication with acetaminophen 650 mg and diphenhydramine 50 mg is given prior to the dosimetric and radiolabeled doses. To prevent uptake of I[131] by the thyroid gland, patients are given SSKI (saturated solution of potassium iodide) at a dose of 2 drops orally three times a day for 14 days. Treatment with SSKI is initiated 24 hours before the dose of I[131] tositumomab.

Administration

Unlabeled tositumomab is administered intravenously over 1 hour followed by a 20-minute infusion of the I[131] radiolabeled tositumomab.

Toxicity

Hematological. Neutropenia (20% of patients exhibited an absolute neutrophil count [ANC] less than 500/mm^3) and thrombocytopenia (approximately 22% of patients developed a platelet count less than 25,000/mm^3). The median absolute neutrophil count (ANC) nadir in one study was 800/mm^3 and the median platelet count in this same study was 50,000/mm^3. The median time to ANC nadir following the radiolabeled dose is 43 days, the median time to platelet nadir is 34 days. Recovery of neutrophil and platelet counts is expected 7 to 9 days after the nadir. Infections occurred in 25% of patients in one study.

In a phase II study of 24 patients who received a dose of 0.3 mCi/kg, 15% of patients developed grade 4 thrombocytopenia.

Gastrointestinal. Nausea (25%), vomiting (13%), anorexia (10%).

Dermatological. Pruritus has been reported in approximately 13% of patients.

Cardiovascular. Hypotension is reported in approximately 10% of patients.

Pulmonary. Lung hemorrhage and dyspnea have been reported.

Metabolic. Elevated levels of thyroid-stimulating hormone have been observed in approximately 7% of patients.

Other. Infusion-related reactions, primarily consisting of fever and chills, occur in most patients with administration of labeled and unlabeled tositumomab. Most of these reactions are grade 1 or grade 2. Grade 3 fever and chills have been observed in approximately 2% of patients. Occasionally hypotension, rigors, wheezing, and/or nasal congestion occur during or following the infusion. Fatigue has been reported in approximately 43% of patients. Arthralgia and myalgia have been reported.

Storage and Stability

Tositumomab is stored in accordance with the manufacturer's recommendations.

Preparation

Doses of tositumomab are to be processed by nuclear medicine facilities in accordance with local, state, and federal regulations for handling of radioactive material and biohazardous waste. Specific preparation and handling guidelines are provided to personnel responsible for radiolabeling these products.

Availability

Tositumomab is an investigational agent that is available from the manufacturer.

Selected Readings

Kaminski MS et al. Pivotal study of iodine I^{131} tositumomab for chemotherapy-refractory low-grade or transformed low-grade B-cell non-Hodgkin's lymphomas. J Clin Oncol 19: 3918–3928, 2001.

Press OW et al. A phase I/II trial of iodine-131-tositumomab (anti-CD20), etoposide, cyclophosphamide, and autologous stem cell transplantation for relapsed B-cell lymphomas. Blood 96: 2934–2942, 2000.

TRASTUZUMAB

Other Names

Herceptin®; anti-HER2neu antibody; NSC-688097.

Indications

FDA approved for the treatment of advanced breast cancer in tumors that overexpress the protein HER2 (human epidermal growth factor receptor 2 protein). Trastuzumab can be used as single agent therapy for patients previously treated with chemotherapy or in combination with a taxane for previously untreated patients.

Classification and Mechanisms of Action

Trastuzumab is a DNA-derived recombinant humanized monoclonal antibody selectively directed against cells that overexpress the human epidermal growth factor

TRASTUZUMAB *(continued)*

receptor 2 protein, commonly referred to as HER2. Trastuzumab binds the extracellular domain of the protein HER2 on the cell surface. This binding triggers a number of potential mechanisms. Trastuzumab down-regulates the HER2/neu receptors, inhibits growth signal pathways, engages natural killer cells of the immune system to attack the tumor, induces cell lysis antibody-dependent cell-mediated cytotoxicity (ADCC), and enhances chemotherapy cytotoxicity.

Pharmacokinetics

At standard dosing, trastuzumab exhibits a half-life of approximately 6 days, with a steady-state serum concentration occurring between weeks 16 and 32. The larger the dose, the longer the half-life, and thus the longer the clearance. Minimal information is available on distribution, metabolism, and excretion of this monoclonal antibody.

Dose

The recommended dose of trastuzumab therapy begins with a load dose consisting of 4 mg/kg/dose in the first week of therapy. Trastuzumab maintenance therapy is dosed at 2 mg/kg/dose in subsequent weeks. Some ongoing studies are utilizing trastuzumab 8 mg/kg/dose for the first dose, followed by 6 mg/kg/dose for subsequent doses given every 3 weeks, instead of weekly.

Administration

Trastuzumab is administered intravenously, diluted in 250 mL of 0.9% sodium chloride. The loading dose is administered as a 90-minute infusion with a post-observation period of 60 minutes. If the loading dose is tolerated, the maintenance doses are administered as 30-minute infusions in 250 mL 0.9% sodium chloride.

Toxicity

The toxicities listed below were observed in patients who received trastuzumab as a single agent, without concomitant chemotherapy. The majority of the side effects listed were reported in higher percentages in the trastuzumab plus paclitaxel and trastuzumab plus doxorubicin/cyclophosphamide arms of the clinical trials.

Hematological. Anemia and leukopenia were observed in less than 5% of patients on single agent trastuzumab therapy. In clinical studies, anemia and leukopenia increased significantly in both the paclitaxel plus trastuzumab and the AC plus trastuzumab arm.

Gastrointestinal. Nausea was reported in 33% of patients, vomiting in 23%, diarrhea in 25%, and anorexia in 14% of patients on trastuzumab alone.

Dermatological. Most commonly observed is rash. Herpes simplex and acne were reported in 2% of patients.

Neurological. Headache (26%), insomnia and dizziness in approximately 14% of patients. Also reported are paresthesia (9%) depression (6%), peripheral neuritis (2%), and neuropathy (1%).

Cardiovascular. Tachycardia was reported in 5% of patients. Congestive heart failure was reported in 7% of patients on single agent trastuzumab. Left ventricular dysfunction should be monitored in all patients prior to and during trastuzumab therapy. The incidence of the cardiac events reported was significantly higher when the trastuzumab is combined with anthracycline or cyclophosphamide therapy. The congestive heart failure reported has been severe and disabling, at times resulting in stroke or death.

Pulmonary. Most commonly reported (>20%) are cough and dyspnea. Also reported are rhinitis (14%), pharyngitis (12%), and sinusitis (9%).

Infusion reactions. For mild to moderate reactions the most common symptoms are chills and fever. Also observed are nausea, vomiting, rigors, headache, dizziness, dyspnea, hypotension, rash, asthenia, and pain at disease sites. The infusion-related symptom complex reaction is most common with the first infusion (40%); the incidence decreased with subsequent infusion. Symptoms can be managed with administration of acetaminophen, diphenhydramine, and meperidine as clinically indicated. Rarely, severe hypersensitivity/anaphylactic reactions have occurred with trastuzumab therapy within 24 hours of administration. If severe hypotension, angioedema, urticaria, bronchospasm, or shortness of breath occur, stop trastuzumab therapy and treat with appropriate emergency medications. Rechallenging a patient after a severe hypersensitivity reaction is based on physician clinical judgement. Portions of reactive patients have been rechallenged and have tolerated therapy, others have been rechallenged and the hypersensitivity reaction occurred once again, despite premedication.

Other. Fever (36%), pain (47%), asthenia (42%), chills (32%), abdominal and back pain (22%), infection (20%), flu-like symptoms (10%), peripheral edema (10%) and edema (8%), bone pain (7%), arthralgia (6%), and urinary tract infections (5%). Pregnancy category B.

Drug Interactions

Trastuzumab administered concomitantly with anthracyclines resulted in an increase in cardiotoxicity.

Storage and Stability

Intact vials are stored in the refrigerator at temperatures of 2° to 8°C. Once reconstituted, trastuzumab is a multidose vial and is stable for 28 days at refrigerated temperatures.

Preparation

Trastuzumab is reconstituted with 20 mL of bacteriostatic water for injection. The diluent is provided with the product. Withdraw **only** 20 mL of the diluent and inject it into the sidewall of the lyophilized trastuzumab to provide a 21 mg/mL solution. Gently swirl the vial, do not shake. Allow the entire contents of the drug to go into solution before withdrawing the dose. The desired dose is added to a 250-mL polyvinylchloride or polyethylene bag of 0.9% sodium chloride. Date the vial with the appropriate 28-day expiration date and store any remaining drug in the refrigerator until it expires.

Availability

Trastuzumab is commercially available as a 440-mg vial of lyophilized powder. It is packaged with a 30-mL vial of bacteriostatic water for injection with 1.1% benzyl alcohol.

Selected Readings

Goldenberg MM. Trastuzumab, a recombinant DNA-derived humanized monoclonal antibody, a novel agent for the treatment of metastatic breast cancer. Clin Therap 21: 309–317, 1999.

Shak S. Overview of the trastuzumab (Herceptin) anti-HER2 monoclonal antibody clinical program in HER2-overexpressing metastatic breast cancer. Herceptin multinational investigator study group. Semin Oncol 26(suppl 12): 71–77, 1999.

TUMOR NECROSIS FACTOR

Other Names

Tasonermin; Beromun; FK-516; rTNF-alfa; TNF-alfa; cachectin.

Indications

Tumor necrosis factor (TNF) has not been shown to be a useful antitumor agent when administered by intravenous or intramuscular injection. Some activity is observed against Kaposi's sarcoma after intralesional injection. TNF has been shown to be very active against malignant melanoma when the TNF is administered by isolated limb perfusion in combination with interferon gamma and melphalan.

Mechanisms of Action

TNF is a naturally occurring protein that is secreted by macrophages in response to infection. In combination with IL-1 and IL-6, TNF is an important factor in the acute phase reaction to an infection. TNF is a polypeptide cytokine that mediates inflammation and immune effector cell regulation. The direct cytotoxic effects of TNF appear to be cell-cycle dependent with prolonged exposure yielding greater cell kill in vitro. Other actions may account for some of the antitumor activity of TNF, such as endothelial cell effects and procoagulation (hemorrhagic necrosis), enhanced macrophage cytotoxicity, activation of NK cells, or as a part of an inflammatory reaction. Synergism with TNF and gamma interferon has been demonstrated.

Pharmacokinetics

Peak levels of TNF occur 30 minutes after IV injection and 2 to 3 hours after initiation of a continuous IV infusion. Despite continued infusion, levels of TNF are undetectable within 6 to 12 hours. TNF has an elimination half-life of 10 to 16 minutes after systemic administration of 25 to 100 microg/m^2. The half-life after administration of higher doses (e.g., 150 to 727 microg/m^2) is 40 to 80 minutes.

Dose

Systemically administered TNF has been utilized on varied regimens, including daily for 5 days, twice daily for 5 days, and 3 times weekly. The maximum tolerated dose is approximately 200 to 300 microg/m^2/day. Intralesional injections are usually given at a dose of 25 to 300 microg/m^2 3 times weekly. When given by isolated limb perfusion, 3 to 6 mg is added to the perfusate of crystalloid (700 mL) and packed red blood cells (1 unit). Intraperitoneal and intravesical doses ranging from 50 to 1,800 microg/m^2 have been evaluated.

Administration

TNF has been given by isolated limb and organ perfusion, IV bolus, IV infusion over 24 hours or longer, intraperitoneally, and by subcutaneous, intramuscular, intra-arterial, intravesical, and intralesional injection.

Toxicity

The toxicities seen after administration with TNF are dependent on dose and schedule of administration, although similar toxicities are seen in patients receiving TNF by IV bolus or continuous infusion.

Hematological. Mild leukopenia (after high doses or repeated IV administration); thrombocytopenia is not common or severe; eosinophilia; transient leukocytosis is dose-related and lasts approximately 24 hours after a single dose; immune thrombocytopenia in patients also receiving IL-2 has been reported. Disseminated intravascular coagulation has been reported in patients receiving systemic TNF. After large intravenous doses, thrombocytosis may be observed.

Dermatological. Tenderness, erythema, induration, and inflammation at the site of subcutaneous or intramuscular injection. Local (regional) toxicities after isolated limb perfusion include mild chronic edema (56%), muscle tenderness with atrophy (8%), blistering (50%), paresthesia (40%), and arterial occlusion requiring amputation in one patient.

Gastrointestinal. Abdominal pain, dose-related nausea and vomiting, anorexia, diarrhea. Abdominal pain and peritonitis are dose-limiting when TNF is administered intraperitoneally. Hemorrhagic gastritis (11%) was reported in an intravenous phase I study of solid tumor patients.

Hepatic. The following effects are usually mild and transient: hyperbilirubinemia, elevated hepatic transaminase levels (40%), and elevated alkaline phosphatase levels.

Neurological. Headache, confusion, speech disorders, somnolence, lethargy, hallucinations, seizures. Peripheral neuropathy has been reported in up to 67% of patients with isolated limb perfusion.

Cardiovascular. Hypotension occurs frequently and has been dose-limiting in most phase I studies. Hypotension usually occurs within 12 or 24 hours after initiation of a continuous IV infusion. Intravenous vasopressors are necessary in some patients. Hypotension also occurs when TNF is administered by isolated limb perfusion. In one study, 4 to 6 mg of TNF was administered by isolated limb perfusion. The incidence of grade 3 or 4 hypotension was 39%. Other cardiovascular adverse effects include fluid retention, tachycardia, and hypertension (often related to a febrile episode).

Pulmonary. Dyspnea (rare), wheezing, pulmonary edema, and pulmonary embolism were reported in patients who exhibited DIC (disseminated intravascular coagulation).

Renal. Mild elevation of serum creatinine and BUN levels.

Other. Fever occurs in all patients regardless of the route of administration or dose and generally resolves within a few hours; chills, rigor, myalgia, fatigue, malaise, phlebitis, hypophosphatemia, hyperglycemia, and hypertriglyceridemia.

Storage and Stability

Vials are shipped frozen on dry ice and must be stored in the refrigerator. If TNF is received thawed, **do not use**. Small perturbations in storage temperature are tolerable (e.g., several hours at 25°C). Small colorless particles of protein may be visible, are not unusual, and do not alter the potency of TNF. Vigorous handling results in aggregation of the protein and may create cloudy solutions that should not be used.

Preparation

Before use the vial should be gently swirled to ensure uniform mixing of the contents. TNF is sensitive to shear-induced stress; do not shake vials. TNF is diluted only in normal saline. Adsorption of TNF to glassware, plastic IV sets, and syringes occurs when delivered intravenously or diluted to concentrations of less than 10 microg/mL. To prevent adsorption, it is recommended that human albumin be added at a final concentration of 2 mg/mL. Human albumin effectively reduces adsorption at TNF concentrations as low as 0.1 microg/mL.

Availability

TNF-alfa is available from the NCI.

Selected Reading

Fraker DL et al. Treatment of patients with melanoma of the extremity using hyperthermic isolated limb perfusion with melphalan, tumor necrosis factor, and interferon gamma: results of a tumor necrosis factor dose-escalation study. J Clin Oncol 14: 479–489, 1996.

GENERAL REFERENCES

Chabner BA, Longo DL, eds. Cancer Chemotherapy and Biotherapy Principles and Practice, 3rd ed. Philadelphia, Lippincott Williams and Wilkins, 2001.

Dillman RO. Monoclonal antibody therapy for lymphoma, an update. Cancer Practice 9: 71–80, 2001.

Geller RB. The use of cytokines in the treatment of acute myelocytic leukemia: a critical review. J Clin Oncol 14: 1371–1382, 1996.

Hutchinson TA, Shahan DR, eds. DRUGDEX System. MICROMEDEX, Greenwood Village, Colorado (Edition expires 3/2002).

Isaacs A, Lindemann JJ. Virus interference: the interferon. Proc R Soc Lond 147: 258–267, 1957.

Kirkwood JM. Pharmacology of cancer biotherapeutics: interferons. In DeVita VT Jr, Hellman S, Rosenberg SA, eds. Principles and Practice of Oncology, 6th ed. Philadelphia, Lippincott Williams and Wilkins, 2001.

Maloney DG, McLaughlin P. Rituximab for the treatment of patients with B-cell non-Hodgkin's lymphoma. In DeVita VT Jr, Hellman S, Rosenberg SA, eds. Progress in Oncology, Boston, Jones and Bartlett, 2001, pp204–227.

Rieger PT, ed. Biotherapy: A Comprehensive Overview, 2nd ed. Boston, Jones and Bartlett, 2001, pp3–37, 85–122.

Rosenberg SA. The immunotherapy and gene therapy of cancer. J Clin Oncol 10: 180–199, 1992.

Rosenberg SA. Principles of cancer management: biologic therapy. In DeVita VT Jr, Hellman S, Rosenberg SA, eds. Principles and Practice of Oncology, 6th ed. Philadelphia, Lippincott Williams and Wilkins, 2001.

Weiner LM. An overview of monoclonal antibody therapy of cancer. Semin Oncol 26(suppl 12): 41–51, 1999.

Weiner LM, Adams GP, Von Mehren M. Pharmacology of cancer biotherapeutics: therapeutic monoclonal antibodies: general principles. In DeVita VT Jr, Hellman S, Rosenberg SA, eds. Principles and Practice of Oncology, 6th ed. Philadelphia, Lippincott Williams and Wilkins, 2001.

CANCER CHEMOTHERAPY ADMINISTRATION

Higher patient volume and acuity levels, combined with increasingly complex and more intensive therapy, have significantly challenged provider resources and those of the patient and family. The changing healthcare environment has eliminated participation in care as a decision choice for patients; it has become an essential expectation. Patients and their identified caregivers must be adequately prepared with the knowledge and skill required to fulfill their designated roles in cancer care. This chapter provides information and guidelines for nursing, physician, and pharmacy staff in the delivery of cancer chemotherapy across various clinical settings: in the hospital, clinic, private office, and home. The first and most important factor for safe drug delivery and quality patient care is knowledge. Comprehensive knowledge, from the initial drug indication through predicted side effects and supportive care, provides the basis for patient teaching, safe drug administration, prevention of complications, and interventions for adverse effects.

Oncology physicians, nurses, and pharmacists are the members of the healthcare team primarily responsible for safe chemotherapy drug delivery (see Chapter 3). Each team member is responsible for standards unique to his/her discipline and for collaboration as a multidisciplinary team in their setting for the prescription, admixture, administration, and disposal of drugs, as well as care of the patient receiving chemotherapy. National guidelines and recommendations for controlling exposure to antineoplastic agents have been provided by the Occupational Safety and Health Administration (OSHA) of the Department of Labor of the United States (1999). Standards for nursing education, practice, and administration of therapy are provided by the Oncology Nursing Society (Brown et al, 2001) and guidelines for handling of chemotherapy are provided by the American Society of Hospital Pharmacists (1990). National recommendations provide a framework for oncology personnel at the work site to design policies and procedures for safe delivery of antineoplastic drugs. Most hospitals have educational programs that certify nurses and pharmacy personnel for the handling and delivery of cancer chemotherapy drugs and policies for writing orders, verification, and dose modifications (Fischer et al, 1996). The recommendations for controlling exposure to chemotherapy drugs, however, apply to all settings (i.e., physician offices) and strategies need to be identified in order to reduce the risks associated with exposure (Carmignani & Raymond, 1997, OSHA, 1999).

CONTROLLING EXPOSURE TO ANTINEOPLASTIC DRUGS

Inhalation, absorption, and ingestion are the three major sources of exposure to antineoplastic drugs. Exposure to antineoplastic agents is considered a risk based on four drug characteristics that are considered hazardous:

- carcinogenicity
- genotoxicity
- teratogenicity
- fertility impairment and organ system toxicity (ASHP, 1990).

Animal and human data support the carcinogenic risks of alkylating agents and observations of chromosomal aberrations, gonadal dysfunction, organ system toxicity, and second malignancies suggest that chemotherapy drugs carry broad potential hazardous risk. In addition to chemotherapy, other anticancer agents are considered as hazardous, including the biological agent interferon-alfa and some hormonal therapies (e.g., leuprolide, tamoxifen). Assessment of investigational and new drugs for hazard risk is an ongoing process (OSHA, 1999).

Assessment of airborne levels, biological absorption, and human effects (cytogenetic and reproductive) have been three targeted areas of research attempting to establish occupational exposure risk from chemotherapy drugs. Aerosolization has been documented in the admixture process, which poses the largest risk for inhalation or absorption via contamination of work surfaces. Urinary mutagenicity, thioethers, or metabolites as markers of absorption exposure were the focus of a great deal of research in the 1980s following the first report by Falck et al (1979). While some early studies reported significant increases in urine mutagenicity in nurses handling cytotoxic drugs, a similar number of investigations failed to show any difference between nurses who were or were not exposed to these drugs.

Later, markers for cytogenetic abnormalities (e.g., sister chromatid exchanges, structural aberrations, micronuclei in peripheral blood lymphocytes) were measured in workers with and without chemotherapy drug exposure. These studies similarly produced conflicting results and suggested that compliance with safety standards against drug exposure results in minimal or no cytogenetic changes (Hessel et al, 2001; Jakab et al, 2001; Pilger et al, 2000).

Chemotherapy, specifically alkylating agents, produces known gonadal toxicity in men and women who receive therapeutic doses of these drugs. Recent studies suggest that exposed workers may have an increased risk for menstrual abnormalities, infertility, and miscarriages (OSHA, 1999; Valanis et al, 1997, 1999). Exposure of pregnant workers, especially in the first trimester (or men trying to procreate), should be considered a risk and compliance with recommended safety precautions is essential to prevent any adverse reproductive outcomes.

The first step to prevent employee exposure is education of all personnel about occupational exposure, potential risk of exposure to hazardous drugs, explanation and rationale for measures to reduce exposure, and plans for monitoring and assessing the effectiveness of protective measures. Important factors for individuals at risk include the environment in which the employee works, tasks performed (e.g., preparation, administration, or both), the average number of drug exposures per week, the number of consecutive days with drug exposure, the type of protective measures utilized, the percentage of reported accidental skin contacts, and adherence to recommended protective measures.

Work-practice guidelines to reduce exposure are no longer optional, and the employer is responsible for education, implementation, assessment, and periodic re-evaluation. Individual health protection is the responsibility of the employee, who should be well informed and adhere to protective guidelines and institutional policies. Each institution must integrate the OSHA recommendations together with the available scientific evidence into its policies to minimize any occupational hazardous drug risk. A policy for the protection of employees is critical but requires institutional support to implement it in all sites and must include available resources, education, and routine surveillance. The current OSHA (1999) recommendations are presented in Box 6-1.

BOX 6-1

RECOMMENDATIONS: PREVENTION OF EMPLOYEE EXPOSURE TO HAZARDOUS DRUGS (ASHP, 1990; OSHA, 1999)

1. HAZARDOUS DRUG SAFETY AND HEALTH PLAN

Develop a plan according to the ASHP (1990) criteria that is available and accessible to all employees. Designate personnel responsible for implementation of the plan and review effectiveness at least annually. This will minimize exposure and protect the employee from health hazards associated with handling hazardous drugs.

2. DRUG PREPARATION PRECAUTIONS

Work area: A restricted, preferably centralized area is recommended for preparation of hazardous drugs. Eating, drinking, smoking, chewing gum, applying cosmetics, and storing food prohibited.

Biological safety cabinets (BSC): Class II (type B) or III are recommended. The blower should be on at all times; if turned off, the BSC should be decontaminated and covered until airflow is resumed. The BSC should be serviced and certified by a qualified technician every six months or any time the BSC is moved or repaired. If a BSC is not available, preparation can be performed in another location and transported to the area where the drug will be administered.

Personal protective equipment (PPE): Wear protective gloves, latex is preferable unless an allergy exists. Thickness of gloves provides best protection against exposure, which was the rationale for the latex recommendation. Because of latex allergy concerns, the use of vinyl or nitrile gloves or glove liners has been more recently considered. Use gloves with minimal or no powder since powder may absorb contamination. Change gloves hourly or immediately if torn, punctured, or contaminated with a spill. Wash hands before gloves are put on and after removal. All gloves are permeable to some extent, and permeability increases with time. Wear disposable, lint-free, low permeability fabric gown with closed front, long sleeves, and elastic or knot-closed cuffs. Gowns provide an additional barrier to potential skin contact (direct or aerosol). No ideal material has been identified, but some gowns have reinforced sleeves to minimize permeability in the most exposure-prone area. Remove gown and gloves (last) before leaving area. Face and eye protection must be provided whenever splashes, sprays, or aerosols from hazardous drugs may be generated to prevent or minimize eye, nose, or mouth contamination.

Work equipment: Place absorbent plastic-backed paper liner on work surface; use Luer lock fittings; have covered disposable container to contain excess solution and have hazardous drug-labeled plastic bags for disposal of used protective equipment contaminated materials. Change liner every shift (hospital) or at the end of the day (ambulatory settings).

Work practices: Use aseptic technique for drug preparation; put on protective equipment before working in the BSC; label all drugs according to standard pharmacy labeling practices and for identification as a hazardous drug. Whenever possible, prime drug administration sets in the BSC before addition of the drug. If priming must occur outside the BSC, prime with non-drug-containing fluid or use a back-flow closed system. Avoid positive and negative pressures in medication vials. Use of venting devices is recommended, along with appropriate employee education to reduce aerosol exposure. An alternative to venting devices is adding diluent slowly in small amounts, allowing displaced air to escape into the syringe. For ampules, wrap a sterile gauze around ampule

(cont'd)

BOX 6-1

RECOMMENDATIONS: PREVENTION OF EMPLOYEE EXPOSURE TO HAZARDOUS DRUGS (ASHP, 1990; OSHA, 1999)—cont'd

2. DRUG PREPARATION PRECAUTIONS—cont'd

neck before breaking; if diluent is needed, inject slowly down the side wall of the ample. This helps to prevent cuts, aerosolization, and skin contamination. Tablets that may produce dust or potential exposure to the handler should be counted in the BSC.

For prepared drugs to be transported, the outside of the bag or bottle needs to be wiped with a moist gauze; entry ports must be wiped with alcohol and capped.

3. DRUG ADMINISTRATION

Wash hands before and after; wear protective gloves and gown; discard gloves after each use. Infusion sets should have Luer lock fittings; use plastic-back absorbent pad under tubing during administration; use sterile gauze at injection sites. Do not clip needles or syringes; place in puncture-resistant container. This helps to minimize possible contamination from needle sticks or aerosol exposure. Dispose of administration sets intact. Have spill and emergency and eye decontamination kits available and accessible. Administration of aerosolized hazardous drugs requires special engineering controls for employee protection.

4. CARING FOR PATIENTS RECEIVING HAZARDOUS DRUGS

Observe universal precautions, according to the Blood Borne Pathogens Standard, to prevent contact with blood or other potentially infectious material. Wear protective gloves and gowns when dealing with excreta, specifically urine, of patients who have received hazardous drugs within the past 48 hours. Linen contaminated by hazardous drugs or excreta from patients (as above) is a potential source of exposure; use gloves during handling and place in marked laundry bags. Contents should be prewashed and then added to other laundry for a second wash.

5. WASTE DISPOSAL

Use thick, leak-proof, labeled plastic bags for discarded protective equipment and materials. Keep waste bag inside a covered waste container labeled *HD Waste Only*; have one receptacle located in each area of drug preparation and administration; do not move from one area to another. Hazardous drug-related wastes should be handled separately from other trash and disposed of according to appropriate regulations for hazardous waste. Check current regulations and institutional policy.

6. SPILLS

Personal contamination: Immediately remove protective clothing and wash affected skin with soap and water. If eye exposure has occurred, flush at eye-wash fountain area or with isotonic eyewash for 5 minutes; seek prompt medical attention; document exposure in the employee's record.

Small spills (<5 mL): Immediately clean up spill while wearing protective gowns, double gloves, and splash goggles. Wipe liquids with absorbent gauze pads and solids with wet absorbent gauze; clean spill area three times with detergent solution followed by clean water; pick up broken glass with a small scoop and place in sharps container.

Large spills: Isolate area and avoid aerosol generation. Limit liquid spread by covering with absorbent sheets or spill-control pads. Use NIOSH approved respirator if airborne powder or aerosol has been created.

Spills in the BSC: If greater than 150 mL or the contents of one vial, decontamination of the interior BSC is recommended after spill cleanup.

(cont'd)

BOX 6-1

RECOMMENDATIONS: PREVENTION OF EMPLOYEE EXPOSURE TO HAZARDOUS DRUGS (ASHP, 1990; OSHA, 1999)—cont'd

7. STORAGE AND TRANSPORT

Signs should restrict entry to storage area of HD to authorized personnel; damaged HD packages should be opened in a BSC or isolated area only by an individual trained in processing damaged packages. Transport of HD should be in a clear plastic bag in a container designed to avoid breakage.

8. MEDICAL SURVEILLANCE

Workers with potential exposure to hazardous drugs should be monitored in a systematic program, such as preplacement, periodic, and exit medical examinations, postexposure evaluation, and maintenance of exposure records for all employees. The purpose is to identify biologic effects at the earliest and most reversible point and take action to minimize or eliminate exposure.

Reproductive toxicity of hazardous drugs should be explained to all employees with potential exposure. Although the data on reproductive risks are inconclusive with the current recommended use of BSCs and PPE, each setting should have a policy for worker exposure in male and female employees.

9. HAZARD COMMUNICATION

Employers are responsible for developing, implementing, and maintaining a written hazard communication program, which should include all drugs that represent a health hazard to employees.

10. INFORMATION DISSEMINATION AND TRAINING

All employees must be informed of drugs that may present a hazard, and knowledge and competence of those workers should be evaluated on a regular basis; updated information should be provided as it evolves.

11. RECORD KEEPING

Workplace exposure records associated with handling hazardous drugs are to be kept and made available for the duration of employment plus 30 years; training records should be maintained for three years from the date of training.

DRUG ADMINISTRATION

A comprehensive physical and psychosocial assessment of the patient (Table 6-1) is indicated before initiation of therapy to establish baseline information, determine appropriateness of the treatment and setting, evaluate venous access, and identify patient and family resources and needs. Adequate preparation of the patient and staff for treatment decreases the risk of unpredictable problems and unnecessary time delays, reduces potential protocol violations, minimizes emotional distress, and enhances the patient-caregiver relationship.

Administration of chemotherapeutic drugs requires knowledge and, in most cases, skill. Cancer chemotherapy treatment follows the five basic pharmacological principles: right patient, right drug, right dose, right route, and right time. Orders should always be verified and drug doses recalculated and checked against the order (Brown et al, 2001). A written policy defining verification (e.g., knowledge of the protocol regimen and correct drugs for day in the cycle of the drug regimen) and personnel responsibility for order writing and verification is strongly recommended. Assessment should also include evaluating appropriate laboratory values, checking the need for pretreatment medications or supportive therapy such as hydration, and ensuring the patient's understanding and readiness for the therapy.

TABLE 6-1

PRETREATMENT ASSESSMENT CHECKLIST

History and physical	Social	Psychological	Sexual
Extent of disease	Role responsibilities	Emotional status	Sexual preference
Comorbid conditions	Financial resources	Handling of past crises	Significant other
Systems review	Health insurance coverage	Informational needs	Sexual activity
Current medications	Employment	Available support	Reproductive status
Allergies	Family structure/ relationship	Body image	Birth control
Prior cancer treatment	Cultural factors	Spirituality	

DOSING

Drug doses are most often calculated according to the patient's body surface area (meter squared, or m^2) and occasionally by weight (kilograms). Calculating drug doses using body surface area (BSA) was initially introduced for phase I trials in order to derive a safe starting dose in the transition from animal to human testing. The use of BSA for drug dosing of chemotherapy agents beyond the phase I trials emerged as standard practice despite lack of scientific evidence for any clinical relevance or utility. The formula has not been sufficiently evaluated and has an estimated relative error (over- or underestimation) of 15–17% (Sawyer & Ratain, 2001). More importantly, it fails to achieve the purpose of standardizing drug dosing, which is to reduce inter-patient pharmacokinetic variability and to produce consistent drug exposure (Baker et al, 1995). Drug effectiveness and organ system toxicity are the critical parameters in dosing and assessing outcome of anticancer therapy. Drug effectiveness is dependent on the pharmacokinetics and individual sensitivity to the therapy. Several investigators have explored the relationship between pharmacokinetics of specific drugs and BSA. With the exception of docetaxel (Bruno et al, 1996), high interpatient variability and either weak or no correlation to BSA have been reported for cisplatin (deJongh et al, 2001), epirubicin (Dobbs & Twelves, 1998; Gurney et al, 1998), topotecan (Loos et al, 2000), irinotecan (Mathijssen et al, 2001), busulfan (Gibbs et al, 1999), and a variety of other drugs (Gurney, 1996). These data suggest that the use of BSA does not reduce interpatient variability in drug exposure, and thus there is little supporting evidence for BSA dosing.

Furthermore, research to date has failed to support an advantage to BSA drug dosing related to predicted or actual organ system toxicity. Cardiac output is correlated with BSA, but liver and renal clearance are not correlated or have reported weak correlations (Sawyer & Ratain, 2001). Exploring alternative methods for drug dosing has been strongly encouraged, including developing dosing for new drugs differently (Ratain, 1998), and using fixed dosing based on phase I trial data, AUC estimations, or pharmacokinetic data (Gurney, 1996; deJongh et al, 2001; Loos et al, 2000). Because of the significant barriers to alternative methods to BSA dosing in everyday clinical practice (SWOG, 2001), BSA will likely remain the standard approach for the next decade (see Appendix A, Table A-1, Table A-2). One exception to using BSA for drug calculation is carboplatin dosing, for which the Calvert formula (Calvert et al, 1989, 1992) is recommended. The Calvert formula uses a combination of factors that correlate a desired level of drug exposure, expressed by Area Under the [time and concentration] Curve (AUC), with factors that predict the drug's elimination from the body (i.e., estimated creatinine clearance). The Calvert formula is provided in the carboplatin section of the Chemotherapy Drugs chapter (see page 76). Other exceptions are drugs that are dosed as "one size fits all." Most of the drugs that are dosed in this way are cytostatic agents with a relatively wide range between effective dose and toxic dose (e.g., some of the EGFR inhibitors).

Calculation of Weight: Ideal Body Weight versus Actual Body Weight

The proper dose for obese patients is controversial. Some clinicians suggest that the dose should be calculated on the basis of the patient's ideal (or lean body) weight, or based upon body mass index (BMI). Controversy over use of ideal weight (see Appendix A, Table A-3) versus actual weight is based on concerns for increased toxicity in overweight patients. The concern is based on the relationship of body size and physiologic organ function. Factors that may influence drug distribution in obese patients include increased blood volume, cardiac output, lean body mass, organ size, and amount of adipose tissue (Baker et al, 1995), but pharmacokinetics of obese individuals are poorly understood (Morgan & Bray, 1994; Smith & Desch, 1991). Gelman et al (1987) reported that drugs calculated on actual versus ideal body weight would result in an increased amount of drug delivered but this would not result in any significant increase in hematologic toxicity, although only 8% of that sample were categorized as overweight. Nonetheless, more recent investigations have confirmed that toxicity is not increased if dosing is based on actual weight regardless of body size or degree of obesity (Georgiadis et al, 1995; Poikonen et al, 2001; Rosner et al, 1996). The policy of at least one large cooperative oncology group (SWOG, 2001) is that the initial doses of chemotherapy **always** be calculated using the patient's actual body weight. Two studies with over 1,600 patients reported that using actual body weight does not lead to increased toxicity, even in patients whose actual weight was 180% of their ideal weight (Georgiadis et al, 1995; Rosner et al, 1996). Until there is clear evidence to the contrary, the following patients should receive their initial course of therapy based on their actual body weight: patients on a clinical trial, and patients not on a clinical trial who are receiving treatment that is likely to extend their survival (e.g., testicular cancer, Hodgkin's disease, etc.). Patients who are receiving palliative treatment that is not likely to lead to extended survival or significant palliation should receive doses calculated based upon the method their physician feels is appropriate based upon current knowledge.

High-dose chemotherapy has increased clinicians' concerns about obesity and potential increased toxicity and survival outcomes. In a survey of 52 bone marrow transplant institutions, Grigg et al (1997) received responses from 33 institutions. Dose calculations fell into five categories: ideal weight, actual weight, lowest of ideal or actual, and two adjusting for overweight or large-framed individuals. Although there was considerable variability across institutions, actual weight was used by 24% for busulfan dosing and by 30% of the institutions for cyclophosphamide dosing. Another 21–24% reported adjusting doses for busulfan and cyclophosphamide for patients who exceeded their ideal body weight by 20%. In addition, Grigg et al (1997) retrospectively reviewed 169 patients in their institution and reported that only 24% of their patients had >20% disparity from ideal weight. The authors concluded that adjusting doses for wide disparities between actual and ideal weight may be reasonable, although there are no data supporting a specific method for calculating the adjusted dose for high-dose chemotherapy.

6

DRUG ADMINISTRATION

In addition to toxicity outcomes, Petros et al (2002) raised concerns about lower systemic drug absorption in obese patients when doses are adjusted for weight. Dickson et al (1999) conducted a retrospective analysis of 473 patients who underwent autologous bone marrow transplantation. The chemotherapy was dosed based on actual body weight at the time of admission unless the patient was over-weight, defined as ≥15 kg above IBW. For those patients, the dose was calculated by a 40% adjustment between the actual and ideal body weight. To evaluate the impact of weight and dose adjustment, patients were classified into five groups of age-adjusted body mass index (aBMI). Using multivariate analysis, a significant increase in relative risk of nonrelapse mortality in the two highest weight groups (102–139% aBMI $p = 0.003$; 140–199% aBMI $p = 0.05$) was reported, but there was no relation between aBMI and event-free survival or relapse. In addition, while not statistically significant ($p = 0.08$), patients in the underweight group (70–79% aBMI) also had an increased relative risk for nonrelapse mortality. Based on concerns of increased risk of relapse and drug toxicity, the authors concluded that dose adjustments should be con-sidered for patients who vary substantially from ideal weight (< 80%, > 120% aBMI) yet recognize that there is sparse evidence to support what that adjustment should be, and pharmacokinetic studies in obese patients who receive dose-intense therapy are clearly needed.

HYPERSENSITIVITY REACTIONS

Chemotherapy drugs have been associated with all four types of hypersensitivity reactions (HSR), but Type I reactions are observed most frequently in clinical practice. Type I HSR is an allergic reaction that is IgE-mediated and can produce an anaphylac-tic (antibody response to sensitization of an antigen) or anaphylactoid reaction (no antigen sensitization required, different physiologic response mechanism). The rapid release of various mediators of the HSR (i.e., histamine, chemotactins, prostaglandins) is responsible for the symptoms produced primarily affecting the cardiovascular, gastrointestinal, cutaneous, and respiratory systems (Table 6-2).

Factors influencing the incidence and degree of HSR include the route of entry, amount of antigen introduced, rate of antigen absorption, specific chemotherapy drug known to produce HSR, prior exposure to the drug, and the hypersensitivity of the individual to the drug (Labovich, 1999). Chemotherapy drugs associated with HSR include carboplatin, chlorambucil, cisplatin, cyclophosphamide, cytarabine, daunoru-bicin, docetaxel, doxorubicin, fluorouracil, ifosfamide, L-asparaginase, melphalan, methotrexate, oxaliplatin, paclitaxel, procarbazine, and teniposide. While most chemotherapy drugs have a low HSR risk, carboplatin, docetaxel, L-asparaginase, and paclitaxel are associated with a somewhat higher, more predictable risk.

Carboplatin

The incidence of HSR with carboplatin rises significantly once patients have received six or more courses of therapy. Markman et al (1999) initially reported a 12% incidence, with the first HSR episode occurring after a median of eight courses. Moderately severe reactions were observed in one-half of the patients. These HSRs included diffuse erythroderma, tachycardia, chest tightness, wheezing, facial swelling, dyspnea, and/or hypo- or hypertension. Symptoms were reported after approximately 50% of the drug was infused. Women with minor reactions continued with therapy but only one-third of those with more severe reactions were successfully retreated. Subsequently, Zanotti et al (2001) reported a 27–28% incidence of HSR in women with gynecologic malignancies who were treated with carboplatin. Skin testing was

TABLE 6-2

CLINICAL SIGNS AND SYMPTOMS OF IMMEDIATE HYPERSENSITIVITY REACTIONS

Organ system	Subjective complaints	Objective findings
Respiratory	Dyspnea, inability to speak, tightness in chest	Stridor, bronchospasm, decreased air movement
Skin	Pruritus, urticaria	Cyanosis, urticaria, angioedema
Cardiovascular	Chest pain, increased heart rate	Tachycardia, hypotension, arrhythmias
CNS	Dizziness, agitation	Decreased sensorium, anxiety, loss of consciousness
Gastrointestinal	Abdominal pain, nausea	Increased bowel sounds, diarrhea, vomiting

From Craig JB, Capizzi RL. The prevention and treatment of immediate hypersensitivity reactions from cancer chemotherapy. Semin Oncol Nurs 1: 285–291, 1985.
CNS=Central nervous system.

initiated prior to each course in the patients who had received seven or more courses of carboplatin in an attempt to predict HSR risk. In 44 women, 181 skin tests were performed resulting in 168 negative reactions and 13 positive responses. Of the negative reactions, 166/168 accurately predicted the lack of HSR. In the 13 women who tested positive, nine were eventually retreated resulting in eight who had another HSR, despite desensitization in five. The authors cite skin testing as a promising tool to identify carboplatin HSR risk, but more data are required before it can be accepted into standard clinical practice.

L-Asparaginase

A 5% to 8% incidence of anaphylaxis has been reported for L-asparaginase, which increases to nearly a 33% incidence in all patients with subsequent courses (Albanell & Baselga, 2000). Patients generally begin therapy with the *Escherichia coli* form of L-asparaginase and substitution with either the *Erwinia chrysanthemi* (also known as *carotovora*) or *pegaspargase* forms may decrease, although not eliminate, the risk for an HSR. The risk of a reaction to L-asparaginase is much greater with intravenous administration. Thus, to reduce the risk of HSR, subcutaneous or intramuscular injection is recommended with pretreatment with intravenous diphenhydramine (Weiss, 1992).

Paclitaxel

The risk of paclitaxel-induced HSR is estimated to be approximately 30%, but recommended prophylactic regimens have been reported to reduce the incidence to 1% to 3% (Albanell & Baselga, 2000). Yet current clinical data suggest that up to 10% of patients who receive paclitaxel are at risk (Markman et al, 2000; Olson et al, 1998). The wide spectrum of indications for paclitaxel in current practice translates this risk into a significant issue in the administration and monitoring of patients. Although the mechanism of the HSR is not fully understood, it is likely to be an anaphylactoid reaction because more than half of patients demonstrate hypersensitivity on the first administration (Markman et al, 2000; Weiss et al, 1990). It is strongly speculated that the drug vehicle cremophor EL is responsible, producing a release of histamine and other reactive mediators. Most patients react within the first 5 to 10 minutes, symptoms are consistent with a true Type I HSR, and risk factors include initial dosing (e.g., first or second course), high doses, shorter infusions, and faster infusion rates. The standard prophylactic regimen recommended to decrease the HSR includes dexamethasone 20 mg administered orally 12 and 6 hours before the paclitaxel (with/without an additional 20 mg intravenous dose 30 minutes before infusion), and diphenhydramine 50 mg and a histamine-2 blocker (e.g., cimetidine 300 mg, ranitidine 50 mg, or famotidine 20 mg) administered intravenously 30 minutes before the paclitaxel. Replacing the two doses of oral dexamethasone with a 20-mg intravenous dose 30 minutes before paclitaxel administration has been reported as a safe alternative (Gennari et al, 1996; Koppler et al, 2001; Markman et al, 2000). With the exception of severe hypersensitivity reactions to paclitaxel, most patients can be successfully retreated the same day. Upon resolution of symptoms of HSR, Olson et al (1998) reported a successful rechallenge, consisting of reinstitution of the original paclitaxel solution at an initial slow rate (1 to 2 mg/hour) and increasing the rate so that the infusion was completed within a 24-hour period. Markman et al (2000) reported successful retreatment as soon as 30 minutes after stopping the infusion in 38 of 43 patients, but reported that 5 of the 43 patients had another HSR to the reinfusion. A desensitization protocol was designed and the treatment was successfully reinitiated in those women. Docetaxel hypersensitivity reactions have been reported in approximately 12% to 29% of patients. However, severe HSRs have only been reported in 2.8% of patients who received a 3-day course of dexamethasone starting one day before administration of docetaxel.

Intervention Guidelines for HSR

The following clinical guidelines are recommended for patients who receive chemotherapy drugs with a known potential risk of Type I hypersensitivity reactions (Albanell & Baselga, 2000; Labovitch, 1999; Brown et al, 2001):

- Carefully assess patients for clinical signs and symptoms (Table 6-2). Review medication history for beta-blockers and ACE-inhibitors, as they can enhance the HSR reaction, reduce the effectiveness of epinephrine, or challenge reversal of hypotension.
- Have emergency drugs available and accessible. Consider developing a protocol for pharmacologic management of HSR. Many clinicians recommend administration of epinephrine first followed by diphenhydramine (Albanell & Baselga, 2000; Labovich, 1999) while others recommend diphenhydramine and hydrocortisone as first-line therapy specifically for paclitaxel reactions (Markman et al, 2000). Histamine blockers (H1 and H2) should be considered as well.
- Once a reaction occurs, immediately stop the infusion. Notify the physician or emergency team.
- Assess airway, breathing, and circulation.
- Maintain intravenous access with normal saline; closely monitor the patient's vital signs; administer emergency drugs per standing order or physician order; have quick access to life-support therapies in case of failure to respond to initial pharmacologic interventions.
- Administer oxygen as needed and intravenous fluids for hypotension that does not respond to epinephrine.
- If wheezing or respiratory distress persist despite initial pharmacologic intervention, consider administering nebulized albuterol.

- Administer hydrocortisone 100 mg or methylprednisolone 125 mg to prevent prolonged or biphasic anaphylactic reaction.
- Document the reaction, treatment, and patient response.

DRUG DELIVERY

The goal of therapy and the available form of the drug are primary factors dictating the route of drug administration. The routes of chemotherapy drug administration include systemic (oral, subcutaneous, intramuscular, and intravenous) and regional approaches (intraperitoneal, intravesical, intrathecal, intra-arterial, intrapleural, and topical). Systemic drug administration is the most common method of drug delivery.

ORAL, SUBCUTANEOUS, INTRAMUSCULAR

Drugs may be prescribed in the oral form alone or in combination with other drugs. It is important to emphasize that oral drug delivery requires the same attentiveness to dose calculation, patient teaching, monitoring of side effects, follow-up, and compliance evaluation. To maximize safety, review the brand and generic drug names with the patient and prescribe only one course of therapy at a time (Goodman, 2001). Follow-up evaluation is critical to assess side effects, which may influence level of adherence to the prescribed regimen. While administration of chemotherapy by subcutaneous and intramuscular routes is relatively uncommon, the administration of biologicals by the subcutaneous route is very common. Nurses need to assess the receptivity and resources of the patient and family for participation in subcutaneous drug delivery. Many written and audiovisual teaching guides are available to complement the initial verbal instruction. Intramuscular administration and subcutaneous injection of implants (i.e., goserelin acetate implant, Zoladex®) are relatively uncommon and the manufacturer's instructions should be followed for special precautions and procedural guidelines.

INTRAVENOUS DRUG DELIVERY

The intravenous route is the dominant method for delivering systemic cancer therapy. Successful intravenous drug administration is dependent on patient factors and the knowledge and skill of the nurse or physician in vascular access and drug administration procedures. Intravenous drug delivery is accomplished through peripheral insertion of a steel needle or plastic catheter or through a central venous access device.

Peripheral Venous Access

The patient should be well informed and comfortably positioned. The clinician should have easy access to both arms and minimize or avoid potential occupational exposure by following universal precautions and recommendations for handling of hazardous drugs. The following procedural guidelines are provided to optimize safe, effective drug delivery by peripheral venous access:

1. Thoroughly wash hands and put on protective gloves.
2. Exercise patience in vein selection; begin distally and work proximally. Avoid extremities with lymphedema, impaired circulation, edema, sites where venipuncture has been performed within the previous 24 hours, hematomas, axillary lymph node dissections, local infection, and phlebitis. To minimize potential patient morbidity from drugs capable of producing tissue necrosis, avoid the antecubital fossa, wrist, and dorsum of the hand. Warm soaks for

10 to 15 minutes may enhance detection of a potential site in patients with limited vascular access.

3. Choose a cannula based on the purpose, rate of flow, and duration of therapy, the size and availability of the patient's veins, and your own experience and success with each type of cannula. If a short-term infusion (i.e., less than 24-hour infusion) is planned, either a steel needle or an appropriate plastic catheter can be used.

4. Prepare the skin with povidone-iodine solution and allow it to dry. An alternative to iodine is 70% alcohol alone, rubbed vigorously for 1 minute, or 2% tincture of iodine.

5. Once the cannula is successfully placed, apply enough tape to secure it but not to obscure the end so that infiltration of fluid can be immediately detected, especially if a known vesicant is to be given.

6. Test the patency of the cannula with 5% dextrose in water or normal saline, which should flow freely. If the flow is slow or intermittent, recheck the cannula, taping, and IV system (if used), and then recheck patency.

7. If venipuncture has been unsuccessful after two attempts, ask a colleague for assistance.

8. Drugs should be administered as ordered and according to protocol directions. For bolus injections and drugs infused through the side arm of IV tubing, infuse the drug slowly to prevent leakage around the needle and pressure on the wall of the vein. Blood return should be checked frequently.

9. The cannula and tubing should be flushed with solution between drugs and after completion of the last drug administered.

10. Heed any patient complaints. Stop the drug administration for any complaints that might indicate extravasation (see Chapter 11). Evaluate with a saline flush. If there is any doubt, restart the infusion. Venous irritation or phlebitis, which may produce varying degrees of local pain, have been associated with several drugs, including but not limited to: amsacrine, carmustine, dacarbazine, daunorubicin, docetaxel, doxorubicin, etoposide, idarubicin, mechlorethamine, mitomycin, mitoxantrone, paclitaxel, teniposide, vinblastine, vincristine, and vinorelbine tartrate. Ice applied above the IV site may alleviate the acute discomfort during drug administration for some of the drugs, such as dacarbazine, whereas for others, such as vinorelbine tartrate, adherence to the infusion time recommendations is the most important intervention (Rittenberg et al, 1995). If discomfort persists from venous irritation or phlebitis, apply warm soaks daily to the affected area and conduct a follow-up assessment, including careful evaluation of the level of discomfort and effectiveness of interventions.

11. Record drug administered, dose, route of administration, type and volume of solution, start and stop times, and any adverse reactions.

Central Venous Access

Limited vascular access, intensive chemotherapy, parenteral nutrition, continuous drug delivery, and projected long-term need for venous access are the major indications for central venous catheters in cancer patients. Technological advances in the plastics industry have diminished the incidence and severity of catheter complications with the introduction of polyurethane and silastic elastomer materials for catheter construction (Camp-Sorrell, 1996; Hadaway, 1995). Catheter materials are also radiopaque, which is a critically important feature in determining correct placement and evaluation of catheter malfunction. The cited improvements in catheter construction have diminished but not eliminated catheter-associated complications. Thrombosis and fibrin sheath formation producing partial or complete catheter occlusion are persistent catheter problems faced daily by clinicians. Guidelines for catheter care in conjunction with algorithms for determining and managing catheter complications provide consistent approaches to maintaining patent functional catheters.

Three major types of central venous access devices used in cancer therapy are nontunneled, tunneled, and implanted ports. Nontunneled catheters include short-term percutaneously inserted catheters, peripherally inserted catheters, and apheresis catheters. The percutaneous short-term catheters are most frequently used in the acute-care setting for immediate need for central venous access or high acuity patients who require multilumen infusional therapies. Exit-site care and restriction of activities limit the utility of these catheters beyond the short-term or acute-care indications. Midline catheters refer to peripherally inserted catheters that terminate in the upper arm at the axillary vein, not at the superior vena cava, which is the usual endpoint for a central venous catheter. Similarly, catheters that terminate before or at the subclavian vein and not at the superior vena cava should be described as long-line catheters, not central catheters.

The peripherally inserted catheter, referred to as a PICC or PIC catheter, offers an alternative to the existing short-term peripheral catheters and tunneled catheters. These catheters are peripherally inserted into the basilic or cephalic vein and advanced centrally, terminating at the superior vena cava. Although some of these catheters have been used as long-line catheters, terminating in the subclavian or axillary vein, the optimal tip location is the superior vena cava, and radiologic examination is recommended after placement (James et al, 1993). Radiologic confirmation of correct tip position will also minimize or eliminate complications associated with tip malposition, especially in the asymptomatic patient (LaFortune, 1993). Educational programs have been designed to qualify clinicians – specifically, registered nurses – to insert and manage these catheter lines.

The most common indication for a PICC line is antibiotics, but these lines are also used for parenteral nutrition, hydration, chemotherapy, pain control, and blood products. These catheters can be inserted at the bedside, are used for hospital or home infusion, are easily removed, are economical, are available with dual lumens, have been used successfully with immunosuppressed patients, and have been reported to remain in place up to several months (Goodwin & Carlson, 1993). A month or less is the most common duration of catheter placement in the majority of patients. Disadvantages of PICC lines include daily to weekly care requirements, occlusive exit-site dressing, careful attention to prevent dislodgment (may be sutured), availability of a qualified nurse for insertion, difficulty or inability to draw blood, and body image concerns (Winslow et al, 1995). Complications are similar to other central lines and include occlusion, phlebitis, insertion malposition, dislodgment, infection, and breakage.

Tunneled central venous catheters are available in single, double, or triple lumens with either a Dacron or collagen matrix cuff, which provides a mechanical barrier to organisms (Hadaway, 1995) (Figure 6-1). These catheters are either open at the end or are the Groshong type, with a closed distal tip with a three-way slit valve. The type of valve construction of the Groshong catheter is unique and eliminates the need for heparin flushes or external clamps because it restricts the backflow of blood. Physicians insert tunneled central catheters under general or local anesthesia into one of the central veins, with the catheter tip resting in the right atrium. The catheter is tunneled for several inches through subcutaneous tissue to a separate incision, usually on the chest wall, allowing the catheter to exit at a site that is easy to see and care for and distanced from the entry point into the major vein (Figure 6-2). After insertion, the

6

DRUG DELIVERY

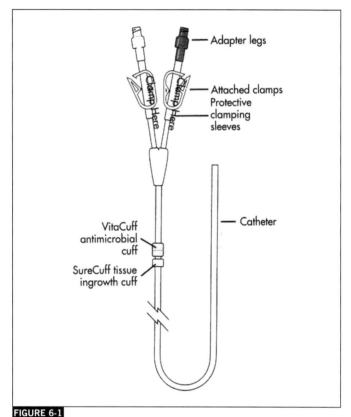

FIGURE 6-1

Multilumen tunneled catheter. (Courtesy of Bard Access System, Salt Lake City, Utah.)

type, length, size, length of external portion of the catheter, and confirmation of the catheter tip position should be documented. All catheters should flush easily and have adequate blood return immediately after insertion, and patients should be observed at the insertion, exit, and tunnel sites.

Scientific evidence is lacking for a definitive standard of catheter care and maintenance. The major components of care include exit-site care, cap change, flushing, and dressing change (Table 6-3).

Guidelines for care are based on available clinical literature and scientific principles related to skin integrity, risk of infection, and hemostasis (Camp-Sorrell, 1996). The guidelines for prevention of intravascular device-related infections represents a consensus of the evidence for practice by the Hospital Infection Control Practices Advisory Committee (Pearson et al, 1996). Despite this more recent overview, unresolved issues remain and it is imperative to have agreement on policies, procedures, and teaching for catheter care for continuity of both patients and staff in the hospital and

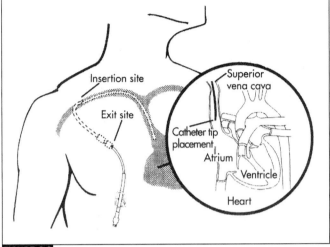

FIGURE 6-2
Placement of tunneled central venous access catheter. (Courtesy of Bard Access System, Salt Lake City, Utah.)

ambulatory care settings. It is equally important to have a mechanism established for periodic review and revision of policies to incorporate changes as new information evolves from practice and research.

Implanted Ports

An infusion port is a subcutaneous device that consists of a portal body, septum, reservoir, and catheter (Figure 6-3). Ports can be placed for venous, intra-arterial, intraperitoneal, intrapleural, or epidural access and are available from multiple manufacturers. The portal body is made from stainless steel, titanium, plastic, or polysulfone, with heights of 9.8 mm to 17 mm, diameters of 16.5 mm to 40 mm, internal body volumes of 0.2 mL to 1.47 mL, and weights ranging from 2.1 g to 28.8 g. Within the portal body is a self-sealing silicone septum that requires a noncoring needle for access (Camp-Sorrell, 1992). Ports are manufactured with attachable or preattached catheters made of silicone or polyurethane; multiple lumens are available, and the ports are available in pediatric and low-profile styles. The venous infusion ports are the most commonly used port devices in practice. The port is placed under the skin with the incision above or below the septum of the device. For easy access and stability, ports are implanted between the chest midline and distal third of the clavicle. A needle can be inserted for access immediately if use is critical. If not, a 2- to 5-day delay is recommended to allow resolution of postoperative tenderness and edema. New types of ports continue to be designed and it is critical to consult the manufacturer's product brochure for specifications and guidelines for use.

The basic principles for access and maintenance include using Huber needles for access; flushing the system for patency; maintaining positive pressure when withdrawing the needle; and heparinizing once monthly and after each use. The Huber-point

TABLE 6-3

CLINICAL PARAMETERS FOR TUNNELED CATHETER CARE AND USE

Care component	Procedure
Saline flush for Groshong-type catheters	Flush briskly with 5 mL before and after each use and weekly in-between use; use 10 to 20 mL after blood sampling or infusion of viscous fluids.
Flush for open-end catheters	Flush with 5 to 10 mL of normal saline before and after use, followed by a 3 to 5 mL of a 10 to 100 units/mL heparin flush. (Camp-Sorrell, 1996). Maintain positive pressure at end of procedure to minimize reflux of blood. The frequency of heparin flush varies from daily to weekly.
Exit-site care	Consider sterile technique initially after insertion until site is healed, generally 3 to 4 weeks, and for immunocompromised patients. Cleanse with effective antiseptic solution (70% alcohol, 10% povidine-iodine, 2% tincture of iodine). If tincture of iodine is used, remove with alcohol prior to access (Pearson et al, 1996).
Ointment at exit site	Do not routinely apply antimicrobial ointment (Pearson et al, 1996).
Dressing change, occlusive (gauze/tape or transparent)	For oncology patients, dressing changes are recommended every 5 to 7 days (Camp-Sorrell, 1996) but current evidence does not fully support any specific frequency of dressing changes (Pearson et al, 1996).
No dressing	Controversial, may consider for non-immunosuppressed patient following complete healing of exit site.
Cap change	Change weekly (Winslow et al, 1995) and whenever there are signs of blood, precipitates, or leaks.
Clamping	Use for accessing and de-accessing open-ended catheters; if clamp is not available, have patient perform the Valsalva maneuver at the time the catheter is open to air; do not use clamps for Groshong catheters.
Blood sampling	Discard 5 to 10 mL of blood from catheter before your blood sample for laboratory analysis except for specimens for blood cultures. Coagulation values may be altered when drawn through a heparinized catheter; other factors, such as specific drug levels, may alter laboratory results drawn from a central catheter.

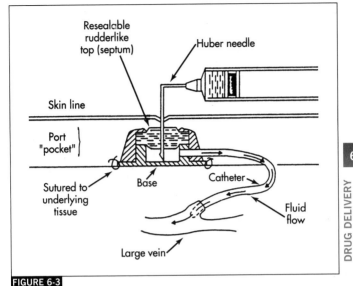

FIGURE 6-3
Port design. (From Camp-Sorrell D: Implantable ports: everything you always wanted to know. J Intrav Nurs 15: 264, 1992.)

6

DRUG DELIVERY

needles are designed with a deflected point that prevents coring of the septum and are available as a single needle that can be attached to a syringe or extension tubing or as a single device (Figure 6-3). The extension tubing or single device (Huber needle with preattached tubing) offers a closed system, decreases the risk of compromising sterility, has a self-sealing rubber cap or Y site, and facilitates changing of syringes, blood drawing, and flushing.

Before a port is accessed, it is important to identify the type of device and characteristics of the specific product. Verification from the patient's record or confirmation from the surgeon is essential. If the patient is in a nonhospital setting, a policy to record the type of device should be established.

Guidelines for access procedures for ports generally adhere to aseptic technique (Camp-Sorrell, 1996):

1. Assemble all necessary equipment.
2. Wash hands thoroughly.
3. Stabilize port with index finger and thumb of nondominant hand, and palpate septum of port with opposite hand.
4. Prepare skin over port with povidone-iodine or 70% alcohol.
5. Using aseptic technique, fill the extension tubing and Huber needle with saline, expelling all air.
6. Stabilize port and access with Huber needle at a 90-degree angle (Figure 6-3).
7. Flush with 5 to 10 mL of normal saline to check for patency.
8. If resistance is met, try to advance the needle farther into the septum until it hits the needle stop. If unsuccessful, try another needle and re-enter port.

9. If withdrawal of blood is required, discard the first 5 mL to 10 mL, except for specimens for blood cultures (Moore et al, 1986). A syringe for withdrawing blood can be used, exerting very slow, steady pressure, or, preferably, the Vacutainer blood-drawing method can be used. The latter is time-efficient and decreases the risk of blood exposure to the caregiver. After blood withdrawal or blood administration, flush the port with 20 mL of normal saline.

10. For long-term or continuous infusions, secure the needle hub with a small pad and sterile strips or tape, and secure with an occlusive, transparent dressing. The transparent dressing allows close observation of the site for any signs of erythema, irritation, or infiltration.

11. When therapy or access is completed, flush with 3 mL to 5 mL of 10 units/mL or 100 units/mL of heparin flush. When 0.5 mL is remaining, withdraw the needle, maintaining slight pressure to heparin lock the system. This will decrease the risk of backflow of blood into the catheter or reservoir.

Advantages of the implanted venous access ports include excellent patient acceptance, no dressing changes, less frequent heparinization, no activity restrictions, long functional life, low maintenance costs, and indicated for intermittent or continuous therapy. Disadvantages include high initial cost, surgical procedure for placement and removal, risk of pocket infection, risk of drug extravasation due to needle dislodgment or backtracking of the drug (due to a fibrin sheath or clot) and needle puncture for access.

Access of ports for other placement sites and routes of administration follows the same principles for venous access. Flushing recommendations vary by type of port and system accessed (Camp-Sorrell, 1996). For arterial ports, flush before and after medication with 5 to 10 mL of normal saline; for final flush, use a 5 mL flush of 100 units heparin/mL or 1000 units heparin/mL (monitor coagulation values if higher heparin flush is used), which should also be done weekly for nonaccessed ports (Camp-Sorrell, 1996). For peritoneal ports, flush before and after medication with 20 mL of compatible solution followed by 5 mL to 10 mL of normal saline flush. Competency-based nursing check-off forms for access of the various devices are available in the Oncology Nursing Society's *Access Device Guidelines* (Camp-Sorrell, 1996, Appendices 2–8).

COMPLICATIONS OF CENTRAL VENOUS CATHETERS

Complications associated with central venous catheters include infection, occlusion, migration, venous thrombosis, malposition, air embolism, vessel perforation, breakage, and extravasation of medication. Nurses must be alert to signs and symptoms associated with potential catheter complications (Table 6-4).

Local and systemic infection is a common complication. Local infection may occur at the exit site, subcutaneous tunnel, or port pocket for implanted ports. Stringent site

TABLE 6-4

POTENTIAL COMPLICATIONS OF CENTRAL VENOUS CATHETERS

Complication	Frequency	Signs and symptoms
Infection	Common	
Local		Induration, erythema, exudate, tenderness
Systemic		Fever, chills, malaise, diaphoresis, tachycardia

cont'd

TABLE 6-4

POTENTIAL COMPLICATIONS OF CENTRAL VENOUS CATHETERS—cont'd

Complication	Frequency	Signs and symptoms
Withdrawal occlusion	Common	Ability to flush catheter but unable to withdraw blood
Complete occlusion	Occasional	Inabilities to flush catheter or withdraw blood
Migration or malposition	Uncommon	Lack of blood return; flushing problems; swelling in ipsilateral extremity; dyspnea; discomfort with infusion
Extravasation	Uncommon	Swelling in the area of port pocket or subcutaneous tunnel; local symptom complaints, such as pain or burning; slow infusion rate
Separation of catheter from port	Rare	Lack of blood return; local swelling; change in ability to infuse fluids; patient complains of altered sensation in portal site
Venous perforation	Rare	Symptom related to site of perforation but shortness of breath common
Twiddler's syndrome	Rare	A flipped portal body resulting in an inability to determine hub, port, or septal area, intentional or unintentional manipulation of port
Pinch-off syndrome: anatomic, mechanical compression of the catheter at the costoclavicular space between the clavicle and first rib	Rare	Withdrawal occlusion, resistance to infusion; irregular flushing pattern with patient positioning; may lead to catheter fracture, which has been associated with cardiac arrhythmias and potential for drug extravasation (Ingle, 1995).
Venous thrombosis	Rare	Discomfort, pain, or swelling in chest wall, scapula, or shoulder area; pattern of venous distention in neck, shoulder, or chest wall; inability to flush device
Breakage: internal or external	Rare	Leakage; reflux of blood into catheter or extension tubing; unexplained drainage on dressing; air embolism (Ingle, 1995)
Dislodgment of needle in septum of port or inadequate needle length	Uncommon, rare	Inability to infuse; local swelling; inability to withdraw blood; potential for extravasation

care and a 10- to 14-day course of oral or intravenous antibiotics is usually a successful strategy to eliminate local infection and preserve the function and utility of the catheter (Rumsey & Richardson, 1995). Catheter-related septicemia is a major risk. Blood cultures (two sets) should be drawn through the central catheter except if the patient presents with obvious signs and symptoms of a port pocket infection (Mermel et al, 2001; Viale, 2002). However, if the central catheter is already accessed when the pocket infection develops, blood cultures can be drawn and antibiotics infused through the catheter. Initially, catheter-related sepsis should not dictate catheter removal until a trial of IV antibiotics is administered through the catheter. If the catheter is a double or triple lumen, administration of antibiotics should be alternated among each of the lumens. Removal of a catheter is generally indicated when associated symptoms of sepsis do not resolve after IV antibiotics are given through the catheter, the causative organism is fungi or bacilli, the patient experiences chills and hypotension after irrigation of the catheter, or there is evidence of endocarditis (Rumsey & Richardson, 1995).

Partial or complete catheter occlusion is a very common clinical problem. The causes include position of the catheter tip against the vessel wall, a fibrin sheath, thrombus in the lumen or at the catheter tip, lipid or drug precipitate, or malposition. Partial occlusions are often related to tip position, fibrin sheath formation, or a clot at the tip of the catheter, the latter two resulting in blood withdrawal occlusion ("one-way catheter"). Brisk irrigations with 10 mL to 30 mL of normal saline or changing the patient's position to reposition the catheter tip (turning side to side, leaning forward, elevating arms, coughing, deep breathing, lying supine) are often successful interventions. If blood withdrawal occlusion persists despite vigorous flushing, consult with the physician to consider a chest radiograph or dye study to confirm the position of the catheter (and/or document presence of a fibrin sheath) or instillation of a fibrinolytic agent.

Completely occluded catheters prevent administration of any fluids or withdrawal of blood. All possible causes should be evaluated to determine the most appropriate intervention. If the patient has an implanted port, the needle placement should be checked or changed. If complete occlusion persists, attempt a gentle flush/aspiration using a 10-mL syringe filled with 5 mL of saline. If unsuccessful and a clot is suspected, consult with the physician about instillation of alteplase, a tissue plasminogen activator (CathFlo Ativase®, Genentech, Inc.). Timoney et al (2002) reported an 81% success rate, with 71% of the catheters cleared on the first try, with a mean dwell time of 45 minutes. Alteplase is reconstituted to a concentration of 1 mg/mL with a total vial dose of 2 mg/2 mL. Alteplase is instilled and allowed to dwell for 30 minutes; aspiration of the alteplase and clot is attempted, repeated every 30 minutes until patency is restored; once patency is restored, withdraw 5 to 10 mL of blood and follow by a saline flush (Luptak, 2001; Timoney et al, 2002). For occlusion secondary to suspected drug precipitate, catheter patency can be restored, if the solubility of the fluid can be changed by altering the pH, resulting in returning the precipitate into solution. Instillation of 0.1 N hydrochloric acid has been used successfully in restoring patency in catheters obstructed by precipitates such as lipids or calcium and phosphorus incompatibilities with total parenteral nutrition (Rumsey & Richardson, 1995).

REGIONAL DRUG DELIVERY

Infusion of chemotherapeutic drugs directly into the area of the tumor has theoretical advantages over the systemic route of administration. The most common approaches to regional drug perfusion include intra-arterial, intraperitoneal, and intraventricular.

Intra-arterial

The intra-arterial route for regional drug delivery has been attempted in several malignancies such as head and neck tumors and limb perfusions for melanoma, but liver metastasis has been the primary target for intra-arterial drug delivery. Arterial perfusion with chemotherapy can be delivered through an externally placed percutaneous catheter, an implanted port-catheter system, or an implanted infusion pump. Percutaneous catheters are inserted under local anesthesia and placement is confirmed by angiography. Patients usually require hospitalization and bedrest with femoral artery access (Lynes, 1993).

Subcutaneously implanted intra-arterial ports are similar to the venous access ports. The most common indication is hepatic metastases, and catheters are usually placed in the common hepatic artery with the port body on either side of the rib cage. Totally implantable infusion pumps are used in practice and permit safe, reliable, and prolonged delivery of chemotherapy. Camp-Sorrell (1996) provides a detailed comparison of the two infusion pumps (Infusaid, Medtronics), including description, indications, use, advantages, disadvantages, access procedures, and complications.

Intraventricular

Prophylaxis or treatment of the central nervous system (CNS) can be performed via lumbar puncture, an implanted pump, or Ommaya reservoir. The Ommaya reservoir is the preferred device for obtaining cerebrospinal fluid (CSF) specimens and for delivering drugs into the CSF (Figure 6-4). The design of this device is a mushroom-shaped dome that has a reservoir attached to a ventricular catheter. There are several models with reservoir sizes of 1.5 cm and 3.5 cm, with either bottom burr hole inlet or flat bottom side inlet designs (Almadrones et al, 1995). The approximate volume of the reservoir is 1.5 to 2.5 mL. An Ommaya reservoir is inserted by a neurosurgeon into the right frontal region under the scalp, and the catheter is positioned into the lateral ventricle through a burr hole. The reservoir can be used 48 hours after insertion, even though sutures remain until 7 to 10 days after surgical placement. Patients should be instructed to avoid trauma to the area, and hair is allowed to regrow except for a 2.5- to 3-cm area that will be shaved for access procedures (Esparza & Weyland, 1982).

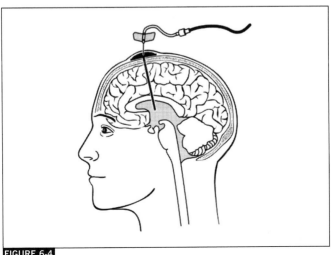

FIGURE 6-4
The Ommaya reservoir.

Infection, malfunction, catheter displacement, and spread of tumor cells by catheter placement are potential but uncommon complications.

Infection is an ongoing potential complication of reservoir usage. The patient should be routinely monitored for tenderness, erythema, drainage, fever, neck stiffness, and headache. Careful adherence to aseptic technique for access of the reservoir is the best preventive strategy against infection. Depending on institutional policy, physicians or nurses who have received specialized instruction may access the Ommaya reservoir. With maintenance of strict aseptic technique, the following procedural guidelines are recommended (Camp-Sorrell, 1996; Goodman, 2001; Kosier & Minkler, 1999):

1. Educate the patient and obtain informed consent.
2. Place the patient in a supine or semi-Fowler's position. Examine the site for any potential signs of infection.
3. With aseptic technique, prepare the skin over the area with povidone-iodine and alcohol. Allow to dry or remove any moist povidone-iodine with a sterile gauze.
4. With a 2 x 2-in. gauze, **gently** place finger on top of the reservoir and push and release once or twice. If the reservoir does not refill or fills very slowly, a physician should be notified, and radiologic confirmation of placement may be indicated.
5. Access the reservoir obliquely with a 23–25-gauge scalp vein needle with attached tubing.
6. Remove fluid by gravity. Never forcefully aspirate. The amount of fluid removed must equal what is to be returned. Gently remove 2 to 3 mL CSF and set aside if your procedure is to use this for a flush return. Obtain additional CSF specimen for cytology. The CSF should be clear; if not, do not proceed with medication injection but wait for cytologic analyses.
7. Attach medication syringe and inject medication **slowly** into the reservoir. Time recommendations vary from 1 mL/min for 3 to 5 minutes to 5 to 10 minutes. Solution for the drug admixture should be normal saline **without preservative**.
8. Although generally recommended, flushing with the initial 2 to 3 mL of removed CSF is controversial. If your policy is not to use the CSF to flush, gentle pressure to the top of the reservoir, repeated once or twice, will aid in drug dispersement.
9. Dress the site with a sterile gauze.
10. The patient should remain in a supine position without a pillow for at least 30 minutes.
11. Instruct the patient/family or other caregiver to call for tenderness, redness or drainage from the site, fever greater than 101°F, neck stiffness, or headache with/without vomiting (Esparza & Weyland, 1992).

Intraperitoneal

Delivery of chemotherapy into the peritoneal cavity has been investigated in patients with malignant ascites and intra-abdominal metastases primarily from carcinomas of the colon and ovary. The major advantage of intraperitoneal chemotherapy is pharmacological; that is, higher concentrations of some drugs can be delivered to the tumor than could be safely administered by other routes. Cytotoxicity is enhanced by direct drug contact with the cells in the peritoneal cavity and by very high drug concentrations.

Access can be achieved with a semipermanent Tenckhoff catheter or a Tenckhoff catheter attached to a subcutaneous implanted port. Instituting therapy involves surgical implantation of a catheter. Postoperative procedures vary from no flushing to intermittent dialysis exchanges through the catheter. Postoperative complications of catheter placement include intestinal perforation, bleeding, ileus, and incisional discomfort (Jenkins et al, 1982). The Tenckhoff catheter attached to a subcutaneously implanted port has become the device of choice for intraperitoneal drug delivery. The implanted port has eliminated exit-site care, potential exit-site infection, and restriction on patient activity. To access the implanted port, the same guidelines as described for intravenous port access should be followed with the exception of a larger volume flush (20-mL heparin flush of 100 units/mL).

Intraperitoneal drug delivery follows the same basic principles as peritoneal dialysis (Doane et al, 1990). The solution should be allowed to reach room temperature or may be warmed to body temperature, and fluids run in and out by gravity. For chemotherapy, patency should be assessed by a 10- to 20-mL flush with normal saline before drug administration. The prescribed dose of chemotherapy is usually prepared in 2 L of solution. The fluid is instilled by gravity, and it usually takes at least 30 to 40 minutes with the implanted systems. Patients are instructed to change position periodically to permit optimal drug distribution in the abdominal cavity. Drainage is by gravity, but outflow problems are common. They may be caused by malposition of the catheter, a fibrin sheath at the tip of the catheter, or kinking of the catheter. Aspiration with a syringe, irrigation with normal saline, or changing the patient's position are often successful interventions used to institute outflow.

Outflow problems occur in one-third to one-half of patients and result in less than 50% recovery of fluid instilled (Almadrones & Yerys, 1990). This does not present a significant clinical problem for most treatment patients because most drugs are removed via the portal circulation and metabolized by the liver before entering the systemic circulation and the fluid is absorbed over a few days. For patients with ascites, however, outflow obstruction may be a problem, and a percutaneous paracentesis may be needed. Other complications that occur much less frequently include bacterial or chemical phlebitis, leakage of the chemotherapeutic agent, and infection.

Symptoms associated with treatment include abdominal distention and drug-related side effects. The increase in abdominal pressure from fluid volume can produce a variety of clinical symptoms such as pain, nausea, anorexia, shortness of breath, diarrhea, constipation, and esophageal reflux (Swenson & Eriksson, 1986). Pain is the most common symptom. In a review of 137 patients who received intraperitoneal therapy, 25% reported mild discomfort (no analgesia required), 12% had moderate pain (analgesia given), and 11% reported severe pain during instillation that required narcotics and discontinuance of the procedure (Almadrones & Yerys, 1990). The mild discomfort was described as bloating or fullness and disappeared within 1 to 2 days after treatment.

Drug-related side effects are agent-specific and similar to those observed with systemic intravenous therapy. It is important to remember that drugs are eliminated from the body by usual routes after absorption from the peritoneal cavity. Thus intraperitoneal cisplatin is associated with the same long-term and short-term toxicity as intravenous administration, although timing of onset may differ because of delayed absorption from the peritoneal cavity.

Intrapleural

Management of malignant pleural effusions has historically included insertion of a chest tube, drainage of the fluid, and administration of a sclerosing agent. The goal of pleural sclerosis is pleurodesis, the fusion of the visceral and parietal pleurae, which prevents further accumulation of fluid (Little, 1994). The thoracostomy or chest tube remains in place until daily drainage is in the range of 100 to 250 mL to maximize the goal of pleural adherence. At this point, a chemical agent (a known pleural irritant) is instilled, which produces pleural inflammation. Pain during the procedure is common, but severity is dependent on the chemical irritant chosen for the procedure. Sedation, lidocaine administered through the chest tube, and systemic pain medication after the procedure, are recommended to maintain patient comfort.

The use of pleuroperitoneal shunts for patients with malignant effusions has been evaluated as an alternative to a thoracostomy tube placement with pleurodesis or for those patients who have been refractory. The shunt consists of a double-valved pump chamber with connecting pleural and peritoneal catheters. While it has been associated with palliation of symptoms, the complication rate limits its utility (Ponn et al, 1991). More recently, the indwelling pleural catheter (Pluerx Pleural Catheter, Denver, Denver Biomedical) has emerged as a cost-effective, successful intervention for management of pleural effusions. This catheter is placed in the pleural space and tunneled subcutaneously with the catheter and valve external for drainage. The valve is designed to prevent leakage or air from entering the catheter. The Pluerx drainage kit provides all the necessary equipment for ambulatory or home drainage. Putnam et al (1999) compared the indwelling pleural catheter to doxycycline pleurodesis and reported that fewer patients with the catheter had recurrent effusions, hospitalization was shorter (1 day versus 6.5 days), and nearly half of the patients with the indwelling catheter achieved spontaneous pleurodesis at a median of 27 days. Insertion of these catheters has predominantly become an outpatient procedure, the majority of patients and caregivers easily learn the drainage procedure, and it allows patients to manage their respiratory symptom distress. Once the effusion has been resolved, the catheter can be simply removed.

REFERENCES

Albanell J, Baselga J. Systemic therapy emergencies. Semin Oncol 27: 347–361, 2000.

Almadrones L, Yerys C. Problems associated with administration of intraperitoneal therapy using the Port-A-Cath system. Oncol Nurs Forum 17: 75–80, 1990.

Almadrones L, Campana P, Dantis EC. Arterial, peritoneal and intraventricular access devices. Semin Oncol Nurs 11: 194–202, 1995.

American Society of Hospital Pharmacists. Technical assistance bulletin on handling cytotoxic and hazardous drugs. Am J Hosp Pharm 47: 1033–1049, 1990.

Baker SD, Grochow LB, Donehower RC. Should anticancer drug doses be adjusted in the obese patient? J Natl Cancer Inst 87: 333–334, 1995.

Brown KA et al. Chemotherapy and Biotherapy: Guidelines and Recommendations for Practice. Pittsburgh, PA, Oncology Nursing Press, 2001.

Bruno R et al. A population pharmacokinetic model for docetaxel (Taxotere): model building and validation. J Pharmacokinet Biopharm 24: 153–172, 1996.

Calvert AH et al. Carboplatin dosage: prospective evaluation of a simple formula based on renal function. J Clin Oncol 7: 1748–1756, 1989.

Calvert AH, Newell DR, Gore ME. Future directions with carboplatin: can therapeutic monitoring, high dose administration and hematologic support with growth factors expand the spectrum compared with cisplatin? Semin Oncol 19: 155–163, 1992.

Camp-Sorrell D. Implantable ports. J Intrav Nurs 15: 262–272, 1992.

Camp-Sorrell D. Access Device Guidelines. Pittsburgh, PA, Oncology Nursing Press, 1996.

Carmignani SS, Raymond GG. Safe handling of cytotoxic drugs in the physician office: a procedure manual model. Oncol Nurs Forum 24: 41–48, 1997.

Craig JB, Capizzi RL. The prevention and treatment of immediate hypersensitivity reactions from cancer chemotherapy. Semin Oncol Nurs 1: 285–291, 1985.

deJongh FE et al. Body-surface area based dosing does not increase accuracy of predicting cisplatin exposure. J Clin Oncol 19: 3733–3739, 2001.

Dickson TM et al. Impact of admission body weight and chemotherapy dose adjustment on the outcome of autologous bone marrow transplantation. Biol Blood Marrow Transplant 5: 299–305, 1999.

Doane LS, Fisher LM, McDonald W. How to give peritoneal chemotherapy. Am J Nurs 4: 58–66, 1990.

Dobbs NA, Twelves CJ. What is the effect of adjusting epirubicin doses for body surface area? Br J Cancer 78: 662–666, 1998.

Esparza DM, Weyland JB. Nursing care of the patient with an Ommaya reservoir. Oncol Nurs Forum 9: 17–20, 1982.

Falck K et al. Mutagenicity in urine of nurses handling cytotoxic drugs. Lancet 1: 1250–1251, 1979.

Fischer DS et al. Improving the chemotherapy use process. J Clin Oncol 14: 3148–3155, 1996.

Gelman RS et al. Actual versus ideal weight in the calculation of surface area effects on dose of 11 chemotherapy agents. Cancer Treat Rep 71: 907–911, 1987.

Gennari A et al. Rapid intravenous premedication with dexamethasone prevents hypersensitivity reactions. J Clin Oncol 7: 978–979, 1996.

Georgiadis MS et al. Obesity and therapy-related toxicity in patients treated for small cell lung cancer. J Natl Cancer Inst 87: 361–366, 1995.

Gibbs JP et al. The impact of obesity and disease on busulfan oral clearance in adults. Blood 93: 4436–4440, 1999.

Goodman M. Chemotherapy: principles of administration. In: Yarbro CH, Frogge M, Goodman M, Groenwald S, eds. Cancer Nursing Principles and Practice. Boston: Jones and Bartlett, 2001, pp 385–443.

Goodwin ML, Carlson I. The peripherally inserted central catheter. J Intrav Nurs 16: 92–103, 1993.

Grigg A, Harun MH, Szer J. Variability in determination of body weight used for dosing busulphan and cyclophosphamide in adult patients: results of an international survey. Leuk Lymph 25: 487–491, 1997.

Gurney HP. Dose calculation of anticancer drugs: a review of the current practice and introduction of an alternative. J Clin Oncol 14: 2590–2611, 1996.

Gurney HP et al. Factors affecting epirubicin pharmacokinetics and toxicity: evidence against using body surface area for dose calculation. J Clin Oncol 16: 2299–2304, 1998.

Hadaway LC. Comparison of vascular access devices. Semin Oncol Nurs 11: 154–166, 1995.

Hessel H et al. The genotoxic risk of hospital, pharmacy and medical personnel occupationally exposed to cytostatic drugs – evaluation by micronucleus assay. Mutat Res 497: 101–109, 2001.

Ingle, RJ. Rare complications of vascular access devices. Semin Oncol Nurs 11: 184–193, 1995.

Jakab MG, Major J, Tompa A. Followup genotoxicological monitoring of nurses handling antineoplastic drugs. J Tox Environ Health 62: 307–318, 2001.

James L, Bledsoe L, Hadaway LC. A retrospective look at tip location and complications of peripherally inserted central catheter lines. J Intrav Nurs 16: 104–109, 1993.

Jenkins J et al. Technical considerations in the use of intraperitoneal chemotherapy administered by Tenckhoff catheter. Surg Gynecol Obstet 154: 858–864, 1982.

Koppler H, Heymanns J, Weide R. Dose reduction of steroid premedication for paclitaxel: no increase of hypersensitivity reactions. Oncologie 24: 283–285, 2001.

Kosier MB, Minkler P. Nursing management of patients with an implanted Ommaya reservoir. Clin J Oncol Nurs 3: 63–67, 1999.

Labovich TM. Acute hypersensitivity reactions to chemotherapy. Semin Oncol Nurs 15: 222–231, 1999.

LaFortune S. The use of confirming x-rays to verify tip position for peripherally inserted catheters. J Intrav Nurs 16: 246–250, 1993.

Little AG. Malignant pleural effusion. In: McKenna RJ, Murphy GP, eds. Cancer Surgery. Philadelphia, JB Lippincott, 1994, pp 351–356.

Loos WJ et al. Inter- and intrapatient variability in oral topotecan pharmacokinetics: implications for body surface area dosage regimens. Clin Cancer Res 6: 2685–2689, 2000.

Luptak P. Management of catheter occlusion with Cathflo Activase. Spectrum 13: 1–19, 2001.

Lynes AC. Percutaneous hepatic arterial chemotherapy and chemoembolization. Cancer Nurs 16: 283–287, 1993.

Markman M et al. Clinical features of hypersensitivity reactions to carboplatin. J Clin Oncol 17: 1141–1145, 1999.

Markman M et al. Paclitaxel-associated hypersensitivity reactions: experience of the gynecologic oncology program of the Cleveland Clinic Cancer Center. J Clin Oncol 18: 102–105, 2000.

Mathijssen RH et al. Impact of body-size measures on irinotecan clearance: alternative dosing recommendations. J Clin Oncol 20: 81–87, 2001.

6

Mermel LA et al. Guidelines for the management of intravascular catheter-related infections. Clin Infect Dis 32: 1249–1272, 2001.

Moore CL et al. Nursing care and management of venous access ports. Oncol Nurs Forum 13: 35–39, 1986.

Morgan DJ, Bray KM. Lean body mass as a predictor of drug dosage. Clin Pharmacol Concepts 26: 294–307, 1994.

Occupational Safety and Health Administration. Controlling occupational exposure to hazardous drugs (OSHA Instruction CPL 2-2.20B). Washington, DC, 1999.

Olson JK et al. Taxol hypersensitivity: rapid re-treatment is safe and cost effective. Gynecol Oncol 68: 25–28, 1998.

Pearson ML et al. Guideline for prevention of intravascular device-related infections. Am J Infect Control 24: 262–293, 1996.

Petros WP et al. Association of high-dose cyclophosphamide, cisplatin and carmustine pharmaco-kinetics with survival, toxicity and dosing weight in patients with primary breast cancer. Clin Cancer Res 8: 698–705, 2002.

Pilger A et al. Long term monitoring of sister chromatid exchanges and micronucleus frequencies in pharmacy personnel occupationally exposed to cytostatic drugs. Int Arch Occup Environ Health 73: 442–448, 2000.

Poikonen P, Blommqvist C, Joensuu H. Effect of obesity on the leukocyte nadir in women treated with adjuvant cyclophosphamide, methotrexate and flourouracil dosed according to body surface area. Acta Oncol 40: 67–71, 2001.

Ponn RB et al. Pleuroperitoneal shunting for intractable pleural effusions. Ann Thoracic Surg 51: 605–609, 1991.

Putnam JB et al. A randomized comparison of indwelling pleural catheter and doxycycline pleurodesis in the management of malignant pleural effusions. Cancer 86: 1992–1999, 1999.

Ratain MJ. Body-surface area as a basis for dosing anticancer agents: science, myth or habit? J Clin Oncol 16: 2297–2298, 1998.

Rittenberg CN, Gralla R, Rehmeyer TA. Assessing and managing venous irritation associated with vinorelbine tartrate (Navelbine). Oncol Nurs Forum 22: 707–710, 1995.

Rosner GL et al. Relationship between toxicity and obesity in women receiving adjuvant chemotherapy for breast cancer: results from Cancer and Leukemia Group B study 8541. J Clin Oncol 14: 3000–3008, 1996.

Rumsey KA, Richardson DK. Management of infection and occlusion associated with vascular access devices. Semin Oncol Nurs 11: 174–183, 1995.

Sawyer M, Ratain MJ. Body surface area as a determinant of pharmacokinetics and drug dosing. Investig New Drugs 19: 171–177, 2001.

Smith TJ, Desch CE. Neutropenia wise and pound foolish: safe and effective chemotherapy in massively obese patients. South Med J 84: 883–885, 1991.

Swenson KK, Eriksson JH. Nursing management of intraperitoneal chemotherapy. Oncol Nurs Forum 13: 33–39, 1986.

SWOG (2001) www.swog.org, policy #38 Dosing principles.

Timoney JP et al. Safe and cost effective use of alteplase for the clearance of occluded central venous access devices. J Clin Oncol 20: 1918–1922, 2002.

Valanis B et al. Occupational exposure to antineoplastic agents and self reported infertility among nurses and pharmacists. J Occup Environ Med 39: 574–580, 1997.

Valanis B, Vollmer WM, Steele P. Occupational exposure to antineoplastic agents: self-reported miscarriages and stillbirths among nurses and pharmacists. J Occup Environ Med 41: 632–638, 1999.

Viale PH. To draw or not to draw: drawing blood cultures from a potentially infected port site. Clin J Oncol Nurs 6: 232, 2002.

Weiss RB. Hypersensitivity reactions. Semin Oncol 19: 458–477, 1992.

Weiss RB et al. Hypersensitivity reactions from taxol. J Clin Oncol 8: 1263–1268, 1990.

Winslow MN, Trammell L, Camp-Sorrell D. Selection of vascular access devices and nursing care. Semin Oncol Nurs 11: 167–173, 1995.

Zanotti et al. Carboplatin skin-testing protocol for predicting hypersensitivity to carboplatin chemotherapy. J Clin Oncol 19: 3126–3129, 2001.

CANCER CHEMOTHERAPY AND BIOTHERAPY

During the 1950s, drugs were used mainly as single agents and yielded only a few complete responses with short durations. Choriocarcinoma was one of the few malignancies cured by single-agent chemotherapy (Berkowitz et al, 1982). Later, hairy-cell leukemia was added to the list (Piro et al, 1990). The 1960s marked the beginning of the era of combination chemotherapy and was dominated by the "cell kill hypothesis" (Skipper et al, 1964). Combination chemotherapy regimens have been designed on the basis of cell cycle specificity, drugs with different modes of action, varied toxicities, effectiveness of drugs, and synergy between drugs. In recent years there has been a renewed interest in some single-agent therapy and in sequential therapy instead of concomitant chemotherapy. Hence, some single-agent therapies of interest are listed in this section with relevant references. Individual drugs and their use in a more general way are listed in the sections on chemotherapy and biotherapy drugs. Although combination chemotherapy and biotherapy regimens comprise the bulk of this chapter, single agents may sometimes yield responses equal to combinations and they are usually less toxic.

Literally hundreds of combination chemotherapy regimens have been developed. Many of them are listed in the on-line computer service Physician's Data Query (PDQ) system operated by the National Cancer Institute (NCI) or in other on-line sources that we have provided in Chapter 2 of this book. As a quick reference for those who use combination chemotherapy, we have compiled a selection of completed studies with references to the original or follow-up report by the investigators. This is not meant as a "cookbook," but as a resource for oncology professionals who are familiar with the therapy. With this in mind, we have selected articles in English and in journals or proceedings more readily available to oncology professionals. A few abstracts have been included, but in general we have tried to avoid abstracts because they are not peer reviewed, often have little or no toxicity data, dosages sometimes are changed in the final full publication, and many are never published as full reports (see comments on abstracts in Chapter 8). Additional treatment options are to be found in oncology textbooks.

When the compilation of chemotherapy protocols in this book is used as a guide, it is imperative to consult the original or cited literature to verify dosage (transcription or printing errors do occur), to check timing and sequencing, for suggested dose-reduction schedules, and to ascertain the need for ancillary support such as hydration or antiemetics or prophylaxis of allergic reactions. When we refer to repetition of a chemotherapy combination at a stated interval, we frequently use the terms course or cycle interchangeably, as they often are in the literature. If combined modality therapy is being used with radiation, dose reduction is usually necessary and should be stated in the original report of combined modality therapy. In addition, appropriate antiemetics, hydration, and colony-stimulating factors are occasionally mentioned in commenting on a particular regimen, but these would be too repetitive to list with every regimen. Clinicians should be familiar with these supportive measures, most of which are detailed in other relevant chapters.

The patient's quality of life is a central consideration in all therapy and is deservedly receiving more attention in the literature. Patients will generally accept more toxic side effects in an attempt to cure them or significantly prolong their lives, but may be unwilling to tolerate much discomfort for brief prolongation or slight palliation. That is a decision that belongs to the patient and should be made as part of informed decision-making. Every patient is entitled to full information before agreeing to therapy, whether that therapy is considered "routine" or "standard" or is part of an investigational protocol approved by an Institutional Review Board (IRB)/Ethics Committee with a formalized informed consent form.

Regimens for children's cancers have been deleted because more than 80% of children with systemic cancer are treated on a national cooperative group protocol.

New combinations are being developed every week and will require critical evaluation. As we predicted, biological response modifiers, targeted therapies, radiation sensitizers, hormones, antihormones, and monoclonal antibodies are being used with chemotherapy in many combinations and permutations. We do not endorse any regimen as being necessarily superior, but attempted to reflect the current literature.

The concept of the standard or best therapy for any condition is really a "moving target" that changes with time, new knowledge, and consensus opinions. The protocols that we list here are in rough alphabetic order of name or acronym. The acronyms are composed of arbitrary letters from generic and trade names of drugs, and occasionally include numbers to indicate scheduling. The listing reflects **NO** preferential order. The knowledgeable oncologist will recognize the common and popular regimens of the moment that are most frequently used for initial therapy. The larger group of less commonly used regimens may be of value for salvage therapy or special situations therapy to compensate for comorbidities or organ system deficiencies.

We have not included in this chapter any preparative high-dose chemotherapy regimens for use with bone marrow or peripheral blood stem cell transplantation. We have intentionally placed Chapter 10, High-Dose Chemotherapy with Stem Cell Support, at some distance to avoid confusion and potentially life-threatening errors.

What therapeutic regimen should be used for the patient? Time, experience, and prospective randomized trials will eventually select the better regimens for the general patient population. Participation in clinical trials should be encouraged when appropriate for the patient (see Chapter 2).

Many of the regimens listed here are "salvage regimens" to be used after failure of initial therapy for the patient who wants to "keep fighting." Many are second-line alternatives for the patient who has organ disease that contraindicates the use of a superior regimen (e.g., cardiac disease with an abnormal left ventricular ejection fraction or renal disease with an abnormal creatinine clearance). However, it is just as important for the oncologist to know when not to treat and when to stop treatment as it is to know when and how to treat. Determining what is best for a particular patient will always be the job of the experienced, conscientious clinician. Since so much progress needs to be made in the fight against so many different cancers, patients, whenever possible, should be offered the opportunity to enter into an appropriate research study to generate the data to make future treatment decisions.

REFERENCES

Berkowitz RA et al. Methotrexate with citrovorum factor rescue as primary therapy for gestational trophoblastic disease. Cancer 50: 2024–2027, 1982.

Piro LD et al. Lasting remissions in hairy-cell leukemia induced by a single infusion of 2-chlorodeoxyadenosine. N Engl J Med 322: 1117–1121, 1990.

Skipper HE et al. Experimental evaluation of potential anti-cancer agents. XII. On the criteria and kinetics associated with "curability" of experimental leukemia. Cancer Chemother Rep 35: 1–111, 1964.

ADRENAL CORTICAL CARCINOMA

Adrenal cortical carcinoma is a rare tumor that is functional in about half of all cases. Its incidence is highest in the fourth and fifth decades and it is seen more often in women than in men. When localized, it may be surgically curable. Recurrent or metastatic disease may be palliated with radiation or chemotherapy. There is no evidence that chemotherapy increases survival, but palliation may be achieved with single-agent mitotane or doxorubicin or one of several combination chemotherapy regimens. Neither adjuvant radiation nor adjuvant chemotherapy has been shown to improve survival.

CAP—CYCLOPHOSPHAMIDE-DOXORUBICIN-CISPLATIN

Cyclophosphamide. 600 mg/m^2 intravenously on day 1.
Doxorubicin. 40 mg/m^2 intravenously on day 1.
Cisplatin. 50 mg/m^2 intravenously on day 1.
NOTE: Repeat the cycle every 21 days.

Selected Reading

van Slooten H, van Oosterom AT. CAP (cyclophosphamide, doxorubicin and cisplatin) regimen in adrenal cortical carcinoma. Cancer Treat Rep 67: 377–379, 1983.

CE—CISPLATIN-ETOPOSIDE

Cisplatin. 40 mg/m^2 intravenously on days 1 to 3.
Etoposide. 100 mg/m^2 intravenously on days 1 to 3.
NOTE: Repeat the cycle every 3 weeks. Although the report is of two cases, the responses after failure of mitotane are impressive.

Selected Reading

Johnson DH, Greco FA. Treatment of metastatic adrenal cortical carcinoma with cisplatin and etoposide (VP-16). Cancer 58: 2198–2202, 1986.

CM—CISPLATIN-MITOTANE

Cisplatin. 100 mg/m^2 (good risk) or 75 mg/m^2 (poor risk) intravenously every 3 weeks.
Mitotane. 1,000 mg orally 4 times a day with escalation as tolerated.
Cortisone acetate. 25 mg orally twice a day.
Fludrocortisone acetate. 0.1 mg orally daily.

Selected Readings

Bukowski RM et al. Phase II trial of mitotane and cisplatin in patients with adrenal carcinoma: a Southwestern Oncology Group study. J Clin Oncol 11: 161–165, 1993.

EDP—ETOPOSIDE-DOXORUBICIN-CISPLATIN PLUS MITOTANE

Etoposide. 100 mg/m^2 intravenously on days 5 to 7.
Doxorubicin. 20 mg/m^2 intravenously on days 1 and 8.
Cisplatin. 40 mg/m^2 intravenously on days 1 and 9.
Mitotane. 1,000 mg orally 4 times a day or the maximum tolerated dose.
NOTE: Regimen is repeated every four weeks. Mitotane is given without interruption between chemotherapy cycles.

Selected Reading

Berruti A et al. Mitotane associated with etoposide, doxorubicin, and cisplatin in the treatment of advanced adrenocortical carcinoma. Cancer 83: 2194–2200, 1998.

FDC—FLUOROURACIL-DOXORUBICIN-CISPLATIN

5-Fluorouracil. 500 mg/m^2 by 1-hour IV infusion on days 1 to 3.
Doxorubicin. 60 mg/m^2 intravenously on day 2.
Cisplatin. 120 mg/m^2 intravenously on day 2.
NOTE: Hydration and mannitol diuresis are essential on day 2. Repeat every 4 weeks.

Selected Reading

Schlumberger M et al. 5-Fluorouracil, doxorubicin, and cisplatin as treatment for adrenal cortical carcinoma. Cancer 67: 2997–3000, 1991.

SINGLE-AGENT THERAPY

Mitotane. 1,000 to 6,000 mg/day orally in 3 or 4 divided doses until regression of tumor, absence of clinical benefit, or adverse clinical reactions.

Selected Reading

Lubitz JA et al. Mitotane use in inoperable adrenal cortical carcinoma. JAMA 223: 1109–1112, 1973.

Doxorubicin. 60 mg/m^2 every 3 weeks until regression of tumor, absence of clinical benefit, a maximum safe dose of doxorubicin, or adverse clinical reactions.

Selected Reading

Decker RA et al. Eastern Cooperative Oncology Group study 1879: mitotane and adriamycin in patients with advanced adrenocortical carcinoma. Surgery 110: 1006–1013, 1991.

ANAL CARCINOMA

Anal carcinoma is an uncommon but often curable disease. Traditionally, surgery was the treatment of choice and remains so in some cases. In an increasing percentage of cases, radiation therapy with fluorouracil and mitomycin has been proved to have a comparable cure rate with preservation of a functioning anus and rectum. Studies are in progress to determine whether equivalent results can be obtained with radiation and fluorouracil and elimination of the added toxicity of mitomycin or the substitution of the less toxic porfiromycin.

FC—FLUOROURACIL-CISPLATIN

5-Fluorouracil. 750 mg/m^2/day by continuous intravenous infusion on days 1 through 4.
Cisplatin. 100 mg/m^2 by a 60-minute intravenous infusion on day 1.
NOTE: Two or three cycles of chemotherapy are given beginning on days 1 and 21 and concurrent radiotherapy at a daily dose of 1,800 cGy up to a total dose of 3,600 to 3,800 cGy in 4 weeks delivered to the anal region, perineum, middle and lower pelvis, and inguinal and external iliac nodes. Radiotherapy was then delivered to the anoperineal region and metastatic inguinal nodes to a total dose of 1,800 to 2,400 cGy in 10 fractions.

Selected Reading

Doci R et al. Primary chemoradiation therapy with fluorouracil and cisplatin for cancer of the anus: results in 35 consecutive patients. J Clin Oncol 14: 3121–3125, 1996.

FLUOROURACIL-MITOMYCIN

5-Fluorouracil. 1,000 mg/m^2/day by continuous intravenous infusion on days 1 through 4 (maximum dose, 1,500 mg/day).

Mitomycin. 10 mg/m^2 intravenously on day 1.

NOTE: Radiation may be delivered in a single course of 250 cGy/day 5 days a week for 4 weeks (5,000 cGy) or in a split course with 2,500 cGy in 2 weeks and an additional 2,500 cGy beginning on day 43, in which case the above chemotherapy is repeated.

Selected Reading

Cummings BJ et al. Epidermoid anal cancer: treatment by radiation alone or by radiation and 5-fluorouracil with and without mitomycin. Int J Radiat Oncol Biol Phys 21: 1115–1125, 1991.

MITOMYCIN-FLUOROURACIL

5-Fluorouracil. 1,000 mg/m^2/day by continuous IV infusion on days 1 through 4 and on days 29 through 32.

Mitomycin. 10 mg/m^2 (20 mg maximum) intravenously on days 1 and 29.

NOTE: Radiation therapy, 180 cGy/day, is administered for 5 days a week to a total dose of 4,500 cGy.

Selected Reading

Flam M et al. Role of mitomycin in combination with fluorouracil and of radiotherapy, and of salvage chemoradiation in the definitive nonsurgical treatment of epidermoid carcinoma of the anal canal. J Clin Oncol 14: 2527–2539, 1996.

BLADDER (TRANSITIONAL CELL) CARCINOMA

Transitional cell carcinoma is the second most common tumor of the genitourinary tract. Treatment of superficial disease is by cautery, topical chemotherapy, and biologicals. Active topical intravesical agents include BCG, doxorubicin, epirubicin, mitomycin, and thiotepa. Invasive disease is treated with surgery with or without radiation and adjuvant chemotherapy. Metastatic disease is treated with palliative systemic cytotoxic chemotherapy. For many years, three- and four-drug combinations have been popular because of their efficacy. Now, single-agent and two- and three-drug combinations are being used to reduce toxicity while trying to maintain efficacy. There are many contenders, but the leaders have not yet established their superiority.

CD—CISPLATIN-DOCETAXEL

Cisplatin. 75 mg/m^2 intravenously on day 1.

Docetaxel. 75 mg/m^2 intravenously on day 1.

NOTE: Remember hydration and premedication. Repeat the cycle every 21 days.

Selected Reading

Sengelov L et al. Docetaxel and cisplatin in metastatic urothelial cancer: a phase II study. J Clin Oncol 16: 3392–3397, 1998.

CMV—CISPLATIN-METHOTREXATE-VINBLASTINE

Methotrexate. 30 mg/m² intravenously on days 1 and 8.
Vinblastine. 4 mg/m² intravenously on days 1 and 8.
Cisplatin. 100 mg/m² intravenously over a 4-hour period on day 2 after vigorous hydration.
NOTE: Repeat the cycle every 3 weeks as tolerated. Wei et al use methotrexate 40 mg/m² on days 1 and 8, with acceptable toxicity.

Selected Readings

Harker WG et al. Cisplatin, methotrexate, and vinblastine (CMV): an effective chemotherapy regimen for metastatic transitional cell carcinoma of the urinary tract. J Clin Oncol 3: 1463–1470, 1985.

Wei CH et al. Adjuvant methotrexate, vinblastine and cisplatin chemotherapy for invasive transitional cell carcinoma: Taiwan experience. J Urol 155: 118–125, 1996.

DGC—DOCETAXEL-GEMCITABINE-CISPLATIN

Docetaxel. 35 mg/m² intravenously on days 1 and 8.
Gemcitabine. 800 mg/m² intravenously on days 1 and 8.
Cisplatin. 35 mg/m² intravenously on days 1 and 8.
NOTE: Prophylactic filgrastim (i.e., G-CSF) is given on days 3 to 6 and 10 to 15. Repeat the cycle every 3 weeks.

Selected Reading

Pectasides D et al. Weekly chemotherapy with docetaxel, gemcitabine and cisplatin in advanced transitional cell urothelial cancer: a phase II trial. Ann Oncol 13: 243–250, 2002.

GC—GEMCITABINE-CISPLATIN

Gemcitabine. 1,000 mg/m² intravenously on days 1, 8, and 15.
Cisplatin. 70 mg/m² intravenously on day 1 after gemcitabine.
NOTE: Cisplatin 70 mg/m² was given by Von der Maase et al one hour after gemcitabine on day 1. It was given on day 2 by Moore et al. Kaufman et al used cisplatin 75 mg/m² on day 1.

All authors repeated the cycle every 28 days. Von der Maase et al compared GC to MVAC and found a similar survival advantage but GC had a better safety profile and tolerability.

Selected Readings

Kaufman D et al. Phase II trial of gemcitabine plus cisplatin in patients with metastatic urothelial cancer. J Clin Oncol 18: 1921–1927, 2000.

Moore MJ et al. Gemcitabine plus cisplatin, an active regimen in advanced urothelial cancer: a phase II trial of the National Cancer Institute of Canada Clinical Trials Group. J Clin Oncol 17: 2876–2881, 1999.

Von der Maase H et al. Gemcitabine and cisplatin versus methotrexate, vinblastine, doxorubicin, and cisplatin in advanced or metastatic bladder cancer: results of a large, randomized, multinational, multicenter, phase III study. J Clin Oncol 18: 3068–3077, 2000.

ITP—IFOSFAMIDE-PACLITAXEL-CISPLATIN

Ifosfamide. 1,500 mg/m² intravenously on days 1, 2, and 3.
Paclitaxel. 200 mg/m² intravenously over 3 hours on day 3.
Cisplatin. 70 mg/m² intravenously on day 1.

NOTE: Repeat cycle every 28 days. Remember to use mesna for ifosfamide and hydration for cisplatin.

Selected Reading
Bajorin DF et al. Treatment of patients with transitional-cell carcinoma of the urothelial tract with ifosfamide, paclitaxel, and cisplatin: a phase II trial. J Clin Oncol 16: 2722–2727, 1998.

MAC—METHOTREXATE-DOXORUBICIN-CYCLOPHOSPHAMIDE

Methotrexate. 30 mg/m^2 intravenously on days 1 and 8.
Doxorubicin. 30 mg/m^2 intravenously on day 1.
Cyclophosphamide. 300 mg/m^2 intravenously on day 1.
NOTE: Repeat the cycle every 21 days.

Selected Reading
Tannock IF et al. Chemotherapy for metastatic transitional carcinoma of the urinary tract: a prospective trial of methotrexate, adriamycin, and cyclophosphamide (MAC) with cisplatinum for failure. Cancer 51: 216–219, 1983.

M-VAC—METHOTREXATE-VINBLASTINE-DOXORUBICIN-CISPLATIN

Methotrexate. 30 mg/m^2 intravenously on days 1, 15, and 22.
Vinblastine. 3 mg/m^2 intravenously on days 2, 15, and 22.
Doxorubicin. 30 mg/m^2 intravenously on day 2.
Cisplatin. 70 mg/m^2 intravenously on day 2 after vigorous hydration.
NOTE: On days 15 and 22, vinblastine (3 mg/m^2 intravenously) and methotrexate (30 mg/m^2 intravenously) are administered only if the white blood cell (WBC) count is greater than 2,500 cells/microL and the platelet count is greater than 100,000 cells/microL. Cycles are repeated every 28 days even if an interim dose is withheld because of myelosuppression or mucositis. The dose of doxorubicin is reduced to 15 mg/m^2 in patients who have received more than 2,000 cGy in 5 days to the pelvis. The use of filgrastim (i.e., granulocyte colony-stimulating factor, G-CSF) has allowed better adherence to the scheduled therapy with less neutropenia and its resulting toxicity.

Selected Readings
Gabrilove JL et al. Effect of granulocyte colony-stimulating factor on neutropenia and associated morbidity due to chemotherapy for transitional-cell carcinoma of the urothelium. N Engl J Med 318: 1414–1422, 1988.
Loehrer PJ et al. A randomized comparison of cisplatin alone or in combination with methotrexate, vinblastine and doxorubicin in patients with metastatic urothelial carcinoma: a cooperative group study. J Clin Oncol 10: 1066–1073, 1992.
Sternberg CN et al. Methotrexate, vinblastine, doxorubicin, and cisplatin for advanced transitional cell carcinoma of the urothelium. Cancer 64: 2448–2458, 1989.

M-VAC: HIGH DOSE

Methotrexate. 30 mg/m^2 intravenously on day 1.
Vinblastine. 4 mg/m^2 intravenously on day 2.
Doxorubicin. 30 mg/m^2 intravenously on day 2.
Cisplatin. 70 mg/m^2 intravenously on day 2.
Filgrastim (i.e., G-CSF). 240 microg/m^2 subcutaneously at alternating sites on days 4 to 10. May be extended to day 14 if necessary.
NOTE: Should be repeated at 14-day intervals for a minimum of 4 cycles or more if indicated and tolerated.

Selected Reading

Sternberg CN et al. Randomized phase III trial of high-dose-intensity methotrexate, vinblastine, doxorubicin, and cisplatin (MVAC) chemotherapy and recombinant human Granuloctye Colony-Stimulating Factor versus classic MVAC in advanced urothelial tract tumors: European Organization for Research and Treatment of Cancer Protocol No. 30924. J Clin Oncol 19: 2638–2646, 2001.

M-VEC—METHOTREXATE-EPIRUBICIN-VINBLASTINE-CISPLATIN

Methotrexate. 30 mg/m^2 intravenously on days 1, 15, and 22.
Vinblastine. 3 mg/m^2 intravenously on days 2, 15, and 22.
Epirubicin. 50 mg/m^2 intravenously on day 2.
Cisplatin. 70 mg/m^2 intravenously on day 2.
NOTE: M-VEC is a modification of M-VAC using epirubicin instead of doxorubicin to reduce cardiac toxicity. M-VECa is a further modification to reduce renal, gastrointestinal, and neural toxicity by substituting carboplatin 250 mg/m^2 on day 2 for cisplatin. The carboplatin regimen had the expected reduced toxicities and had increased hematological toxicity as anticipated but was significantly less effective in this trial. The study has been criticized for selecting a carboplatin dose that many regard as too low and not comparable to the cisplatin dose with which it was compared.

Selected Reading

Petrioli R et al. Comparison between a cisplatin-containing regimen and a carboplatin-containing regimen for recurrent or metastatic bladder cancer patients. Cancer 77: 344–351, 1996.

MVNC—METHOTREXATE-VINBLASTINE-MITOXANTRONE-CARBOPLATIN

Methotrexate. 50 mg/m^2 intravenously on days 1 and 15.
Vinblastine. 3 mg/m^2 intravenously on day 1.
Mitoxantrone. 10 mg/m^2 intravenously on day 1.
Carboplatin. 200 mg/m^2 intravenously on day 1.
NOTE: Repeat every 4 weeks. Leucovorin 15 mg (total) is given orally 24 hours after each dose of methotrexate. Only four courses are administered until there is evidence of incomplete but continuing response, in which case additional courses may be cautiously given.

Selected Reading

Waxman J et al. New combination chemotherapy programme for bladder cancer. Br J Urol 63: 68–71, 1989.

PC—PACLITAXEL-CARBOPLATIN

Paclitaxel. 225 mg/m^2 intravenously over 3 hours on day 1.
Carboplatin. To AUC 6 following paclitaxel on day 1.
NOTE: Repeat every 21 days. Redman et al used paclitaxel 200 mg/m^2 and carboplatin to AUC 5.

Selected Readings

Redman BG et al. Phase II trial of paclitaxel and carboplatin in the treatment of advanced urothelial cancer. J Clin Oncol 16: 1844–1848, 1998.
Vaughn DJ et al. Paclitaxel plus carboplatin in advanced carcinoma of the urothelium: an active and tolerable outpatient regimen. J Clin Oncol 16: 225–260, 1998

PCG—PACLITAXEL-CARBOPLATIN-GEMCITABINE

Paclitaxel. 200 mg/m^2 intravenously on day 1.
Carboplatin. To AUC 5 after paclitaxel on day 1.
Gemcitabine. 800 mg/m^2 on days 1 and 8.
NOTE: Repeat every 21 days.

Selected Reading

Hussain M et al. Combination paclitaxel, carboplatin, and gemcitabine is an active treatment for
  advanced urothelial cancer. J Clin Oncol 19: 2527–2533, 2001.

TG—PACLITAXEL-GEMCITABINE

Paclitaxel. 200 mg/m^2 intravenously over 1 hour on day 1.
Gemcitabine. 1,000 mg/m^2 intravenously on days 1, 8, and 15.
NOTE: Repeat cycles every 21 days for up to 6 courses.

Selected Reading

Meluch AA et al. Paclitaxel and gemcitabine chemotherapy for advanced transitional-cell carcinoma
  of the urothelial tract: a phase II trial of the Minnie Pearl Cancer Research Network. J Clin Oncol
  19: 3018–3024, 2001.

TP—PACLITAXEL-CISPLATIN

Paclitaxel. 175 mg/m^2 intravenously over 3 hours on day 1.
Cisplatin. 75 mg/m^2 intravenously following paclitaxel on day 1.
*NOTE: Repeat cycle every 21 days for up to 6 cycles. Use adequate hydration with
cisplatin.*

Selected Reading

Dreicer R et al. Phase II study of cisplatin and paclitaxel in advanced carcinoma of the urothelium:
  an Eastern Cooperative Oncology Group Study. J Clin Oncol 18: 1058–1061, 2000.

TPG—PACLITAXEL, CISPLATIN-GEMCITABINE

Paclitaxel. 80 mg/m^2 intravenously on days 1 and 8.
Cisplatin. 70 mg/m^2 intravenously on day 1.
Gemcitabine. 1,000 mg/m^2 intravenously on days 1 and 8.
NOTE: Repeat cycles every 21 days to a maximum of 6 cycles.

Selected Reading

Bellmunt J et al. Phase I-II study of paclitaxel, cisplatin, and gemcitabine in advanced transitional-
  cell carcinoma of the urothelium. J Clin Oncol 18: 3247–3255, 2000.

BRAIN TUMORS

Brain tumors are disproportionately devastating to the persona of the victim. They are
treated surgically when possible. Small tumors can sometimes be destroyed by gamma
knife therapy. Radiation therapy given postoperatively frequently prolongs survival. There
is increasing evidence that chemotherapy given concurrently with radiation can add
incrementally to survival. The approach differs somewhat depending on the
histology and whether the tumor is metastatic or primary. Single-agent chemotherapy
with carmustine (BCNU), temozolomide, irinotecan, thalidomide, lomustine (CCNU),
high-dose methotrexate, or cisplatin may be as effective (or ineffective) as combination

chemotherapy and is usually less toxic. Neo-adjuvant therapy is being evaluated. Childhood brain tumors are almost always treated on cooperative group studies. Metastatic brain tumors usually respond better to drugs that are efficacious in treatment of the primary. In the special case of primary CNS lymphoma, a regimen based on high-dose methotrexate appears to be more efficacious than the usual systemic therapy.

CARMUSTINE

Carmustine. 80 mg/m^2 intravenously on days 1 to 3.

NOTE: Carmustine was given concurrently with the first 3 days of a radiation course which consisted of 6,000 cGy given in 30 to 35 fractions, 5 days per week over 6 to 7 weeks to the whole brain through bilateral opposing ports. The drug was repeated every 6 to 8 weeks depending on clinical response, for at least two courses. The dose was reduced to 60 mg/m^2 per day for thrombocytopenia, leukopenia, or severe anemia. An additional dose reduction to 45 mg/m^2 per day was made if the same toxicity was observed after subsequent treatment. Some groups have attempted to simplify the chemotherapy by using carmustine 200 mg/m^2 as a single dose on day 1, extrapolating from a regimen used in gastrointestinal tumors. We know of no peer-reviewed studies using this dose in brain tumors.

Selected Reading

Walker MD et al. Randomized comparisons of radiotherapy and nitroso-ureas for the treatment of malignant glioma after surgery. N Engl J Med 303: 1323–1329, 1980.

IRINOTECAN

Irinotecan. 125 mg/m^2 intravenously over 90 minutes.

NOTE: Drug is repeated once weekly for 4 weeks followed by a 2-week rest period, which comprises one course. The dose of irinotecan will need to be increased in patients who are taking enzyme-inducing anticonvulsants such as phenytoin or phenobarbital.

Selected Reading

Friedman HS et al. Irinotecan therapy in adults with recurrent or progressive malignant glioma. J Clin Oncol 17: 1516–1525, 1999.

TEMOZOLOMIDE

Temozolomide (for chemotherapy-naïve patients). 200 mg/m^2 daily for 5 days.
(for patients previously treated with chemotherapy). 150 mg/m^2 daily for 5 days.
NOTE: Each cycle was repeated every 28 days.

Selected Readings

Chinot O-L et al. Safety and efficacy of temozolomide in patients with recurrent anaplastic oligodendrogliomas after standard radiotherapy and chemotherapy. J Clin Oncol 19: 2449–2455, 2001.

Osoba D et al. Health-related quality of life in patients treated with temozolomide versus procarbazine for recurrent glioblastoma multiforme. J Clin Oncol 18: 1481–1491, 2000.

Yung WKA et al. Multicenter phase II trial of temozolomide in patients with anaplastic astrocytoma or anaplastic oligoastrocytoma at first relapse. J Clin Oncol 17: 2762–2771, 1999.

THALIDOMIDE

Thalidomide. 800 mg daily for initial therapy with increases in dose by 200 mg daily every two weeks until 1,200 mg per day or maximum tolerated dose.

NOTE: This drug must be used with the utmost caution in females of child-bearing potential because of danger of congenital anomalies (refer to the manufacturer's regulated STEPS program for details). The drug is sedating and is best given at bedtime. Used alone, the results are not impressive. It was combined with temozolomide by Hwu et al in a recent study.

Selected Readings

Fine HA et al. Phase II trial of the anti-angiogenic agent thalidomide in patients with recurrent high-grade gliomas. J Clin Oncol 18: 708–715, 2000.

Hwu WJ et al. Treatment of metastatic melanoma in the brain with temozolomide and thalidomide. Lancet 2: 634–635, 2001.

CYCLOPHOSPHAMIDE-VINCRISTINE

Cyclophosphamide. Up to 1,000 mg/m^2 intravenously over a 1-hour period on days 1 and 2 as tolerated.

Vincristine. 1 mg/m^2 intravenously (maximum 2 mg) on day 1.

NOTE: Repeat every 3 or 4 weeks for 12 months or until progression.

Selected Reading

Longee DC et al. Treatment of patients with recurrent gliomas with cyclophosphamide and vincristine. J Neurosurg 72: 583–588, 1990.

PCV PLUS RT—LOMUSTINE-VINCRISTINE-PROCARBAZINE

Whole-brain radiation. 180 to 200 cGy/day to a total of 6,000 cGy.

Hydroxyurea. 400 mg/m^2 orally every other day of radiation therapy.

Within 14 days of completion of radiation therapy, give the following:

Lomustine. 110 mg/m^2 orally on day 1.

Procarbazine. 60 mg/m^2 orally on days 8 to 21.

Vincristine. 1.4 mg/m^2 intravenously (maximum 2 mg) on days 8 and 29.

NOTE: Repeat PCV every 6 to 8 weeks for 1 year or until tumor progression. This regimen apparently prolongs survival in astrocytoma but not in glioblastoma multiforme.

Selected Reading

Levin VA et al. Superiority of post-radiotherapy adjuvant chemotherapy with CCNU, procarbazine and vincristine (PCV) over BCNU for anaplastic gliomas: NCOG 6G61 final report. Int J Radiat Oncol Biol Phys 18: 321–324, 1990.

PRIMARY CNS LYMPHOMA

Methotrexate. 3,500 mg/m^2 intravenously over 2 hours given every other week for a total of 5 doses.

Intra-Ommaya methotrexate (preservative-free). 12 mg total dose given weekly on alternate weeks after systemic methotrexate.

Leucovorin. Rescue begins at 24 hours after each dose of systemic methotrexate (10 mg every 6 hours for at least 12 doses) and intra-Ommaya (10 mg every 12 hours for 8 doses).

Vincristine. 1.4 mg/m^2 (maximum 2.8 mg) concomitant with each dose of systemic methotrexate.

Procarbazine. 100 mg/m^2/day for 7 days with the first, third, and fifth dose of systemic methotrexate.

NOTE: Chemotherapy is followed by 4,500 cGy of whole-brain radiation therapy. Three weeks after completion of radiation therapy, patients receive two courses of high-dose cytarabine. Each course consists of two doses of 3,000 mg/m² intravenously over 3 hours separated by 24 hours. Patients need to be watched for development of neurotoxicity (e.g., cognitive impairment that may progress to ataxia, urinary incontinence, and loss of memory and executive function).

Selected Reading

Abrey LE et al. Treatment for primary CNS lymphoma: the next step. J Clin Oncol 18: 3144–3150, 2000.

BREAST CARCINOMA

Although it is now the second most common cause of cancer death in women, breast carcinoma remains the most frequent cancer in women. Initial therapy is usually surgical and often curative. Depending on stage, age, and receptor status, adjuvant therapy is frequently employed (i.e., radiation, hormonal, or cytotoxic chemotherapy or some combination thereof). Neo-adjuvant therapy is being evaluated for large, bulky tumors and may reduce the tumor size sufficiently to allow breast-conserving surgery and avoid mastectomy. Recurrent or metastatic disease is often palliated with hormonal manipulation if the tumor is estrogen receptor (ER) or progesterone receptor (PR) positive. Tamoxifen has been used for two decades. Several new hormonal agents have recently become available, including antiestrogens (e.g., toremifene, raloxifene), an estrogen receptor antagonist without known agonist effects (fulvestrant), aromatase inhibitors (e.g., anastrozole, letrozole, and exemestane), and luteinizing hormone-releasing hormone (LHRH) analogues (e.g., leuprolide and goserelin). The potential for combinations of some of these agents will open up new vistas for treatment. Many cytotoxic chemotherapeutic drugs have shown varying degrees of activity in the adjuvant or palliative treatment of breast cancer. Activity has more recently been demonstrated for paclitaxel, epirubicin, mitoxantrone, ifosfamide, cisplatin, etoposide, docetaxel, vinorelbine, capecitabine, and gemcitabine. Some of these drugs, e.g., vinorelbine and capecitabine, may be used as single agents (see Chapter 4). Various combinations of these agents have been and are being evaluated in clinical trials and some are in stage III trials with preliminary reports available. We list a few of the available regimens and a few of the early phase II trial combinations for salvage therapy with the caution that more experience with them is needed to establish their efficacy, dosage, and toxicity. In addition, the monoclonal antibody trastuzumab has been shown to be effective (alone and in combination with chemotherapy) in tumors that overexpress HER2 protein as measured by immunohistochemical testing (IHC), or better yet, by fluorescence in situ hybridization (FISH) testing. Finally, the high hopes for the curative potential of high-dose chemotherapy (HDC) with stem cell (bone marrow or peripheral blood stem cell) support have not been realized and the technique needs further experimental study in randomized clinical trials. To avoid the danger of inadvertently using HDC by error when that approach was in vogue, in the previous edition we listed a selection of some of those regimens in a separate chapter for information and perspective. In this edition, we do not list any HDC regimens with stem cell support for breast cancer. Again, we emphasize, as we did once before (Fischer DS. Need randomized clinical trials, not litigation. J Clin Oncol 16: 1237–1238, 1998), high-dose chemotherapy with stem cell support for the treatment of breast cancer should be used only in an IRB-approved, randomized, clinical trial.

ADJUVANT METHOTREXATE-FLUOROURACIL

Methotrexate. 100 mg/m^2 intravenously on days 1 and 8.
5-Fluorouracil. 600 mg/m^2 intravenously 1 hour after methotrexate on days 1 and 8.
Leucovorin. 10 mg/m^2 orally every 6 hours for six doses beginning 24 hours after methotrexate.
NOTE: A course is given every 28 days for 6 months. The original paper called for 12 months, but subsequent data in several studies has led to a consensus that 6 months is sufficient to achieve the same benefits.

Selected Readings

Fisher B et al. A randomized clinical trial evaluating sequential methotrexate and fluorouracil in the treatment of patients with node-negative breast cancer who have estrogen-receptor-negative tumors. N Engl J Med 320: 473–478, 1989.

Fisher B et al. Sequential methotrexate and fluorouracil for the treatment of node-negative breast cancer patients with estrogen receptor-negative tumors: eight-year results from National Surgical Adjuvant Breast and Bowel Project (NSABP) B-13 and first report of findings from NSABP B-19 comparing methotrexate and fluorouracil with conventional cyclophosphamide, methotrexate, and fluorouracil. J Clin Oncol 14: 1982–1992, 1996.

AC—DOXORUBICIN-CYCLOPHOSPHAMIDE

Doxorubicin. 60 mg/m^2 intravenously on day 1.
Cyclophosphamide. 600 mg/m^2 intravenously on day 1.
NOTE: Repeat the cycle every 21 days. Usual course is four cycles.

Selected Reading

Fisher B et al. Two months of doxorubicin-cyclophosphamide with and without interval re-induction therapy compared with six months of cyclophosphamide, methotrexate and fluorouracil in positive-node breast cancer patients with tamoxifen-nonresponsive tumors: results from the National Surgical Adjuvant Breast and Bowel Project B-15. J Clin Oncol 8: 1483–1496, 1990.

ATC—DOXORUBICIN-PACLITAXEL-CYCLOPHOSPHAMIDE

Doxorubicin. 90 mg/m^2 intravenously on days 1, 15, and 29.
Paclitaxel. 250 mg/m^2 intravenously as a 24-hour infusion on days 43, 57, and 71.
Cyclophosphamide. 3,000 mg/m^2 intravenously on days 85, 99, and 113.
NOTE: Each drug is repeated every 14 days for three courses, then the next drug for three courses, etc. For all nine cycles, support with filgrastim (i.e., G-CSF) 5 microg/kg subcutaneously. To avoid hypersensitivity reactions with paclitaxel, premedicate with the usual three-drug regimen of dexamethasone, diphenhydramine, and cimetadine or ranitidine or famotidine.

Selected Reading

Hudis CA et al. Sequential adjuvant therapy with doxorubicin/paclitaxel/cyclophosphamide for resectable breast cancer involving four or more axillary nodes. Semin Oncol 22(6 suppl 15): 18–23, 1995.

AT—DOXORUBICIN-PACLITAXEL

Doxorubicin. 50 mg/m^2 intravenously on day 1.
Paclitaxel. 220 mg/m^2 intravenously as a 3-hour infusion on day 2.
NOTE: Repeat the cycle every 3 weeks for up to 8 cycles. The Intergroup trial E 1193 followed a similar protocol but used a paclitaxel dose of 150 mg/m^2. See Paclitaxel-Doxorubicin, page 346.

Selected Reading

Jassem J et al. Doxorubicin and paclitaxel versus fluorouracil, doxorubicin, and cyclophosphamide as first-line therapy for women with metastatic breast cancer: final results of a randomized phase III multicenter trial. J Clin Oncol 19: 1707–1715, 2001.

CAF—CYCLOPHOSPHAMIDE-DOXORUBICIN-FLUOROURACIL

Cyclophosphamide. 500 mg/m^2 intravenously on day 1.
Doxorubicin. 50 mg/m^2 intravenously on day 1.
5-Fluorouracil. 500 mg/m^2 intravenously on day 1.
NOTE: Repeat the cycle every 21 days. The regimen differs from FAC in that 5-fluorouracil is given on days 1 and 8 in FAC but is given only once per course in this regimen.

Selected Readings

Smalley RV et al. A comparison of cyclophosphamide, Adriamycin, 5-fluorouracil, vincristine, prednisone (CMFVP) in patients with metastatic breast cancer. Cancer 40: 625–632, 1977.
Smalley RV. A comparison of cyclophosphamide, Adriamycin, and 5-fluorouracil (CAF) and cyclophosphamide, methotrexate, 5-fluorouracil, vincristine, and prednisone (CMFVP) in patients with advanced breast cancer. Breast Cancer Res Treat 3: 209–220, 1983.

CAF: HIGH DOSE, CYCLOPHOSPHAMIDE-DOXORUBICIN-FLUOROURACIL

Cyclophosphamide. 600 mg/m^2 intravenously on day 1.
Doxorubicin. 60 mg/m^2 intravenously on day 1.
5-Fluorouracil. 600 mg/m^2 intravenously on days 1 and 8.
NOTE: CAF, high dose produces neutropenia in the majority of cases and this may require G-CSF support. Repeat the courses every 28 days for four courses.

Selected Readings

Budman DR et al. Dose and dose intensity as determinants of outcome in the adjuvant treatment of breast cancer: the Cancer and Leukemia Group B. J Natl Cancer Inst 90: 1205–1211, 1998.
Wood WC et al. Dose and dose intensity of adjuvant chemotherapy for stage II, node-positive breast carcinoma. N Engl J Med 330: 1253–1259, 1994.

CAPECITABINE-DOCETAXEL

Capecitabine. 1,250 mg/m^2 twice daily orally for 14 days.
Docetaxel. 75 mg/m^2 intravenously over one hour on day 1.
NOTE: After 14 days of capecitabine, no treatment is given for one week. Repeat the cycle every 3 weeks.

Selected Reading

Food and Drug Administration. New combination therapy for advanced breast cancer. JAMA 286: 2085, 2001.

CAPECITABINE-PACLITAXEL

Capecitabine. 825 mg/m^2 orally twice daily for 14 days.
Paclitaxel. 175 mg/m^2 intravenously on day 1.
NOTE: After 14 days of capecitabine no treatment is given for one week. Regimen is repeated every 3 weeks.

Selected Reading
Villalona-Calero MA et al. A phase I and pharmacologic study of capecitabine and paclitaxel in breast cancer patients. Ann Oncol 12: 605–614, 2001.

CEF—CYCLOPHOSPHAMIDE-EPIRUBICIN-FLUOROURACIL

Cyclophosphamide. 75 mg/m^2 orally on days 1 to 14.
Epirubicin. 60 mg/m^2 intravenously on days 1 and 8.
Fluorouracil. 500 mg/m^2 intravenously on days 1 and 8.
NOTE: Repeat cycle every 28 days for 6 cycles.

Selected Reading
Levine MN et al. Randomized trial of intensive cyclophosphamide, epirubicin, and fluorouracil chemotherapy compared with cyclophosphamide, methotrexate, and fluorouracil in pre-menopausal women with node positive breast cancer. J Clin Oncol 16: 2651–2658, 1998.

CMF (ADJUVANT)—CYCLOPHOSPHAMIDE-METHOTREXATE-FLUOROURACIL

Below the age of 60 years:
Cyclophosphamide. 100 mg/m^2 orally on days 1 to 14.
Methotrexate. 40 mg/m^2 intravenously on days 1 and 8.
5-Fluorouracil. 600 mg/m^2 intravenously on days 1 and 8.
Above the age of 60 years:
Cyclophosphamide. 100 mg/m^2 orally on days 1 to 14.
Methotrexate. 30 mg/m^2 intravenously on days 1 and 8.
5-Fluorouracil. 400 mg/m^2 intravenously on days 1 and 8.
NOTE: Repeat the cycle every 28 days. Many clinicians make no change in dosage for patients over 60 years of age and use the higher dose for women of all ages.

Selected Readings
Bonadonna G et al. Combination chemotherapy as an adjuvant treatment in operable breast cancer. N Engl J Med 294: 405–410, 1976.
Bonadonna G et al. Adjuvant cyclophosphamide, methotrexate and fluorouracil in node-positive breast cancer: the results of 20 years of follow-up. N Engl J Med 332: 901–906, 1995.

CMF (INTRAVENOUS)—21 DAYS

Cyclophosphamide. 600 mg/m^2 intravenously every 21 days.
Methotrexate. 40 mg/m^2 intravenously every 21 days.
5-Fluorouracil. 600 mg/m^2 intravenously every 21 days.

Selected Reading
Weiss RB et al. Adjuvant chemotherapy after conservative surgery plus irradiation versus modified radical mastectomy. Am J Med 83: 455–463, 1987.

CMF (INTRAVENOUS)—28 DAYS

Cyclophosphamide. 600 mg/m^2 intravenously on days 1 and 8.
Methotrexate. 40 mg/m^2 intravenously on days 1 and 8.
5-Fluorouracil. 600 mg/m^2 intravenously on days 1 and 8.
NOTE: Repeat the cycle every 28 days.

Selected Reading

Bonadonna G et al. Milan adjuvant and neo-adjuvant studies in stage I and II resectable breast cancer. In Salmon SE, ed. Adjuvant Therapy of Cancer VI. Philadelphia, WB Saunders, 1990, pp 169–173.

CMFP—CYCLOPHOSPHAMIDE-METHOTREXATE-FLUOROURACIL-PREDNISONE

Cyclophosphamide. 100 mg/m^2 orally on days 1 to 14.
Methotrexate. 30 to 40 mg/m^2 intravenously on days 1 and 8.
5-Fluorouracil. 400 to 600 mg/m^2 intravenously on days 1 and 8.
Prednisone. 40 mg/m^2 orally on days 1 to 14.
NOTE: The lower dose is for patients over 65 years of age. Repeat the cycle every 28 days.

Selected Reading

Marschke RF et al. Randomized clinical trial of CFP versus CMFP in women with metastatic breast cancer. Cancer 63: 1931–1937, 1989.

CVAP-DOCETAXEL NEO-ADJUVANT

Cyclophosphamide. 1,000 mg/m^2 intravenously on day 1.
Doxorubicin. 50 mg/m^2 intravenously on day 1.
Vincristine. 1.5 mg/m^2 intravenously (maximum 2 mg) on day 1.
Prednisolone. 40 mg/day orally for 5 days on days 1 to 5.
*NOTE: Repeat the cycle every 28 days for 4 cycles. **Then:***
Docetaxel. 100 mg/m^2 is given as a one-hour infusion every 21 days with
Prednisolone. 100 mg/m^2 daily for 5 days orally, beginning one day before the docetaxel. The docetaxel-prednisolone regimen is repeated for a total of 4 cycles.

Suggested Reading

Smith IC et al. Neo-adjuvant chemotherapy in breast cancer: significantly enhanced response with docetaxel. J Clin Oncol 20: 1456–1466, 2002.

DOCETAXEL-AC-DOCETAXEL

Docetaxel. 100 mg/m^2 intravenously every 3 weeks for 4 cycles.
Followed by 4 cycles of AC:
Doxorubicin. 60 mg/m^2 intravenously every 3 weeks for 4 cycles.
Cyclophosphamide. 600 mg/m^2 intravenously every 3 weeks for 4 cycles.
NOTE: The AC cycle may be followed by 4 more cycles of docetaxel at the original dose.

Suggested Reading

Khayat D et al. Phase II study of sequential administration of docetaxel followed by doxorubicin and cyclophosphamide as first-line chemotherapy in metastatic breast cancer. J Clin Oncol 19: 3367–3375, 2001.

DOCETAXEL-DOXORUBICIN

Docetaxel. 75 mg/m^2 intravenously on day 1.
Doxorubicin. 50 mg/m^2 intravenously on day 1.

NOTE: Cycles are generally repeated every 3 weeks. In the study by von Minckwitz et al which was designed as neo-adjuvant therapy prior to surgery, some of the patients had cycles repeated every 2 weeks and received G-CSF on days 5 to 10. Both the 2- and the 3-week cycle group had surgery after 4 cycles. The study by Misset et al was designed for patients with metastatic disease and 6 to 8 cycles were given every 3 weeks and G-CSF was generally not necessary. The study by Miller et al was also neo-adjuvant therapy and gave doxorubicin 56 mg/m^2 and docetaxel 75 mg/m^2 every 3 weeks with G-CSF for 4 cycles prior to surgery.

Selected Readings

Miller KD et al. Combination versus sequential doxorubicin and docetaxel as primary chemotherapy for breast cancer: a randomized pilot trial of the Hoosier Oncology Group. J Clin Oncol 17: 3033–3037, 1999.

Misset JL et al. Dose-finding study of docetaxel and doxorubicin in first-line treatment of patients with metastatic breast cancer. Ann Oncol 10: 553–560, 1999.

Von Minckwitz G et al. Dose-dense doxorubicin, docetaxel, and granulocyte colony-stimulating factor support with or without tamoxifen as pre-operative therapy in patients with operable carcinoma of the breast: a randomized, controlled, open phase IIb study. J Clin Oncol 19: 3506–3515, 2001.

DOCETAXEL-VINORELBINE

Docetaxel. 30 mg/m^2 intravenously on days 1, 8, and 15.
Vinorelbine. 30 mg/m^2 intravenously on days 1 and 15.
NOTE: Repeat the cycle every 28 days for 6 cycles.

Selected Reading

Kornek GV et al. Treatment of advanced breast cancer with vinorelbine and docetaxel with or without human granulocyte colony-stimulating factor. J Clin Oncol 19: 621–627, 2001.

EPIRUBICIN-PACLITAXEL

Epirubicin. 80 mg/m^2 intravenously on day 1.
Paclitaxel. 175 mg/m^2 intravenously over 3 hours on day 1.
NOTE: Repeat the cycles every 21 days for 6 cycles.

Selected Reading

Fountzilas G et al. Dose-dense sequential chemotherapy with epirubicin and paclitaxel versus the combination as first-line chemotherapy, in advanced breast cancer: a randomized study conducted by the Hellenic Cooperative Oncology Group. J Clin Oncol 19: 2232–2239, 2001.

DOXORUBICIN-CMF

Doxorubicin. 75 mg/m^2 intravenously on day 1 every 21 days for four courses.
Then the CMF regimen as listed below is given every 21 days for 8 courses:
Cyclophosphamide. 600 mg/m^2 intravenously on day 1, beginning with course five.
Methotrexate. 40 mg/m^2 intravenously on day 1, beginning with course five.
5-Fluorouracil. 600 mg/m^2 intravenously on day 1, beginning with course five.
NOTE: This protocol is published as adjuvant therapy for patients with four or more involved nodes. Therapy is given every 21 days at full dose unless the patient is severely neutropenic or thrombocytopenic. In such a situation, therapy is postponed a week or, rarely, 2 weeks. The total therapy is 12 cycles, four of doxorubicin and eight of CMF.

Selected Readings

Bonadonna G et al. Sequential or alternating doxorubicin and CMF regimens in breast cancer with more than three positive nodes. JAMA 273: 542–547, 1995.

Buzzoni R et al. Adjuvant chemotherapy with doxorubicin plus cyclophosphamide, methotrexate, and fluorouracil in the treatment of resectable breast cancer with more than three positive axillary nodes. J Clin Oncol 9: 2134–2140, 1991.

DUKE HIGH-DOSE INTENSITY AFM

5-Fluorouracil. 750 mg/m^2 per day by continuous IV infusion on days 1 to 5.

Doxorubicin. 25 mg/m^2 intravenously on days 3 to 5.

Methotrexate. 250 mg/m^2 intravenously on day 15.

Leucovorin. 12.5 mg orally is started 24 hours after methotrexate and taken every 6 hours for six doses (total).

NOTE: Repeat the cycle every 21 days. The treatment can be given with an ambulatory infusion pump. The maximum doxorubicin dose (cumulative) is 400 to 450 mg/m^2. This program had been used for induction before high-dose chemotherapy with autologous bone marrow or peripheral stem cell support when that approach was being evaluated.

Selected Reading

Jones RB et al. The Duke AFM program: intensive induction chemotherapy for metastatic breast cancer. Cancer 66: 431–436, 1990.

FEC ADJUVANT—FLUOROURACIL-EPIRUBICIN-CYCLOPHOSPHAMIDE

5-Fluorouracil. 500 mg/m^2 intravenously on day 1.

Epirubicin. 100 mg/m^2 intravenously on day 1.

Cyclophosphamide. 500 mg/m^2 intravenously on day 1.

NOTE: Repeat the cycle every 21 days for 6 cycles. Radiotherapy was delivered to sites of known disease after completion of chemotherapy.

Selected Reading

French Adjuvant Study Group. Benefit of a high-dose epirubicin regimen in adjuvant chemotherapy for node-positive breast cancer patients with poor prognostic factor: 5-year follow-up results of French Adjuvant Study Group 05 randomized trial. J Clin Oncol 19: 602–611, 2001.

FEC METASTATIC—FLUOROURACIL-EPIRUBICIN-CYCLOPHOSPHAMIDE

5-Fluorouracil. 500 mg/m^2 intravenously on day 1.

Epirubicin. 60 mg/m^2 intravenously on day 1.

Cyclophosphamide. 500 mg/m^2 intravenously on day 1.

NOTE: Repeat the cycle every 28 days to a cumulative maximum epirubicin dose of 1,000 mg/m^2 or to evidence of progression.

Selected Reading

Blomqvist C et al. Influence of treatment schedule on toxicity and efficacy of cyclophosphamide, epirubicin, and fluorouracil in metastatic breast cancer: a randomized trial comparing weekly and every four week administration. J Clin Oncol 11: 467–473, 1993.

FEP—FLUOROURACIL-EPIRUBICIN-CISPLATIN

5-Fluorouracil. 200 mg/m^2 per day by continuous IV infusion on days 1 to 7.

Epirubicin. 50 mg/m^2 intravenously on day 1.
Cisplatin. 60 mg/m^2 intravenously on day 1.
NOTE: The 5-fluorouracil begins 4 hours prior to the cisplatin. The cisplatin is given over 1 hour after 4 hours of pre-hydration, followed by 6 hours of post-hydration. Cycles are repeated every 3 weeks to a maximum of eight cycles (epirubicin 400 mg/m^2). A prophylactic antiemetic regimen is necessary prior to therapy, as well as a delayed antiemetic regimen.

Selected Reading

Jones AL et al. Phase II study of continuous infusion fluorouracil with epirubicin and cisplatin in patients with metastatic and locally advanced breast cancer: an active new regimen. J Clin Oncol 12: 1259–1265, 1994.

GET—GEMCITABINE-EPIRUBICIN-PACLITAXEL

Gemcitabine. 1,000 mg/m^2 intravenously on days 1 and 4.
Epirubicin. 90 mg/m^2 intravenously on day 1.
Paclitaxel. 175 mg/m^2 intravenously over 3 hours on day 1.
NOTE: Grade 4 neutropenia is frequent, but the response rate is high. Repeat the cycle every 21 days for 6 cycles.

Selected Reading

Conte PF et al. Gemcitabine plus epirubicin plus taxol (GET) in advanced breast cancer: a phase II study. Breast Cancer Res Treat 68: 171–179, 2001.

GV—GEMCITABINE-VINORELBINE

Gemcitabine. 1,000 mg/m^2 intravenously on day 1.
Vinorelbine. 25 mg/m^2 intravenously on day 1.
NOTE: Repeat the cycle every 2 weeks for at least 6 cycles.

Selected Reading

Stathopoulos GP et al. Phase II trial of biweekly administration of vinorelbine and gemcitabine in pre-treated advanced breast cancer. J Clin Oncol 20: 37–41, 2002.

IFOSFAMIDE-MITOXANTRONE

Ifosfamide. 2,000 mg/m^2 intravenously over 1 hour on days 1 to 3.
Mesna. 400 mg/m^2 intravenously (bolus) immediately before and 4 hours after ifosfamide administration and 2,000 mg orally 8 hours after ifosfamide on days 1 to 3.
Mitoxantrone. 12 mg/m^2 intravenously on day 3.
NOTE: Repeat the cycle every 21 days.

Selected Reading

Perez JE et al. Ifosfamide and mitoxantrone as first line chemotherapy for metastatic breast cancer. J Clin Oncol 11: 461–466, 1993.

MINI-ICE—IFOSFAMIDE-CARBOPLATIN-ETOPOSIDE

Ifosfamide. 3,000 mg/m^2 intravenously on days 1 to 3.
Carboplatin. 200 mg/m^2 intravenously on days 1 and 2.
Etoposide. 150 mg/m^2 intravenously twice a day for 2 days on days 1 and 2.
Mesna. 1,000 mg/m^2 30 minutes before ifosfamide and 4 and 8 hours after ifosfamide on days 1 to 3.

NOTE: Ifosfamide is begun at time zero, administered over 1 hour, and is followed by etoposide over 11 hours. Then carboplatin is given over 1 hour followed by etoposide over 11 hours. Day 2 is a repetition of day 1. Day 3 involves only the ifosfamide and mesna. Repeat the cycle every 28 days.

Selected Reading

Perkins JB et al. Ifosfamide/carboplatin/etoposide chemotherapy for metastatic breast cancer with or without autologous hematopoietic stem cell transplantation: evaluation of dose response relationship. Semin Oncol 22(3 suppl 7): 5–8, 1995.

NFL—MITOXANTRONE-FLUOROURACIL-HIGH-DOSE LEUCOVORIN

Mitoxantrone. 12 mg/m^2 intravenously on day 1.
Leucovorin (high dose). 300 mg intravenously over 1 hour before 5-fluorouracil on days 1 to 3.
5-Fluorouracil. 350 mg/m^2 intravenously (bolus) by IV push on days 1 to 3.
NOTE: Repeat the cycle every 21 days. Patients older than 65 years receive mitoxantrone, 9 mg/m^2, on day 1 unless the leukocyte count is greater than 2000/microL; if so, they receive the full 12 mg/m^2.

Selected Readings

Hainsworth JD et al. Mitoxantrone, fluorouracil, and high-dose leucovorin: an effective, well-tolerated regimen for metastatic breast cancer. J Clin Oncol 9: 1731–1736, 1991.

Hainsworth JD et al. Mitoxantrone, 5-fluorouracil, and high dose leucovorin (NFL) versus intravenous cyclophosphamide, methotrexate, and 5-fluorouracil (CMF) in first-line chemotherapy for patients with metastatic breast carcinoma: a randomized phase II trial; Cancer 79: 740–748, 1997.

PACLITAXEL-CISPLATIN

Paclitaxel. 90 mg/m^2 intravenously over 3 hours on day 1.
Cisplatin. 60 mg/m^2 intravenously over 3 hours on day 1.
NOTE: Give the cisplatin after the paclitaxel infusion is completed. Repeat the cycle every 2 weeks if the neutrophil count is greater than 750/microL and platelet count greater than 75,000/microL. After a maximum of 8 cycles, patients may receive paclitaxel alone (90 mg/m^2) every other week.

Selected Readings

Sparano JA et al. Phase II trial of biweekly paclitaxel and cisplatin in advanced breast carcinoma: an Eastern Cooperative Oncology Group study. J Clin Oncol 15: 1880–1884, 1997.

Tolcher AW, Gelmon KA. Interim results of a phase I/II study of biweekly paclitaxel and cisplatin in patients with metastatic breast cancer. Semin Oncol 22(4 suppl 8): 28–32, 1995.

PACLITAXEL-DOXORUBICIN

Doxorubicin. 50 mg/m^2 intravenously followed 3 hours later by
Paclitaxel. 150 mg/m^2 intravenously over 24 hours.
NOTE: Repeat the cycle every 3 weeks for a maximum of 8 cycles.

Selected Reading

Sledge GW Jr. Phase III trial of doxorubicin, paclitaxel, and the combination of doxorubicin and paclitaxel as front-line chemotherapy for metastatic breast cancer: An intergroup trial (E1193). J Clin Oncol 21: 588–592, 2003.

PACLITAXEL-VINORELBINE

Vinorelbine. 30 mg/m^2 intravenously over 20 minutes on days 1 and 8.
Paclitaxel. 135 mg/m^2 intravenously over 3 hours. Infusion is given 1 hour after vinorelbine on day 1.
NOTE: Vinorelbine should be given over 6 to 10 minutes unless the patient has a central venous access device. Repeat the cycle every 28 days.

Selected Readings

Klassen U et al. Phase I/II study with paclitaxel in combination with weekly high-dose
   5-fluorouracil/folinic acid in the treatment of metastatic breast cancer: an interim analysis.
   Semin Oncol 22(6 suppl 14): 7–11, 1995.
Romero Acuna L et al. Vinorelbine and paclitaxel as first-line chemotherapy in metastatic breast
   cancer. J Clin Oncol 17: 74–81, 1999.

TRASTUZUMAB-DOCETAXEL

Docetaxel. 35 mg/m^2 intravenously on days 1, 8, and 15.
Trastuzumab. 2 mg/kg intravenously on days 1, 8, and 15.
NOTE: A loading dose of trastuzumab 4 mg/kg is delivered 1 day before the first cycle (day minus one). Repeat the cycle (but not the loading dose) every 28 days.

Selected Reading

Esteva FJ et al. Phase II study of weekly docetaxel and trastuzumab for patients with HER-
   2-overexpressing metastatic breast cancer. J Clin Oncol 20: 1800–1808, 2002.

TRASTUZUMAB-PACLITAXEL

Paclitaxel. 175 mg/m^2 intravenously over 3 hours every 3 weeks.
Trastuzumab. 2 mg/kg intravenously every week.
NOTE: Trastuzumab 4 mg/kg as a loading dose is administered one day before the first cycle. Six cycles or more may be given.

Selected Reading

Slamon DJ et al. Use of chemotherapy plus a monoclonal antibody against HER 2 for metastatic
   breast cancer that overexpresses HER 2. N Engl J Med 344: 783–792, 2001.

TRASTUZUMAB-VINORELBINE

Trastuzumab. 4 mg/m^2 loading dose intravenously over 90 minutes the day preceding the first cycle.
Trastuzumab. 2 mg/m^2 intravenously over 30 to 90 minutes every week as tolerated.
Vinorelbine. 25 mg/m^2 intravenously every week after trastuzumab with dose modifications for toxicity as listed in article.
NOTE: If dose modification causes vinorelbine to be delayed for more than 2 weeks, use G-CSF.

Selected Reading

Burstein HJ et al. Clinical activity of trastuzumab and vinorelbine in women with HER2-overexpress-
   ing metastatic breast cancer. J Clin Oncol 19: 2722–2730, 2001.

VINORELBINE-DOXORUBICIN

Doxorubicin. 50 mg/m^2 intravenously on day 1.
Vinorelbine. 25 mg/m^2 intravenously on days 1 and 8.

NOTE: Repeat the cycle every 3 weeks up to toxicity or a maximum of 9 cycles (450 mg/m² of doxorubicin).

Selected Readings

Hochster HS. A combined doxorubicin/vinorelbine (Navelbine) therapy in the treatment of advanced breast cancer. Semin Oncol 22(2 suppl 5): 55–60, 1995.

Norris B et al. Phase III comparative study of vinorelbine combined with doxorubicin versus doxorubicin alone in disseminated metastatic/recurrent breast cancers: National Cancer Institute of Canada Clinical Trials Group study. J Clin Oncol 18: 2385–2394, 2000.

Spielmann M et al. Phase II trial of vinorelbine/doxorubicin as first-line therapy of advanced breast cancer. J Clin Oncol 12: 1764–1770, 1994.

CARCINOID (MALIGNANT) AND ISLET CELL CARCINOMA

These are not common tumors. The carcinoid syndrome occurs in about 10% of patients with malignant carcinoid. When it occurs, consider the use of the somatostatin analogue octreotide before chemotherapy for carcinoid. For metastatic disease, the active palliative agents include doxorubicin, cisplatin, streptozocin, 5-fluorouracil, cyclophosphamide, and interferon-alfa. There are no convincing randomized studies demonstrating the superiority of combination regimens over single-agent therapy.

FAC-S—FLUOROURACIL-DOXORUBICIN-CYCLOPHOSPHAMIDE-STREPTOZOCIN

5-Fluorouracil. 400 mg/m² (300 mg/m²) intravenously on days 1 and 8.
Doxorubicin. 30 mg/m² (15 mg/m²) intravenously on day 1.
Cyclophosphamide. 75 mg/m² (50 mg/m²) orally on days 1 to 14.
Streptozocin. 400 mg/m² (200 mg/m²) intravenously on days 1 and 8.
NOTE: Poor-risk patients were given the doses in parentheses. Poor risk was defined by any one of the following: age older than 70 years, total bilirubin level greater than 1.5 mg/dL, SGOT level greater than three times normal, 5-hydroxyindoleacetic acid (5-HIAA) level greater than 150 mg/24 hours, carcinoid syndrome, or bone marrow involvement by tumor. Repeat the cycle every 4 weeks.

Patients with heart disease did not receive doxorubicin but were given the following:

5-Fluorouracil. 600 mg/m² (400 mg/m²) intravenously on days 1 and 8.
Cyclophosphamide. 100 mg/m² (75 mg/m²) orally on days 1 to 14.
Streptozocin. 600 mg/m² (400 mg/m²) intravenously on days 1 and 8.

Selected Reading

Bukowski RM et al. A phase 2 trial of combination chemotherapy in patients with metastatic carcinoid tumors: a Southwest Oncology Group study. Cancer 60: 2891–2895, 1987.

OCTREOTIDE

Octreotide acetate. 150 microg subcutaneously 3 times a day for symptomatic relief of severe diarrhea and flushing.
NOTE: Mild symptoms can usually be handled with standard antidiarrheal agents. More debilitating symptoms may be palliated with octreotide. The drug is commercially available as Sandostatin. Within the first 2 weeks of therapy, doses may range from 100 to 600 microg/day in 2 to 4 divided doses, but the mean is about 300 microg/day. When symptoms have improved sufficiently, the long-acting preparation, Sandostatin LAR, may be given as 20 microg intramuscularly intragluteally at 4-week intervals. It is prudent to continue the subcutaneous preparation for 2 to 4 weeks to

be sure that the long-acting preparation is giving adequate control of symptoms before discontinuing it. Then the dose of the long-acting preparation can be increased or decreased according to symptoms.

Suggested Reading

Kvols LK et al. Treatment of the malignant carcinoid syndrome: evaluation of a long-acting somato-statin analogue. N Engl J Med 315: 663–666, 1986.

SC—STREPTOZOCIN-CYCLOPHOSPHAMIDE

Streptozocin. 500 mg/m^2/day intravenously on days 1 to 5.
Cyclophosphamide. 1,000 mg/m^2 intravenously on day 1.
NOTE: Repeat streptozocin every 6 weeks and cyclophosphamide every 3 weeks. If the 5-HIAA level exceeds 150 mg/24 hours or there are florid manifestations of the carcinoid syndrome, begin with half doses and gradually work up to the recommended doses.

Selected Reading

Moertel CG, Hanley JA. Combination chemotherapy trials in metastatic carcinoid syndrome. Cancer Clin Trials 2: 327–334, 1979.

SD—STREPTOZOCIN-DOXORUBICIN (ISLET CELL CARCINOMA OR CARCINOID)

Streptozocin. 500 mg/m^2/day intravenously on days 1 to 5.
Doxorubicin. 50 mg/m^2 intravenously on days 1 and 22.
NOTE: Repeat the cycle every 42 days. The cumulative dose of doxorubicin should not exceed 500 mg/m^2.

Selected Reading

Moertel CG et al. Streptozocin-doxorubicin, streptozocin-fluorouracil, or chlorozotocin in the treatment of advanced islet-cell carcinoma. N Engl J Med 326: 519–523, 1992.

SF—STREPTOZOCIN-FLUOROURACIL

Streptozocin. 500 mg/m^2/day intravenously on days 1 to 5.
5-Fluorouracil. 500 mg/m^2/day intravenously (bolus) on days 1 to 5.
NOTE: Repeat the cycle every 28 days.

Selected Reading

Chernicoff D et al. Combination chemotherapy for islet cell carcinoma and metastatic carcinoid tumors with 5-fluorouracil and streptozotocin. Cancer Treat Rep 63: 795–796, 1979.

CARCINOMA OF UNKNOWN PRIMARY

Carcinoma of unknown primary (CUP) accounts for about 3% to 9% of all cancers. These patients present with biopsy-confirmed metastatic disease, with no known primary organ involved. They should be designated as having neoplasia of unknown primary site. Some are poorly differentiated and with special histochemical studies (e.g., immunoperoxidase staining) will be found to be melanomas, sarcomas, neuroendocrine tumors, mesotheliomas, lymphomas, or germ cell tumors and should be treated as such. Some remain undiagnosed even at autopsy. Other more differentiated tumors that present in the axilla in women are usually breast cancers, whereas those that present in the lymph nodes of the neck are usually of respiratory origin (i.e., lung, esophagus, pharynx, or larynx) or occasionally of thyroid or breast origin and are treated accordingly. Still others are fairly well differentiated adenocarcinomas below the diaphragm and are usually of pancreatic, prostatic, or ovarian origin.

CARBOPLATIN-PACLITAXEL

Carboplatin. At AUC 6, intravenously followed by
Paclitaxel. 200 mg/m^2 intravenously as a 3-hour infusion.
NOTE: Repeat the cycle every 21 days to a maximum of 8 cycles. This regimen was effective in patients with nodal, pleural, and peritoneal disease.

Selected Reading

Briasoulis E et al. Carboplatin plus paclitaxel in unknown primary carcinoma: a phase II Hellenic Cooperative Oncology Group study. J Clin Oncol 18: 3101–3107, 2000.

DOCETAXEL-CISPLATIN OR DOCETAXEL-CARBOPLATIN

Docetaxel. 75 mg/m^2 intravenously.
Cisplatin. 75 mg/m^2 intravenously.
    OR
Docetaxel. 65 mg/m^2 intravenously.
Carboplatin. At AUC of 6 intravenously.
NOTE: Repeat the cycle (either regimen) every 3 weeks to a maximum of 8 courses of therapy.

Selected Reading

Greco FA et al. Carcinoma of unknown primary site: phase II trials with docetaxel plus cisplatin or carboplatin. Ann Oncol 11: 211–215, 2000.

GCP—GEMCITABINE-CARBOPLATIN-PACLITAXEL

Gemcitabine. 1,000 mg/m^2 intravenously on days 1 and 8.
Carboplatin. At AUC 6 intravenouly on day 1.
Paclitaxel. 200 mg/m^2 intravenously over 1 hour on day 1.
NOTE: Repeat the cycle every 21 days for 4 cycles. Responding patients may continue on paclitaxel 70 mg/m^2 weekly for 6 weeks with 2 weeks of no therapy. This 8-week cycle may be given 3 times if response continues.

Selected Reading

Greco FA et al. Gemcitabine, carboplatin, and paclitaxel for patients with carcinoma of unknown primary site: a Minnie Pearl Cancer Research Network study. J Clin Oncol 20: 1651–1656, 2002.

PACLITAXEL-CARBOPLATIN-ETOPOSIDE

Paclitaxel. 200 mg/m^2 intravenously over 1 hour on day 1.
Carboplatin. At AUC 6 intravenously on day 1.
Etoposide. 50 mg/100 mg total dose, orally, alternating on days 1 to 10.
NOTE: Repeat the cycle every 21 days for 4 cycles.

Selected Readings

Greco FA et al. Carcinoma of unknown primary site. Cancer 89: 2655–2660, 2000.
Hainsworth JD et al. Carcinoma of unknown primary site: treatment with 1-hour paclitaxel, carboplatin and extended-schedule etoposide. J Clin Oncol 15: 2385–2393, 1997.

PVB—CISPLATIN-VINBLASTINE-BLEOMYCIN AND
PEB—CISPLATIN-ETOPOSIDE-BLEOMYCIN

Cisplatin. 20 mg/m^2 intravenously on days 1 to 5.
Vinblastine. 0.15 mg/kg intravenously on days 1 and 2.
Bleomycin. 30 units total, intravenously on days 2, 9, and 16 of each course.

OR

Cisplatin. 20 mg/m^2 intravenously on days 1 to 5.
Etoposide. 100 mg/m^2 intravenously on days 1 to 5.
Bleomycin. 30 units total intravenously on day 1, 8 and 15 of each course.
NOTE: Repeat the cycle every 3 weeks for three or four cycles. Many find PEB more efficacious and less toxic.

Selected Readings

Greco FA et al. Advanced poorly differentiated carcinoma of unknown
    primary site: recognition of a treatable syndrome. Ann Intern Med 104: 547–553, 1986.
Hainsworth JD et al. The role of cisplatin/bleomycin-based chemotherapy
    in the treatment of poorly differentiated carcinoma of unknown primary site. Semin Oncol
    19(2 suppl 5): 54–57, 1992.

CERVICAL CARCINOMA

Early diagnosis has dramatically reduced the death rate because early-stage disease is frequently curable by surgery and/or radiation therapy. Current studies suggest that the efficacy of radiation is enhanced by the concomitant use of hydroxyurea or cisplatin. Neo-adjuvant therapy is being evaluated. Recurrent or metastatic disease is treated with chemotherapy for palliation. There are no controlled studies demonstrating a superior response to combination chemotherapy compared with single-drug therapy, but several studies are in progress to evaluate some new combinations. Further considerations include histology, renal function, and the effect of prior radiation therapy, which may change the sensitivity of the tumor to therapeutic agents and can compromise the pelvic bone marrow.

ADENOCARCINOMA REGIMEN

5-Fluorouracil. 500 to 800 mg/m^2 intravenously as a total dose by continuous infusion over a 76-hour period.
Doxorubicin. 40 to 50 mg/m^2 intravenously as a total dose by continuous infusion over a 76-hour period.
Cisplatin. 50 to 60 mg/m^2 intravenously as a total dose by continuous infusion over a 76-hour period.
NOTE: Repeat cycle every 28 days.

Selected Reading

Kavanagh JJ et al. Combination chemotherapy for metastatic or recurrent adenocarcinoma of the
    cervix. J Clin Oncol 10: 1621–1623, 1987.

BIC—BLEOMYCIN-IFOSFAMIDE-CARBOPLATIN

Bleomycin. 30 units intravenously on day 1.
Ifosfamide. 2,000 mg/m^2/day intravenously over 2 hours on days 1 to 3.
Carboplatin. 200 mg/m^2 intravenously on day 1.
Mesna. 400 mg/m^2 intravenously at 15 minutes, at 4 hours, and at 8 hours (800 mg/m^2 if given orally) after the start of each dose of ifosfamide.

NOTE: Repeat the cycle every 28 days. Treatment is usually given on an outpatient basis.

Selected Reading

Murad AM et al. Phase II trial of bleomycin, ifosfamide, and carboplatin in metastatic cervical cancer. J Clin Oncol 12: 55–59, 1994.

BIP—BLEOMYCIN-IFOSFAMIDE-CISPLATIN

Bleomycin. 30 units intravenously in 3 L of 5% dextrose or normal saline over a 24-hour period on day 1.

Cisplatin. 50 mg/m^2 intravenously by slow bolus on day 2.

Ifosfamide. 5,000 mg/m^2 intravenously in 3 L of 5% dextrose or normal saline as a continuous infusion over a 24-hour period on day 2.

Mesna. 6,000 mg/m^2 administered intravenously by continuous infusion concurrent with the ifosfamide and for 12 hours thereafter.

NOTE: During treatment, maintain the urine output at 100 mL/hour. Repeat the cycle every 21 days.

Selected Reading

Buxton EJ et al. Combination bleomycin, ifosfamide, and cisplatin chemotherapy in cervical cancer. J Natl Cancer Inst 81: 359–361, 1989.

CISPLATIN-VINORELBINE

Cisplatin. 80 mg/m^2 intravenously on day 1.

Vinorelbine. 25 mg/m^2 intravenously on days 1 and 8.

NOTE: This therapy is given to women with cancer of the uterine cervix who have not been previously treated with chemotherapy. Repeat the cycle every 3 weeks for 3 courses. For those who had locoregional disease, surgery or radiation therapy may be offered. For stage IVB or recurrent disease, responders may be given up to 6 cycles as tolerated.

Selected Reading

Pignata S et al. Phase II study of cisplatin and vinorelbine as first-line chemotherapy in patients with carcinoma of the uterine cervix. J Clin Oncol 17: 756–760, 1999.

IFOSFAMIDE-CARBOPLATIN

Ifosfamide. 5,000 mg/m^2 intravenously by continuous infusion on day 1.

Carboplatin. 300 mg/m^2 intravenously over 30 minutes on day 1.

Mesna. 9,200 mg total dose intravenously by continuous 36-hour infusion starting on day 1.

NOTE: Repeat the cycle every 4 weeks if WBC count exceeds 3,000/microL, platelet count exceeds 100,000/microL, and the creatinine clearance is greater than or equal to 60 mL/minute. If these levels are not reached, delay up to 2 weeks as necessary.

Selected Reading

Kuhnle H et al. Phase II study of carboplatin/ifosfamide in untreated advanced cervical cancer. Cancer Chemother Pharmacol 26: S33–S35, 1990.

MVAC—METHOTREXATE-VINBLASTINE-DOXORUBICIN-CISPLATIN

Methotrexate. 30 mg/m^2 intravenously on days 1, 15, and 22.

Vinblastine. 3 mg/m^2 intravenously on days 2, 15, and 22.

Doxorubicin. 30 mg/m^2 intravenously on day 2.
Cisplatin. 70 mg/m^2 intravenously on day 2.
NOTE: Repeat the cycle every 28 days to 2 cycles beyond complete regression for a maximum of 6 cycles.

Selected Reading

Long HJ et al. Phase II trial of methotrexate, vinblastine, doxorubicin, and cisplatin in advanced/ recurrent carcinoma of the uterine cervix and vagina. Gynecol Oncol 57: 235–239, 1995.

COLON CARCINOMA

This is a surgically treatable and often curable tumor when confined to the bowel. There is convincing evidence in stage III (Duke's C) that adjuvant chemotherapy with 5-fluorouracil and leucovorin can significantly delay recurrence and may prolong life. It is not yet clear whether this is true of stage II (Duke's B). Metastatic disease (stage IV) may be palliated with chemotherapy with 5-fluorouracil alone or with leucovorin or interferon-alfa, as well as with other modulators in a variety of combinations. Irinotecan and oxaliplatin are drugs that have significant activity in patients who fail 5-fluorouracil therapy. Raltitrexed is an antifolate drug that has been in use in Europe and other countries for several years and shows promise for colon carcinoma. Single-agent intravenous fluorouracil and irinotecan have demonstrated activity and the combination of irinotecan, 5-fluorouracil, and leucovorin has been approved by the FDA as a first-line regimen. The combination of 5-fluorouracil, leucovorin, and oxaliplatin has been approved by the FDA for those failing first-line therapy, but some clinicians use it up-front. Single-agent capecitabine is active orally and is being evaluated in combination regimens. Hepatic artery infusion of floxuridine is useful in patients with predominant liver metastases.

CAPECITABINE—SINGLE AGENT

Capecitabine. 1,250 mg/m^2 orally twice a day.
NOTE: The total daily dose is 2,500 mg/m^2 per day rounded to the nearest dose that can be given with the 500 mg and 150 mg tablets. Treatment is continued for 14 days of a 21-day cycle. Doses should be given about 12 hours apart with water and within 30 minutes of ingestion of a meal, usually breakfast and supper.

Selected Readings

Hoff PM et al. Comparison of oral capecitabine versus intravenous fluorouracil plus leucovorin as first-line treatment in 605 patients with metastatic colorectal cancer: results of a randomized phase III study. J Clin Oncol 19: 2282–2292, 2001.
Van Cutsem E et al. Oral capecitabine compared with intravenous fluorouracil plus leucovorin in patients with metastatic colorectal cancer: results of a large phase III study. J Clin Oncol 19: 4097–4106, 2001.

FLUOROURACIL—SINGLE AGENT, BOLUS

5-Fluorouracil. 500 mg/m^2/day intravenously on days 1 to 5.
NOTE: Repeat the cycle every 5 weeks. In this study 7 different regimens were evaluated, including leucovorin and PALA-modulated regimens. No regimen provided substantial improvement relative to 5-FU bolus or single-agent therapy for either response or survival in the treatment of disseminated colorectal cancer. Single-agent continuous infusion regimens gave similar responses with a more favorable toxicity profile, but required indwelling catheters and ambulatory infusion pumps.

Selected Reading

Leichman CG et al. Phase II study of fluorouracil and its modulation in advanced colorectal cancer: a Southwest Oncology Group study. J Clin Oncol 13: 1303–1311, 1995.

FLUOROURACIL—SINGLE AGENT, CONTINUOUS INFUSION

Fluorouracil. 300 mg/m^2/day intravenously as continuous infusion.
NOTE: The drug is given by ambulatory infusion pump through an indwelling catheter. If significant toxicity develops, the dose is decreased 50 mg/m^2/day to a tolerable level. Therapy is continued for 10 weeks or more as tolerated or until progression of disease.

Selected Reading

Lokich JJ et al. A prospective randomized comparison of continuous infusion fluorouracil with a conventional bolus schedule in metastatic colorectal carcinoma: a Mid-Atlantic Oncology Program study. J Clin Oncol 7: 425–432, 1989.

IMPACT STUDY-FLOUROURACIL-LEUCOVORIN

5-Fluorouracil. 370 to 400 mg/m^2/day intravenously on days 1 to 5.
Leucovorin. 200 mg/m^2/day intravenously on days 1 to 5.
NOTE: Repeat the cycle every 28 days for 6 cycles.

Selected Reading

International Multicentre Pooled Analysis of Colon Cancer Trials (IMPACT) Investigators. Efficacy of adjuvant fluorouracil and folinic acid in colon cancer. Lancet 345: 939–944, 1995.

FLUOROURACIL-INTERFERON ALFA-2a

5-Fluorouracil. 750 mg/m^2/day intravenously by continuous infusion on days 1 to 5 and then 750 mg/m^2/week intravenously by bolus beginning on day 15.
Interferon alfa-2a. 9 million units subcutaneously 3 times weekly beginning on day 1.

Selected Readings

Wadler S et al. Fluorouracil and recombinant alfa-2a-interferon: an active regimen against advanced colorectal carcinoma. J Clin Oncol 7: 1769–1775, 1989.

Wadler S et al. Phase II trial of fluorouracil and recombinant interferon alfa-2a in patients with advanced colorectal carcinoma: an Eastern Cooperative Oncology Group study. J Clin Oncol 9: 1806–1810, 1991.

FLUOROURACIL-LEUCOVORIN: HIGH-DOSE (ROSWELL PARK REGIMEN)

Leucovorin. 500 mg/m^2 intravenously as a 2-hour infusion on days 1, 8, 15, 22, 29, and 36.
5-Fluorouracil. 600 mg/m^2 intravenously by IV bolus 1 hour after the start of leucovorin on days 1, 8, 15, 22, 29, and 36.
NOTE: Repeat the cycle every 8 weeks until progression or excessive toxicity. In the United States, this is a commonly used regimen. Jager et al in Germany compared a regimen of fluorouracil 500 mg/m^2 with either leucovorin 500 mg/m^2 or 20 mg/m^2 and found that the high-dose leucovorin regimen was more toxic but not superior to the low-dose leucovorin regimen in response rate and survival, and therefore preferred the low-dose regimen.

Selected Reading

Jager E et al. Weekly high-dose leucovorin versus low-dose leucovorin combined with fluorouracil in advanced colorectal cancer: results of a randomized multicentre trial. Study Group for Palliative Treatment of Metastatic Colorectal Cancer Study Protocol 1. J Clin Oncol 14: 2274–2279, 1996.

Petrelli N et al. A prospective randomized trial of 5-fluorouracil versus 5-fluorouracil and high-dose leucovorin versus 5-fluorouracil and methotrexate in previously untreated patients with advanced colorectal carcinoma. J Clin Oncol 5: 1559–1565, 1987.

Petrelli N et al. The modulation of fluorouracil with leucovorin in metastatic colorectal carcinoma: a prospective randomized phase III trial of the Gastrointestinal Tumor Study group. J Clin Oncol 7: 1419–1426, 1989.

FLUOROURACIL-LEUCOVORIN: LOW-DOSE (MAYO CLINIC AND NCCTG STUDY GROUP)

5-Fluorouracil. 425 mg/m^2/day intravenously by bolus on days 1 to 5.

Leucovorin. 20 mg/m^2/day intravenously by bolus on days 1 to 5.

NOTE: Repeat the cycle at 4 weeks, 8 weeks, and then every 5 weeks.

Selected Readings

Buroker TR et al. Randomized comparison of two schedules of fluorouracil and leucovorin in the treatment of advanced colorectal cancer. J Clin Oncol 12: 14–20, 1994.

O'Connell MJ et al. Controlled trial of fluorouracil and low-dose leucovorin given for 6 months as postoperative adjuvant therapy for colon carcinoma. J Clin Oncol 15: 245–250, 1997.

Poon MA et al. Biochemical modulation of fluorouracil with leucovorin: confirmatory evidence of improved therapeutic efficacy in advanced colorectal cancer. J Clin Oncol 9: 1967–1972, 1991.

FLUOROURACIL-LEUCOVORIN-OXALIPLATIN—BIMONTHLY (FOLFOX4)

Oxaliplatin. 85 mg/m^2 intravenously over 2 hours on day 1.

Leucovorin. 200 mg/m^2/day intravenously as a 2-hour infusion (on days 1 and 2) followed by

5-Fluorouracil. 400 mg/m^2/day intravenously as a bolus, followed by

5-Fluorouracil. 600 mg/m^2/day as a continuous infusion on days 1 and 2.

NOTE: Repeat the cycle every 2 weeks until disease progression. The oxaliplatin on day 1 may be given concurrently with the leucovorin as long as both drugs are mixed in dextrose 5% water. Oxaliplatin is incompatible with 0.9% sodium chloride.

Selected Readings

Andre T et al. Multicenter phase II study of bimonthly high-dose leucovorin, fluorouracil infusion, and oxaliplatin for metastatic colorectal cancer resistant to the same leucovorin and fluorouracil regimen. J Clin Oncol 17: 3560–3568, 1999.

De Gramont A et al. Leucovorin and fluorouracil with or without oxaliplatin as first-line treatment in advanced colorectal cancer. J Clin Oncol 18: 2938–2947, 2000.

HEPATIC ARTERY INFUSION WITH FLOXURIDINE FOR LIVER METASTASES

Floxuridine (FUDR). 0.30 mg/kg/day.

Leucovorin. 15 mg/m^2/day.

Dexamethasone. 20 mg/day total dose.

NOTE: Infuse all three drugs into the hepatic artery through an implantable pump for 14 days alternating with heparinized isotonic saline. Repeat the cycle every 28 days. In a later publication, this group has modified the way they calculate the floxuridine dose and now uses 0.16 mg/kg/day – pump volume/pump flow rate (total mg = mg/kg × pump volume/pump flow rate). They have also omitted the leucovorin and now give intravenous irinotecan 100 mg/m^2 over 30 minutes every week for 3 weeks of a 28-day cycle.

Selected Readings

Kemeny N et al. Phase I study of hepatic arterial infusion of floxuridine and dexamethasone with systemic irinotecan for unresectable hepatic metastases from colorectal cancer. J Clin Oncol 19: 2687–2695, 2001.

Kemeny N et al. Phase II study of hepatic arterial floxuridine, leucovorin, and dexamethasone for unresectable liver metastases from colorectal cancer. J Clin Oncol 12: 2288–2295, 1994.

IRINOTECAN—SINGLE AGENT

Irinotecan. 125 mg/m^2/week intravenously for 4 weeks followed by a 2-week rest (Pitot et al). In view of frequent need to reduce dose at weeks 3 and 4, some groups are trying this therapy for 2 weeks and resting 1 week for a 3-week cycle instead of a 6-week cycle.

OR

Irinotecan. 350 mg/m^2 intravenously every 3 weeks (Rougier et al).
NOTE: An intensive loperamide regimen is essential for the management of diarrhea.

Selected Readings

Pitot HC et al. Phase II trial of irinotecan in patients with metastatic colorectal carcinoma. J Clin Oncol 15: 2910–2919, 1997.

Rougier P et al. Phase II study of irinotecan in the treatment of advanced colorectal cancer in chemotherapy-naïve patients and patients pretreated with fluorouracil-based chemotherapy. J Clin Oncol 15: 251–260, 1997.

IFL—IRINOTECAN-FLUOROURACIL-LEUCOVORIN (BOLUS—SALTZ)

Irinotecan. 125 mg/m^2/week intravenously on days 1, 8, 15, and 22.
5-Fluorouracil. 500 mg/m^2/week intravenously on days 1, 8, 15, and 22.
Leucovorin. 20 mg/m^2/week intravenously on days 1, 8, 15, and 22.
NOTE: A cycle consists of 4 weeks of therapy followed by a 2-week rest. This 6-week cycle is repeated as tolerated. An intensive loperamide regimen for the management of diarrhea is essential. Nonetheless, 2 NCI-sponsored cooperative group studies reported 44 early deaths using this regimen. Most of the deaths were due to a gastrointestinal syndrome (i.e., diarrhea, nausea, and vomiting) or unexpected cardiovascular and thromboembolic events or neutropenia leading to sepsis. The safety and monitoring boards of the NCCTG and of the CALGB suspended their trials. At a December 6, 2001 meeting of the FDA Oncologic Drugs Advisory Committee (ODAC), it was agreed to continue the approval of this regimen for first-line treatment of patients with metastatic colorectal cancer. The prescribing information was revised to include statements that

> *...patients with diarrhea should be carefully monitored and given fluid and electrolyte replacement if they become dehydrated, or antibiotic therapy if they develop ileus, fever or severe neutropenia...*

In addition,

> *...After the first treatment, subsequent weekly chemotherapy treatments should be delayed in patients with active diarrhea until return of pretreatment bowel function for at least 24 hours without need for antidiarrhea medication. If grade 2, 3, or 4 late diarrhea occurs, subsequent doses of irinotecan should be decreased within the current cycle...*

As the drug is better understood and more widely used, it may be necessary to check for genetic polymorphisms of the UGT1A1 promoter that seems to correlate with pharmacokinetic handling of SN-38, the active metabolite, and toxicity.

Suggested Readings

Ratain MJ. Irinotecan dosing: does the CPT in CPT-11 stand for "cannot predict toxicity?" J Clin Oncol 20: 7–8, 2002.

Rothenberg ML et al. Mortality associated with irinotecan plus bolus fluorouracil/leucovorin: summary findings of an independent panel. J Clin Oncol 19: 3801–3807, 2002.

Saltz LB et al. Phase I clinical and pharmacokinetic study of irinotecan, fluorouracil, and leucovorin in patients with advanced solid tumors. J Clin Oncol 14: 2959–2967, 1996.

Saltz LB et al. Irinotecan plus fluorouracil and leucovorin for metastatic colorectal cancer. N Engl J Med 343: 905–914, 2000.

Sargent DL et al. Recommendations for caution with irinotecan, fluorouracil, and leucovorin for colorectal cancer. N Engl J Med 345: 144–146, 2001.

IRINOTECAN-FLUOROURACIL-LEUCOVORIN (INFUSIONAL—DOUILLARD)

Irinotecan. 180 mg/m^2 intravenously on day 1.
5-Fluorouracil. 400 mg/m^2 intravenously as a bolus.
5-Fluorouracil. 600 mg/m^2/day intravenously as a 22-hour infusion for 2 consecutive days, on days 1 and 2.
Leucovorin. 200 mg/m^2 intravenously on days 1 and 2.
NOTE: Therapy is given every 2 weeks until disease progression or patient decides to stop. Early deaths have been reported with this regimen, but not as many as with the Saltz protocol. An intensive loperamide regimen for the management of diarrhea is essential. Dose reductions may be necessary to ameliorate severe toxicity.

Suggested Reading

Douillard JY et al. Irinotecan combined with fluorouracil compared with fluorouracil alone as first-line treatment for metastatic colorectal cancer: a multicenter randomized trial. Lancet 355: 1041–1047, 2000.

OXALIPLATIN-CAPECITABINE

Oxaliplatin. 130 mg/m^2 intravenously on day 1.
Capecitabine. 1,250 mg/m^2 orally twice a day on days 1 to 14.
NOTE: Repeat the cycle every 3 weeks. In patients who have received prior chemotherapy the capecitabine dose is reduced to 1,000 mg/m^2 twice a day.

Selected Reading

Borner MM et al. Phase II study of capecitabine and oxaliplatin in first- and second-line treatment of advanced or metastatic colorectal cancer. J Clin Oncol 20: 1759–1766, 2002.

OXALIPLATIN-FLUOROURACIL-LEUCOVORIN

Oxaliplatin. 130 mg/m^2 intravenously on day 1.
5-Fluorouracil. 350 mg/m^2 intravenously on days 1 to 5.
Leucovorin. 20 mg/m^2 intravenously on days 1 to 5.
NOTE: Repeat the cycles every 21 days for a maximum of 6 cycles.

Selected Reading

Ravaioli A et al. Bolus fluorouracil and leucovorin with oxaliplatin as first-line treatment in metastatic colorectal cancer. J Clin Oncol 20: 2545–2550, 2002.

OXALIPLATIN-IRINOTECAN

Oxaliplatin. 85 mg/m^2 as a 2-hour infusion on day 1 followed by

Irinotecan. 175 mg/m² as a 2-hour infusion on day 1.
NOTE: Repeat the cycle every 14 days for 6 months as tolerated or until evidence of progressive disease. An intensive course of loperamide for the management of diarrhea is essential.

Suggested Reading

Scheithauer W et al. Randomized multicenter phase II trial of oxaliplatin plus irinotecan versus raltitrexed as first-line treatment in advanced colorectal cancer. J Clin Oncol 20: 165–172, 2002.

ENDOMETRIAL CANCER

Endometrial cancer is the most common malignancy of the female genital tract in the United States. Early disease is usually curable with surgery and/or radiation therapy. For recurrent or metastatic disease, some single agents provide palliative relief. Combination chemotherapy can also be palliative.

CAP—CYCLOPHOSPHAMIDE-DOXORUBICIN-CISPLATIN

Cyclophosphamide. 500 mg/m² intravenously on day 1.
Doxorubicin. 50 mg/m² intravenously on day 1.
Cisplatin. 50 mg/m² intravenously on day 1.
NOTE: Repeat the cycle every 4 weeks for 6 courses.

Selected Readings

Burke TW et al. Postoperative adjuvant cisplatin, doxorubicin, and cyclophosphamide chemotherapy in women with high-risk endometrial carcinoma. Gynecol Oncol 55: 47–50, 1994.
Hancock KC et al. Use of cisplatin, doxorubicin, and cyclophosphamide to treat advanced and recurrent adenocarcinoma of the endometrium. Cancer Treat Rep 70: 789–791, 1986.

CISPLATIN-DOXORUBICIN

Doxorubicin. 50 mg/m² intravenously on day 1.
Cisplatin. 50 mg/m² intravenously on day 1.
NOTE: Repeat every 3 weeks for eight cycles. More toxic than doxorubicin alone for a small, but statistically significant, therapeutic advantage.

Selected Reading

Deppe G et al. Treatment of recurrent and metastatic endometrial carcinoma with cisplatin and doxorubicin. Eur J Gynaecol Oncol 15: 263–266, 1994.

DOXORUBICIN ALONE OR WITH CYCLOPHOSPHAMIDE

Doxorubicin. 60 mg/m² intravenously every 3 weeks for 8 cycles
                                OR
Doxorubicin. 60 mg/m² intravenously with
Cyclophosphamide. 500 mg/m² intravenously.
NOTE: The combination is also given every 3 weeks for 8 cycles and appears to offer a small advantage over doxorubicin alone at the expense of more frequent and severe myelosuppression and gastrointestinal toxicity.

Selected Reading

Thigpen JT et al. A randomized comparison of doxorubicin alone versus doxorubicin plus cyclophosphamide in the management of advanced or recurrent endometrial carcinoma: a Gynecologic Oncology Group study. J Clin Oncol 12: 1408–1414, 1994.

MEDROXYPROGESTERONE ACETATE—ORALLY

Medroxyprogesterone acetate. 200 mg/day (total dose) orally.
NOTE: Continue medication until unacceptable toxicity or disease progression.

Selected Reading

Thigpen JT et al. Oral medroxyprogesterone acetate in the treatment of advanced or recurrent
endometrial carcinoma: a dose-response study by the Gynecologic Oncology Group. J Clin
Oncol 17: 1736–1744, 1999.

PAVM—CISPLATIN-DOXORUBICIN-ETOPOSIDE-MEGESTROL ACETATE

Cisplatin. 20 mg/m^2/day intravenously on days 1, 2, and 3.
Doxorubicin. 40 mg/m^2 intravenously on day 1.
Etoposide. 75 mg/m^2/day intravenously on days 1, 2, and 3.
Megestrol acetate. 40 mg orally 4 times a day.
NOTE: Repeat the cycle every 28 days as tolerated or until recurrence or a maximum of 10 courses.

Selected Reading

Cornelison TL et al. Cisplatin, adriamycin, etoposide, megestrol acetate versus melphalan,
5-fluorouracil, medroxyprogesterone acetate in the treatment of endometrial carcinoma. Gynecol
Oncol 59: 243–248, 1995.

PACLITAXEL—SINGLE AGENT

Paclitaxel. 175 mg/m^2 intravenously every 3 weeks.
*NOTE: The dose recommended has variously been 170 mg/m^2, 175 mg/m^2, and
250 mg/m^2 given over 3 hours or 24 hours for up to a maximum of 10 cycles if the
patient remains responsive or discontinued for toxicity or relapse.*

Selected Readings

Ball HG et al. A phase II trial of paclitaxel in patients with advanced or recurrent adenocarcinoma of the endometrium: a Gynecologic Oncology Group study. Gynecol Oncol
62: 278–281, 1996.
Lissoni A et al. Phase II study of paclitaxel as salvage treatment in advanced endometrial cancer.
Ann Oncol 7: 861–863, 1996.
Thigpen JT et al. Phase II trial of paclitaxel in patients with progressive ovarian carcinoma after platinum-based chemotherapy: a Gynecologic Oncology Group study. J Clin Oncol 12: 1748–1753,
1994.

PACLITAXEL-CARBOPLATIN

Carboplatin. At AUC 6 intravenously.
Paclitaxel. 175 mg/m^2 intravenously over 3 hours.
NOTE: Repeat the cycle every 4 weeks.

Selected Reading

Hoskins PJ et al. Paclitaxel and carboplatin, alone or with irradiation, in advanced or recurrent
endometrial cancer: a phase II study. J Clin Oncol 19: 4048–4053, 2001.

TAMOXIFEN

Tamoxifen. 20 mg orally twice a day.
NOTE: Continue until toxicity or recurrence.

7

ENDOMETRIAL CANCER

Selected Reading

Quinn MA, Campbell JJ. Tamoxifen therapy in advanced/recurrent endometrial carcinoma. Gynecol Oncol 32: 1–3, 1989.

ESOPHAGEAL CARCINOMA

Upper esophageal (cervical) cancer is primarily squamous cell carcinoma and associated with smoking and alcohol consumption. Lower (thoracic and gastroesophageal) cancer is usually adenocarcinoma and is less clearly so associated and may have other etiologies. At presentation, 50% of cases appear to be locoregional and 50% disseminated. After careful staging, about 80% are found to be disseminated. Combination chemotherapy is used as neo-adjuvant, concomitant with radiation, or after recurrence or metastasis.

CISPLATIN-FLUOROURACIL-RADIATION THERAPY

5-Fluorouracil. 1,000 mg/m^2/day for 4 days intravenously by continuous infusion on days 1 to 4 of weeks 1, 5, 8, and 11.
Cisplatin. 75 mg/m^2 intravenously (at 1 mg/min) on day 1 of each cycle on weeks 1, 5, 8, and 11.
NOTE: Radiation therapy is given concurrently as 200 cGy 5 days a week with a total of 3,000 cGy of regional treatment and 2,000 cGy to a boost field (total 5,000 cGy) in 5 weeks.

Selected Reading

Herskovic A et al. Combined chemotherapy and radiotherapy compared with radiotherapy alone in patients with cancer of the esophagus. N Engl J Med 326: 1593–1598, 1992.

CISPLATIN-VINBLASTINE-FLUOROURACIL

Cisplatin. 20 mg/m^2/day for 5 days intravenously by continuous infusion on days 1 to 5 and 17 to 21.
Vinblastine. 1 mg/m^2/day intravenously by bolus on days 1 to 4 and 17 to 20.
5-Fluorouracil. 300 mg/m^2/day for 21 days intravenously by continuous infusion on days 1 to 21.
NOTE: Radiation therapy is given in daily fractions of 250 cGy 5 days per week to a total of 3,750 cGy over a period of 21 days. When possible, radiation therapy may be delivered at 150 cGy twice a day for 5 days a week to a total dose of 4,500 cGy over the 21-day period. After a 3-week rest, surgery (transhiatal esophagectomy) is performed on day 42 if feasible.

Selected Readings

Forastiere AA et al. Concurrent chemotherapy and radiation therapy followed by transhiatal esophagectomy for local-regional cancer of the esophagus. J Clin Oncol 8: 119–127, 1990.

Forastiere AA et al. Preoperative chemoradiation followed by transhiatal esophagectomy for carcinoma of the esophagus: final report. J Clin Oncol 11: 1118–1123, 1993.

ECF—EPIRUBICIN-CISPLATIN-FLUOROURACIL

Epirubicin. 50 mg/m^2 intravenously on day 1.
Cisplatin. 60 mg/m^2 intravenously on day 1.
5-Fluorouracil. 200 mg/m^2/day intravenously by protracted (continuous) venous infusion (PVI).
NOTE: Epirubicin and cisplatin were repeated every 3 weeks. 5-Fluorouracil PVI was given by ambulatory infusion pump. ECF was given as long as tolerated up to 6 months or until progression.

Selected Reading

Ross P et al. Prospective randomized trial comparing mitomycin, cisplatin, and protracted venous-infusion fluorouracil (PVI 5-FU) with epirubicin, cisplatin, and PVI 5-FU in advanced esophago-gastric cancer. J Clin Oncol 20: 1996–2004, 2001.

FAP—FLUOROURACIL-DOXORUBICIN-CISPLATIN

5-Fluorouracil. 600 mg/m^2 intravenously on days 1 and 8.
Doxorubicin. 30 mg/m^2 intravenously on day 1.
Cisplatin. 75 mg/m^2 intravenously on day 1 with hydration and mannitol diuresis.
NOTE: Repeat the cycle every 4 weeks.

Selected Reading

Gisselbrecht C et al. Fluorouracil (F), Adriamycin (A), and cisplatin (P) (FAP): combination chemotherapy of advanced esophageal carcinoma. Cancer 52: 974–977, 1983.

INTERFERON ALFA-FLUOROURACIL

5-Fluorouracil. 750 mg/m^2/day by continuous infusion on days 1 to 5 followed by a weekly outpatient bolus of 750 mg/m^2.
Interferon alfa-2a. 9 million units 3 times a week from day 1.

Selected Reading

Kelsen D et al. Interferon alfa-2a and fluorouracil in the treatment of patients with advanced esophageal cancer. J Clin Oncol 10: 269–274, 1992.

IRINOTECAN-CISPLATIN

Irinotecan. 65 mg/m^2 intravenously on day 1.
Cisplatin. 30 mg/m^2 intravenously on day 1.
NOTE: The drugs were given weekly for 4 weeks followed by a 2-week rest period. Treatment was repeated every 6 weeks.

Selected Reading

Ilson DH et al. Phase II trial of weekly irinotecan plus cisplatin in advanced esophageal cancer. J Clin Oncol 17: 3270–3275, 1999.

NEOADJUVANT FLUOROURACIL-CISPLATIN

Cisplatin. 20 mg/m^2/day for 5 days intravenously over 1 hour on days 1 to 5.
5-Fluorouracil. 1,000 mg/m^2/day intravenously by continuous infusion over 20 hours on days 1 to 5.
NOTE: The first course is given in the hospital. The 5-fluorouracil is given over 20 hours to allow the cisplatin to be administered. Doses are increased or decreased in subsequent courses (some of which may be given as outpatient therapy) depending on predetermined criteria of toxicity, which are outlined in the report. Two preoperative and three or four postoperative courses are given. Repeat the cycle every 21 days for up to six courses maximum. For unresectable disease a radiation therapy course is outlined with concomitant 5-fluorouracil.

Selected Reading

Ajani JA et al. Prolonged chemotherapy for localized squamous carcinoma of the esophagus. Eur J Cancer 28A: 880–884, 1992.

PACLITAXEL-CISPLATIN-FLUOROURACIL

Paclitaxel. 175 mg/m^2 intravenously over 3 hours on day 1.
Cisplatin. 20 mg/m^2/day intravenously on days 1 to 5.
5-Fluorouracil. 750 mg/m^2/day intravenously by continuous infusion on days 1 to 5.
NOTE: Cycle is repeated every 3 weeks for 3 courses and then cisplatin dose is reduced to 15 mg/m^2 for the next 3 courses.

Selected Reading

Ilson DH et al. A phase II trial of paclitaxel, fluorouracil, and cisplatin in patients with advanced carcinoma of the esophagus. J Clin Oncol 16: 1826–1834, 1998.

PREOPERATIVE CHEMORADIATION AND POSTOPERATIVE ADJUVANT CHEMOTHERAPY

Cisplatin. 20 mg/m^2/day for 5 days intravenously by continuous infusion on days 1 to 5 and 26 to 30.
5-Fluorouracil. 225 mg/m^2/day intravenously by continuous infusion on days 1 to 30.
NOTE: Radiation therapy is given at a daily dose of 200 cGy up to a total of 4,400 cGy, with the spinal cord dose limited to 4,000 cGy. Esophagectomy or esophagogastrectomy is performed approximately 4 weeks after completion of chemoradiotherapy if the blood counts are adequate and there is no evidence of untreated metastases. Adjuvant chemotherapy is given to patients who have total gross removal of disease and negative margins (RO resection) about 8 to 12 weeks later, after recovery from surgery and when blood counts are adequate. Chemotherapy consists of:
Paclitaxel. 175 mg/m^2 intravenously over 24 hours on day 1.
Cisplatin. 25 mg/m^2 intravenously on day 2.
Adjuvant chemotherapy is repeated every 3 weeks for 3 cycles.

Selected Reading

Heath EI et al. Phase II evaluation of preoperative chemoradiation and postoperative adjuvant chemotherapy for squamous cell and adenocarcinoma of the esophagus. J Clin Oncol 18: 868–876, 2000.

GASTRIC ADENOCARCINOMA

Treatment of choice is surgical attempt at cure when localized and resectable.
Adjuvant therapy may be radiation or chemotherapy or a combination thereof.

EAP-II—ETOPOSIDE-DOXORUBICIN-CISPLATIN

Etoposide. 100 mg/m^2/day intravenously on days 1 to 3.
Doxorubicin. 40 mg/m^2 intravenously on day 1.
Cisplatin. 80 mg **total** dose intravenously in divided doses over 1 to 3 days.
NOTE: Dose is reduced in patients over 65 years. Repeat the cycle every 21 days. Claimed to be less toxic than original EAP.

Selected Reading

Haim N et al. Treatment of gastric adenocarcinoma with the combination of etoposide, adriamycin and cisplatin (EAP): comparison between two schedules. Oncology 51: 102–107, 1994.

ECF—EPIRUBICIN-CISPLATIN-FLUOROURACIL

Epirubicin. 50 mg/m^2 intravenously on day 1.

Cisplatin. 60 mg/m^2 intravenously on day 1.
5-Fluorouracil. 200 mg/m^2/day for 21 days intravenously by continuous infusion.
NOTE: Epirubicin and cisplatin are given every 3 weeks for up to 8 cycles while 5-fluorouracil is given for 21 weeks or more.

Selected Readings

Findlay M et al. A phase II study in advanced gastro-esophageal cancer using epirubicin and cisplatin in combination with continuous infusion 5-fluorouracil (ECF). Ann Oncol 5: 609–616, 1994.
Waters JS et al. Long-term survival after epirubicin, cisplatin and fluorouracil for gastric cancer: results of a randomized trial. Br J Cancer 80: 269–272, 1999.

ELF—ETOPOSIDE-LEUCOVORIN-FLUOROURACIL

Etoposide. 120 mg/m^2/day intravenously over 1 hour on days 1 to 3.
Leucovorin. 300 mg/m^2/day intravenously over 2 hours on days 1 to 3.
5-Fluorouracil. 500 mg/m^2/day intravenously by IV bolus midway through the leucovorin infusion on days 1 to 3.
NOTE: Give leucovorin immediately after etoposide. Repeat the cycle every 4 or 5 weeks.

Selected Readings

Wilke H et al. Etoposide, folinic acid, and 5-fluorouracil in carboplatin-pretreated patients with advanced gastric cancer. Cancer Chemother Pharmacol 29: 83–84, 1991.
Wilke H et al. New developments in the treatment of gastric carcinoma. Semin Oncol 17(suppl 2): 61–70, 1990.

FAM—FLUOROURACIL-DOXORUBICIN-MITOMYCIN

5-Fluorouracil. 600 mg/m^2 intravenously on days 1, 8, 29, and 36.
Doxorubicin. 30 mg/m^2 intravenously on days 1 and 29.
Mitomycin. 10 mg/m^2 intravenously on day 1.
NOTE: Repeat the cycle every 56 days. The efficacy and therapeutic index of this regimen has been questioned by a prospectively randomized trial showing no improvement in survival versus 5-fluorouracil alone (Cullinan et al).

Selected Readings

Cullinan SA et al. A comparison of three chemotherapeutic regimens in the treatment of advanced pancreatic and gastric carcinoma: fluorouracil versus fluorouracil and doxorubicin versus fluorouracil, doxorubicin, and mitomycin. JAMA 253: 2061–2067, 1985.
Macdonald JS et al. 5-Fluorouracil, doxorubicin, and mitomycin (FAM) combination chemotherapy for advanced gastric cancer. Ann Intern Med 93: 533–536, 1980.

FAMTX—FLUOROURACIL-DOXORUBICIN-METHOTREXATE

5-Fluorouracil. 1,500 mg/m^2 intravenously on day 1 (given 1 hour after the end of the methotrexate infusion).
Methotrexate. 1,500 mg/m^2 intravenously on day 1.
Leucovorin. 15 mg/m^2 orally every 6 hours for 48 hours starting 24 hours after methotrexate.
Doxorubicin. 30 mg/m^2 intravenously on day 15.
NOTE: Repeat the cycle every 4 weeks.

Selected Readings

Kelsen D et al. FAMTX versus etoposide, doxorubicin, and cisplatin: a random assignment trial in gastric cancer. J Clin Oncol 10: 541–548, 1992.

7

GASTRIC ADENOCARCINOMA

Wils J et al. An EORTC Gastrointestinal Group evaluation of the combination of sequential methotrexate and 5-fluorouracil, combined with Adriamycin in advanced measurable gastric cancer. J Clin Oncol 4: 1799–1803, 1986.

FAP—FLUOROURACIL-DOXORUBICIN-CISPLATIN

5-Fluorouracil. 300 mg/m^2/day intravenously by bolus on days 1 to 5.
Doxorubicin. 40 mg/m^2 intravenously on day 1.
Cisplatin. 60 mg/m^2 intravenously, following hydration, on day 1.
NOTE: Repeat the cycle every 5 weeks.

Selected Reading

Moertel CG et al. Phase II study of combined 5-fluorouracil, doxorubicin, and cisplatin in the treatment of advanced upper gastrointestinal adenocarcinoma. J Clin Oncol 4: 1053–1057, 1986.

IRINOTECAN-CISPLATIN

Irinotecan. 70 mg/m^2 intravenously on days 1 and 15.
Cisplatin. 80 mg/m^2 intravenously on day 1.
NOTE: Repeat the cycle every 28 days.

Selected Reading

Boku N et al. Phase II study of a combination of irinotecan and cisplatin against metastatic gastric cancer. J Clin Oncol 17: 319–323, 1999.

PCF—PACLITAXEL-CISPLATIN-FLUOROURACIL

Paclitaxel. 175 mg/m^2 intravenously as a 3-hour infusion on days 1 and 22.
Cisplatin. 50 mg/m^2 intravenously as a 1-hour infusion on days 8 and 29.
5-Fluorouracil. 2,000 mg/m^2 intravenously by 24-hour infusion on days 1, 8, 15, 22, 29, and 36 following leucovorin.
Leucovorin. 500 mg/m^2 intravenously as a 2-hour infusion on days 1, 8, 15, 22, 29, and 36.
NOTE: Six weeks of therapy (days 1, 8, 15, 22, 29, 36) followed by 2 weeks rest is considered a cycle.

Selected Reading

Kollmannsberger C et al. A phase II study of paclitaxel, weekly, 24-hour continuous infusion 5-fluorouracil, folinic acid and cisplatin in patients with advanced gastric cancer. Br J Cancer 83: 458–462, 2000.

PEF—CISPLATIN-ETOPOSIDE-FLUOROURACIL

Cisplatin. 20 mg/m^2/day for 5 days intravenously on days 1 to 5.
Etoposide. 100 mg/m^2 intravenously on days 1, 3 and 5.
5-Fluorouracil. 800 mg/m^2/day for 5 days intravenously by continuous infusion on days 1 to 5.
NOTE: Repeat the cycle every 3 weeks for 3 cycles after a presumed curative gastric or gastro-esophageal resection.

Selected Reading

Ryoo BY et al. Adjuvant (cisplatin, etoposide, and 5-fluorouracil) chemotherapy after curative resection of gastric adenocarcinoma involving the esophagogastric junction. Am J Clin Oncol 22: 253–257, 1999.

TC—DOCETAXEL-CISPLATIN
Docetaxel. 85 mg/m^2 intravenously on day 1.
Cisplatin. 75 mg/m^2 intravenously on day 1.
NOTE: Repeat the cycle every 3 weeks for up to 8 cycles or toxicity or recurrence.

Selected Reading
Roth AD et al. Docetaxel (taxotere)-cisplatin (TC): an effective drug combination in gastric carcinoma.
  Swiss Group for Clinical Cancer Research (SAKK) and the European Institute of Oncology (EIO).
  Ann Oncol 11: 301–306, 2000.

GIST—GASTROINTESTINAL STROMAL TUMORS

IMATINIB (STI 571) (GLEEVEC®)
Imatinib. 400 mg daily or twice daily as tolerated.
NOTE: Therapy is continued for 8 weeks or more to minimal disease as tolerated.

Selected Readings
Joensuu H et al. Effect of the tyrosine kinase inhibitor STI 571 in a patient with metastatic
  gastrointestinal stromal tumor. N Engl J Med 344: 1052–1056, 2001.
Van Oosterom AT et al. Safety and efficacy of imatinib (STI 571) in metastatic gastrointestinal
  stromal tumors: a phase I study. Lancet 358: 1421–1423, 2001.

GESTATIONAL TROPHOBLASTIC DISEASE

Gestational trophoblastic disease (GTD) is a group of diseases that extends over the range of the relatively benign hydatidiform mole, invasive mole, or placental site trophoblastic tumor to the choriocarcinoma with its high potential for widespread metastasis and high mortality without therapy. Fortunately, the tumor is rare. In good-prognosis cases (low-risk), single-agent methotrexate or dactinomycin are usually sufficient. In more aggressive disease (moderate-risk), combination chemotherapy is usually effective using several drugs. In high-risk cases, multidrug combinations including etoposide are necessary but incur a 1.5% risk of a secondary neoplasm (Rustin GJS et al. Combination but not single-agent methotrexate chemotherapy for gestational trophoblastic tumors increases the incidence of second tumors. J Clin Oncol 14: 2769–2773, 1996). Response to therapy can be followed by the fall in the human chorionic gonadotropin level or its beta-subunit, which serves as a marker for residual tumor. In experienced hands and with early therapy, the overall cure rate is 96%. Hence, all patients with GTD should be referred promptly to a center with oncologists experienced in the management of this tumor.

APE—DACTINOMYCIN-CISPLATIN-ETOPOSIDE (HIGH-RISK)
Dactinomycin. 0.3 mg/m^2 intravenously on days 1 to 3 and 14 to 16.
Cisplatin. 100 mg/m^2 intravenously on day 1.
Etoposide. 100 mg/m^2 intravenously (or 200 mg/m^2 orally) on days 1 to 3 and 14 to 16.
NOTE: Repeat the cycle every 4 weeks.

Selected Reading
Theodore C et al. Treatment of high-risk gestational trophoblastic disease with chemotherapy combination containing cisplatin and etoposide. Cancer 64: 1824–1828, 1989.

EMA-CO—ETOPOSIDE-METHOTREXATE-DACTINOMYCIN-CYCLOPHOSPHAMIDE-VINCRISTINE (HIGH-RISK)

Etoposide. 100 mg/m^2 intravenously on days 1 and 2.

Methotrexate. 300 mg/m^2 intravenously as a 12-hour infusion on day 1.

Dactinomycin. 0.5 mg intravenously on days 1 and 2.

Leucovorin. 15 mg orally twice a day on days 2 and 3.

Cyclophosphamide. 600 mg/m^2 intravenously on day 8.

Vincristine. 0.8 mg/m^2 intravenously on day 8 (maximum 2 mg).

NOTE: For high-risk patients, this regimen is repeated every 2 weeks until remission or failure. After 12 courses, a rest period is frequently necessary. In their later publication, this group treated failures by substituting cisplatin 75 mg/m^2 intravenously on day 8 for the cyclophosphamide and adding etoposide 150 mg/m^2 intravenously on day 8 instead of the vincristine. This change caused many patients to develop neutropenia and thrombocytopenia and in those cases, the etoposide and dactinomycin were omitted on day 2.

Selected Readings

Bower M et al. EMA/CO for high-risk gestational trophoblastic tumors: results from a cohort of 272 patients. J Clin Oncol 15: 2636–2643, 1997.

Newlands ES. VP-16 in combinations for first-line treatment of malignant germ-cell tumors and gestational choriocarcinoma. Semin Oncol 12(suppl 2): 37–41, 1985.

EMA—ETOPOSIDE-METHOTREXATE-DACTINOMYCIN (MODERATE-RISK)

Etoposide. 100 mg/m^2 intravenously over 30 minutes on days 1 and 2.

Methotrexate. 100 mg/m^2 intravenously by bolus on day 1 followed by 200 mg/m^2 intravenously over 12 hours.

Dactinomycin. 12 microg/kg intravenously on days 1 and 2.

Leucovorin. 15 mg orally or intramuscularly every 12 hours for 4 doses starting 24 hours after the methotrexate bolus.

NOTE: Repeat the cycle every 14 days. Small risk of second malignancy must be weighed against risk of inadequate response to less aggressive therapy.

Selected Reading

Soto-Wright V et al. The management of gestational trophoblastic tumors with etoposide, methotrexate, and actinomycin-D. Gynecol Oncol 83: 156–159, 1997.

METHOTREXATE-LEUCOVORIN (LOW-RISK)

Methotrexate. 1 mg/kg intramuscularly on days 1, 3, 5, and 7.

Leucovorin. 0.1 mg/kg (i.e., 10% of the methotrexate dose) intramuscularly 24 hours after each methotrexate dose.

NOTE: A second course is given if the HCG titer does not fall by 1 log within 18 days, if the HCG level plateaus for 3 weeks or increases, or if new sites of disease develop. If the response is inadequate, give dactinomycin 12 to 15 microg/kg/day intravenously for 5 days.

Selected Readings

Berkowitz RS et al. Methotrexate with citrovorum factor rescue as primary therapy for gestational trophoblastic disease. Cancer 50: 2024–2027, 1982.

Berkowitz RS et al. Ten years experience with methotrexate and folinic acid as primary therapy for gestational trophoblastic disease. Gynecol Oncol 23: 111–118, 1986.

PEBA—CISPLATIN-ETOPOSIDE-BLEOMYCIN-DOXORUBICIN (HIGH-RISK)

Cisplatin. 20 mg/m^2/day intravenously on days 1 to 4.
Etoposide. 100 units/m^2/day intravenously on days 1 to 4.
Bleomycin. 10 units/m^2/day intravenously on days 1 to 4.
Doxorubicin. 40 mg/m^2 intravenously day 1.
NOTE: Repeat the cycle every 21 days for up to 6 or 8 cycles.

Selected Reading

Chen LP et al. PEBA regimen (cisplatin, etoposide, bleomycin, and adriamycin) in the treatment of drug-resistant choriocarcinoma. Gynecol Oncol 56: 231–234, 1995.

PVB—CISPLATIN-VINBLASTINE-BLEOMYCIN

Vinblastine. 0.3 mg/kg intravenously on day 1.
Bleomycin. 15 units/day intravenously by continuous infusion on days 1 to 3.
Cisplatin. 100 mg/m^2 intravenously on day 2.
NOTE: Repeat the cycle every 21 days.

Selected Reading

Azab M et al. Cisplatin, vinblastine, and bleomycin combination in the treatment of resistant high-risk gestational trophoblastic tumors. Cancer 64: 1829–1832, 1989.

HEAD AND NECK CARCINOMA

Head and neck squamous cell carcinoma accounts for 5% of all malignancies. The larynx is the most common site, followed by the oral cavity, pharynx, and salivary gland. Frequency is closely correlated with smoking and heavy alcohol intake (particularly the combination). Smokeless tobacco is an important factor in the cause of oral cancer, whereas pipe smoking and chronic sun exposure are linked to an increased incidence of lip cancer. Epstein-Barr virus is associated with nasopharyngeal carcinoma (NPC), which tends to be a lympho-epithelioma and does not usually behave the way squamous cell carcinomas do. NPC is frequently treated with local and regional radiation therapy, but chemoradiotherapy is superior.

Surgery is the treatment of first choice when it can be curative. The exception to this is laryngeal cancer where chemotherapy combined with radiation therapy gives equivalent results with preservation of the organ and of normal speech. Chemotherapy may be used as neo-adjuvant (therapy given before surgery or radiation), synchronous with radiation, or post-definitive (as adjuvant after surgery or radiation).

CABO—CISPLATIN-METHOTREXATE-BLEOMYCIN-VINCRISTINE

Cisplatin. 50 mg/m^2 intravenously on day 4.
Methotrexate. 40 mg/m^2 intravenously on days 1 and 15.
Bleomycin. 10 units intravenously on days 1, 8, and 15.
Vincristine. 2 mg intravenously on days 1, 8, and 15.
NOTE: Repeat the cycle every 3 weeks. After three cycles, weekly maintenance methotrexate is given. Vincristine therapy may be discontinued after 6 doses.

Selected Reading

Clavel M et al. Randomized comparison of cisplatin, methotrexate, bleomycin and vincristine (CABO) versus cisplatin and 5-FU (CF) versus cisplatin in recurrent or metastatic squamous cell

carcinoma of the head and neck: a phase III study of the EORTC Head and Neck Cancer
Cooperative Group. Ann Oncol 5: 521–526, 1994.

CARBOPLATIN-FLUOROURACIL

Carboplatin. 300 mg/m^2 intravenously on day 1.
5-Fluorouracil. 1,000 mg/m^2/day for 4 days (96 hours) intravenously by continuous
infusion on days 1 to 4.
*NOTE: Repeat the cycle every 28 days. Response rates are superior to methotrexate
40 mg/m^2 intravenously weekly, but toxicity is greater and there is no improvement in
overall survival.*

Selected Reading

Forastiere AA et al. Randomized comparison of cisplatin plus fluorouracil and carboplatin plus fluorouracil versus methotrexate in advanced squamous cell carcinoma of the head and neck: a
Southwest Oncology Group study. J Clin Oncol 10: 1245–1251, 1992.

CISPLATIN-FLUOROURACIL

Cisplatin. 100 mg/m^2 intravenously on day 1.
5-Fluorouracil. 1,000 mg/m^2/day for 4 days (96 hours) intravenously by continuous
infusion on days 1 to 4.
NOTE: Repeat the cycle every 3 weeks.

Selected Reading

Jacobs C et al. A phase III randomized study comparing cisplatin and fluorouracil as single agents
and in combination for advanced squamous cell carcinoma of the head and neck. J Clin Oncol
10: 257–263, 1992.

HYPERFRACTIONATED IRRADIATION—WITH CISPLATIN-FLUOROURACIL

Cisplatin. 12 mg/m^2/day for 5 days (total dose 60 mg/m^2) intravenously on days 1 to 5.
5-Fluorouracil. 600 mg/m^2/day for 5 days intravenously by continuous infusion on
days 1 to 5.
*NOTE: Patients with advanced head and neck cancers are treated with 125 cGy
twice daily for a total of 7,000 cGy. The chemotherapy is given on weeks
1 and 6. Two additional cycles of chemotherapy are given after the completion of
all local therapy, with the cisplatin divided into 5 daily doses of 16 mg/m^2 (total
dose 80 mg/m^2) for the 3rd cycle and 5 daily doses of cisplatin 20 mg/m^2 (total
dose 100 mg/m^2) for the 4th cycle. The fluorouracil dose remains the same for
each cycle.*

Selected Reading

Brizel DM et al. Hyperfractionated irradiation with or without concurrent chemotherapy for locally
advanced head and neck cancer. N Engl J Med 338: 1798–1804, 1998.

NASOPHARYNGEAL CANCER—CHEMORADIOTHERAPY

Cisplatin. 100 mg/m^2 intravenously during radiation therapy on days 1, 22, and 43.
*NOTE: Radiotherapy is given as 180 to 200 cGy 5 days per week for 35 to 39 frac-
tions over 7 to 8 weeks to a total dose of 7,000 cGy. Post-radiotherapy, chemotherapy with cisplatin 80 mg/m^2 on day 1 and fluorouracil 1,000 mg/m^2/day on days 1
to 4 is administered every 4 weeks for 3 cycles.*

Selected Reading

Al-Sarraf M et al. Chemoradiotherapy versus radiotherapy in patients with advanced nasopharyngeal cancer: phase III randomized Intergroup study 0099. J Clin Oncol 16: 1310–1317, 1998.

PACLITAXEL-CISPLATIN

Paclitaxel. 135 or 200 mg/m² intravenously over 3 hours on day 1.
Cisplatin. 75 or 100 mg/m² intravenously over 1 hour on day 1.
NOTE: Paclitaxel should always be given before cisplatin to avoid excess toxicity. Repeat the cycle every 3 weeks. Hanauske et al recommend cisplatin 100 mg/m² whereas Hitt et al and Forastiere et al recommend 75 mg/m² and tend to give fil-grastim (G-CSF). Even using only 135 mg/m² paclitaxel over 24 hours and cisplatin 75 mg/m², Forastiere et al found such excessive hematological toxicity that they could not recommend the regimen.

Selected Readings

Forastiere AA et al. Phase III comparison of high-dose paclitaxel + cisplatin + granulocyte colony-stimulating factor versus low-dose paclitaxel + cisplatin in advanced head and neck cancer: Eastern Cooperative Oncology Group study E 1393. J Clin Oncol 19: 1088–1095, 2001.

Hanauske AR et al. Clinical phase I study of paclitaxel followed by cisplatin in advanced head and neck squamous cell carcinoma. Semin Oncol 22(6 suppl 14): 35–39, 1995.

Hitt R et al. A phase I/II study of paclitaxel plus cisplatin as first line therapy for head and neck cancers: preliminary results. Semin Oncol 22(6 suppl 15): 50–54, 1995.

PFL—CISPLATIN-FLUOROURACIL-LEUCOVORIN

Cisplatin. 25 mg/m²/day for 5 days intravenously on days 1 to 5.
5-Fluorouracil. 800 mg/m²/day for 5 days intravenously on days 2 to 6.
Leucovorin. 500 mg/m²/day for 6 days intravenously on days 1 to 6.
NOTE: All drugs are administered by continuous infusion. Repeat the cycle every 28 days.

Selected Reading

Dreyfuss AI et al. Continuous infusion high-dose leucovorin with 5-fluorouracil and cisplatin for untreated stage IV carcinoma of the head and neck. Ann Intern Med 112: 167–172, 1990.

RADIATION THERAPY—CARBOPLATIN-FLUOROURACIL

Carboplatin. 70 mg/m²/day for 4 days intravenously on days 1 to 4, 22 to 25, and 43 to 46.
5-Fluorouracil. 600 mg/m²/day for 4 days by continuous infusion on days 1 to 4, 22 to 25, and 43 to 46.
NOTE: Radiation therapy was 7,000 cGy in 35 fractions.

Selected Reading

Calais G et al. Randomized trial of radiation therapy versus concomitant chemotherapy and radiation therapy for advanced-stage oropharynx carcinoma. J Natl Cancer Inst 91: 2081–2086, 1999.

SIMULTANEOUS FLUOROURACIL-CISPLATIN-RADIATION

5-Fluorouracil. 1,000 mg/m²/day intravenously as a continuous infusion beginning on days 1 to 4 and days 22 to 26 of the radiation (total dose is 4,000 mg/m² as a 96-hour infusion in each 4-day segment).
Cisplatin. 20 mg/m²/day intravenously as a continuous infusion beginning on days 1 to 4 and days 22 to 26 of the radiation (total dose is 80 mg/m² as a 96-hour infusion in each 4-day segment).

NOTE: Simultaneous radiation of 6,600 to 7,200 cGy at 180 to 200 cGy/day.
Primary site resection may be performed for patients with residual or recurrent local
disease and cervical lymph node resection for persistent or recurrent disease.

Selected Reading

Adelstein DJ et al. Mature results of phase III randomized trial comparing concurrent chemoradiotherapy with radiation therapy alone in patients with stage III and IV squamous cell carcinoma of
the head and neck. Cancer 88: 876–883, 2000.

TIC—PACLITAXEL-IFOSFAMIDE-CARBOPLATIN

Paclitaxel. 175 mg/m^2 intravenously over 3 hours on day 1.
Ifosfamide. 1,000 mg/m^2/day for 3 days intravenously over 2 hours on days 1 to 3.
Mesna. 600 mg/m^2/day for 3 days intravenously on days 1 to 3.
Carboplatin. At AUC 6 intravenously over 30 minutes on day 1.
NOTE: Repeat the cycle every 3 to 4 weeks.

Selected Reading

Shin DM et al. Phase II study of paclitaxel, ifosfamide, and carboplatin in patients with recurrent or
metastatic head and neck squamous cell carcinoma. Cancer 91: 1316–1323, 2001.

TIP—PACLITAXEL-IFOSFAMIDE-CISPLATIN

Paclitaxel. 175 mg/m^2 intravenously over 3 hours on day 1.
Ifosfamide. 1,000 mg/m^2/day for 3 days intravenously over 2 hours on days 1 to 3.
Mesna. 600 mg/m^2/day for 3 days intravenously on days 1 to 3.
Cisplatin. 60 mg/m^2 intravenously on day 1.
NOTE: Repeat the cycle every 3 to 4 weeks.

Selected Reading

Shin DM et al. Phase II trial of paclitaxel, ifosfamide, and cisplatin in patients with recurrent head
and neck squamous cell carcinoma. J Clin Oncol 16: 1325–1330, 1998.

TPF—DOCETAXEL-CISPLATIN-FLUOROURACIL—INDUCTION

Docetaxel. 75 mg/m^2 intravenously on day 1.
Cisplatin. 100 mg/m^2 intravenously on day 1.
5-Fluorouracil. 1,000 mg/m^2/day for 4 days (96 hours) by continuous infusion on
days 1 to 4.
*NOTE: Repeat the cycle every 21 days for 3 cycles. Then give definitive therapy
according to institutional or group preference.*

Selected Reading

Posner MR et al. Multicenter phase I-II trial of docetaxel, cisplatin, and fluorouracil induction
chemotherapy for patients with locally advanced squamous cell cancer of the head and neck.
J Clin Oncol 19: 1096–1104, 2001.

KAPOSI'S SARCOMA

Kaposi's sarcoma (KS) may present in any of five different modes:

1. Classic KS in elderly males of Italian or East European Jewish extraction; follows
   a relatively indolent course.
2. African KS in young or middle-aged males; may be indolent or aggressive.
3. Immunosuppressive treatment-related KS in patients with renal or other organ
   transplant on immunosuppressive drugs.

4. Epidemic KS in young male homosexuals with HIV and usually aggressive and disseminated disease.
5. Nonepidemic homosexual-related KS, which is usually indolent.

Local skin lesions may be treated with intralesional injections of drugs such as vinblastine or interferon-alfa or with electron beam radiation therapy. Systemic disease is treated with active single agents such as vinblastine, etoposide, vincristine, bleomycin, liposomal daunorubicin, liposomal doxorubicin, or interferon-alfa or with combination chemotherapy. Aggressiveness of the therapy is dependent on the extent of the underlying disease and residual immunocompetency.

SINGLE AGENTS

Etoposide. 60 mg/m^2/day orally for 3 consecutive days of the first cycle, 4 consecutive days of the 2nd cycle, and 5 consecutive days of the 3rd cycle. Repeat the cycle every 3 weeks.

Selected Reading

Brambilla L et al. Mediterranean Kaposi's sarcoma in the elderly. A randomized study of oral etoposide versus vinblastine. Cancer 74: 2873–2878, 1994.

Gemcitabine. 1,200 mg intravenously on days 1 and 8 of a 21-day cycle to maximum response or toxicity.

Selected Reading

Brambilla L et al. Treatment of classical Kaposi's sarcoma with gemcitabine. Dermatology 202: 119–222, 2001.

Interferon-alfa. 35 million units (MU) daily, and reduced by 5 to 10 MU as needed for management of toxicity. Maintain therapy for 12 weeks.

Selected Reading

Lane HC et al. Anti-retroviral effects of interferon-alfa in AIDS-associated Kaposi's sarcoma. Lancet 2: 1218–1222, 1988.

Liposomal daunorubicin (Daunoxome®). 40 mg/m^2 intravenously every 2 weeks continued until complete response, disease progression, or toxicity.

Selected Reading

Gill PS et al. Randomized phase III trial of liposomal daunorubicin versus doxorubicin, bleomycin, and vincristine in AIDS-related Kaposi's sarcoma. J Clin Oncol 14: 2353–2364, 1996.

Paclitaxel. 135 mg/m^2 intravenously over 3 hours every 21 days as tolerated or until progression.

Selected Reading

Saville MW et al. Treatment of HIV-associated Kaposi's sarcoma with paclitaxel. Lancet 346: 26–28, 1995.

OR

Paclitaxel. 100 mg/m^2 intravenously over 3 hours every 2 weeks until complete remission or unacceptable toxicity.

Selected Reading

Gill PS et al. Paclitaxel is safe and effective in the treatment of advanced AIDS-related Kaposi's sarcoma. J Clin Oncol 17: 1876–1883, 1999.

Pegylated liposomal doxorubicin (Doxil®). 20 mg/m^2 intravenously every 3 weeks for 6 cycles.

Selected Reading

Stewart S et al. Randomized comparative trial of pegylated liposomal doxorubicin versus bleomycin and vincristine in the treatment of AIDS-related Kaposi's sarcoma. International Pegylated Liposomal Doxorubicin Study Group. J Clin Oncol 16: 683–691, 1998.

Vinblastine. 4 to 8 mg/week with modification for neutropenia.

Selected Reading

Volberding PA et al. Vinblastine therapy for Kaposi's sarcoma in the acquired immunodeficiency syndrome. Ann Int Med 103: 335–338, 1985.

DOXORUBICIN-BLEOMYCIN-VINCRISTINE

Doxorubicin. 10 mg/m^2 intravenously on days 1 and 15.
Bleomycin. 15 units/m^2 intravenously on days 1 and 15.
Vincristine. 1 mg/m^2 (maximum 2 mg) intravenously on days 1 and 15.
NOTE: Repeat the cycle every 28 days to complete remission or 2 cycles beyond maximum response. Do not exceed cumulative doxorubicin dose 450 mg/m^2 or bleomycin dose 300 units.

Selected Reading

Gill PS et al. Randomized phase III trial of liposomal daunorubicin versus doxorubicin, bleomycin, and vincristine in AIDS-related Kaposi's sarcoma. J Clin Oncol 14: 2353–2364, 1996.

VINCRISTINE-VINBLASTINE ALTERNATING

Vincristine. 2 mg total intravenously during odd-numbered weeks.
Vinblastine. 0.1 mg/kg intravenously during even-numbered weeks.
NOTE: Alternate therapy as long as effective. Reduce dose of vinblastine for WBC counts less than 3,000/microL or platelet counts less than 50,000/microL. Discontinue for detectable to moderate muscle weakness or severe paresthesias.

Selected Reading

Kaplan L et al. Treatment of Kaposi's sarcoma in acquired immunodeficiency syndrome with an alternating vincristine-vinblastine regimen. Cancer Treat Rep 70: 1121–1122, 1986.

LEUKEMIA: ACUTE LYMPHOBLASTIC

About 80% of acute lymphoblastic leukemia (ALL) is seen in children and it accounts for about one-third of childhood malignancies. Fortunately, over the past 30 years the prognosis has changed from 100% fatal within 3 or 4 months of diagnosis to approximately 85% curable today. The major instruments of that progress have been new and improved drugs used more effectively in systematic studies by cooperative groups. To get closer to the goal of a 100% cure rate with less toxicity, it is important to continue the systematic study of new and better therapies through the cooperative group mechanism. Hence no protocols are listed here for childhood ALL. All patients should be placed on a protocol of one of the national cooperative study groups.

About 20% of ALL occurs in adults and does not respond as well to therapy. Treatment involves remission induction followed by an aggressive consolidation and maintenance program as well as central nervous system prophylaxis. Response is related to age and other risk factors. After remission induction, further short-term intensive consolidation chemotherapy is given for one or more courses and then longer-term maintenance therapy at lower dose. For those in the high-risk group but

younger than 55 years of age, high-dose marrow ablative chemotherapy (with or
without radiation) followed by allogeneic transplantation is a consideration in first or
second remission if there is a compatible donor. Autologous transplantation for
those without a suitable donor is being evaluated because there is no convincing
proof that the results thus far are superior to a good, intensive chemotherapy program. For the group with standard-risk ALL, there is, as yet, no demonstrable survival advantage to the transplantation program, allogeneic or autologous. Because
the optimal therapy for patients with ALL is still unclear, participation in clinical trials should be considered.

DVPA—DAUNORUBICIN-VINCRISTINE-PREDNISONE-ASPARAGINASE—LINKER PROTOCOL

Induction 1A (DVPAsp)
Daunorubicin. 60 mg/m^2 intravenously on days 1 to 3 (and day 15 if day-14 bone
marrow has residual leukemia).
Vincristine. 1.4 mg/m^2 intravenously on days 1, 8, 15, and 22 (capped at 2 mg if
age >40 years).
Prednisone. 60 mg/m^2/day orally on days 1 to 28.
L-Asparaginase. 6,000 units/m^2/day subcutaneously on days 17 to 28.
Consolidation: 1B, 2B (HADC/etoposide)
Cytarabine. 2,000 mg/m^2/day intravenously over 2 hours on days 1 to 4.
Etoposide. 500 mg/m^2/day intravenously over 3 hours on days 1 to 4.
Consolidation: 2A (DVPAsp)
Daunorubicin. 60 mg/m^2/day intravenously on days 1 to 3.
Vincristine. 2 mg intravenously on days 1, 8, and 15.
Prednisone. 60 mg/day orally on days 1 to 21.
L-Asparaginase. 12,000 units/m^2 subcutaneously on days 2, 4, 7, 9, 11, and 14
(a day earlier or later is acceptable scheduling).
Consolidation: 1C, 2C, 3C (HDMTX/6-MP)
Methotrexate. 220 mg/m^2 intravenously as a bolus followed by 60 mg/m^2/hour intra-
venously for 36 hours on days 1 to 2 and 15 to 16.
Leucovorin. 50 mg/m^2 intravenously every 6 hours for 3 doses, then oral leucovorin
until methotrexate level is less than 0.05 micromol.
6-Mercaptopurine. 75 mg/m^2/day orally on days 1 to 28.
*NOTE: Treatment consists of a total of 7 courses given in the order 1A, 1B, 1C,
2A, 2B, 2C, and 3C (as above) followed by maintenance chemotherapy. Patients
not in remission at the end of 1A receive 1B. Those who do not then achieve a
complete remission are taken off this therapeutic program. Post-remission therapy
includes 6 cycles of consolidation chemotherapy. Maintenance chemotherapy with
oral methotrexate 20 mg/m^2 weekly and oral 6-mercaptopurine 75 mg/m^2 is given
until complete remission for 30 months. Then all treatment is stopped unless
patients are at high risk [adverse cytogenetics defined as t(9,22) or t(4,11),
requirement of 2 courses of treatment to achieve remission, or B-precursor
patients with WBC counts more than 100,000/microL] and they are referred for
transplantation when possible.*

Selected Reading

Linker CA et al. Intensified and shortened cyclic chemotherapy for adult acute lymphoblastic
leukemia. J Clin Oncol 20: 2464–2471, 2002.

HYPER-CVAD—CYCLOPHOSPHAMIDE-VINCRISTINE-DOXORUBICIN-DEXAMETHASONE

Cyclophosphamide. 300 mg/m^2 intravenously over 3 hours every 12 hours for 6 doses on days 1 to 3.

Mesna. 1,800 mg/m^2 total dose intravenously by continuous infusion starting with cyclophosphamide infusion and ending 6 hours after last dose.

Vincristine. 2 mg intravenously on days 4 and 11.

Doxorubicin. 50 mg/m^2 intravenously on day 4.

Dexamethasone. 40 mg/day intravenously or orally on days 1 to 4 and 11 to 14.

HD MTX-ARA-C—METHOTREXATE-CYTARABINE-LEUCOVORIN

Methotrexate. 200 mg/m^2 intravenously over 2 hours followed by 800 mg/m^2 intravenously by continuous infusion over 24 hours on day 1.

Leucovorin. 15 mg orally or intravenously starting 24 hours after completion of MTX infusion and given every 6 hours for 8 doses and increased to 50 mg every 6 hours until MTX levels are less than 0.1 microM.

Cytarabine. 3,000 mg/m^2 intravenously over 2 hours every 12 hours for 4 doses on days 2 and 3.

Methylprednisolone. 50 mg intravenously twice daily on days 1 to 3.

NOTE: Induction consists of 8 cycles of alternating intensive chemotherapy. Cycles 1, 3, 5, and 7 are HYPER-CVAD and cycles 2, 4, 6, and 8 are HD MTX-ARA-C. Maintenance chemotherapy and CNS prophylaxis depend on the degree of risk and subtype of ALL and are described in detail in the original reports.

Selected Readings

Kantarjian HM et al. Results of treatment with hyper-CVAD, a dose-intensive regimen, in adult acute lymphocytic leukemia. J Clin Oncol 18: 547–561, 2000.

Koller CA et al. The hyper-CVAD regimen improves outcome in relapsed acute lymphoblastic leukemia. Leukemia 11: 2039–2044, 1997.

FIVE-DRUG CANCER AND LEUKEMIA GROUP B INDUCTION REGIMEN

Cyclophosphamide. 1,200 mg/m^2 intravenously on day 1.

Daunorubicin. 45 mg/m^2/day for 3 days intravenously on days 1 to 3.

Vincristine. 2 mg total intravenously on days 1, 8, 15, and 22.

Prednisone. 60 mg/m^2/day orally on days 1 to 21.

L-Asparaginase. 6,000 units/m^2 intravenously on days 5, 8, 11, 15, 18, and 22.

NOTE: Doses of cyclophosphamide, daunorubicin, and prednisone are reduced for patients over 60 years of age. Treatment lasts 24 months. Consolidation over 8 weeks is with cyclophosphamide, 6-mercaptopurine, cytarabine, vincristine, and L-asparaginase. CNS prophylaxis is given with 2,400 cGy brain radiation and intrathecal methotrexate. Late intensification is with doxorubicin, vincristine, dexamethasone, cyclophosphamide, cytarabine, and 6-thioguanine. Maintenance is with vincristine, prednisone, 6-mercaptopurine, and methotrexate.

Selected Reading

Larson RA et al. A five-drug remission induction regimen with intensive consolidation for adults with acute lymphoblastic leukemia: Cancer and Leukemia Group B study 8811. Blood 85: 2025–2037, 1995.

GERMAN MULTISTUDY GROUP

Induction: Phase I

Prednisone. 60 mg/m^2/day orally on days 1 to 28.

Vincristine. 1.5 mg/m^2 (maximum, 2 mg) intravenously on days 1, 8, 15, and 22.

Daunorubicin. 25 mg/m^2 intravenously on days 1, 8, 15, and 22.

L-Asparaginase. 5,000 units/m^2/day intravenously on days 1 to 14.

Induction: Phase II

Cyclophosphamide. 650 mg/m^2 intravenously on days 29, 43, and 57.

Cytarabine. 75 mg/m^2/day for 4 days intravenously on days 31 to 34, 38 to 41, 45 to 48, and 52 to 55.

6-Mercaptopurine. 60 mg/m^2/day orally on days 29 to 57.

Methotrexate. 10 mg/m^2 (maximum, 15 mg) intrathecally on days 31, 38, 45, and 52.

Reinduction: Phase I

Dexamethasone. 10 mg/m^2/day orally on days 1 to 28.

Vincristine. 1.5 mg/m^2 (maximum, 2 mg) intravenously on days 1, 8, 15, and 22.

Doxorubicin. 25 mg/m^2 intravenously on days 1, 8, 15, and 22.

Reinduction: Phase II

Cyclophosphamide. 650 mg/m^2 (maximum, 1,000 mg) intravenously on day 29.

Cytarabine. 75 mg/m^2/day for 4 days intravenously on days 31 to 34 and 38 to 41.

Thioguanine. 60 mg/m^2/day for 6 days orally on days 29 to 34.

Maintenance

6-Mercaptopurine. 60 mg/m^2/daily for 7 days orally during weeks 10 to 18 and 29 to 130.

Methotrexate. 20 mg/m^2/week orally or intravenously during weeks 10 to 18 and 29 to 130.

NOTE: Cranial irradiation at 2,400 cGy is instituted after remission is achieved.

Selected Readings

Freund M et al. Treatment of relapsed or refractory adult acute lymphocytic leukemia. Cancer 69: 709–716, 1992. (This protocol is from the same group but somewhat more intense as befits relapsed or refractory disease.)

Hoelzer D et al. Prognostic factors in a multicenter study for treatment of acute lymphoblastic leukemia in adults. Blood 71: 123–131, 1988.

LEUKEMIA: ACUTE MYELOID

Acute myeloid leukemia (AML) includes the eight subtypes as defined by the French-American-British (FAB) classification based on morphological, histochemical, and immunological criteria. Response depends on prognostic factors and therapy. Adverse prognostic factors include older age, central nervous system involvement, systemic infection at diagnosis, WBC count greater than 100,000/microL, certain cytogenetic abnormalities and the evolution of the AML from chronic myelocytic leukemia, the myelodysplastic syndrome, polycythemia vera, alkylating agent or radiation therapy, and the development of multiple drug resistance. Effective induction therapy involves at least two or more active drugs. Once complete remission (CR) is achieved, consolidation therapy is critical to survival. Whether long-term maintenance therapy is necessary remains to be clarified. The development of the monoclonal antibody gemtuzumab ozogamicin for treatment of patients with CD33-positive AML opens up new vistas of therapy for more specific biological approaches. The role of high-dose chemotherapy with stem cell transplantation remains a subject of intense study and is discussed more fully in Chapter 10, devoted to stem cell transplantation. Suffice it to point out here that patients 15 to 55 years old with de novo AML in first CR who received either high-dose chemotherapy and allotransplantation or autotransplantation or intensive consolidation chemotherapy had comparable 4-year disease-free survival and overall survival (Harousseau J-L et al. Comparison of autologous bone marrow transplantation and intensive chemotherapy as post-remission therapy in adult acute myeloid leukemia. Blood 90: 2978–2986, 1997 and Cassileth PA et al. Chemotherapy compared with autologous or allogeneic bone marrow transplantation in the management of acute myeloid leukemia in first remission. N Engl J Med 339: 1649–1656, 1998). Allogeneic bone marrow transplantation can be considered in poor prognosis patients younger than 55 in first remission if a histocompatible sibling is available as a potential donor. It is the only potentially curative therapy after relapse of poor prognosis patients.

Acute promyelocytic leukemia (APL) therapy runs a high probability of severe hemorrhagic complications with disseminated intravascular coagulation, often in spite of low-dose heparinization. The use of all-trans-retinoic acid (ATRA, tretinoin) in induction therapy of APL and arsenic trioxide in recurrences has increased the response rate and reduced the incidence of hemorrhagic complications. Tretinoin can be used initially and then followed by combination chemotherapy to induce and maintain a remission or it can be used concomitantly, perhaps providing an advantage.

ALL-TRANS-RETINOIC ACID (ATRA, TRETINOIN) IN ACUTE PROMYELOCYTIC LEUKEMIA

Tretinoin. 45 mg/m^2/day orally until complete remission (CR) or 90 days.
Daunorubicin. 60 mg/m^2/day intravenously on days 1 to 3 after CR.
Cytarabine. 200 mg/m^2/day intravenously on days 1 to 7 after CR.
NOTE: A randomized group of patients who received the ATRA regime as above and began the daunorubicin and cytarabine on day 3 for the same number of doses indicated, had a statistically significant decrease in relapse-free survival at 2 years. Those patients who achieved a CR with the first course get a second course of the same therapy. When CR is achieved, a consolidation or third course is given with daunorubicin 45 mg/m^2 on days 1 to 3 and cytarabine 1,000 mg/m^2 every 12 hours for 4 days. Patients placed on a two-year maintenance program of tretinoin 45 mg/m^2/day orally for 15 days every 3 months and continued chemotherapy with 6-mercaptopurine 90 mg/m^2/day orally and methotrexate 15 mg/m^2 weekly seemed to have a decreased rate of relapse compared to those who did not have the maintenance program.

Selected Readings

Fenaux P et al. Effect of all transretinoic acid in newly diagnosed acute promyelocytic leukemia: results of a multicenter randomized trial. Blood 82: 3241–3249, 1993.

Fenaux P et al. Prolonged follow-up confirms that all transretinoic acid followed by chemotherapy reduces the risk of relapse in newly diagnosed acute promyelocytic leukemia. Blood 84: 666–667, 1994.

Fenaux P et al. A randomized comparison of all transretinoic acid (ATRA) followed by chemotherapy with ATRA plus chemotherapy and the role of maintenance therapy in newly diagnosed acute promyelocytic leukemia. Blood 94: 1192–1200, 1999.

AIDA—ATRA (TRETINOIN)-IDARUBICIN

Tretinoin. 45 mg/m^2/day orally until complete remission or 90 days.
Idarubicin. 12 mg/m^2 intravenously on days 2, 4, 6, and 8.

Three consolidation courses (after recovery from the previous course when PMN >1,500/microL and platelets >100,000/microL):

1. *Cytarabine.* 1,000 mg/m^2/day intravenously over 6 hours on days 1, 2, 3, and 4.
   Idarubicin. 5 mg/m^2/day intravenously on days 1, 2, 3, and 4 (3 hours after the end of the cytarabine).
2. *Mitoxantrone.* 10 mg/m^2/day intravenously on days 1, 2, 3, and 4.
   Etoposide. 100 mg/m^2/day intravenously over 60 minutes on days 1, 2, 3, and 4 (12 hours after the start of the mitoxantrone).
3. *Idarubicin.* 12 mg/m^2 intravenously on day 1.
   Cytarabine. 150 mg/m^2 every 8 hours subcutaneously on days 1, 2, 3, and 4.
   6-Thioguanine. 70 mg/m^2 orally every 8 hours on days 1, 2, 3, and 4.

NOTE: Patients who remained RAR alfa-positive after all therapy, were referred for allogeneic stem cell transplantation.

Selected Readings

Avvisati G et al. AIDA (all-trans retinoic acid + idarubicin) in newly diagnosed acute promyelocytic leukemia: a Gruppo Italiano Malattie Ematologiche Maligna dell'Adulto (GIMEMA) pilot study. Blood 88: 1390–1398, 1996.

Mandelli F et al. Molecular remission in PML/RAR alfa-positive acute promyelocytic leukemia by combined all-trans retinoic acid and idarubicin (AIDA) therapy. Blood 90: 1014–1021, 1997.

ARSENIC TRIOXIDE FOR PROMYELOCYTIC LEUKEMIA

Arsenic trioxide. 10 or 15 mg/day intravenously over 2 to 4 hours until complete remission (less than 5% marrow blasts or promyelocytes).

NOTE: Patients in complete remission were eligible for treatment with additional cycles 3 to 6 weeks after the preceding cycle. Cycles were generally no longer than 25 days for a maximum of 6 (total) cycles over 10 months.

Selected Reading

Soignet SL et al. Complete remission after treatment of acute promyelocytic leukemia with arsenic tri-oxide. N Engl J Med 339: 1341–1348, 1998.

BF-12—IDARUBICIN-HIGH-DOSE CYTARABINE-ETOPOSIDE

Idarubicin. 5 mg/m^2/day for 5 days intravenously on days 1 to 5.
Cytarabine. 2,000 mg/m^2 every 12 hours for 5 days (10 doses total) intravenously over 3 hours on days 1 to 5.
Etoposide. 100 mg/m^2/day for 5 days intravenously over 1 hour on days 1 to 5.
NOTE: After induction of a complete remission, consolidation chemotherapy is indicated.

Selected Reading

Mehta J et al. Idarubicin, high-dose cytarabine, and etoposide for induction of remission in acute leukemia. Semin Hematol 33(4 suppl I3): 18–23, 1996.

CD—CYTARABINE-DAUNORUBICIN

Cytarabine. 100 mg/m^2/day intravenously by continuous infusion for 7 days on days 1 to 7.
Daunorubicin. 45 mg/m^2/day for 3 days intravenously on days 1 to 3.
NOTE: Repeat the courses for further induction or consolidation, with cytarabine for 5 days and daunorubicin for 2 days.

Selected Readings

Yates JW et al. Cytosine arabinoside and daunorubicin therapy in acute nonlymphocytic leukemia. Cancer Chemother Rep 57: 485–488, 1973.

Yates J et al. Cytosine arabinoside with daunorubicin or Adriamycin for therapy of acute myelocytic leukemia: a CALGB study. Blood 60: 454–462, 1982.

DAUNORUBICIN-CYTARABINE–HIGH-DOSE CYTARABINE

Induction

Daunorubicin. 45 mg/m^2/day intravenously for 3 days on days 1 to 3.

Cytarabine. 200 mg/m^2/day by continuous infusion for 7 days on days 1 to 7.

Consolidation

Cytarabine. 3,000 mg/m^2 every 12 hours intravenously over a 3-hour period for 6 doses on days 1, 3, and 5 for four cycles.

Maintenance

Cytarabine. 100 mg/m^2 subcutaneously every 12 hours for 10 doses on days 1 to 5.

Daunorubicin. 45 mg/m^2 intravenously on day 1.

NOTE: If the day-14 bone marrow after induction shows persistent disease, a second induction course is given with daunorubicin for 2 days and cytarabine for 5 days in the same doses as in the original induction.

Selected Readings

Dillman RO et al. A comparative study of 2 different doses of cytarabine for acute myeloid leukemia: a phase III trial of CALGB. Blood 78: 2520–2526, 1991.

Mayer RJ et al. Intensive post-remission chemotherapy in adults with acute myeloid leukemia. N Engl J Med 331: 896–903, 1994.

GEMTUZUMAB OZOGAMICIN IN CD33-POSITIVE ACUTE MYELOID LEUKEMIA

Gemtuzumab ozogamicin (Mylotarg®). 9 mg/m^2 intravenously over 2 hours and repeated 2 weeks later.

NOTE: About half the patients received the treatment as outpatients. Those who did not go into remission or relapsed were referred for other therapy.

Selected Readings

Sievers EL et al. Selective ablation of acute myeloid leukemia using antibody-targeted chemotherapy: a phase I study of an anti-CD33 calicheamicin immunoconjugate. Blood 93: 3678–3684, 1999.

Sievers EL et al. Efficacy and safety of gemtuzumab ozogamicin in patients with CD33-positive acute myeloid leukemia in first relapse. J Clin Oncol 19: 3244–3254, 2001.

ICE—IDARUBICIN-CYTARABINE-ETOPOSIDE

Idarubicin. 6 mg/m^2/day for 5 days intravenously on days 1 to 5.

Cytarabine. 600 mg/m^2/day for 5 days intravenously over 2 hours on days 1 to 5.

Etoposide. 150 mg/m^2/day for 3 days intravenously over 2 hours on days 1 to 3.

NOTE: Patients who achieve a complete remission should go on to consolidation therapy. If this salvage therapy fails, patients should be considered for other protocols and transplantation if otherwise suitable.

Selected Reading

Carella AM et al. Idarubicin in combination with intermediate-dose cytarabine and VP-16 in the treatment of refractory or rapidly relapsed patients with acute myeloid leukemia. The GIMEMA Cooperative Group. Leukemia 7: 196–199, 1993.

IDARUBICIN-CYTARABINE

Induction

Idarubicin. 13 mg/m^2/day for 3 days intravenously on days 1 to 3.
Cytarabine. 100 mg/m^2/day for 7 days intravenously by continuous infusion on days 1 to 7.

Post-remission Therapy

Idarubicin. 13 mg/m^2/day for 2 days intravenously on days 1 to 2.
Cytarabine. 100 mg/m^2/day for 5 days intravenously by continuous infusion on days 1 to 5.

NOTE: If remission is not achieved with the first cycle, a second induction cycle is given. Two post-remission cycles are given as consolidation.

Selected Reading

Wiernik PH et al. Cytarabine plus idarubicin or daunorubicin as induction and consolidation therapy for previously untreated adult patients with acute myeloid leukemia. Blood 79: 313–319, 1992.

INTENSIVE FIVE-DRUG THERAPY

Remission Induction

Daunorubicin. 70 mg/m^2/day for 3 days intravenously on days 1 to 3.
Cytarabine. 100 mg/m^2 intravenously every 12 hours on days 1 to 7.
6-Thioguanine. 100 mg/m^2 orally every 12 hours on days 1 to 7.
Prednisone. 40 mg/m^2/day for 7 days orally on days 1 to 7.
Vincristine. 1 mg/m^2 intravenously on days 1 and 7.

Consolidation

Daunorubicin. 70 mg/m^2/day for 2 days intravenously on days 1 and 2.
Cytarabine. 100 mg/m^2 intravenously every 12 hours on days 1 to 5.
6-Thioguanine. 100 mg/m^2 orally every 12 hours on days 1 to 5.
Prednisone. 40 mg/m^2/day for 5 days orally on days 1 to 5.
Vincristine. 1 mg/m^2 intravenously on day 1.

Monthly Maintenance

Cytarabine. 20 to 25 mg/m^2 subcutaneously every 6 hours on days 1 to 5.
6-Thioguanine. 100 mg/m^2 orally every 12 hours on days 1 to 5.
Prednisone. 40 mg/m^2/day for 5 days orally on days 1 to 5.
Vincristine. 1 mg/m^2 intravenously on day 1.

Intensification (Courses 6 and 12)

Same as remission induction.

Selected Reading

Glucksberg H. Intensification therapy for acute nonlymphoblastic leukemia in adults. Cancer 52: 198–205, 1983.

MITOXANTRONE-CYTARABINE

Mitoxantrone. 12 mg/m^2/day for 3 days intravenously on days 1 to 3.
Cytarabine. 100 mg/m^2/day intravenously for 7 days as a continuous infusion on days 1 to 7.

NOTE: If not in bone marrow CR by day 10, the cycle is repeated with mitoxantrone for 2 days and cytarabine for 5 days. Consolidation begins when peripheral blood is normal, usually 6 weeks after induction. Consolidation consists of two cycles given 4 weeks apart of mitoxantrone for 2 days and cytarabine for 5 days.

Selected Reading

Arlin Z et al. Randomized multicenter trial of cytosine arabinoside with mitoxantrone or daunorubicin in previously untreated adult patients with acute nonlymphocytic leukemia. Leukemia 4: 177–183, 1990.

MEC—MITOXANTRONE-ETOPOSIDE-CYTARABINE

Mitoxantrone. 12 mg/m^2/day for 3 days intravenously on days 1 to 3.
Etoposide. 200 mg/m^2/day intravenously for 3 days by continuous infusion on days 8 to 10.
Cytarabine. 500 mg/m^2/day intravenously for 3 days by continuous infusion on days 1 to 3 and 8 to 10.
NOTE: Patients who have a partial or complete remission can receive a second course for reinduction or consolidation, respectively, or may be considered for bone marrow transplantation. Only patients younger than 60 years of age are treated with this regimen.

Selected Reading

Archimbaud E et al. Intensive sequential chemotherapy with mitoxantrone and continuous infusion etoposide and cytarabine for previously treated myelogenous leukemia. Blood 77: 1894–1900, 1991.

MITOXANTRONE-ETOPOSIDE-INTERDOSE CYTARABINE

Mitoxantrone. 6 mg/m^2/day intravenously on days 1 to 6.
Etoposide. 80 mg/m^2/day intravenously over a 1-hour period on days 1 to 6.
Cytarabine. 1,000 mg/m^2/day intravenously over a 6-hour period on days 1 to 6.
NOTE: Etoposide was given first each day over a 1-hour period and followed immediately by the 6-hour cytarabine infusion, which was followed 3 hours later by a bolus of mitoxantrone. Complete responders were given a 4-day repeat course as consolidation and then individualized for long-term therapy.

Selected Reading

Amadori S et al. Mitoxantrone, etoposide, and intermediate-dose cytarabine: an effective and tolerable regimen for the treatment of refractory acute myeloid leukemia. J Clin Oncol 9: 1210–1214, 1991.

LEUKEMIA: CHRONIC LYMPHOCYTIC

Chronic lymphocytic leukemia (CLL) is the most common of the lymphoid leukemias. Early-stage disease is frequently indolent and is not actively treated with cytotoxic drugs, but patients must avoid immunization with live vaccines, are advised to be immunized against pneumococcal pneumonia, and are treated vigorously for infections. In more advanced stages, therapy is indicated. Active drugs include chlorambucil, cyclophosphamide, prednisone, fludarabine, cladribine, vincristine, pentostatin, and more recently the monoclonal antibody, alemtuzumab (Campath-1H®). The monoclonal antibody rituximab (Rituxan®), widely used in lymphoma, is now being used in CLL, alone or in combination. Whether combination chemotherapy is more efficacious than single-agent therapy is not yet resolved.

ALEMTUZUMAB (CAMPATH-1H®)

Alemtuzumab. 30 mg intravenously over 2 hours 3 times a week.

NOTE: This therapy is for patients who relapsed after initial response or were refractory. Maximum duration of therapy is 12 weeks.

Selected Readings

Keating MJ et al. Therapeutic role of alemtuzumab (Campath-1H) In patients who have failed fludarabine: results of a large international study. Blood 99: 3554–3561, 2002.
Osterborg A et al. Phase II multicenter study of human CD 52 antibody in previously treated chronic lymphocytic leukemia. European Study Group of Campath-1H treatment In chronic lymphocytic leukemia. J Clin Oncol 15: 1567–1574, 1995.

CLADRIBINE

Cladribine. 0.1 mg/kg/day intravenously on days 1 to 7.
NOTE: Repeat the cycle every 28 to 35 days depending on white blood cell counts until complete response or excessive toxicity.

Selected Reading

Saven A et al. 2-Chlorodeoxyadenosine activity in patients with untreated chronic lymphocytic leukemia. J Clin Oncol 13: 570–574, 1995.

CP VERSUS CVP—CHLORAMBUCIL-PREDNISONE VERSUS CYCLOPHOSPHAMIDE-VINCRISTINE-PREDNISONE

Chlorambucil. 30 mg/m^2 orally on day 1.
Prednisone. 80 mg/day for 5 days orally on days 1 to 5.
versus
Cyclophosphamide. 300 mg/m^2/day for 5 days orally on days 1 to 5.
Vincristine. 1.4 mg/m^2 intravenously on day 1.
Prednisone. 100 mg/m^2/day for 5 days orally on days 1 to 5.
NOTE: Repeat the CP cycle every 2 weeks and the CVP cycle every 3 weeks for up to 18 months or maximal response. There are no significant differences between these two regimens in complete remission or duration of remission.

Selected Reading

Raphael B et al. Comparison of chlorambucil and prednisone versus cyclophosphamide, vincristine and prednisone as initial treatment for chronic lymphocytic leukemia: long-term follow-up of an Eastern Cooperative Oncology Group randomized clinical trial. J Clin Oncol 9: 770–776, 1991.

FLUDARABINE

Fludarabine. 25 mg/m^2/day for 5 days intravenously on days 1 to 5.
NOTE: Repeat the cycle every 28 days for a maximum of 12 cycles. Although this drug is more effective than chlorambucil, it severely depresses the bone marrow, and one must be extremely cautious after 6 cycles because of infection, especially Pneumocystis carinii pneumonia, which is seen in a significant percentage of patients. Adding prednisone to fludarabine did not improve the overall response rate or survival but did decrease the complete response rate.

Selected Readings

Keating MJ et al. Long-term follow-up of patients with chronic lymphocytic leukemia (CLL) receiving fludarabine regimens as initial therapy. Blood 92: 1165–1171, 1998.
Rai KR et al. Fludarabine compared with chlorambucil as primary therapy for lymphocytic leukemia. N Engl J Med 343: 1750–1757, 2000.

FLUDARABINE-CYCLOPHOSPHAMIDE

Fludarabine. 20 mg/m^2/day for 5 days intravenously on days 1 to 5.
Cyclophosphamide. 600 mg/m^2 intravenously on day 1.
NOTE: Repeat the cycle every 28 days for a maximum of 6 cycles. O'Brien et al used fludarabine 30 mg/m^2/day for 3 days and cyclophosphamide 300 mg/m^2/day for 3 days.

Selected Readings

Flinn IW et al. Fludarabine and cyclophosphamide with filgrastim support in patients with previously untreated indolent lymphoid malignancies. Blood 96: 71–75, 2000.

O'Brien SM et al. Results of the fludarabine and cyclophosphamide combination regimen in chronic lymphocytic leukemia. J Clin Oncol 19: 1414–1420, 2001.

RITUXIMAB

Rituximab. 375 mg/m^2 intravenously over 6 hours with premedication and a slow infusion rate of 50 mg/hour for the first dose.
NOTE: Subsequent doses were administered at a more rapid rate and over a shorter period of time. A total of 4 doses at weekly intervals was given and dose escalation was tested. Byrd et al gave rituximab 100 mg intravenously over 4 hours (25 mg/hour) without dose escalation on day 1. On day 3, rituximab 375 mg/m^2 was given intravenously beginning at 50 mg/hour and increased by 100 mg/hour every 30 minutes to a maximum of 400 mg/hour. On day 5 and thereafter, rituximab 375 mg/m^2 was administered at 50 mg/hour for 15 minutes and then increased to administer the entire dose in 1 hour. The drug was continued 3 times a week for 4 cycles. Combinations of rituximab with fludarabine are in clinical trials.

Selected Readings

Byrd JC et al. Rituximab using a thrice weekly dosing schedule in B-cell chronic lymphocytic leukemia and small lymphocytic lymphoma demonstrates clinical activity and acceptable toxicity. J Clin Oncol 19: 2153–2164, 2001.

O'Brien SM et al. Rituximab dose-escalation trial in chronic lymphocytic leukemia. J Clin Oncol 19: 2165–2170, 2001.

LEUKEMIA: CHRONIC MYELOGENOUS

Chronic myelogenous leukemia (myelocytic) (CML) is the most common of the myeloproliferative disorders. Average survival is 3 or 4 years in the chronic phase; after development of an accelerated phase, survival is usually less than a year, and after blastic transformation it is only a few months. The treatment of CML has been revolutionized by the development and use of imatinib mesylate (Gleevec®), a tyrosine kinase inhibitor of Bcr-Abl and c-kit. Previously, treatment of CML for cure was initiated early in the chronic phase for patients who had an appropriate stem cell donor. Stem cell transplantation is less successful in the accelerated phase and almost never in the blastic phase. For standard-dose chemotherapy, active drugs include interferon-alfa, hydroxyurea, busulfan, and cytarabine. They are frequently used as single agents and sometimes in combination. Interferon-alfa will often induce a disappearance of the Ph chromosome and a clinical remission for a time. Hydroxyurea may prolong survival but never achieves a cure. Busulfan was once standard therapy but is difficult to use safely and has more toxicity than the other two agents. Combination chemotherapy seems to give some increased palliation in small series but needs more study. Therapy with imatinib mesylate may replace these in the future. Whether it will be curative, alone or in combination, remains to be seen.

HYDROXYUREA

Hydroxyurea. 40 mg/kg/day orally.
NOTE: When the white count is very high, it may take a higher dose to bring the count down to a more manageable level. The usual dose range is about 1,000 to 5,000 mg/day or whatever is needed to keep the WBC in the 5,000 to 10,000/microL range.

Selected Reading
Hehlmann R et al. Randomized comparison of interferon-alfa with busulfan and hydroxyurea in chronic myelogenous leukemia. The German CML Study Group. Blood 84: 4064–4077, 1994.

IMATINIB MESYLATE

Imatinib mesylate. 400 mg/day orally.
NOTE: Usual dose in chronic phase disease is 400 mg/day. In accelerated phase or blast crisis 600 mg/day is recommended, but 800 mg/day has been used in some studies.

Selected Readings
Druker BJ et al. Efficacy and safety of a specific inhibitor of the BCR-ABL tyrosine kinase in chronic myeloid leukemia. N Engl J Med 344: 1031–1037, 2001.
Kantarjian HM et al. Hematologic and cytogenetic responses to imatinib mesylate in chronic myelogenous leukemia. N Engl J Med 346: 645–652, 2002.

INTERFERON-ALFA

Interferon-alfa. 5 million units/m^2/day subcutaneously.
NOTE: This dose was given daily until a cytogenetic response or toxicity. The results with imatinib are so superior that it is likely to supplant interferon-alfa use as first-line therapy so that it will be used only for salvage for those without a transplant donor.

Selected Reading
Kantarjian HM et al. Prolonged survival in chronic myelogenous leukemia after cytogenetic response to interferon-alfa therapy. The Leukemia Service. Ann Intern Med 122: 254–261, 1995.

INTERFERON-ALFA PLUS LOW-DOSE CYTARABINE

Interferon-alfa. 5 milllion units/m^2/day subcutaneously.
Cytarabine. 10 mg/day subcutaneously.
NOTE: Therapy is continued until cytogenetic response or toxicity. On a similar regimen, Hensley et al noted a significant risk of neuropsychiatric toxicity for patients with previous neuropsychiatric risk. Toxicity resolved after withdrawal but recurred with rechallenge. The results with imatinib are so superior that it is likely to supplant interferon-alfa use as first-line therapy so that it will be used only for salvage for those without a transplant donor.

Selected Readings
Hensley ML et al. Risk factors for severe neuropsychiatric toxicity in patients receiving interferon alfa-2b and low-dose cytarabine for chronic myelogenous leukemia: analysis of Cancer and Leukemia Group B 9013. J Clin Oncol 18: 1301–1308, 2000.
Kantarjian HM et al. Treatment of Philadelphia chromosome-positive early chronic phase chronic myelogenous leukemia with daily doses of interferon alfa and low-dose cytarabine. J Clin Oncol 17: 284–292, 1999.

LEUKEMIA: HAIRY CELL

Hairy-cell leukemia is an uncommon B-cell leukemia that presents with leukocytosis, pancytopenia, splenomegaly, frequent opportunistic infections, and lytic bone abnormalities. It is distinguished from other lymphocytic leukemias by the characteristic cytoplasmic projections and the positive tartrate-resistant acid phosphatase (TRAP) stain. Response to therapy may be as high as 95% with cladribine, and somewhat less with pentostatin and interferon-alfa. Splenectomy is necessary only when all other therapies fail. Infection is the great danger during and after therapy.

CLADRIBINE

Cladribine. 0.1 mg/kg/day intravenously for 7 days.
NOTE: A single cycle usually produces a complete response. Patients with a partial response need a second cycle.

Selected Readings

Piro LD et al. Lasting remissions in hairy-cell leukemia induced by a single infusion of 2-chlorodeoxyadenosine. N Engl J Med 322: 1117–1121, 1990.
Saven A et al. Long-term follow-up of patients with hairy cell leukemia after cladribine treatment. Blood 92: 1918–1926, 1998.

INTERFERON-ALFA

Interferon alfa-2a. 2 million units/m² subcutaneously 3 times a week
OR
Interferon alfa-2b. 3 million units (total dose) subcutaneously 3 times a week.
NOTE: Repeat therapy for at least 8 weeks or until complete remission, which may take 30 weeks of treatment.

Selected Reading

Ratain MJ et al. Treatment of hairy cell leukemia with recombinant alfa 2 interferon. Blood 65: 644–648, 1985.

PENTOSTATIN (2′-DEOXYCOFORMYCIN)

Pentostatin. 4 mg/m² intravenously on day 1.
NOTE: Repeat cycle every 14 days as tolerated for 6 cycles or complete remission or progression.

Selected Readings

Cassileth PA et al. Pentostatin induces durable remissions in hairy cell leukemia. J Clin Oncol 9: 243–246, 1991.
Spiers AS et al. Remissions in hairy-cell leukemia with pentostatin (2′–deoxycoformycin). N Engl J Med 316: 825–830, 1987.

LUNG CANCER: NON-SMALL-CELL CARCINOMA

Non-small-cell lung carcinoma (NSCLC) is the designation that is used to include squamous cell carcinoma, adenocarcinoma, and large-cell undifferentiated carcinoma of the lung when considering therapy because these diseases tend to respond similarly to treatment. They account for about 80% of lung cancers, whereas small-cell cancers comprise almost all of the rest. Unlike many cancers, the cause of lung cancer is clear – 85% to 87% of cases are the result of the direct effects of smoking tobacco, 3% to 5% are caused by passive smoke, 3% to 4% are caused by radon, and 4% to

9% are the result of other causes. Thus, 90% of lung cancer cases are preventable by avoiding tobacco.

NSCLC is staged by the TNM staging system; stages I and II are surgically resectable and frequently curable but account for only 25% of cases at diagnosis. There is no evidence that chemotherapy is indicated after surgery for stage I disease. However, several studies demonstrate that platinum-based adjuvant chemotherapy increases the time to tumor recurrence and prolongs survival in stage II disease. About 35% of cases are stage III. Platinum-based neo-adjuvant chemotherapy plus radiation therapy in ambulatory patients with good performance in this stage sometimes makes previously inoperable lesions surgically resectable, with prolongation of survival. Stage IV patients are incurable but may derive some palliative benefit from systemic chemotherapy or local radiation therapy to painful metastatic sites or brain metastases.

Single agents that have demonstrated efficacy include cisplatin, ifosfamide, mitomycin, vinblastine, etoposide, paclitaxel, vinorelbine, and carboplatin. New drugs that show promise and are being evaluated include irinotecan, gemcitabine, docetaxel, and topotecan. Various combination chemotherapy regimens include two or three drugs used concurrently or in sequence. For several years, all regimens used as first line were platinum-based. Four such drug regimens were compared in a phase III ECOG study and showed no significant advantage of one over the others. In several phase II studies, a series of nonplatinum doublets appear to have approximately equal efficacy as first-line therapy. In second-line therapy, docetaxel, paclitaxel and gemcitabine appear to have significant activity while vinorelbine is sufficiently active to suggest its use for salvage therapy in the elderly.

CAP—CYCLOPHOSPHAMIDE-DOXORUBICIN-CISPLATIN

Cyclophosphamide. 400 mg/m^2 intravenously on day 1.
Doxorubicin. 40 mg/m^2 intravenously on day 1.
Cisplatin. 60 mg/m^2 intravenously on day 1.
Mannitol. 25 g intravenously with cisplatin.
NOTE: Repeat the cycle every 4 weeks.

Selected Readings

Eagan RT et al. Phase II trial of cyclophosphamide, Adriamycin, and cis-dichloro-diammine-platinum II by infusion in patients with adenocarcinoma and large cell carcinoma of the lung. Cancer Treat Rep 64: 1589–1591, 1979.

Feld R, Rubenstein L, Thomas PA. Adjuvant chemotherapy with cyclophosphamide, doxorubicin and cisplatin in patients with completely resected stage I non-small cell lung cancer. Chest 106(6 suppl): 307S–309S, 1994.

CARBOPLATIN-IFOSFAMIDE-ETOPOSIDE

Carboplatin. 300 to 350 mg/m^2 intravenously on day 1.
Ifosfamide. 1,500 mg/m^2 intravenously on days 1, 3, and 5.
Mesna. 2,000 mg (400-mg IV bolus and 1,600 mg intravenously as a continuous infusion over 24 hours) on days 1, 3, and 5.
Etoposide. 60 to 100 mg/m^2 intravenously on days 1, 3, and 5.
NOTE: Repeat the cycle every 28 days until progression or a maximum of 6 courses. Chang et al gave ifosfamide 1,250 mg/m^2/day and mesna on days 1 to 3 and etoposide 80 mg/m^2/day on days 1 to 3.

Selected Readings

Chang AY et al. Ifosfamide/carboplatin/etoposide chemotherapy in patients with metastatic non-small cell lung cancer. Semin Oncol 22(3 suppl 7): 9–12, 1995.

van Zandwijk N et al. Dose-finding studies with carboplatin, ifosfamide, etoposide, and mesna in non-small cell lung cancer. Semin Oncol 17(suppl 2): 16–19, 1990.

CISPLATIN-CYCLOPHOSPHAMIDE-MITOMYCIN

Cisplatin. 75 mg/m^2 intravenously on day 1.
Mitomycin. 10 mg/m^2 intravenously on day 1.
Cyclophosphamide. 400 mg/m^2 intravenously on day 1.
NOTE: Repeat the cycle every 3 weeks with attention to adequate hydration and antiemetics. A maximum of 6 cycles is given if there is no progression or unacceptable toxicity. No dose reductions are made, but supportive care is active. This careful, prospective, randomized study showed a highly statistically significant prolongation of survival in the chemotherapy group compared with the supportive care group. Most of the chemotherapy patients were treated as outpatients and had only mild toxicity.

Selected Reading

Cartei G et al. Cisplatin-cyclophosphamide-mitomycin combination chemotherapy with supportive care versus supportive care alone for treatment of metastatic non-small cell lung cancer. J Natl Cancer Inst 85: 794–800, 1993.

CISPLATIN-VINBLASTINE

Cisplatin. 100 mg/m^2 intravenously on days 1 and 29.
Vinblastine. 5 mg/m^2 intravenously on days 1, 8, 15, 22, and 29.
NOTE: Begin radiation therapy on day 50, and give 6,000 cGy over a 6-week period. The chemotherapy plus radiation arm showed a survival advantage over the radiation therapy alone arm.

Selected Reading

Dillman RO et al. A randomized trial of induction chemotherapy plus high-dose radiation versus radiation alone in stage III non-small cell lung cancer. N Engl J Med 323: 940–945, 1990.

DOCETAXEL

Docetaxel. 75 mg/m^2/day intravenously every 3 weeks.
NOTE: Docetaxel was used as second-line therapy.

Selected Readings

Fossella FV et al. Randomized phase III trial of docetaxel versus vinorelbine or ifosfamide in patients with advanced non-small-cell lung cancer previously treated with platinum-containing chemotherapy regimens. J Clin Oncol 18: 2354–2362, 2000.
Shepherd FA et al. Prospective randomized trial of docetaxel versus best supportive care in patients with non-small-cell lung cancer previously treated with platinum-based chemotherapy. J Clin Oncol 18: 2095–2103, 2000.

DOCETAXEL-CARBOPLATIN

Docetaxel. 80 mg/m^2 intravenously every 3 weeks.
Carboplatin. At AUC 6 intravenously every 3 weeks.

Selected Reading

Belani CP et al. Multicenter phase II trial of docetaxel and carboplatin in patients with stage IIIB and IV non-small-cell lung cancer. Ann Oncol 1: 673–678, 2000.

DOCETAXEL-GEMCITABINE

Docetaxel. 100 mg/m^2 intravenously on day 8.
Gemcitabine. 900 mg/m^2 intravenously on days 1 and 8.
NOTE: Repeat the cycle every 3 weeks.

Selected Reading

Georgoulias V et al. Front-line treatment of advanced non-small-cell lung cancer with docetaxel and gemcitabine: a multicenter phase II trial. J Clin Oncol 17: 914–920, 1999.

DOCETAXEL-IRINOTECAN

Docetaxel. 50 mg/m^2 intravenously on day 2.
Irinotecan. 50 mg/m^2 intravenously on days 1, 8, and 15.
NOTE: Repeat the cycle every 28 days.

Selected Reading

Masuda N et al. Phase I and pharmacologic study of docetaxel and irinotecan in advanced non-small-cell lung cancer. J Clin Oncol 18: 2996–3003, 2000.

ECOG COMPARISON OF 4 PLATINUM-BASED 2-DRUG REGIMENS

CISPLATIN-PACLITAXEL 3-WEEK CYCLE

Paclitaxel. 135 mg/m^2 intravenously over 24 hours on day 1.
Cisplatin. 75 mg/m^2 intravenously on day 2.

CISPLATIN-GEMCITABINE 4-WEEK CYCLE

Gemcitabine. 1,000 mg/m^2 intravenously on days 1, 8, and 15.
Cisplatin. 100 mg/m^2 intravenously on day 1.

CISPLATIN-DOCETAXEL 3-WEEK CYCLE

Docetaxel. 75 mg/m^2 intravenously on day 1.
Cisplatin. 75 mg/m^2 intravenously on day 1.

CARBOPLATIN-PACLITAXEL 3-WEEK CYCLE

Paclitaxel. 225 mg/m^2 intravenously over 3 hours on day 1.
Carboplatin. At AUC 6 intravenously on day 1.
NOTE: None of the four regimens offered a significant advantage over the others.

Selected Reading

Schiller JH et al. Comparison of four chemotherapy regimens for advanced non-small-cell lung cancer. N Engl J Med 346: 92–98, 2002.

ETOPOSIDE WITH CISPLATIN OR CARBOPLATIN

Cisplatin. 120 mg/m^2 intravenously on day 1.
Etoposide. 100 mg/m^2/day intravenously on days 1 to 3.
OR

Carboplatin. 325 mg/m^2 intravenously on day 1.
Etoposide. 100 mg/m^2/day intravenously on days 1 to 3.
NOTE: Repeat the cycle every 3 to 4 weeks.

Selected Reading

Klastersky J et al. A randomized study comparing cisplatin or carboplatin with etoposide in patients with advanced non-small-cell lung cancer: European Organization for Research and Treatment of Cancer protocol 07861. J Clin Oncol 8: 1556–1562, 1990.

GEMCITABINE

Gemcitabine. 1,250 mg/m^2 intravenously over 30 minutes on days 1, 8, and 15.
NOTE: Repeat the cycle every 28 days. Some patients do not do well with the day 15 treatment and sometimes therapy is given on days 1 and 8 every 21 days. Manegold et al used gemcitabine 1,000 mg/m^2 intravenously over 30 minutes on days 1, 8, and 15 of a 28-day cycle.

Selected Readings

Manegold C et al. Single-agent gemcitabine versus cisplatin-etoposide: early results of a randomised phase II study in locally advanced or metastatic non small-cell lung cancer. Ann Oncol 8: 525–529, 1997.

Perng RP et al. Gemcitabine versus the combination of cisplatin and etoposide in patients with inoperable non-small-cell lung cancer in a phase II randomized study. J Clin Oncol 15: 2097–2102, 1997.

GEMCITABINE-CARBOPLATIN

Carboplatin. At AUC 5.2 intravenously on day 1.
Gemcitabine. 1,000 mg/m^2 intravenously on days 1 and 8.
NOTE: Repeat the cycle every 21 days.

Selected Reading

Langer CJ et al. Gemcitabine and carboplatin in combination: an update of phase I and phase II studies in non-small-cell lung cancer. Semin Oncol 26(1 suppl 4): 12–18, 1999.

GEMCITABINE-CISPLATIN-PACLITAXEL

Cisplatin. 50 mg/m^2 intravenously on days 1 and 8.
Gemcitabine. 1,000 mg/m^2 intravenously on days 1 and 8.
Paclitaxel. 125 mg/m^2 intravenously over 1 hour on days 1 and 8.
NOTE: Repeat the cycle every 3 weeks.

Selected Reading

Frasci G et al. Cisplatin, gemcitabine, and paclitaxel in locally advanced or metastatic non small-cell lung cancer: a phase I-II study. J Clin Oncol 17: 2316–2325, 1999.

GEMCITABINE-CISPLATIN-VINORELBINE

Cisplatin. 50 mg/m^2 intravenously on days 1 and 8.
Gemcitabine. 1,000 mg/m^2 intravenously on days 1 and 8.
Vinorelbine. 25 mg/m^2 intravenously on days 1 and 8.
NOTE: Repeat the cycle every 3 weeks.

Selected Reading

Comella P et al. Randomized trial comparing cisplatin, gemcitabine and vinorelbine with either cisplatin and gemcitabine or cisplatin and vinorelbine in advanced non-small-cell lung cancer: interim analysis of a phase III randomized study of the Southern Italy Cooperative Oncology Group. J Clin Oncol 18: 1451–1457, 2000.

GIN—GEMCITABINE-IFOSFAMIDE-VINORELBINE

Gemcitabine. 1,000 mg/m^2 intravenously on day 1 and 1,000 mg/m^2 or 800 mg/m^2 on day 4.

Ifosfamide. 3,000 mg/m^2 intravenously (with mesna) on day 1.
Vinorelbine. 25 mg/m^2 intravenously on day 1 and 25 mg/m^2 or 20 mg/m^2
on day 4.
NOTE: Repeat the cycle every 3 weeks for up to 6 cycles.

Selected Reading

Baldini E et al. Gemcitabine, ifosfamide and navelbine (GIN): activity and safety of a non-platinum-based triplet in advanced non-small-cell lung cancer (NSCLC). Br J Cancer 85: 1452–1455, 2001.

GEMCITABINE-VINORELBINE

Gemcitabine. 1,200 mg/m^2 intravenously on days 1 and 8.
Vinorelbine. 30 mg/m^2 intravenously on days 1 and 8.
NOTE: Repeat the cycle every 3 weeks.

Selected Reading

Frasci G et al. Gemcitabine plus vinorelbine versus vinorelbine alone in elderly patients with advanced non-small-cell lung cancer. J Clin Oncol 18: 2529–2536, 2000.

IRINOTECAN-CISPLATIN

Irinotecan. 60 mg/m^2 intravenously on days 1, 8, and 15.
Cisplatin. 80 mg/m^2 intravenously (after irinotecan) on day 1.
NOTE: Repeat the cycle every 28 days.

Selected Reading

DeVore RF et al. Phase II study of irinotecan plus cisplatin in patients with advanced non-small-cell lung cancer. J Clin Oncol 17: 2710–2720, 1999.

IRINOTECAN-PACLITAXEL-CARBOPLATIN

Irinotecan. 100 mg/m^2 intravenously over 90 minutes on day 1.
Paclitaxel. 175 mg/m^2 intravenously over 90 minutes on day 1.
Carboplatin. At AUC 5 intravenously on day 1.
NOTE: Repeat the cycle every 3 weeks.

Selected Reading

Socinski MA et al. Phase I trial of the combination of irinotecan, paclitaxel, and carboplatin in patients with advanced non-small-cell lung cancer. J Clin Oncol 19: 1078–1087, 2001.

MVP—MITOMYCIN-VINBLASTINE-CISPLATIN

Mitomycin. 8 mg/m^2 intravenously on day 1 every other cycle.
Vinblastine. 6 mg/m^2 (maximum 10 mg) intravenously on day 1.
Cisplatin. 50 mg/m^2 intravenously on day 1.
NOTE: Repeat the cycle every 21 days for 3 cycles, but mitomycin is given only every other cycle.

Selected Readings

Ellis PA et al. Symptom relief with MVP (mitomycin C, vinblastine and cisplatin) chemotherapy in advanced non-small-cell lung cancer. Br J Cancer 71: 366–370, 1995.
Smith IE et al. Duration of chemotherapy in advanced non-small-cell lung cancer: a randomized trial of three versus six courses of mitomycin, vinblastine and cisplatin. J Clin Oncol 19: 1336–1343, 2001.

ORAL ETOPOSIDE-CYCLOPHOSPHAMIDE

Etoposide. 50 mg/m^2/day orally on days 1 to 14.
Cyclophosphamide. 50 mg/m^2/day orally on days 1 to 14.
NOTE: Repeat the cycle every 28 days and adjust for myelosuppression. This out-patient treatment is well tolerated in stage IV patients with survival rates comparable to those with more intensive regimens.

Selected Reading

Grunberg SM et al. Extended administration of oral etoposide and oral cyclophosphamide for the treatment of advanced non-small-cell lung cancer: a Southwest Oncology Group study. J Clin Oncol 11: 1598–1601, 1993.

OXALIPLATIN-VINORELBINE

Oxaliplatin. 130 mg/m^2 intravenously on day 1.
Vinorelbine. 26 mg/m^2 intravenously on days 1 and 8.
NOTE: Repeat the cycle every 21 days.

Selected Reading

Monnet I et al. Oxaliplatin plus vinorelbine in advanced non-small-cell lung cancer: final results of a multicenter phase II study. Ann Oncol 13: 103–107, 2002.

PACLITAXEL

Paclitaxel. 200 mg/m^2 intravenously over 3 hours every 21 days for a maximum of 6 cycles.

Selected Reading

Tester WJ et al. Phase II study of patients with metastatic non-small-cell carcinoma of the lung treated with paclitaxel by a 3-hour infusion. Cancer 79: 724–729, 1997.

PACLITAXEL-CARBOPLATIN

Paclitaxel. 135 mg/m^2 intravenously over 24 hours on day 1.
Carboplatin. Dose targeted to AUC 7.5 intravenously on day 1.
Filgrastim (G-CSF). 5 microg/kg subcutaneously on days 3 to 17 in cycles 2 to 6.
NOTE: Paclitaxel can be gradually escalated in increments of 40 mg/m^2 to a maximum of 215 mg/m^2 if well tolerated. Repeat the cycle every 3 weeks to a total of 6 cycles unless the relapse occurs sooner. Thirty minutes before starting the paclitaxel infusion, give hypersensitivity prophylaxis with dexamethasone 20 mg intravenously, diphenhydramine 50 mg orally, and an H-2 blocking agent orally. Give carboplatin after the paclitaxel.

Selected Reading

Langer CJ et al. Paclitaxel and carboplatin in combination in the treatment of advanced non-small-cell lung cancer: a phase II toxicity response and survival analysis. J Clin Oncol 13: 1860–1870, 1995.

VINBLASTINE-CISPLATIN

Vinblastine. 4 mg/m^2 intravenously on days 1 and 2.
Cisplatin. 20 mg/m^2/day for 3 days intravenously on days 1 to 3.
NOTE: Cisplatin is given over a 2-hour period in 1,000 mL of 5% dextrose in 0.45% normal saline with appropriate antiemetics. Repeat the cycle every 3 weeks to relapse or limiting toxicity.

Selected Reading

Blum RH et al. Cisplatin and vinblastine chemotherapy for metastatic non-small-cell carcinoma followed by irradiation in patients with regional disease. Cancer Treat Rep 70: 333–337, 1986.

VINORELBINE

Vinorelbine. 25 mg/m^2/week intravenously for at least 4 weeks to evaluate desired response or clear failure.

Selected Reading

Furuse K et al. Randomized study of vinorelbine (VRB) versus vindesine (VDS) in previously untreated stage IIIB or IV non-small-cell lung cancer (NSCLC). The Japan Vinorelbine Lung Cancer Cooperative Study Group. Ann Oncol 7: 815–820, 1996.

VINORELBINE-CISPLATIN

Vinorelbine. 30 mg/m^2/week intravenously over 20 minutes.
Cisplatin. 120 mg/m^2 intravenously over 1 hour on days 1 and 29, then every 6 weeks.

Selected Reading

LeChevalier T et al. Randomized study of vinorelbine and cisplatin versus vindesine and cisplatin versus vinorelbine alone in advanced non-small-cell lung cancer: results of a European multicenter trial including 612 patients. J Clin Oncol 12: 360–367, 1994.

LUNG CANCER: SMALL-CELL CARCINOMA

Small-cell lung cancer (SCLC) comprises 20% of new lung cancer cases and is primarily the result of smoking tobacco. Because it spreads so rapidly, the majority of cases are metastatic at the time of diagnosis. Hence the TNM system has not generally been used, and patients are classified as having limited disease (confined to one lung and the ipsilateral lymph nodes that can be included in a reasonable radiation field) or extensive disease (anything beyond the definition of limited stage). The natural history of untreated SCLC is 4-month survival in limited-stage disease and 2-month survival in extensive-stage disease. The tumor is very sensitive to multiple chemotherapy drugs and to radiation, with a complete response (CR) rate of 40% to 70% and an overall response (OR) rate of 80% to 95% in limited-stage disease, and a 15% to 30% CR and a 65% to 85% OR rate in extensive-stage disease. In spite of these encouraging response rates, the median survival is 12 to 20 months in limited-stage disease with a 2-year survival of 10% to 40% and a 5-year survival of 6% to 12%. In extensive-stage disease, median survival is 5 to 7 months and a 2-year survival of up to 5% and only anecdotal 5-year survivals.

Active drugs include cisplatin, carboplatin, etoposide, cyclophosphamide, ifosfamide, vincristine, vinblastine, gemcitabine, paclitaxel, vinorelbine, docetaxel, irinotecan, and topotecan. Chemotherapy is used as a single agent as radiation sensitizer or as second-line therapy. First-line chemotherapy is used therapeutically in combinations of two to four drugs concomitantly or sequentially. Platinum-based regimens have been standard, but irinotecan, paclitaxel, gemcitabine, and topotecan have demonstrated efficacy alone or in combination. In limited-stage disease, concurrent radiation appears to be more effective than sequential radiation therapy. Prophylactic cranial radiation used to be given routinely, but since the recognition of postradiation cognitive impairment, radiation is given less frequently to the brain and usually only if the patient has a CR and understands the potential for cognitive impairment. In extensive-stage disease, radiation is used for palliation of bone pain, for bronchial obstruction, for superior vena cava syndrome not responsive to chemotherapy, and for brain metastases.

CAE—CYCLOPHOSPHAMIDE-DOXORUBICIN-ETOPOSIDE

Cyclophosphamide. 1,000 mg/m^2 intravenously on day 1.
Doxorubicin. 45 mg/m^2 intravenously on day 1.
Etoposide. 50 mg/m^2/day for 5 days intravenously on days 1 to 5.
NOTE: Repeat the cycle every 3 weeks. Patients achieving a complete response receive 3,000 cGy of whole-brain irradiation. Patients with limited-stage disease who are not in complete remission after four courses receive 3,000 cGy to residual intrathoracic tumor.

Selected Reading

Bunn PA Jr et al. Cyclophosphamide, doxorubicin, and etoposide as first line therapy in the treatment of small-cell lung cancer. Semin Oncol 13(3 suppl 3): 45–53, 1986.

CARBOPLATIN-ETOPOSIDE

Carboplatin. 300 mg/m^2 intravenously on day 1.
Etoposide. 100 mg/m^2/day for 3 days intravenously on days 1 to 3.
NOTE: Repeat the cycle every 28 days for 4 cycles. Bishop et al gave carboplatin 100 mg/m^2 intravenously on days 1 to 3 and etoposide 120 mg/m^2 intravenously on days 1 to 3 and gave up to 6 cycles if progression-free.

Selected Readings

Bishop JF et al. Carboplatin (CBDCA, JM-8) and VP 16-213 in previously untreated patients with small-cell lung cancer. J Clin Oncol 5: 1574–1578, 1987.
Smith IE et al. Carboplatin (Paraplatin; JM-8) and etoposide (VP-16) as first-line combination therapy for small-cell lung cancer. J Clin Oncol 5: 185–189, 1987.

CARBOPLATIN-ETOPOSIDE-VINCRISTINE

Carboplatin. 300 mg/m^2 intravenously on day 1.
Etoposide. 140 mg/m^2/day for 3 days intravenously on days 1 to 3.
Vincristine. 1.4 mg/m^2 intravenously (maximum, 2 mg) on days 1, 8, and 15.
NOTE: Repeat the cycle every 4 weeks for 6 cycles.

Selected Reading

Gatzemeier U et al. Combination chemotherapy with carboplatin, etoposide, and vincristine as first-line treatment in small-cell lung cancer. J Clin Oncol 10: 818–823, 1992.

CAV—CYCLOPHOSPHAMIDE-DOXORUBICIN-VINCRISTINE

Cyclophosphamide. 1,000 mg/m^2 intravenously on day 1.
Doxorubicin. 40 mg/m^2 intravenously on day 1.
Vincristine. 1 mg/m^2 (maximum, 2 mg) intravenously on day 1.
NOTE: Repeat the cycle every 3 weeks for 6 cycles.

Selected Reading

Roth BJ et al. Randomized study of cyclophosphamide, doxorubicin, and vincristine versus etoposide and cisplatin versus alternation of these two regimens in extensive small-cell lung cancer: a phase III trial of the Southeastern Cancer Study Group. J Clin Oncol 10: 282–291, 1992.

CISPLATIN-ORAL ETOPOSIDE

Cisplatin. 100 mg/m^2 intravenously on day 1.
Etoposide. 50 mg/m^2/day orally for 21 days.
NOTE: *Repeat the cycle every 28 days. Since etoposide is only available as a 50-mg capsule, dose "rounding" is necessary.*

Selected Reading

Murphy PB et al. A phase II trial of cisplatin and prolonged administration of oral etoposide in extensive-stage small cell lung cancer. Cancer 69: 370–375, 1992.

CISPLATIN-ETOPOSIDE

Etoposide. 80 mg/m^2/day for 3 days intravenously on days 1 to 3.
Cisplatin. 80 mg/m^2 intravenously on day 1.
NOTE: *Repeat the cycle every 3 weeks. The high-dose schedule with etoposide given for 5 days increases toxicity but not the response or survival rates.*

Selected Reading

Ihde DC et al. Prospective randomized comparison of high-dose and standard-dose etoposide and cisplatin chemotherapy in patients with extensive-stage small-cell lung cancer. J Clin Oncol 12: 2022–2034, 1994.

CISPLATIN-ETOPOSIDE-PACLITAXEL

Cisplatin. 75 mg/m^2 intravenously on day 1.
Etoposide. 80 mg/m^2/day for 3 days intravenously on days 1 to 3.
Paclitaxel. 130 mg/m^2 intravenously over 3 hours on day 1.
NOTE: *Repeat the cycle every 3 weeks for 6 cycles. Kelly et al used cisplatin 80 mg/m^2, paclitaxel 175 mg/m^2, and etoposide 80 mg/m^2 on day 1 and etoposide 160 mg/m^2 on days 2 and 3, with cycles repeated every 3 weeks for 6 cycles.*

Selected Readings

Glisson BS et al. Cisplatin, etoposide, and paclitaxel in the treatment of patients with extensive small-cell lung carcinoma. J Clin Oncol 17: 2309–2315, 1999.

Kelly K et al. Cisplatin, etoposide, and paclitaxel with granulocyte colony-stimulating factor in untreated patients with extensive-stage small-cell lung cancer: a phase II trial of the Southwest Oncology Group. Clin Cancer Res 7: 2325–2329, 2001.

CPE—CARBOPLATIN-PACLITAXEL-ETOPOSIDE

Paclitaxel. 135 mg/m^2 intravenously over 1 hour on day 1.
Carboplatin. To AUC 5 intravenously on day 1.
Etoposide. 50 mg alternating with 100 mg orally on days 1 to 10.
NOTE: *Always give paclitaxel before carboplatin. Premedicate with usual paclitaxel hypersensitivity regimen. Repeat the cycle every 21 days for 4 cycles. Patients with limited-stage disease receive concurrent radiation therapy (4,500 cGy/25 fractions) beginning with the third chemotherapy cycle (week 6). Better survival with this regimen may be achieved with escalation of the dose of paclitaxel to 200 mg/m^2 and the carboplatin to AUC 6, but the incidence of neutropenia also rises.*

Selected Reading

Hainsworth JD et al. Paclitaxel, carboplatin, and extended-schedule etoposide in the treatment of small-cell lung cancer: comparison of sequential phase II trials using different dose-densities. J Clin Oncol 15: 3464–3470, 1997.

ECCO—ETOPOSIDE-CARBOPLATIN-CYCLOPHOSPHAMIDE-VINCRISTINE

Etoposide. 120 mg/m^2/day for 3 days intravenously on days 1 to 3.
Carboplatin. 100 mg/m^2/day for 3 days intravenously on days 1 to 3.
Cyclophosphamide. 750 mg/m^2 intravenously on day 1.
Vincristine. 1.4 mg/m^2 intravenously on day 1.
NOTE: Repeat the cycle every 28 days for 6 cycles.

Selected Reading

Bishop JF et al. Etoposide, carboplatin, cyclophosphamide and vincristine in previously untreated patients with small-cell lung cancer. Cancer Chemother Pharmacol 25: 367–370, 1990.

ETOPOSIDE-IFOSFAMIDE-CISPLATIN

Etoposide. 75 mg/m^2/day intravenously on days 1 to 4.
Ifosfamide. 1,200 mg/m^2/day intravenously on days 1 to 4.
Cisplatin. 20 mg/m^2/day intravenously on days 1 to 4.
Mesna. 300 mg/m^2 by IV bolus just before ifosfamide and then 1,200 mg/m^2/day by continuous IV infusion on days 1 to 4.
NOTE: Repeat the cycle every 21 days for 4 cycles.

Selected Readings

Loehrer PJ et al. Etoposide, ifosfamide, and cisplatin in extensive small cell lung cancer. Cancer 69: 669–673, 1992.

Loehrer PJ et al. Cisplatin plus etoposide with and without ifosfamide in extensive small-cell lung cancer: a Hoosier Oncology Group study. J Clin Oncol 13: 2594–2599, 1995.

GEMCITABINE

Gemcitabine. 1,250 mg/m^2 intravenously over 30 minutes on days 1, 8, and 15 of a 28-day cycle as long as tolerated or until relapse.

Selected Reading

Perng RP et al. Gemcitabine versus the combination of cisplatin and etoposide in patients with inoperable non-small-cell lung cancer in a phase II randomized study. J Clin Oncol 15: 2097–2102, 1997.

IRINOTECAN-CISPLATIN

Irinotecan. 60 mg/m^2 intravenously on days 1, 8, and 15.
Cisplatin. 60 mg/m^2 intravenously on day 1.
NOTE: Repeat the cycle every 28 days for 4 cycles.

Selected Reading

Noda K et al. Irinotecan plus cisplatin compared with etoposide plus cisplatin for extensive small-cell lung cancer. N Engl J Med 346: 85–91, 2002.

IRINOTECAN-ETOPOSIDE

Irinotecan. 70 mg/m^2 intravenously on days 1, 8, and 15.
Etoposide. 80 mg/m^2/day for 3 days intravenously on days 1 to 3.
NOTE: Repeat the cycles every 28 days. Irinotecan dose may be increased as tolerated.

Selected Reading

Masuda N et al. Combination of irinotecan and etoposide for treatment of refractory or relapsed small-cell lung cancer. J Clin Oncol 16: 3329–3334, 1998.

PACLITAXEL-CISPLATIN-ETOPOSIDE

Paclitaxel. 170 mg/m^2 intravenously over 3 hours on day 1.
Cisplatin. 60 mg/m^2/day intravenously on days 1 to 3.
Etoposide. 80 mg/m^2/day intravenously on days 1 to 3.
NOTE: Repeat the cycle every 21 days. Complete response rate is low.

Selected Reading

Dowlati A et al. Paclitaxel added to the cisplatin/etoposide regimen in extensive-stage small cell lung cancer – the use of complete response rate as the primary endpoint in phase II trials. Lung Cancer 32: 155–162, 2001.

TOPOTECAN

Topotecan. 1.5 mg/m^2/day intravenously over 30 minutes on days 1 to 5.
NOTE: Repeat the cycle every 3 weeks for 5 cycles. Von Pawel et al obtained similar results with an oral dose of 2.3 mg/m^2 daily for 5 days.

Selected Readings

Ardizzoni A et al. Topotecan, a new active drug in the second-line treatment of small-cell lung cancer: a phase II study in patients with refractory and sensitive disease. The European Organization for Research and Treatment of Cancer Early Clinical Studies Group and New Drug Development Office, and the Lung Cancer Cooperative Group. J Clin Oncol 15: 2090–2096, 1997.

Von Pawel et al. Phase II comparator study of oral versus intravenous topotecan in patients with chemosensitive small-cell lung cancer. J Clin Oncol 19: 1743–1749, 2001.

LYMPHOMA: HODGKIN'S DISEASE

The treatment regimen for Hodgkin's disease (HD) is one of the great success stories of combination chemotherapy. The development of the four-drug regimen with the acronym MOPP produced long-lasting, disease-free intervals that appeared to be cures. This set the stage for the evaluation of combination chemotherapy, and ABVD is now the standard to which other therapies must be compared.

Staging is very important in directing therapy, and the Cotswold revision of the Ann Arbor modification of the Rye staging system is generally used. In addition to the four stages, disease is also described as A or B, the latter characterized by fever, night sweats, and a 10% loss of body weight without obvious other cause. The stages are sometimes modified with the designation E to indicate that an organ has been directly invaded by disease from a lymph node. Since the tumor is contiguous and can be included in a reasonable radiation field, it does not downstage the condition. However, one must be sure that the disease in the organ is an extension from the node; otherwise, involvement of a nonlymphoid organ indicates stage IV disease and a worse prognosis. Even in stage III–IV disease, combination chemotherapy can lead to cure in 75% of cases.

The usual treatment for stage I and stage IIA is radiation therapy to the area of involvement and one lymph node group beyond, as it is thought that HD spreads in an orderly fashion. Treatment of stage IIB is controversial because the condition is rare and there are no large randomized trials of treatment of this stage. It is important to emphasize, however, that initial therapy should aim for cure and that it should not be compromised to minimize toxicity with the idea that relapse can be salvaged later with aggressive chemotherapy. It is true that combination chemotherapy cures about two-thirds of those who relapse after radiation therapy and a lesser percentage of those who relapse after induction chemotherapy, but it ultimately results in more toxicity and a lower cure rate than initial curative therapy. Combined modality therapy is being widely used, but one must consider balancing its immediate benefits against the long-term survivors' risk of a higher incidence of leukemia, non-Hodgkin's lymphoma, and secondary solid neoplasms.

When using chemotherapy, one must be aware of the potential lung damage from bleomycin, carmustine, and radiation and of the potential cardiac damage of anthracyclines and high-dose cyclophosphamide and radiation therapy. In case of relapse, salvage regimens are used to try to induce another complete response. Failing that, it may be used to demonstrate sensitivity to chemotherapy for cytoreduction, and for priming for a peripheral blood stem cell (PBSC) collection for high-dose chemotherapy with stem cell and cytokine support. Some regimens for high-dose therapy with autologous bone marrow transplantation (ABMT) or PBSC support are listed in Chapter 10, High-Dose Chemotherapy with Stem Cell Support.

ABVD—DOXORUBICIN-BLEOMYCIN-VINBLASTINE-DACARBAZINE

Doxorubicin. 25 mg/m^2 intravenously on days 1 and 15.
Bleomycin. 10 units/m^2 intravenously on days 1 and 15.
Vinblastine. 6 mg/m^2 intravenously on days 1 and 15.
Dacarbazine. 375 mg/m^2 intravenously on days 1 and 15.
NOTE: In the original 1975 report, dacarbazine was given at 150 mg/m^2 intravenously on days 1 to 5. Cycles are repeated every 4 weeks. For patients with poor prognoses, alternating ABVD and MOPP at 4-week intervals has been effective.

Selected Readings

Bonadonna G et al. Combination chemotherapy of Hodgkin's disease with Adriamycin, bleomycin, vinblastine and imidazole carboxamide (ABVD) vs. MOPP. Cancer 36: 252–259, 1975.
Santoro A et al. Salvage chemotherapy with ABVD in MOPP-resistant Hodgkin's disease. Ann Intern Med 96: 139–143, 1982.

B-CAVe—BLEOMYCIN-LOMUSTINE-DOXORUBICIN-VINBLASTINE

Bleomycin. 2.5 units/m^2 intravenously on days 1, 28, and 35.
Lomustine. 100 mg/m^2 orally on day 1.
Doxorubicin. 60 mg/m^2 intravenously on day 1.
Vinblastine. 5 mg/m^2 intravenously on day 1.
NOTE: Cycles are repeated every 6 weeks (if blood cell counts permit) to a total of 9 cycles.

Selected Readings

Harker GW et al. Combination chemotherapy for advanced Hodgkin's disease after failure of MOPP: ABVD and B-CAVe. Ann Intern Med 101: 440–446, 1984.
Porzig KJ et al. Treatment of advanced Hodgkin's disease with B-CAVe following MOPP failure. Cancer 41: 1670–1675, 1978.

BCVPP—CARMUSTINE-CYCLOPHOSPHAMIDE-VINBLASTINE-PROCARBAZINE-PREDNISONE

Carmustine. 100 mg/m^2 intravenously on day 1.
Vinblastine. 5 mg/m^2 intravenously on day 1.
Cyclophosphamide. 600 mg/m^2 intravenously on day 1.
Procarbazine. 100 mg/m^2 orally on days 1 to 10.

Prednisone. 60 mg/m^2 orally on days 1 to 10.
NOTE: Repeat the cycle every 28 days.

Selected Readings

Bakemeier RF et al. BCVPP chemotherapy for advanced Hodgkin's disease: evidence for greater duration of complete remission, greater survival, and less toxicity than with a MOPP regimen. Results
   of the Eastern Cooperative Oncology Group study. Ann Intern Med 101: 447–456, 1984.
Durant JR et al. BCNU, velban, cyclophosphamide, procarbazine and prednisone (BVCPP) in
   advanced Hodgkin's disease. Cancer 42: 2101–2110, 1978.

BEACOPP—BLEOMYCIN-ETOPOSIDE-DOXORUBICIN-CYCLOPHOS-PHAMIDE-VINCRISTINE-PROCARBAZINE-PREDNISONE

Bleomycin. 10 units/m^2 intravenously on day 8.
Etoposide. 100 mg/m^2/day intravenously on days 1 to 3.
Doxorubicin. 25 mg/m^2 intravenously on day 1.
Cyclophosphamide. 650 mg/m^2 intravenously on day 1.
Vincristine. 1.4 mg/m^2 (maximum 2 mg) intravenously on day 8.
Procarbazine. 100 mg/m^2/day orally on days 1 to 7.
Prednisone. 40 mg/m^2/day orally on days 1 to 14.
*NOTE: Repeat the cycle every 21 days. A more aggressive regimen, BEACOPP
Escalated, increases the dose of etoposide to 200 mg/m^2/day, of doxorubicin to
35 mg/m^2, of cyclophosphamide to 1,200 mg/m^2, and uses filgrastim (G-CSF)
starting on day 8.*

Selected Readings

Diehl V et al. BEACOPP, a new dose-escalated and accelerated regimen, is at least as effective as
   COPP/ABVD in patients with advance-stage Hodgkin's lymphoma: interim report from a trial of
   the German Hodgkin's Lymphoma Study Group. J Clin Oncol 16: 3810–3821, 1998.
Tesch H et al. Moderate dose escalation for advanced Hodgkin's disease using the bleomycin, etoposide, adriamycin, cyclophosphamide, vincristine, procarbazine, and prednisone scheme and adjuvant radiotherapy: a study of the German Hodgkin's Lymphoma Study Group. Blood 92:
   4560–4567, 1998.

ChIVPP/EVA HYBRID—CHLORAMBUCIL-VINCRISTINE-PROCAR-BAZINE-PREDNISOLONE-ETOPOSIDE-VINBLASTINE-DOXORUBICIN

Chlorambucil. 6 mg/m^2/day orally on days 1 to 7.
Vincristine. 1.4 mg/m^2 intravenously on day 1.
Procarbazine. 90 mg/m^2 orally on days 1 to 7.
Prednisolone. 50 mg/day (total) orally on days 1 to 7.
Etoposide. 75 mg/m^2/day orally on days 1 to 5 in first course.
Vinblastine. 6 mg/m^2 intravenously on day 8.
Doxorubicin. 50 mg/m^2 intravenously on day 8.
*NOTE: Repeat the cycle every 28 days for 6 cycles. Etoposide is escalated to
100 mg/m^2 orally for second and subsequent courses if oral mucositis is no worse
than common toxicity criteria grade 1 after exposure at 75 mg/m^2. Maximum of
2 mg vincristine for patients 60 years and over, and 50% of m^2 dose for patients
aged 70 years and older. Prednisone mg for mg can be substituted for prednisolone.
The investigators had previously demonstrated that this regimen is superior to MVPP
and in this report demonstrate that it is superior in freedom from progression (FFP),
event-free survival (EFS), and overall survival (OS) to VAPEC-B (which is described in
the article with doses) in all but the best prognosis cases where it is equivalent.*

Selected Reading

Radford JA et al. ChlVPP/EVA hybrid versus the weekly VAPEC-B regimen for previously untreated Hodgkin's disease. J Clin Oncol 20: 2988–2994, 2002.

DEXA-BEAM—DEXAMETHASONE-CARMUSTINE-ETOPOSIDE-CYTARABINE-MELPHALAN

Dexamethasone. 8 mg orally every 8 hours on days 1 to 10.
Carmustine. 60 mg/m^2 intravenously on day 2.
Etoposide. 100 mg/m^2/day intravenously on days 4 to 7.
Cytarabine. 100 mg/m^2 intravenously every 12 hours on days 4 to 7.
Melphalan. 20 mg/m^2 intravenously on day 3.
NOTE: Repeat the cycle every 28 days.

Selected Reading

Pfreundschuh MG et al. Dexa-BEAM in patients with Hodgkin's disease refractory to multidrug chemotherapy regimens: a trial of the German Hodgkin's Disease Study Group. J Clin Oncol 12: 580–586, 1994.

MINI-BEAM—CARMUSTINE-ETOPOSIDE-CYTARABINE-MELPHALAN

Carmustine. 60 mg/m^2 intravenously on day 1.
Etoposide. 75 mg/m^2/day intravenously on days 2 to 5.
Cytarabine. 100 mg/m^2 intravenously twice a day on days 2 to 5.
Melphalan. 30 mg/m^2 intravenously on day 6.
NOTE: Repeat the cycle every 6 weeks to maximum response.

Selected Reading

Colwill R et al. Mini-BEAM as salvage therapy for relapsed or refractory Hodgkin's disease before intensive therapy and autologous bone marrow transplantation. J Clin Oncol 13: 396–402, 1995.

MOPP—MECHLORETHAMINE-VINCRISTINE-PROCARBAZINE-PREDNISONE

Mechlorethamine. 6 mg/m^2 intravenously on days 1 and 8.
Vincristine. 1.4 mg/m^2 intravenously on days 1 and 8.
Procarbazine. 100 mg/m^2 orally on days 1 to 14.
Prednisone. 40 mg/m^2/day orally on days 1 to 14.
NOTE: Repeat the cycle every 28 days. Usually 6 cycles are given or 2 cycles beyond complete remission. C-MOPP simply replaces the mechlorethamine with cyclophosphamide, 650 mg/m^2, on days 1 and 8.

Selected Reading

DeVita VT Jr et al. Combination chemotherapy in the treatment of advanced Hodgkin's disease. Ann Intern Med 73: 881–895, 1970.

MOPP/ABV HYBRID

Mechlorethamine. 6 mg/m^2 intravenously on day 1.
Vincristine. 1.4 mg/m^2 (maximum dose 2 mg) intravenously on day 1.
Procarbazine. 100 mg/m^2/day orally on days 1 to 7.
Prednisone. 40 mg/m^2/day orally on days 1 to 14.
Doxorubicin. 35 mg/m^2 intravenously on day 8.

Bleomycin. 10 units/m^2 intravenously on day 8.

Vinblastine. 6 mg/m^2 intravenously on day 8.

NOTE: Repeat the cycle every 28 days. Each dose of bleomycin is preceded by 100 mg of hydrocortisone intravenously. If chemical phlebitis occurs from mechlorethamine, 600 mg/m^2 of cyclophosphamide may be substituted.

Selected Reading

Klimo P, Connors JM. MOPP/ABV hybrid program: combination chemotherapy based on early introduction of seven effective drugs for advanced Hodgkin's disease. J Clin Oncol 3: 1174–1182, 1985.

STANFORD V REGIMEN

Doxorubicin. 25 mg/m^2 intravenously on days 1 and 15.

Vinblastine. 6 mg/m^2 intravenously on days 1 and 15.

Mechlorethamine. 6 mg/m^2 intravenously on day 1.

Vincristine. 1.4 mg/m^2 (maximum 2 mg) on days 8 and 22.

Bleomycin. 5 units/m^2 intravenously on days 8 and 22.

Etoposide. 60 mg/m^2 intravenously on days 15 and 16.

Prednisone. 40 mg/m^2 orally every other day.

NOTE: Repeat the cycle every 28 days for 3 cycles. In the third cycle, the vinblastine dose is decreased to 4 mg/m^2 and vincristine to 1 mg/m^2 for patients 50 years and older. Prednisone is tapered for all patients by 10 mg every other day starting at week 10. All patients receive co-trimoxazole, acyclovir, and ketoconazole as prophylaxis against infection. An H-2 blocker is used to prevent corticosteroid gastritis, and stool softeners prevent constipation from vinca alkaloids. Two weeks after the completion of chemotherapy, radiation (3,600 cGy) is given to areas of initially bulky disease.

Selected Readings

Bartlett NL et al. Brief chemotherapy, Stanford V, and adjuvant radiotherapy for bulky or advanced stage Hodgkin's disease: a preliminary report. J Clin Oncol 13: 1080–1088, 1996.

Horning SJ et al. Stanford V and radiotherapy for locally extensive and advanced Hodgkin's disease: mature results of a prospective clinical trial. J Clin Oncol 20: 630–637, 2002.

VBM—VINBLASTINE-BLEOMYCIN-METHOTREXATE

Vinblastine. 6 mg/m^2 intravenously on days 1 and 8.

Bleomycin. 10 units/m^2 intravenously on days 1 and 8.

Methotrexate. 30 mg/m^2 intravenously on days 1 and 8.

NOTE: Repeat the cycle every 28 days for 6 cycles.

Selected Reading

Horning SJ et al. Vinblastine, bleomycin, and methotrexate: an effective adjuvant in favorable Hodgkin's disease. J Clin Oncol 6: 1822–1831, 1988.

VEBEP—ETOPOSIDE-EPIRUBICIN-BLEOMYCIN-CYCLOPHOSPHAMIDE-PREDNISOLONE

Etoposide. 120 mg/m^2 intravenously on days 1 and 2.

Epirubicin. 40 mg/m^2 intravenously on days 1 and 2.

Bleomycin. 10 units/m^2 intravenously on day 1.

Cyclophosphamide. 500 mg/m^2 intravenously on days 1 and 2.

Prednisolone. 50 mg/day (total daily dose) orally on days 1 to 7.

NOTE: Repeat the cycle every 21 days for 6 to 8 cycles or progression.

Selected Reading

Viviani S et al. Long-term results of an intensive regimen: VEBEP plus involved-field radiotherapy in advanced Hodgkin's disease. Cancer J Sci Am 5: 275–282, 1999.

VEEP—VINCRISTINE-EPIRUBICIN-ETOPOSIDE-PREDNISOLONE

Vincristine. 1.4 mg/m^2 (maximum 2 mg) intravenously on days 1 and 8.

Epirubicin. 50 mg/m^2 intravenously on day 1.

Etoposide. 100 mg/m^2/day intravenously on days 1 to 4, or 200 mg/day orally on days 1 to 4.

Prednisolone. 100 mg/day (total daily dose) orally on days 1 to 8.

NOTE: Prednisone may be substituted for prednisolone. Epirubicin was selected for its reputed lesser toxicity compared with doxorubicin. If the WBC count is greater than 1,500/microL and the platelet count greater than 100,000/microL on days 8 and 15, then etoposide is given for 5 days in the next cycle. If the WBC count is less than 1,000/microL or platelets less than 50,000/microL, then etoposide is given for only 3 days in the next cycle. Therapy is given for 2 cycles beyond a complete remission.

Selected Reading

Hill M et al. Evaluation of the efficacy of the VEEP regimen in adult Hodgkin's disease with assessment of gonadal and cardiac toxicity. J Clin Oncol 13: 387–395, 1995.

LYMPHOMA: NON-HODGKIN'S DISEASE

Non-Hodgkin's lymphoma (NHL) is the fifth most common cause of cancer and the sixth most common cause of cancer deaths in the United States. There will be an estimated 61,000 new cases in 2003 with 25,800 deaths. Survival is improving, but better treatments are needed.

Treatment is based on accurate staging and pathology. As the understanding of lymphoma pathology improved with the characterization of B and T cells and the antibodies that are raised to them, new classification schemes have evolved. The current international classification is the Revised European-American Lymphoma (REAL) Classification (Harris NL et al. A revised European-American classification of lymphoid neoplasms: a proposal from the International Lymphoma Study Group. Blood 84: 1361–1392, 1994).

Progress in therapy has been slow in the last decade. A large four-arm intergroup cooperative study showed no significant difference in response rate, time to treatment failure, or overall survival between CHOP, m-BACOD, ProMACE-CytaBOM, and MACOP-B (Fisher RI et al. Comparison of a standard regimen (CHOP) with three intensive chemotherapy regimens for advanced non-Hodgkin's lymphoma. N Engl J Med 328: 1002–1006, 1993). Since then, there have been many new active drugs, monoclonal antibodies, and combinations thereof. In addition, radiolabeled monoclonal antibodies have become available including yttrium^{90} ibritumomab and iodine^{131} tositumomab. The role in therapy of these new agents is still being defined.

Therapy has been based largely on stage and pathology. To develop a more accurate prognostic index, an international group pooled its case material and evaluated outcomes after doxorubicin-based combination chemotherapy. They found that prognosis was most predictable if based on pathological stage, level of lactic dehydrogenase (LDH), performance status, and age (under or over 60 years). This helps in selecting initial therapy and salvage therapy when necessary. Various attempts to salvage patients for whom initial therapy has failed, led to large numbers of salvage regimens.

A few of them are listed because they offer opportunities to treat patients who may have cardiac, renal, or pulmonary contraindications to the use of some of the drugs. In addition, some of the salvage regimens are used to debulk relapsed disease and demonstrate continued drug sensitivity before an attempt at high-dose chemotherapy with autologous bone marrow transplantation or stem cell support to reinduce a sustained remission. The high-dose transplantation-associated regimens, with or without radiation therapy, vary from one transplantation center to another and their role in therapy is still being defined. Some of them are listed in Chapter 10, High-Dose Chemotherapy with Stem Cell Support. The plethora of regimens indicates a lack of clear superiority of any one at this time.

When treating bulky and aggressive lymphomas, such as Burkitt's or T-cell non-Hodgkin's lymphoma, or high-count acute leukemias, one must be prepared to deal with tumor lysis syndrome (Cohen LF et al. Acute tumor lysis syndrome. Am J Med 68: 486–491, 1980). The syndrome is characterized by hyperuricemia, hyperkalemia, and hyperphosphatemia resulting from cell lysis, and can lead to renal failure and death. Uric acid levels can be lowered with aggressive hydration, urine alkalinization, and prophylactic allopurinol, which blocks xanthine oxidase. It should be noted that once cytotoxic therapy is begun, alkalinization should be discontinued lest the high phosphate level predispose to excess formation of calcium phosphate, which is less soluble in an alkaline environment and could injure the kidney. For patients with high-risk tumors or those who present with a high uric acid prior to cytotoxic therapy, the FDA has approved rasburicase (Elitek®), a recombinant form of urate oxidase, for the intravenous management of hyperuricemia in pediatric patients (Medical Letter 44: 96–97, 2002). Rasburicase oxidizes uric acid to form allantoin, a water-soluble metabolite that is eliminated in the urine. After intravenous administration, it begins to lower serum uric acid levels within 4 hours, and is occasionally indicated in adults who present with very high uric acid levels.

Although cures can be achieved in about 50% of patients with intermediate and high-grade lymphoma, cures are rare in low-grade lymphoma. They may be indolent and progress slowly over 5 to 8 years, but eventually kill the patient. It is not yet clear what therapeutic approach is best. Some patients are best observed until they show signs of progression. Others are well served with single-agent chemotherapy including chlorambucil, fludarabine, cladribine, pentostatin, rituximab, denileukin diftitox, alemtuzumab, and some new drugs still in the experimental stage. Many are treated with mild combination chemotherapy, and several regimens are listed for that purpose. High-dose chemotherapy with stem cell support is still being evaluated in this setting.

High-grade B-cell non-Hodgkin's lymphoma in HIV-infected patients is an AIDS-defining morbidity, just as an opportunistic infection is. Because these patients are generally immunosuppressed from their HIV infection, the therapy of their aggressive lymphoma is particularly difficult. Highly active antiretroviral therapy must be given along with the chemotherapy.

The problems of lymphoblastic lymphoma and Burkitt's lymphoma are not addressed with detailed regimens here. They are seen more frequently in children, and although very aggressive, they are fortunately uncommon and potentially curable. Useful regimens are long and complex and include some used in the acute lymphoblastic leukemia section. Some additional references include the following.

Selected Readings
Lymphoblastic lymphoma and Burkitt's lymphoma
Bernstein JI et al. Combined modality therapy for adults with small non-cleaved cell lymphoma (Burkitt's and non-Burkitt's type), J Clin Oncol 4: 847–858, 1986.

Hoelzer D et al. Outcomes of adult patients with T-lymphoblastic lymphoma treated according to protocols for acute lymphoblastic leukemia. Blood 99: 4379–4385, 2001.

Magrath IT et al. An effective therapy for both undifferentiated (including Burkitt's) lymphomas and lymphoblastic lymphomas in children and young adults. Blood 63: 1102–1111, 1984.

Magrath I et al. Adults and children with small non-cleaved-cell lymphoma have a similar excellent outcome when treated with the same chemotherapy regimen. J Clin Oncol 14: 925–934, 1996.

McMaster ML et al. Effective treatment of small non-cleaved-cell lymphoma with high density, brief duration chemotherapy. J Clin Oncol 9: 941–946, 1991.

Millot F et al. Value of high-dose cytarabine during interval therapy of a Berlin-Frankfurt-Münster-based protocol in increased-risk children with acute lymphoblastic leukemia and lymphoblastic lymphoma: results of the European Organization for Research and Treatment of Cancer 58881 randomized phase III trial. J Clin Oncol 19: 1935–1942, 2001.

Reiter A et al. Non-Hodgkin's lymphomas of childhood and adolescence: results of a treatment stratified for biologic subtypes and stage—a report of the Berlin-Frankfurt-Münster group. J Clin Oncol 13: 359–372, 1995.

Reiter A et al. Intensive ALL therapy without local radiotherapy provides a 90% event-free survival for children with T-cell lymphoblastic lymphoma: a BFM Group report. Blood 95: 416–421, 2000.

Seidemann K et al. Short-pulse B-non-Hodgkin lymphoma-type chemotherapy is efficacious treatment for pediatric large cell lymphoma: a report of the Berlin-Frankfurt-Münster Group Trial NHL-BFM 90. Blood 97: 3699–3706, 2001.

Sweetenham JW et al. High-dose therapy and autologous bone marrow transplantation for adult patients with lymphoblastic lymphoma: results of the European Group for Bone Marrow Transplantation. J Clin Oncol 12: 1358–1365, 1994.

Sweetenham JW et al. Adult Burkitt's and Burkitt-like non-Hodgkin's lymphoma – outcome for patients treated with high-dose therapy and autologous stem-cell transplantation in first remission or at relapse: results from the European Group for Blood and Marrow Transplantation. J Clin Oncol 14: 2465–2472, 1996.

Sweetenham JW et al. High-dose therapy and autologous stem-cell transplantation versus conventional dose consolidation/maintenance therapy as post-remission therapy for adult patients with lymphoblastic lymphoma: results of a randomized trial of the European Group for Blood and Marrow Transplantation and the United Kingdom Lymphoma Group. J Clin Oncol 19: 2927–2936, 2001.

Thomas DA et al. Hyper-CVAD program in Burkitt's-type adult acute lymphoblastic leukemia. J Clin Oncol 17: 2461–2470, 1999.

ACOMLA—DOXORUBICIN-CYCLOPHOSPHAMIDE-VINCRISTINE-METHOTREXATE-LEUCOVORIN-CYTARABINE

Doxorubicin. 40 mg/m^2 intravenously on day 1.

Cyclophosphamide. 1,000 mg/m^2 intravenously on day 1.

Vincristine. 2 mg intravenously on days 1, 8, and 15.

Methotrexate. 120 mg/m^2 intravenously on days 22, 29, 36, 43, 50, 57, 64, and 71.

Cytarabine. 300 mg/m^2 intravenously 1 hour after the methotrexate on days 22, 29, 36, 43, 50, 57, 64, and 71.

Leucovorin. 25 mg orally every 6 hours for 6 doses starting 24 hours after each methotrexate dose.

NOTE: Administer three cycles, each lasting 3 months.

Selected Reading

Newcomer LN et al. Randomized study comparing doxorubicin, cyclophosphamide, vincristine, methotrexate with leucovorin rescue, and cytarabine (ACOMLA) with cyclophosphamide, doxorubicin, vincristine, prednisone, and bleomycin (CHOP-B) in the treatment of diffuse histiocytic lymphoma. Cancer Treat Rep 66: 1279–1284, 1982.

AIDS-RELATED ORAL REGIMEN

Lomustine (CCNU). 100 mg/m^2 orally on day 1 of cycles 1, 3, and 5.
Etoposide. 200 mg/m^2/day orally on days 1 to 3.
Cyclophosphamide. 100 mg/m^2/day orally on days 22 to 31.
Procarbazine. 100 mg/m^2/day orally on days 22 to 31.
NOTE: Repeat the cycle every 42 days.

Selected Reading

Remick SC et al. Novel oral combination chemotherapy in the treatment of intermediate-grade and high-grade AIDS-related non-Hodgkin's lymphoma. J Clin Oncol 11: 1691–1702, 1993.

AIDS-RELATED INTRAVENOUS REGIMEN

Cyclophosphamide. 300 mg/m^2 intravenously on day 1.
Doxorubicin. 25 mg/m^2 intravenously on day 1.
Vincristine. 1.4 mg/m^2 intravenously (maximum 2 mg) on day 1.
Bleomycin. 4 units/m^2 intravenously on day 1.
Dexamethasone. 3 mg/m^2/day orally on days 1 to 5.
Methotrexate. 500 mg/m^2 intravenously on day 15.
Leucovorin. 25 mg orally every 6 hours for 4 doses beginning 6 hours after the completion of methotrexate.
Cytarabine. 50 mg intrathecally on days 1, 8, 21, and 28.
NOTE: For patients with known CNS involvement, give helmet-field radiotherapy to 4,000 cGy; with known marrow involvement alone, give 2,400 cGy to same field. Chemotherapy cycles are given at 28-day intervals for 4 to 6 cycles. Zidovudine may be resumed after chemotherapy. Protease drugs need not be interrupted.

Selected Reading

Levine AM et al. Low-dose chemotherapy with central nervous system prophylaxis and zidovudine maintenance in AIDS-related lymphoma. JAMA 266: 84–88, 1991.

AIDS-RELATED INFUSIONAL REGIMEN

Cyclophosphamide. 187.5 mg/m^2/day intravenously by continuous infusion on days 1 to 4.
Doxorubicin. 12.5 mg/m^2/day intravenously by continuous infusion on days 1 to 4.
Etoposide. 60 mg/m^2/day intravenously by continuous infusion on days 1 to 4.
NOTE: Repeat the cycle every 28 or more days for up to 6 cycles.

Selected Readings

Sparano JA et al. Infusional cyclophosphamide, doxorubicin, and etoposide in human immunodeficiency virus and human T-cell leukemia virus type I-related non-Hodgkin's lymphoma: a highly active regimen. Blood 81: 2810–2815, 1993.

Sparano JA et al. Infusional cyclophosphamide, doxorubicin, and etoposide in relapsed and resistant non-Hodgkin's lymphoma: evidence for a schedule-dependent effect favoring infusional administration of chemotherapy. J Clin Oncol 11: 1071–1079, 1993.

CEPP(B)—CYCLOPHOSPHAMIDE-ETOPOSIDE-PROCARBAZINE-PREDNISONE-(BLEOMYCIN)

Cyclophosphamide. 600 mg/m^2 intravenously on days 1 and 8.
Etoposide. 70 mg/m^2 intravenously on days 1 to 3.
Procarbazine. 60 mg/m^2/day orally on days 1 to 10.

Prednisone. 60 mg/m^2/day orally on days 1 to 15.
NOTE: Repeat the cycle every 28 days for 4 cycles. Results were the same with or without bleomycin. Some patients may need filgrastim (G-CSF) for the second and subsequent cycles. This regimen may be used for relapsed patients or those requiring cytoreduction before ablative therapy and stem cell transplantation.

Selected Reading

Chao NJ et al. CEPP(B): an effective and well-tolerated regimen in poor-risk, aggressive non-Hodgkin's lymphoma. Blood 76: 1293–1298, 1990.

CHOP—CYCLOPHOSPHAMIDE-DOXORUBICIN-VINCRISTINE-PREDNISONE

Cyclophosphamide. 750 mg/m^2 intravenously on day 1.
Doxorubicin. 50 mg/m^2 intravenously on day 1.
Vincristine. 1.4 mg/m^2 (maximum 2 mg) intravenously on day 1.
Prednisone. 100 mg/m^2/day orally on days 1 to 5.
NOTE: Repeat the cycle every 3 weeks. Elderly patients generally tolerate this regimen reasonably well, although many clinicians prefer a regimen with mitoxantrone or epirubicin because of the lesser cardiac toxicity of those drugs at equivalent therapeutic doses.

Selected Reading

McKelvey EM et al. Hydroxydaunomycin (Adriamycin) combination chemotherapy in malignant lymphoma. Cancer 38: 1484–1493, 1976.

CHOP-BLEO—CYCLOPHOSPHAMIDE-DOXORUBICIN-VINCRISTINE-PREDNISONE-BLEOMYCIN

Cyclophosphamide. 750 mg/m^2 intravenously on day 1.
Doxorubicin. 50 mg/m^2 intravenously on day 1.
Vincristine. 2 mg/day intravenously on days 1 and 5.
Prednisone. 100 mg/day orally on days 1 to 5.
Bleomycin. 15 units intravenously on days 1 and 5.
NOTE: Repeat the cycle every 21 to 28 days.

Selected Reading

Rodriguez V et al. Combination chemotherapy (CHOP-Bleo) in advanced (non-Hodgkin's) malignant lymphoma. Blood 49: 325–333, 1977.

CHOP-RITUXIMAB—CYCLOPHOSPHAMIDE-DOXORUBICIN-VINCRISTINE-PREDNISONE-RITUXIMAB

Cyclophosphamide. 750 mg/m^2 intravenously on day 1.
Doxorubicin. 50 mg/m^2 intravenously on day 1.
Vincristine. 1.4 mg/m^2 (maximum 2 mg) intravenously on day 1.
Prednisone. 40 mg/m^2/day orally on days 1 to 5.
Rituximab. 375 mg/m^2 intravenously on day 1.
NOTE: Repeat the cycle every 3 weeks for 8 cycles. Vose et al give rituximab on day 1 of each cycle but begin the other drugs on day 3. Czuczman et al give a total of 6 infusions of rituximab and 6 cycles of CHOP every 3 weeks, but give the rituximab on days 1 and 6 before the first CHOP cycle, which they start on day 8. Rituximab infusions 3 and 4 are given 2 days before the third and fifth CHOP cycles and infusions 5 and 6 are given on days 134 and 141, respectively, after the sixth CHOP cycle.

Selected Readings

Coiffier B et al. CHOP chemotherapy plus rituximab compared with CHOP alone in elderly patients with diffuse large-B-cell lymphoma. N Engl J Med 346: 235–242, 2002.

Czuczman MS et al. Treatment of patients with low-grade B-cell lymphoma with the combination of the chemeric anti-CD20 monoclonal antibody and CHOP chemotherapy. J Clin Oncol 17: 268–276, 1999.

Vose JM et al. Phase II study of rituximab in combination with CHOP chemotherapy in patients with previously untreated, aggressive non-Hodgkin's lymphoma. J Clin Oncol 19: 389–397, 2001.

C-MOPP—CYCLOPHOSPHAMIDE-VINCRISTINE-PROCARBAZINE-PREDNISONE

Cyclophosphamide. 650 mg/m^2 intravenously on days 1 and 8.
Vincristine. 1.4 mg/m^2 intravenously on days 1 and 8.
Procarbazine. 100 mg/m^2/day orally on days 1 to 14.
Prednisone. 40 mg/m^2/day orally on days 1 to 14.
NOTE: Repeat the cycle every 28 days (i.e., 14 days of treatment followed by a 14-day rest period).

Selected Reading

DeVita VT Jr et al. Advanced diffuse histiocytic lymphoma, a potentially curable disease. Lancet 1: 248–250, 1975.

CNOP—CYCLOPHOSPHAMIDE-MITOXANTRONE-VINCRISTINE-PREDNISONE

Cyclophosphamide. 750 mg/m^2 intravenously on day 1.
Mitoxantrone. 10 mg/m^2 intravenously on day 1.
Vincristine. 1.4 mg/m^2 (maximum 2 mg) intravenously on day 1.
Prednisone. 50 mg/m^2/day orally on days 1 to 5.
NOTE: Repeat the cycle every 28 days for 6 cycles or 2 cycles beyond a complete remission. In the 1995 paper, Sonneveld et al found that CHOP was relatively well tolerated and gave a higher CR rate, and was to be preferred over CNOP. But considering the complete group of patients alive and disease-free at 3 years, there was no significant difference. Others have found mitoxantrone superior for therapy of the elderly (see Mainwaring et al reference in PMitCEBO regimen).

Selected Readings

Pavlovsky S et al. Results of a randomized study of previously-untreated intermediate and high grade lymphoma using CHOP versus CNOP. Ann Oncol 3: 205–209, 1992.

Sonneveld P, Michiels JJ. Full dose chemotherapy in elderly patients with non-Hodgkin's lymphoma: a feasibility study using a mitoxantrone containing regimen. Br J Cancer 62: 105–108, 1990.

Sonneveld P et al. Comparison of doxorubicin and mitoxantrone in the treatment of elderly patients with advanced diffuse non-Hodgkin's lymphoma using CHOP versus CNOP chemotherapy. J Clin Oncol 13: 2530–2539, 1995.

COP-BLAM—CYCLOPHOSPHAMIDE-VINCRISTINE-PREDNISONE-BLEOMYCIN-DOXORUBICIN-PROCARBAZINE

Cyclophosphamide. 400 mg/m^2 intravenously on day 1.
Vincristine. 1 mg/m^2 (maximum 2 mg) intravenously on day 1.
Prednisone. 40 mg/m^2 orally on days 1 to 10.

Bleomycin. 15 units (total) intravenously on day 14.
Doxorubicin. 40 mg/m^2 intravenously on day 1.
Procarbazine. 100 mg/m^2/day orally on days 1 to 10.
NOTE: Repeat the cycle every 21 days. Graded intensification of the induction phase is described in the report below. Cumulative maximum doses are 550 mg/m^2 of doxorubicin and 250 units/m^2 of bleomycin.

Selected Reading

Laurence J et al. Combination chemotherapy of advanced diffuse histiocytic lymphoma with the six-drug COP-BLAM regimen. Ann Intern Med 97: 190–195, 1982.

COP-BLAM III

COP-BLAM III is a more intensive modification of COP-BLAM, incorporates continuous daily IV infusions of vincristine and bleomycin for up to 5 days, and thus requires considerable periods of hospitalization.

Selected Reading

Coleman M et al. The COP-BLAM programs: evolving chemotherapy concepts in large cell lymphoma. Semin Hematol 23(2 suppl 2): 23–33, 1988.

COPP—CYCLOPHOSPHAMIDE-VINCRISTINE-PROCARBAZINE-PREDNISONE

Cyclophosphamide. 600 mg/m^2 intravenously on days 1 and 8.
Vincristine. 1.4 mg/m^2/day intravenously on days 1 and 8.
Procarbazine. 100 mg/m^2/day orally on days 1 to 10.
Prednisone. 40 mg/m^2/day intravenously on days 1 to 14.
NOTE: Repeat the cycle every 28 days (i.e., 14 days of treatment followed by a 14-day rest period).

Selected Reading

Stein RS et al. Combination chemotherapy of lymphomas other than Hodgkin's disease. Ann Intern Med 81: 601–609, 1974.

CVP—CYCLOPHOSPHAMIDE-VINCRISTINE-PREDNISONE

Cyclophosphamide. 400 mg/m^2/day orally on days 1 to 5.
Vincristine. 1.4 mg/m^2 intravenously on day 1.
Prednisone. 100 mg/m^2/day orally on days 1 to 5.
NOTE: Repeat the cycle every 21 days.

Selected Reading

Bagley CM Jr et al. Advanced lymphosarcoma: intensive cyclical combination chemotherapy with cyclophosphamide, vincristine, and prednisone. Ann Intern Med 76: 227–234, 1972.

DHAP—CISPLATIN-CYTARABINE-DEXAMETHASONE

Cisplatin. 100 mg/m^2 intravenously as a continuous infusion for 24 hours on day 1.
Cytarabine. 2,000 mg/m^2/dose intravenously every 12 hours on day 2 (two doses for a total dose of 4,000 mg/m^2).
Dexamethasone. 40 mg/day intravenously or orally on days 1 to 4.
NOTE: DHAP requires vigorous hydration and adequate antiemetic support. Repeat the cycle every 3 to 4 weeks. For patients over 70 years of age, use only 1,000 mg/m^2 of cytarabine per dose.

Selected Readings

Cabanillas F et al. Results of recent salvage chemotherapy regimens for lymphoma and Hodgkin's disease. Semin Hematol 25(suppl 2): 47–50, 1988.

Velasquez WS et al. Effective salvage therapy for lymphoma with cisplatin in combination with high-dose ara-C and dexamethasone (DHAP). Blood 71: 117–122, 1988.

DICE—DEXAMETHASONE-IFOSFAMIDE-CISPLATIN-ETOPOSIDE

Dexamethasone. 10 mg intravenously every 6 hours on days 1 to 4.

Ifosfamide. 1,000 mg/m^2/day (maximum 1,750 mg/day) intravenously on days 1 to 4.

Cisplatin. 25 mg/m^2/day intravenously on days 1 to 4.

Etoposide. 100 mg/m^2/day on days 1 to 4.

Mesna. 200 mg/m^2 1 hour before each ifosfamide infusion on days 1 to 4. Immediately after the first ifosfamide dose, give mesna, 900 mg/m^2/24 hours (i.e., mesna, 300 mg/m^2 per liter of normal saline), and continue mesna for 12 hours after the last dose of ifosfamide.

NOTE: Repeat the cycle every 3 to 4 weeks, CBC, platelet count, and creatinine clearance values permitting.

Selected Readings

Goss PE et al. Dexamethasone/ifosfamide/cisplatin/etoposide (DICE) as therapy for patients with advanced refractory non-Hodgkin's lymphoma: preliminary report of a phase II study. Ann Oncol 2(suppl 1): 43–46, 1991.

Goss PE. New perspectives in the treatment of non-Hodgkin's lymphoma. Semin Oncol 19(suppl 12): 23–30, 1992.

DICEP—DOSE-INTENSIVE CYCLOPHOSPHAMIDE-ETOPOSIDE-CISPLATIN

Cyclophosphamide. 2,500 mg/m^2/day intravenously on days 1 and 2.

Etoposide. 500 mg/m^2/day intravenously on days 1 to 3.

Cisplatin. 50 mg/m^2/day intravenously on days 1 to 3.

NOTE: Repeat the cycle every 5 weeks for 4 cycles. Hydration, antibacterial, antifungal, antidiarrheal, and antiemetic therapy are essential. GM-CSF or G-CSF may be used to control neutropenia.

Selected Readings

Neidhardt JA et al. Granulocyte colony stimulating factor (rhG-CSF) stimulates recovery of granulocytes in patients receiving dose-intensive chemotherapy without bone marrow transplantation. J Clin Oncol 7: 1685–1692, 1989.

Neidhart JA et al. Multiple courses of dose-intensive cyclophosphamide, etoposide and cisplatinum (DICEP) produce durable responses in refractory non-Hodgkin's lymphoma. Cancer Invest 12: 1–11, 1994.

EPIC—ETOPOSIDE-PREDNISOLONE-IFOSFAMIDE-CARBOPLATIN

Etoposide. 100 mg/m^2/day intravenously on days 1 to 4.

Ifosfamide. 1,000 mg/m^2/day intravenously on days 1 to 5.

Mesna. 1,000 mg/m^2/day intravenously with 3 L normal saline on days 1 to 5.

Prednisolone. 100 mg/day (total daily dose) orally on days 1 to 5.

Carboplatin. 240 mg/m^2 intravenously on day 12.

NOTE: Prednisone can be used in place of prednisolone. This program is for patients for whom induction chemotherapy has failed and for patients who relapse and need to have their tumor mass reduced to benefit from subsequent high-dose ablative chemotherapy with ABMT or PBSC support. Supportive measures include allopurinol, hydration, antiemetics, antifungal agents, and H-2 blockers. Carboplatin is not given on day 12 if the WBC count is less than 1,000/microL or the platelet count less than 100,000/microL. A similar EPIC program using cisplatin instead of carboplatin has been reported by Hickish et al.

Selected Readings

Hickish T et al. EPIC: an effective low toxicity regimen for relapsing lymphoma. Br J Cancer 68: 599–604, 1993.

Richardson DS et al. Salvage chemotherapy for relapsed and resistant lymphoma with a carboplatin containing schedule—EPIC. Hematol Oncol 12: 125–128, 1994.

EPOCH—ETOPOSIDE-PREDNISONE-VINCRISTINE-CYCLOPHOSPHAMIDE-DOXORUBICIN-(RITUXIMAB)

Etoposide. 50 mg/m^2/day intravenously by continuous infusion on days 1 to 4.
Vincristine. 0.4 mg/m^2/day intravenously by continuous infusion on days 1 to 4.
Doxorubicin. 10 mg/m^2/day intravenously by continuous infusion on days 1 to 4.
Cyclophosphamide. 750 mg/m^2 intravenously on day 5.
Prednisone. 60 mg/m^2/day orally on days 1 to 5.
(Rituximab. 375 mg/m^2 intravenously on day 1.)
NOTE: Repeat the cycle every 21 days. In a small experiment, rituximab was added on day 1 of each cycle with a significant increase in apparent response.

Selected Readings

Gutierrez M et al. Role of a doxorubicin-containing regimen in relapsed and resistant lymphomas: an 8-year follow-up of EPOCH. J Clin Oncol 18: 3633–3642, 2000.

Wilson WH et al. Chemotherapy sensitization by rituximab: experimental and clinical evidence. Semin Oncol 27(suppl 12): 30–36, 2000.

FLUDARABINE-CYCLOPHOSPHAMIDE

Fludarabine. 20 mg/m^2/day intravenously on days 1 to 5.
Cyclophosphamide. 600 mg/m^2 intravenously on day 1.
NOTE: Use filgrastim as needed. Repeat the cycle every 28 days to a maximum response or a maximum of 6 cycles. Consider prophylaxis for Pneumocystis carinii following this therapy.

Selected Reading

Flinn IW et al. Fludarabine and cyclophosphamide with filgrastim support in patients with previously untreated indolent lymphoid malignancies. Blood 96: 71–75, 2000.

FMP—FLUDARABINE-MITOXANTRONE-PREDNISONE

Fludarabine. 25 mg/m^2/day intravenously on days 1 to 3.
Mitoxantrone. 10 mg/m^2 intravenously on day 1.
Prednisone. 40 mg/day (total daily dose) orally on days 1 to 5.
NOTE: The regimen of McLaughlin et al (FND) differs from FMP only in the substitution of dexamethasone 20 mg/day orally or intravenously on days 1 to 5 for the prednisone. Repeat the cycle every 4 weeks. Give co-trimoxazole double strength twice a day as prophylaxis.

Selected Readings

McLaughlin P et al. Fludarabine, mitoxantrone, and dexamethasone: an effective new regimen for indolent lymphoma. J Clin Oncol 14: 1262–1268, 1996.

Zinzani PL et al. FMP regimen (fludarabine, mitoxantrone, prednisone) as therapy in recurrent low-grade non-Hodgkin's lymphoma. Eur J Haematol 55: 262–266, 1995.

HYPER-CVAD—CYCLOPHOSPHAMIDE-DOXORUBICIN-VINCRISTINE-DEXAMETHASONE-METHOTREXATE-CYTARABINE

Cyclophosphamide. 300 mg/m^2 intravenously every 12 hours for 6 doses beginning on day 1.

Doxorubicin. 25 mg/m^2/day intravenously on days 4 and 5.

Vincristine. 2 mg administered 12 hours after the last dose of cyclophosphamide on days 4 and 11.

Dexamethasone. 40 mg/day (total daily dose) intravenously or orally on days 1 to 4 and 11 to 14.

Methotrexate. 200 mg/m^2 bolus intravenously followed by a 24-hour infusion of 800 mg/m^2.

Cytarabine. 3,000 mg/m^2/dose every 12 hours for 4 doses on days 2 and 3.

NOTE: Leucovorin 50 mg is given orally 24 hours after completion of methotrexate infusion followed 6 hours later by 15 mg orally every 6 hours for 8 doses. Repeat the cycle every 21 days for 4 cycles. Patients 55 years or younger receive an HLA-identical or a one antigen-mismatch related donor stem cell transplant if there is a suitable donor. Those younger than 65 without a suitable donor receive an autologous transplant provided the bone marrow has less than 10% malignant cells and less than 30% clonal cells by immunophenotyping.

Selected Reading

Khouri IF et al. Hyper-CVAD and high-dose methotrexate/cytarabine followed by stem-cell transplantation: an active regimen for aggressive mantle-cell lymphoma. J Clin Oncol 16: 3803–3809, 1998.

ICE—IFOSFAMIDE-CARBOPLATIN-ETOPOSIDE

Ifosfamide. 5,000 mg/m^2 intravenously over 24 hours starting on day 2.

Carboplatin. To AUC 5 (maximum 800 mg) on day 2.

Etoposide. 100 mg/m^2/day intravenously on days 1 to 3.

Mesna. 5,000 mg/m^2 intravenously by continuous infusion (mixed with the ifosfamide).

NOTE: Repeat the cycle every 14 days. We have modified this regimen for outpatient use by administering the ifosfamide and mesna (mixed) as 1,500 mg/m^2/day (each) intravenously as a 2-hour infusion on days 1, 2, and 3.

Selected Reading

Moskowitz CH et al. Ifosfamide, carboplatin, and etoposide: a highly effective cytoreduction and peripheral-blood progenitor-cell mobilization regimen for transplant-eligible patients with non-Hodgkin's lymphoma. J Clin Oncol 17: 3776–3785, 1999.

MACOP-B—METHOTREXATE-DOXORUBICIN-CYCLOPHOSPHAMIDE-VINCRISTINE-PREDNISONE-BLEOMYCIN

Methotrexate. 400 mg/m^2 intravenously on week 2, 6, and 10.

Leucovorin. 15 mg orally every 6 hours for six doses given 24 hours after each dose of methotrexate.

Doxorubicin. 50 mg/m^2 intravenously on weeks 1, 3, 5, 7, 9, and 11.

Cyclophosphamide. 350 mg/m^2 intravenously on weeks 1, 3, 5, 7, 9, and 11.

Vincristine. 1.4 mg/m^2 (maximum 2 mg) intravenously on weeks 2, 4, 6, 8, 10, and 12.
Bleomycin. 10 units/m^2 intravenously on weeks 4, 8, and 12.
Prednisone. 75 mg/day orally; dose tapered over last 15 days.
Co-trimoxazole. One double-strength tablet orally twice daily throughout.
Ketoconazole. 200 mg/day orally throughout.
Hydrocortisone. 100 mg intravenously given just before each dose of bleomycin.
NOTE: The methotrexate is given as a 100 mg/m^2 IV bolus with the remaining 300 mg/m^2 infused over a 4-hour period. If the creatinine clearance is less than 60 mL/min, bleomycin replaces methotrexate for that course. Do not allow the use of astemizole (Hismanal$^®$) when using ketoconazole.

Selected Readings

Klimo P, Connors JM. MACOP-B chemotherapy for the treatment of advanced diffuse large cell lymphoma. Ann Intern Med 102: 596–602, 1985.

Klimo P, Connors JM. Updated clinical experience with MACOP-B. Semin Hematol 24(suppl 1): 26–34, 1987.

M-BACOD—METHOTREXATE-BLEOMYCIN-DOXORUBICIN-CYCLOPHOSPHAMIDE-VINCRISTINE-DEXAMETHASONE

Methotrexate. 200 mg/m^2 intravenously on days 8 and 15.
Leucovorin. 10 mg/m^2 orally every 6 hours for 8 doses beginning on days 9 and 16.
Bleomycin. 4 units/m^2 intravenously on day 1.
Doxorubicin. 45 mg/m^2 intravenously on day 1.
Cyclophosphamide. 600 mg/m^2 intravenously on day 1.
Vincristine. 1 mg/m^2 intravenously on day 1.
Dexamethasone. 6 mg/m^2/day orally on days 1 to 5.
NOTE: Repeat the cycle every 3 weeks (on day 22) for 10 cycles.

Selected Reading

Shipp MA et al. Identification of major prognostic subgroups of patients with large-cell lymphoma treated with m-BACOD or M-BACOD. Ann Intern Med 104: 757–765, 1986.

MINE-ESHAP

MINE—MESNA-IFOSFAMIDE-MITOXANTRONE-ETOPOSIDE

Mesna. 1,330 mg/m^2/day intravenously on days 1 to 3, and 500 mg orally 4 hours after the ifosfamide dose.
Ifosfamide. 1,330 mg/m^2/day intravenously on days 1 to 3.
Mitoxantrone. 8 mg/m^2 intravenously on day 1.
Etoposide. 65 mg/m^2/day intravenously on days 1 to 3.
NOTE: Repeat the cycle every 21 days for 6 cycles, and then start ESHAP.

ESHAP—ETOPOSIDE-METHYLPREDNISOLONE-HIGH-DOSE CYTARABINE-CISPLATIN

Etoposide. 60 mg/m^2/day intravenously on days 1 to 4.
Methylprednisolone. 500 mg/day (total daily dose) intravenously on days 1 to 4.
High-dose cytarabine. 2,000 mg/m^2 intravenously over 2 hours on day 5. Administer after cisplatin infusion is completed.
Cisplatin. 25 mg/m^2/day intravenously by continuous infusion on days 1 to 4.

NOTE: If complete remission is achieved with MINE, consolidate with 3 cycles of ESHAP. If there is only a partial MINE response, then give 6 cycles of ESHAP.

Many clinicians use ESHAP every 3 weeks as a stand-alone regimen for salvage and debulking prior to marrow ablation and transplantation.

Selected Reading

Rodriguez MA et al. Results of a salvage treatment program for relapsing lymphoma: MINE consolidated with ESHAP. J Clin Oncol 13: 1734–1741, 1995.

M-BNCOD—METHOTREXATE-BLEOMYCIN-MITOXANTRONE-VINCRISTINE-DEXAMETHASONE

Cyclophosphamide. 600 mg/m^2 intravenously on day 1.
Bleomycin. 4 units/m^2 intravenously on day 1.
Vincristine. 1 mg/m^2 intravenously (maximum 2 mg) on day 1.
Mitoxantrone. 10 mg/m^2 intravenously on day 1.
Dexamethasone. 6 mg/m^2/day orally on days 1 to 5.
Methotrexate. 200 mg/m^2/day intravenously on days 8 and 15.
Leucovorin. 15 mg/m^2 orally every 6 hours on days 9, 10, 16, and 17.
NOTE: Repeat the cycle every 21 days. Patients treated with this regimen had less alopecia and no episodes of adverse cardiac events in contrast to 8% in CHOP patients. The two groups had no significant differences in complete remission rate, disease-free survival, and overall survival.

Selected Reading

Guglielmi C et al. A phase III comparative trial of m-BACOD vs. m-BNCOD in the treatment of stage II–IV diffuse non-Hodgkin's lymphomas. Haematologica 74: 563–569, 1989.

PMitCEBO—PREDNISOLONE-MITOXANTRONE-CYCLOPHOS-PHAMIDE-ETOPOSIDE-VINCRISTINE-BLEOMYCIN

Prednisolone. 50 mg/day (total daily dose) orally on days 1 to 14.
Mitoxantrone. 7 mg/m^2 intravenously on day 1.
Cyclophosphamide. 300 mg/m^2 intravenously on day 1.
Etoposide. 150 mg/m^2 intravenously on day 1.
Vincristine. 1.4 mg/m^2 on day 8.
Bleomycin. 10 units/m^2 intravenously on day 8.
NOTE: Repeat the cycle every 2 weeks for a minimum of 8 weeks. Overall and complete response rates and overall survival were better than with the identical regimen using doxorubicin instead of mitoxantrone.

Selected Reading

Mainwaring PN et al. Mitoxantrone is superior to doxorubicin in a multi-agent weekly regimen for patients older than 60 with high-grade lymphoma: results of a BNLI randomized trial of PAdriaCEBO versus PMitCEBO. Blood 97: 2991–2997, 2001.

Pro-MACE-CytaBOM—METHOTREXATE-DOXORUBICIN-CYCLOPHOSPHAMIDE-ETOPOSIDE-CYTARABINE-VINCRISTINE

Cyclophosphamide. 650 mg/m^2 intravenously on day 1.
Doxorubicin. 25 mg/m^2 intravenously on day 1.
Etoposide. 120 mg/m^2 intravenously on day 1.
Prednisone. 60 mg/m^2/day orally on days 1 to 14.

Cytarabine. 300 mg/m^2 intravenously on day 8.
Bleomycin. 5 units/m^2 intravenously on day 8.
Vincristine. 1.4 mg/m^2 intravenously on day 8.
Methotrexate. 120 mg/m^2 intravenously on day 8.
Leucovorin. 25 mg/m^2 orally every 6 hours for 4 doses beginning on day 9.
NOTE: The next cycle begins on day 22. At least 6 cycles are given, 2 cycles beyond a complete remission. This regimen was associated with an increased incidence of diffuse interstitial pneumonia with four deaths. Hence, all patients now receive prophylactic co-trimoxazole, one double-strength tablet twice daily.

Selected Readings

Fisher RI et al. Long-term follow-up of Pro-MACE-CytaBOM in non-Hodgkin's lymphomas. Ann Oncol 2(suppl 1): 33–35, 1991.

Longo DL et al. Superiority of Pro-MACE-CytaBOM over ProMACE-MOPP in the treatment of advanced diffuse aggressive lymphoma: results of a prospective randomized trial. J Clin Oncol 9: 25–38, 1991.

VNCOP-B—ETOPOSIDE-MITOXANTRONE-CYCLOPHOSPHAMIDE-VINCRISTINE-PREDNISONE-BLEOMYCIN

Etoposide. 150 mg/m^2 intravenously on day 1 of weeks 2 and 6.
Mitoxantrone. 10 mg/m^2 intravenously on day 1 of weeks 1, 3, 5, and 7.
Cyclophosphamide. 300 mg/m^2 intravenously on day 1 of weeks 1, 3, 5, and 7.
Vincristine. 2 mg (total) intravenously on day 1 of weeks 2, 4, 6, and 8.
Bleomycin. 10 units/m^2 intravenously on day 1 of weeks 4 and 8.
Prednisone. 40 mg/day orally with dose tapered over the last 2 weeks.
NOTE: This regimen is completed in 8 weeks and is given entirely as an outpatient.

Selected Reading

Zinzani PL et al. Elderly aggressive-histology non-Hodgkin's lymphoma: first-line VNCOP-B regimen experience on 350 patients. Blood 94: 33–38, 1999.

VIM—ETOPOSIDE-IFOSFAMIDE-MITOXANTRONE

Etoposide. 65 mg/m^2/day intravenously on days 1 to 3.
Ifosfamide. 650 mg/m^2/day intravenously on days 1 to 3.
Mesna. 650 mg/m^2/day intravenously on days 1 to 3.
Mitoxantrone. 3 mg/m^2/day intravenously on days 1 to 3.
NOTE: Repeat the cycle every 3 weeks.

Selected Reading

Hopfinger G et al. Ifosfamide mitoxantrone and etoposide (VIM) as salvage therapy of low toxicity in non-Hodgkin's lymphoma. Eur J Haematol 55: 223–227, 1995.

MALIGNANT MESOTHELIOMA

Malignant mesothelioma afflicts about 2,200 and kills 2,000 patients yearly in the United States. A history of asbestos exposure is reported in about 70% to 80% of all cases. Pleural mesothelioma may progress more slowly than peritoneal mesothelioma, but this difference may reflect earlier diagnosis by chest x-ray studies. In many cases the tumor grows through the diaphragm, making the site of origin difficult to assess. Major prognostic factors are age, stage, performance status, histology, and nodal status. Aggressive surgical approaches may provide long-term survival (without cure) when performed in centers with experienced teams. Intracavitary chemotherapy or palliative radiotherapy may follow resection. In general, combination chemotherapy gives response rates only marginally better than single agents (Ong ST, Vogelzang NJ.

Chemotherapy in malignant pleural mesothelioma: a review. J Clin Oncol 14: 1007–1017, 1996).

ALDESLEUKIN (INTERLEUKIN-2)

Aldesleukin. 9 million IU intrapleurally twice a week for 4 weeks.
Aldesleukin. 3 million IU subcutaneously 3 times a week for 6 months.
NOTE: Therapy with subcutaneous aldesleukin is continued for 6 months or as long as the patient is stable and can tolerate the toxicity.

Selected Reading

Castagneto B et al. Palliative and therapeutic activity of IL-2 immunotherapy in unresectable malignant pleural mesothelioma with pleural effusion: results of a phase II study on 31 consecutive patients. Lung Cancer 31: 303–310, 2001.

CISPLATIN-GEMCITABINE

Cisplatin. 100 mg/m^2 intravenously on day 1.
Gemcitabine. 1,000 mg/m^2 intravenously on days 1, 8, and 15.
NOTE: Repeat the cycle every 28 days for 6 cycles.

Selected Reading

Byrne JM et al. Cisplatin and gemcitabine treatment for malignant mesothelioma: a phase II study. J Clin Oncol 17: 25–30, 1999.

CISPLATIN-MITOMYCIN

Cisplatin. 75 mg/m^2 intravenously every 4 weeks.
Mitomycin. 10 mg/m^2 intravenously every 4 weeks.
NOTE: Hydration and antiemetics are important. Maximum cumulative dose of mitomycin is 50 mg/m^2.

Selected Reading

Chahinian AP et al. Randomized phase II trial of cisplatin with mitomycin or doxorubicin for malignant mesothelioma by the Cancer and Leukemia Group B. J Clin Oncol 11: 1559–1565, 1993.

CD—CYCLOPHOSPHAMIDE-DOXORUBICIN

Cyclophosphamide. 400 mg/m^2 intravenously on days 1 and 8.
Doxorubicin. 40 mg/m^2 intravenously on days 1 and 8.
NOTE: Repeat the cycle every 28 days. Discontinue doxorubicin therapy after 450 mg/m^2.
Alternative program given every 21 days:
Cyclophosphamide. 1,000 mg/m^2 intravenously on day 1.
Doxorubicin. 45 mg/m^2 intravenously on day 1.

Selected Reading

Antman KH et al. Peritoneal mesothelioma: natural history and response to chemotherapy. J Clin Oncol 1: 386–391, 1983.

CYCLOPHOSPHAMIDE-DOXORUBICIN-CISPLATIN

Cyclophosphamide. 500 mg/m^2 intravenously on day 1.
Doxorubicin. 50 mg/m^2 intravenously on day 1.
Cisplatin. 80 mg/m^2 intravenously on day 1.

MALIGNANT MESOTHELIOMA

7

NOTE: Repeat the cycle every 3 weeks for 3 cycles. The cisplatin dose was reduced to 50 mg/m² in subsequent cycles. Vigorous hydration and antiemetics are needed.

Selected Reading

Shin DM et al. Prospective study of combination chemotherapy with cyclophosphamide, doxorubicin and cisplatin for unresectable or metastatic malignant pleural mesothelioma. Cancer 76: 2230–2236, 1995.

DOXORUBICIN-CISPLATIN (PLUS/MINUS MITOMYCIN OR INTERFERON ALFA-2B)

Doxorubicin. 60 mg/m² intravenously on day 1.

Cisplatin. 60 mg/m² intravenously on day 1.

NOTE: Repeat the cycle every 3 or 4 weeks. Pennucci et al added mitomycin 10 mg/m² intravenously and repeated cycles every 28 days. The level of increased activity above that of the two drug regimens is minimal. Parra et al added interferon alfa-2b, 6 million IU subcutaneously 3 times a week for a total of 6 cycles or until progression. It is doubtful that the small increment in efficacy is worth the substantial increase in toxicity.

Selected Readings

Ardizzoni A et al. Activity of doxorubicin and cisplatin combination chemotherapy in patients with diffuse malignant pleural mesothelioma. Cancer 67: 2984–2987, 1991.

Parra HS et al. Combined regimen of cisplatin, doxorubicin, and alfa-2b interferon in the treatment of advanced malignant pleural mesothelioma: a phase II multicenter trial of the Italian Group on Rare Tumors (GITR) and the Italian Lung Cancer Task Force (FONICAP). Cancer 92: 650–656, 2001.

Pennucci MC et al. Combined cisplatin, doxorubicin, and mitomycin for the treatment of advanced pleural mesothelioma: a phase II FONICAP trial. Italian Lung Cancer Task Force. Cancer 79: 1897–1902, 1997.

PEMETREXED-CISPLATIN

Pemetrexed. 500 mg/m² intravenously over 10 minutes on day 1.

Cisplatin. 75 mg/m² intravenously on day 1 given 30 minutes after the pemetrexed.

NOTE: Repeat the cycle every 3 weeks for 6 courses. To reduce toxicity, give leucovorin 0.35 to 1 mg/day orally prior to and during therapy and vitamin B₁₂ 1 mg intramuscularly prior to and every 9 weeks. Give dexamethasone prophylaxis for skin rash.

Selected Readings

Fizazi K et al. The emerging role of antifolates in the treatment of malignant pleural mesothelioma. Semin Oncol 29: 77–81, 2002.

Vogelzang NJ et al. Phase III single-blinded study of pemetrexed + cisplatin vs. cisplatin alone in chemonaive patients with malignant pleural mesothelioma, Proc ASCO 21: 2a (abstract 5), 2002.

MELANOMA (CUTANEOUS)

Melanoma accounts for about 4% of all new cancer cases in the United States, and 1.4% of deaths. It is associated with genetic predisposition, somatic mutations, and with increased sun exposure (primarily the ultraviolet light). Prognosis is affected by clinical and histological factors and by anatomical location of the lesion. Thickness (Breslow depth) of the melanoma, ulceration or bleeding at the primary site, and involvement of regional lymph nodes all affect the prognosis, which correlates with the stage (see the 2002 AJCC Cancer Staging Manual, 6th edition, which will be effective after January 1, 2003). Wide local excision and in some cases sentinel node dissection is indicated. Adjuvant immunotherapy with interferon alfa-2 can prolong disease-free survival but with considerable toxicity. Once distant metastases occur, cure is unlikely, but palliation with immunotherapy and/or chemotherapy may be worthwhile. There are many regimens because none has demonstrated superiority, but they have variable toxicities and difficulties of administration. At present, response rates and survival are only marginally improved by combination chemotherapy with or without immunotherapy. However, new vaccines, monoclonal antibodies, and new chemoimmunotherapy approaches are in clinical trials. In the absence of any high response rates in current therapy, patients should be encouraged to participate in clinical trials to evaluate new therapeutic approaches.

ADJUVANT INTERFERON ALFA-2B

Interferon alfa-2b. 20 million international units/m^2 intravenously 5 days a week for 4 weeks.
Interferon alfa-2b. 10 million international units/m^2 subcutaneously 3 times a week for 48 weeks.
NOTE: Dose modifications are made for toxicity. Depression raises the risk of suicide and therapy should be discontinued until a psychiatrist evaluates the patient and agrees that therapy can be safely resumed. Lower doses of interferon have not demonstrated the statistically significant benefits of high-dose therapy.

Selected Readings

Kirkwood JM et al. Interferon alfa-2b adjuvant therapy of high-risk resected cutaneous melanoma: The Eastern Cooperative Oncology Group Trial EST 1684. J Clin Oncol 14: 7–17, 1966.
Kirkwood JM et al. High-dose interferon alfa-2b significantly prolongs relapse-free and overall survival compared with the GM2-KLH/QS-21 vaccine in patients with resected stage IIB–III melanomas: results of Intergroup Trial E1694/S9512/C50901. J Clin Oncol 19: 2370–2380, 2001.

CVD—CISPLATIN-VINBLASTINE-DACARBAZINE

Cisplatin. 20 mg/m^2 intravenously on days 2 to 5.
Vinblastine. 1.6 mg/m^2/day intravenously on days 1 to 5.
Dacarbazine. 800 mg/m^2 intravenously on day 1.
NOTE: Repeat the cycle every 3 weeks as tolerated to maximum benefit or progression.

Selected Reading

Legha SS et al. A prospective evaluation of a triple-drug regimen containing cisplatin, vinblastine, and dacarbazine (CVD) for metastatic melanoma. Cancer 64: 2024–2029, 1989.

CHEMOIMMUNOTHERAPY (BIOCHEMOTHERAPY)

Dacarbazine. 750 mg/m^2 intravenously on day 1 of weeks 1 and 4.
Carboplatin. 400 mg/m^2 intravenously on day 1 of weeks 1 and 4.
Interleukin-2. 4.8 million IU/m^2 subcutaneously 3 times/day, on day 1 of weeks 7 and 10.
Interleukin-2. 2.4 million IU/m^2 subcutaneously 2 times/day, on days 3 to 5 of weeks 7 and 10.
Interleukin-2. 2.4 million IU/m^2 subcutaneously 2 times/day, on days 1 to 5 of weeks 8, 9, 11, and 12.

Interferon-alfa. 3 million IU/m^2 subcutaneously on days 3 and 5 of weeks 7 and 10; 6 million IU/m^2 subcutaneously on days 1, 3, and 5 of weeks 8, 9, 11, and 12.
NOTE: Therapy can be given as outpatient treatment. Toxicity is severe but tolerable with adequate antiemetics. Many other groups have similar programs with 2 or 3 chemotherapy drugs plus or minus tamoxifen and with variable doses of aldesleukin and interferon alfa-2. Legha et al claimed high response rates but with admittedly high toxicity in an uncontrolled trial using CVD plus aldesleukin and interferon alfa-2. Ridolfi et al used cisplatin and dacarbazine with and without interferon alfa-2 and a somewhat lower dose of aldesleukin and found no significant differences in overall survival, time to progression, or overall response between the two groups. Rosenberg et al used cisplatin, dacarbazine, and tamoxifen with or without high-dose aldesleukin and interferon alfa-2a and found that the addition of the immunotherapy increased the toxicity but did not increase survival, and they recommended its use only in well-designed, prospective, randomized protocols. O'Day et al used biochemotherapy in an uncontrolled study and attempted to decrease toxicity by using decrescendo dosing of the aldesleukin. Eton et al compared sequential biochemothrapy with CVD and found increased antitumor activity at the expense of considerable toxicity. Flaherty et al used cisplatin and dacarbazine plus aldesleukin and interferon alfa-2b in an uncontrolled outpatient program and reported activity with acceptable toxicity.

Selected Readings

Atzpodien J et al. Chemo-immunotherapy of advanced malignant melanoma: sequential administration of subcutaneous interleukin-2 and interferon-alfa after intravenous dacarbazine and carboplatin or intravenous dacarbazine, cisplatin, carmustine and tamoxifen. Eur J Cancer 31A: 876–881, 1995.

Eton O et al. Sequential biochemotherapy versus chemotherapy for metastatic melanoma: results from a phase III randomized trial. J Clin Oncol 20: 2045–2052, 2002.

Flaherty LE et al. Outpatient biochemotherapy with interleukin-2 and interferon alfa-2b in patients with metastatic malignant melanoma: results of two phase II Cytokine Working Group trials. J Clin Oncol 19: 3194–3202, 2001.

Legha SS et al. Development of a biochemotherapy regimen with concurrent administration of cisplatin, vinblastine, dacarbazine, interferon alfa, and interleukin-2 for patients with metastatic melanoma. J Clin Oncol 16: 1752–1759, 1998.

O'Day SJ et al. Advantages of concurrent biochemotherapy modified by decrescendo interleukin-2, granulocyte colony-stimulating factor, and tamoxifen for patients with metastastic melanoma. J Clin Oncol 17: 2752–2761, 1999.

Ridolfi R et al. Cisplatin, dacarbazine with or without subcutaneous interleukin-2, and interferon alfa-2b in advanced melanoma outpatients: results from an Italian multicenter phase III randomized clinical trial. J Clin Oncol 20: 1600–1607, 2002.

Rosenberg SA et al. Prospective randomized trial of the treatment of patients with metastatic melanoma using chemotherapy with cisplatin, dacarbazine, and tamoxifen alone or in combination with interleukin-2 and interferon alfa-2b. J Clin Oncol 17: 968–975, 1999.

DACARBAZINE

Dacarbazine. 1,000 mg/m^2 intravenously every 3 weeks.
NOTE: Middleton et al used 250 mg/m^2/day intravenously for 5 days every 21 days. This is the more usual but less convenient dosing.

Selected Readings

Chapman PB et al. Phase II multicenter randomized trial of the Dartmouth regimen versus dacarbazine in patients with metastatic melanoma. J Clin Oncol 17: 2745–2751, 1999.

Middleton MR et al. Randomized phase III study of temozolomide versus dacarbazine in the treatment of patients with advanced metastatic malignant melanoma, J Clin Oncol 18: 158–166, 2000.

DARTMOUTH REGIMEN—DACARBAZINE-CARMUSTINE-CISPLATIN-TAMOXIFEN

Dacarbazine. 220 mg/m^2/day intravenously on days 1 to 3.
Carmustine. 150 mg/m^2 intravenously on day 1.
Cisplatin. 25 mg/m^2/day intravenously on days 1 to 3.
Tamoxifen. 10 mg orally twice a day.
NOTE: Repeat treatment with dacarbazine and cisplatin every 3 weeks. Repeat treatment with carmustine every 6 weeks. Rusthoven et al have called into question the value of adding tamoxifen to this regimen. Creagan et al found no meaningful clinical advantage from the addition of tamoxifen to the 3 chemotherapy drugs.

Selected Readings

Creagan ET et al. Phase III clinical trial of the combination of cisplatin, dacarbazine, and carmustine with or without tamoxifen in patients with advanced malignant melanoma. J Clin Oncol 17: 1884–1890, 1999.
DelPrete SA et al. Combination chemotherapy with cisplatin, carmustine, dacarbazine, and tamoxifen in metastatic melanoma. Cancer Treat Rep 68: 1403–1405, 1984.
Rusthoven JJ et al. Randomized, double-blind, placebo-controlled trial comparing the response rates of carmustine, dacarbazine and cisplatin with and without tamoxifen in patients with metastatic melanoma. J Clin Oncol 14: 2083–2090, 1996.

GM-CSF (SARGRAMOSTIM) AS ADJUVANT

Sargramostim. 125 microg/m^2/day subcutaneously for 14 days.
NOTE: Repeat the cycle every 28 days. Treatment is continued for a year or until disease recurrence.

Selected Reading

Spitler LE et al. Adjuvant therapy of stage III and IV malignant melanoma using granulocyte-macrophage colony-stimulating factor. J Clin Oncol 18: 1614–1621, 2000.

INTERLEUKIN-2 (ALDESLEUKIN)

Aldesleukin. 600,000 IU/kg or 720,000 IU/kg intravenously every 8 hours for up to 14 consecutive doses over 5 days.
NOTE: Give to clinical tolerance with maximum support, including pressors. Repeat the cycle after a 6- to 9-day rest and repeat every 6 to 12 weeks in stable responding patients. Although the response rate is only about 16%, the 6% who had a complete response rate had a long progression-free survival.

Selected Reading

Atkins MB et al. High-dose recombinant interleukin-2 therapy for patients with metastatic melanoma: analysis of 270 patients treated between 1985 and 1993. J Clin Oncol 17: 2105–2116, 1999.

TEMOZOLOMIDE

Temozolomide. 200 mg/m^2/day orally on days 1 to 5.
NOTE: Repeat the cycle every 28 days.

Selected Reading

Middleton MR et al. Randomized phase III study of temozolomide versus dacarbazine in the treatment of patients with advanced metastatic malignant melanoma. J Clin Oncol 18: 158–166, 2000.

TEMOZOLOMIDE-DOCETAXEL

Temozolomide. 150 mg/m^2/day orally on days 1 to 5.
Docetaxel. 80 mg/m^2 intravenously on day 1.
NOTE: Repeat the cycle every 4 weeks for a maximum of 6 cycles.

Selected Reading

Bafaloukos D et al. Temozolomide in combination with docetaxel in patients with advanced melanoma: a phase II study of the Hellenic Cooperative Oncology Group. J Clin Oncol 20: 420–425, 2002.

TEMOZOLOMIDE-THALIDOMIDE

Temozolomide. 75 mg/m^2/day orally for 6 weeks with a 4-week break and repeat.
Thalidomide. 200 mg/m^2/day orally with escalation to 400 mg/m^2/day as tolerated.
NOTE: Thalidomide at 400 mg/m^2/day is well tolerated in patients younger than 70, but older patients are given 200 mg/m^2/day. Risk of fetal damage.

Selected Reading

Hwu W-J et al. Temozolomide plus thalidomide in patients with advanced melanoma: results of a dose-finding trial. J Clin Oncol 20: 2610–2615, 2002.

MULTIPLE MYELOMA (PLASMA CELL NEOPLASM)

A solitary plasmacytoma is sometimes curable by resection or radiation therapy, but multiple myeloma, although highly treatable, is rarely curable. Staging is important in selecting therapy. Benign monoclonal gammopathy requires no therapy unless or until it converts to active myeloma. Indolent myeloma is often observed carefully to determine when and if to treat. Active disease requires therapy, but there is controversy over what that therapy should be, ranging from single agents like dexamethasone or thalidomide, to melphalan-prednisone, to combinations of 3, 4, or 5 drugs, to high-dose chemotherapy with stem cell transplantation. Although it appears that high-dose chemotherapy with stem cell and cytokine support can frequently prolong life, there is no convincing evidence that it is curative in a high proportion of cases. For further information, see Chapter 10, which discusses high-dose chemotherapy with stem cell support. Over time, randomized clinical trials should bring a closer consensus. Bone destruction can often be decreased or slowed with the use of bisphosphonates such as pamidronate or zoledronic acid. Aggressive treatment of infection is essential because major causes of death in myeloma are infection and renal failure.

ABCM—DOXORUBICIN-CARMUSTINE-CYCLOPHOSPHAMIDE-MELPHALAN

Carmustine. 30 mg/m^2 intravenously on day 1.
Doxorubicin. 30 mg/m^2 intravenously on day 1.
Cyclophosphamide. 100 mg/m^2/day orally on days 22 to 25.
Melphalan. 6 mg/m^2/day orally on days 22 to 25.
NOTE: Repeat the cycle every 6 weeks to remission or relapse. Do not exceed doxorubin cumulative dose of 450 mg/m^2.

Selected Reading

MacLennan IC et al. Combined chemotherapy with ABCM versus melphalan for treatment of myelomatosis. The Medical Research Council Working Party for Leukemia in Adults. Lancet 339: 200–205, 1992.

BAP—CARMUSTINE-DOXORUBICIN-PREDNISONE

Carmustine. 75 mg/m^2 intravenously on day 1.
Doxorubicin. 30 mg/m^2 intravenously on days 1 and 22.
Prednisone. 0.6 mg/kg orally in three equally divided doses daily for 7 days every 3 weeks.
NOTE: Repeat the cycle every 6 weeks.

Selected Reading

Kyle RA et al. Multiple myeloma resistant to melphalan: treatment with doxorubicin, cyclophosphamide, carmustine (BCNU) and prednisone. Cancer Treat Rep 66: 451–456, 1982.

CYCLOPHOSPHAMIDE-PREDNISONE

Cyclophosphamide. 150 to 250 mg/m^2 (500 mg maximum) intravenously or orally weekly.
Prednisone. 100 mg orally every other day.

Selected Reading

Wilson K et al. Weekly cyclophosphamide and alternate-day prednisone: an effective secondary therapy in multiple myeloma. Cancer Treat Rep 71: 981–982, 1987.

DEXAMETHASONE

Dexamethasone. 20 mg/m^2 daily for 4 days, beginning on days 1, 9 and 17.
NOTE: After a rest period of 14 days, the cycle is repeated with downward adjustments of dose for toxicity.

Selected Reading

Alexanian R et al. Primary dexamethasone treatment of multiple myeloma. Blood 80: 887–890, 1992.

HYPER-CVAD—CYCLOPHOSPHAMIDE-VINCRISTINE-DOXORUBICIN-DEXAMETHASONE

Cyclophosphamide. 300 mg/m^2 intravenously every 12 hours for 6 doses (total 1,800 mg/m^2).
Mesna. 600 mg/m^2/day intravenously for 3 days simultaneous with the cyclophosphamide.
Vincristine. 2 mg intravenously by continuous infusion over 48 hours beginning 12 hours after completion of cyclophosphamide.
Doxorubicin. 50 mg/m^2 intravenously by 48-hour continuous infusion beginning 12 hours after completion of cyclophosphamide.
Vincristine. 2 mg intravenously by bolus injection on day 11.
Dexamethasone. 20 mg/m^2/day orally in the morning for 5 days beginning on day 1 and again for 4 days beginning on day 11.
NOTE: If there is a 50% reduction of myeloma protein, a second course of Hyper-CVAD is given when the blood counts recover. Responding patients are maintained on oral cyclophosphamide 125 mg/m^2 every 12 hours and dexamethasone 20 mg/m^2

every morning for 5 days every 5 weeks. Appropriate patients may be considered for autologous stem cell transplantation for either persistent resistant disease or to consolidate remission. Supportive care may include filgrastim, ciprofloxacin, fluconazole, and acyclovir.

Selected Reading

Dimopoulos MA et al. HyperCVAD for VAD-resistant multiple myeloma. Am J Hematol 52: 77–81, 1996.

MP—MELPHALAN-PREDNISONE

Melphalan. 10 mg/m^2/day orally on days 1 to 4.
Prednisone. 60 mg/m^2/day orally on days 1 to 4.
NOTE: Repeat the cycle every 6 weeks.

Selected Reading

Southwest Oncology Group Study. Remission maintenance therapy for multiple myeloma. Arch Intern Med 135: 147–152, 1975.

THAL-CED-THALIDOMIDE-CYCLOPHOSPHAMIDE-ETOPOSIDE-DEXAMETHASONE

Thalidomide. 400 mg orally daily until toxic side effects or disease progression.
Cyclophosphamide. 400 mg/m^2/day intravenously by continuous infusion on days 1 to 4.
Etoposide. 40 mg/m^2/day intravenously by continuous infusion on days 1 to 4.
Dexamethasone. 40 mg/day orally on days 1 to 4.
NOTE: Repeat the cycle every 28 days for 3 to 6 cycles until best response or progression.

Selected Reading

Moehler TM et al. Salvage therapy for multiple myeloma with thalidomide and CED chemotherapy. Blood 98: 3846–3848, 2001.

THALIDOMIDE-DEXAMETHASONE

Thalidomide. 200 mg/day orally for 2 weeks, then increase as tolerated in 200-mg increments at 2-week intervals to maximum 800 mg/day.
Dexamethasone. 40 mg/day orally on days 1 to 4, 9 to 12, and 17 to 20.
NOTE: Repeat the cycle every 28 days with these doses in odd-numbered cycles; in even-numbered cycles give dexamethasone only on days 1 to 4.

Selected Reading

Kyle RA, Rajkumar SV. Therapeutic application of thalidomide in multiple myeloma. Semin Oncol 28: 583–587, 2001.

VAD—VINCRISTINE-DOXORUBICIN-DEXAMETHASONE

Vincristine. 0.4 mg/day intravenously by continuous infusion on days 1 to 4.
Doxorubicin. 9 mg/m^2/day intravenously by continuous infusion on days 1 to 4.
Dexamethasone. 40 mg/day orally on days 1 to 4, 9 to 12, and 17 to 20.
NOTE: All patients receive prophylactic antacid treatment with an H2 blocker or a proton pump inhibitor and antibiotic prophylaxis with co-trimoxazole. Repeat the cycle every 25 days until a maximum reduction in myeloma protein levels has occurred. Four additional cycles are given after the myeloma protein levels disappear or stabilize.

Selected Reading

Barlogie B et al. Effective treatment of advanced multiple myeloma refractory to alkylating agents. N Engl J Med 310: 1353–1356, 1984.

VBMCP—VINCRISTINE-CARMUSTINE-CYCLOPHOSPHAMIDE-MELPHALAN-PREDNISONE

Vincristine. 1.2 mg/m² (maximum 2 mg) intravenously on day 1.
Carmustine. 20 mg/m² intravenously on day 1.
Cyclophosphamide. 400 mg/m² intravenously on day 1.
Melphalan. 8 mg/m²/day orally for 4 days, on days 1 to 4.
Prednisone. 40 mg/m²/day orally on days 1 to 7 during all cycles, and 20 mg/m²/day orally on days 8 to 14 during the first 3 cycles only.
NOTE: Repeat the cycle every 35 days for 10 cycles. Thereafter, patients in continuing objective remission are placed on a maintenance program detailed in Oken reference. This regimen is nearly identical to the M-2 regimen of Case et al.

Selected Readings

Case BC Jr et al. Improved survival times in multiple myeloma treated with melphalan, prednisone, cyclophosphamide, vincristine, and BCNU: M-2 protocol. Am J Med 63: 897–903, 1977.
Oken MM et al. Comparison of melphalan and prednisone with vincristine, carmustine, melphalan, cyclophosphamide, and prednisone in the treatment of multiple myeloma: results of Eastern Cooperative Oncology Study Group E2479. Cancer 79: 1561–1567, 1997.

VMCP ALTERNATING WITH VBAP OR VCAP

VMCP—VINCRISTINE-MELPHALAN-CYCLOPHOSPHAMIDE-PREDNISONE

Vincristine. 1 mg/m² (maximum 1.5 mg) intravenously on day 1.
Melphalan. 6 mg/m²/day orally on days 1 to 4.
Cyclophosphamide. 125 mg/m²/day orally on days 1 to 4.
Prednisone. 60 mg/m²/day orally on days 1 to 4.
NOTE: Alternate every 3 weeks with either the VBAP or VCAP regimen.

VBAP—VINCRISTINE-CARMUSTINE-DOXORUBICIN-PREDNISONE

Vincristine. 1 mg intravenously on day 1.
Carmustine. 30 mg/m² intravenously on day 1.
Doxorubicin. 30 mg/m² intravenously on day 1.
Prednisone. 100 mg/day orally on days 1 to 4.
NOTE: Alternate the cycle every 21 days with VMCP.

VCAP—VINCRISTINE-CYCLOPHOSPHAMIDE-DOXORUBICIN-PREDNISONE

Vincristine. 1 mg/m² (maximum 1.5 mg) intravenously on day 1.
Cyclophosphamide. 125 mg/m²/day orally on days 1 to 4.
Doxorubicin. 30 mg/m² intravenously on day 1.
Prednisone. 60 mg/m²/day orally on days 1 to 4.
NOTE: Alternate the cycle every 21 days with VMCP.

Selected Readings

Bonnet J et al. Vincristine, BCNU, doxorubicin, and prednisone (VBAP) combination in the treatment of relapsing or resistant multiple myeloma: a Southwest Oncology Group study. Cancer Treat Rep 66: 1267–1271, 1982.

Salmon SE et al. Alternating combination chemotherapy and levamisole improves survival in multiple myeloma: a Southwest Oncology Group study. J Clin Oncol 1: 453–461, 1983.

Salmon SE et al. Chemotherapy is superior to sequential hemibody irradiation for remission consolidation in multiple myeloma: a Southwest Oncology Group study. J Clin Oncol 8: 1575–1584, 1990.

OSTEOSARCOMA

Osteosarcoma is a malignant spindle cell tumor that produces osteoid and is the most common primary malignant adult bone tumor (with the exception of multiple myeloma, which is usually grouped with the hematopoietic malignancies). Site of the primary tumor is a significant prognostic factor. Distal tumors have a more favorable prognosis, whereas axial skeleton primaries have a poor prognosis. Other prognostic factors include age, histology, duration of symptoms, size of tumor, LDH level, alkaline phosphatase level, and tumor ploidy.

Patients whose tumors can be resected and whose metastases (primarily to lung) can be removed may have a long survival, especially with adjuvant chemotherapy. Activity is significantly enhanced by the use of combination chemotherapy regimens, which may permit limb-sparing surgery.

CARBOPLATIN-IFOSFAMIDE

Carboplatin. 560 mg/m^2 intravenously on day 1.

Ifosfamide. 2,650 mg/m^2/day intravenously for 3 days (with mesna uroprotection) on days 1 to 3.

NOTE: Repeat the cycle in 21 days. Reassess at day 63 and if there is no progression, give a third cycle. After recovery from the chemotherapy, limb-sparing surgery is performed when feasible. After resection of the primary tumor, patients receive doxorubicin (5 treatments at 25 mg/m^2/day for 3 consecutive days as a 72-hour continuous infusion administered in the ambulatory setting) and high-dose methotrexate (9 treatments at 12,000 mg/m^2/dose with leucovorin rescue). Patients whose tumors demonstrated clinical and radiological progression during the 9-week presurgical phase, receive cisplatin (100 mg/m^2/dose) in substitution for the carboplatin-ifosfamide cycles. All other patients receive 2 additional cycles of carboplatin-ifosfamide.

Selected Reading

Meyer WH et al. Carboplatin–ifosfamide window therapy for osteosarcoma: results of the St Jude Children's Research Hospital OS-91 Trial. J Clin Oncol 19: 171–182, 2001.

CISPLATIN-DOXORUBICIN

Cisplatin. 100 mg/m^2 intravenously by 4-hour infusion.

Doxorubicin. 25 mg/m^2 intravenous bolus on days 1, 2, and 3.

NOTE: Pretreatment and post-treatment hydration is an essential element of the protocol. Treatments are repeated at 3-week intervals for 6 cycles.

Selected Readings

Bramwell VHC et al. A comparison of two short intensive adjuvant chemotherapy regimens in operable osteosarcoma of limbs in children and young adults: the first study of the European Osteosarcoma Intergroup. J Clin Oncol 10: 1579–1591, 1992.

Souhami RL et al. Randomised trial of two regimens of chemotherapy in operable osteosarcoma: a study of the European Osteosarcoma Intergroup. Lancet 350: 911–917, 1997.

DFCI-TCH STUDY III

Vincristine. 2 mg/m^2 intravenously; 30 minutes later, give the drugs below.

Methotrexate. 7,500 mg/m^2 intravenously over a 6-hour period.

Leucovorin. 15 mg intravenously (beginning 2 hours after the methotrexate dose is completed) every 3 hours for eight doses and then 15 mg orally every 6 hours for 8 doses.

Doxorubicin. 75 mg/m^2 intravenously every 3 weeks for 6 cycles beginning with the fifth cycle of vincristine-methotrexate.

NOTE: The vincristine-methotrexate-leucovorin (VML) regimen is administered every week for 4 weeks, then every 3 weeks with the addition of doxorubicin for 6 cycles, then VML every week for 4 weeks, then every 3 weeks for 6 cycles, and then every week for a final 4 weeks.

Selected Reading

Goorin AM et al. Weekly high dose methotrexate and doxorubicin for osteosarcoma: the Dana-Farber Cancer Institute/The Children's Hospital—Study III. J Clin Oncol 5: 1178–1184, 1987.

T-10

Methotrexate. 8,000 to 12,000 mg/m^2 on days 1, 8, 15, 22, 64, 71, 99, and 106.

Leucovorin. 10 to 15 mg orally every 6 hours for 10 doses starting 20 hours after each methotrexate dose.

Bleomycin. 15 units/m^2 on days 43 and 44.

Cyclophosphamide. 600 mg/m^2 on days 43 and 44.

Dactinomycin. 0.6 mg/m^2 on days 43 and 44.

Doxorubicin. 30 mg/m^2 on days 78, 79, and 80.

NOTE: On day 29, resection or amputation is performed if indicated; otherwise an endoprosthesis is placed on day 113. If tissue then shows grade I or II tumor (see the references for a definition), the patient's chemotherapy consists of 3 cycles of cisplatin plus doxorubicin, bleomycin, cyclophosphamide, and dactinomycin (T-10A). If the tumor is grade III or IV after chemotherapy, 3 cycles of bleomycin, cyclophosphamide, dactinomycin, methotrexate, and doxorubicin (T-10B) are given. This program requires extensive facilities and experience to perform it safely and successfully. In some later trials, cisplatin was sometimes added and the regimen individualized.

Selected Readings

Meyers PA et al. Chemotherapy for nonmetastatic osteogenic sarcoma: the Memorial Sloan-Kettering experience. J Clin Oncol 10: 5–15, 1992.

Rosen G et al. Preoperative chemotherapy for osteogenic sarcoma: selection of postoperative adjuvant chemotherapy based on the response of the primary tumor to preoperative chemotherapy. Cancer 49: 1221–1230, 1982.

ETOPOSIDE-CYCLOPHOSPHAMIDE-CISPLATIN-DOXORUBICIN

Etoposide. 200 mg/m^2/day intravenously for 3 consecutive days as a 72-hour continuous infusion during weeks 0, 3, 13, 19, 25, and 31.

Cyclophosphamide. 300 mg/m^2 intravenously every 12 hours for 6 doses during weeks 0, 3, 13, 19, 25, and 31.

Cisplatin. 100 mg/m^2 intravenously in weeks 6, 8, 16, 22, 28, and 34.

Doxorubicin. 40 mg/m^2 intravenously in weeks 6, 8, 16, 22, 28, and 34.

NOTE: Chemotherapy is begun on day 1 of each week. Surgery is performed during week 10.

Selected Reading

Cassano WF et al. Etoposide, cyclophosphamide, cisplatin, and doxorubicin as neoadjuvant chemotherapy for osteosarcoma. Cancer 68: 1899–1902, 1991.

OVARIAN CARCINOMA

Ovarian carcinoma is the fourth most common cause of cancer death in women and the leading cause of all female genital cancer deaths in the United States. One in 70 women will develop ovarian cancer in her lifetime. Favorable prognosis in ovarian cancer is associated with younger age; good performance status; cell type other than mucinous and clear-cell; lower-stage, well-differentiated tumor; smaller disease volume before surgical debulking; absence of ascites; and platinum-based therapy. Because the disease is often asymptomatic in its early stages, most patients have widespread disease at the time of diagnosis. Early stages of the disease are curable in a high percentage of patients.

Therapy involves surgical exploration by an experienced gynecological oncologist with debulking of all grossly visible tumor, including the area just under the diaphragm, and leaving minimal tumor – lesions less than 1 cm. This is followed by chemotherapy as soon as adequate surgical healing has taken place. As a result of multiple controlled trials, it seems that the best therapy for advanced ovarian epithelial cancer is a platinum-based regimen, perhaps as a single agent, but more commonly with a taxane. Carboplatin is easier to administer and less toxic than cisplatin. Paclitaxel is less myelotoxic but more neurotoxic than docetaxel. For patients who fail first-line regimens, there are a variety of salvage regimens, some of which are listed. High-dose chemotherapy with bone marrow or peripheral stem cell support is the subject of several experimental trials. The role of radiation therapy is controversial, but is generally reserved for palliation or special situations. For patients who have low-volume disease or minimum residual disease after debulking and systemic chemotherapy, intraperitoneal chemotherapy with cisplatin, paclitaxel, cytarabine, or a combination thereof is frequently successful in prolonging disease-free survival.

Ovarian germ cell tumor is a clinically and histologically different disease, although it afflicts the same organ. It has a different clinical course, prognosis, and therapy. It is discussed in a separate section.

CYCLOPHOSPHAMIDE WITH CISPLATIN OR CARBOPLATIN

Cisplatin-Cyclophosphamide
Cisplatin. 75 mg/m^2 or 100 mg/m^2 intravenously on day 1.
Cyclophosphamide. 600 mg/m^2 intravenously on day 1.

Carboplatin-Cyclophosphamide
Carboplatin. 300 mg/m^2 intravenously on day 1.
Cyclophosphamide. 600 mg/m^2 intravenously on day 1.

NOTE: Repeat the cycle every 28 days for 6 cycles. There is evidence to suggest that the equivalence ratio of carboplatin to cisplatin is 4 to 1. The Southwest Oncology Group used 100 mg/m^2 cisplatin, and the Canadian group used 75 mg/m^2. Neither regimen is optimal, and a taxane with carboplatin is superior.

Selected Readings

Albert D et al. Improved therapeutic index of carboplatin plus cyclophosphamide versus cisplatin plus cyclophosphamide: final report by the Southwest Oncology Group of phase III, randomized trial in stages III and IV ovarian cancer. J Clin Oncol 10: 706–717, 1992.

Swenerton K et al. Cisplatin-cyclophosphamide versus carboplatin-cyclophosphamide in advanced ovarian cancer: a randomized phase III study of the National Cancer Institute of Canada Clinical Trials Group. J Clin Oncol 10: 718–726, 1992.

DOCETAXEL-CARBOPLATIN

Docetaxel. 60 mg/m^2 intravenously on day 1.
Carboplatin. At AUC 6 intravenously on day 1.
NOTE: *This protocol requires appropriate premedication and support for the severe neutropenia. It is highly active. Repeat the cycle every 3 weeks for 6 cycles. A similar program with cisplatin 75 mg/m^2 and docetaxel 75 mg/m^2 was used by Vasey et al but had severe neutropenia and an unacceptably high incidence of neurotoxicity.*

Selected Readings
Markman M et al. Combination chemotherapy with carboplatin and docetaxel in the treatment of cancers of the ovary and fallopian tube and primary carcinoma of the peritoneum. J Clin Oncol 19: 1901–1905, 2001.
Vasey PA et al. Docetaxel and cisplatin in combination as first-line chemotherapy for advanced epithelial ovarian cancer. J Clin Oncol 17: 2069–2080, 1999.

H-CAP—ALTRETAMINE-CYCLOPHOSPHAMIDE-DOXORUBICIN-CISPLATIN

Altretamine. 150 mg/m^2/day orally on days 1 to 14.
Cyclophosphamide. 350 mg/m^2 intravenously on days 1 and 8.
Doxorubicin. 20 mg/m^2 intravenously on days 1 and 8.
Cisplatin. 60 mg/m^2 intravenously on day 1.
NOTE: *Repeat the cycle every 4 weeks.*

Selected Readings
Greco FA et al. A comparison of hexamethylmelamine (altretamine), cyclophosphamide, doxorubicin, and cisplatin (H-CAP) vs cyclophosphamide, doxorubicin, and cisplatin (CAP) in advanced ovarian cancer. Cancer Treat Rev 18(suppl A): 47–55, 1991.
Hainsworth JD et al. Advanced ovarian cancer: long-term results of treatment with intensive cisplatin-based chemotherapy of brief duration. Ann Intern Med 108: 165–170, 1988.

INTRAPERITONEAL CARBOPLATIN

Carboplatin. 200 mg/m^2 intraperitoneally in 2 L 1.5% dextrose solution with a 4-hour dwell time. Dose may be escalated as tolerated.
NOTE: *Repeat the cycle every 28 days for 6 cycles. Escalate very gradually for creatinine clearance less than 60 mL/min.*

Selected Reading
Speyer JL et al. Intraperitoneal carboplatin: favorable results in women with minimal residual ovarian cancer after cisplatin therapy. J Clin Oncol 8: 1335–1341, 1990.

INTRAPERITONEAL CISPLATIN-CYTARABINE

Cisplatin. 200 mg/m^2 intraperitoneally on day 1.
Cytarabine. 2,000 mg/m^2 intraperitoneally on day 1.
Sodium thiosulfate. 4,000 mg/m^2 intravenously by bolus followed by 12,000 mg/m^2 intravenously over 6 hours.

NOTE: Repeat the cycle every 28 days. The cisplatin is mixed with the cytarabine in 2 L of normal saline over a 30- to 50-minute period and drained over a 4-hour span. Alberts et al gave intraperitoneal cisplatin 100 mg/m² and intravenous cyclophosphamide 600 mg/m² at 3-week intervals and had a significantly better survival than a similar cohort who received both drugs intravenously at the same respective doses at the same interval.

Selected Readings

Alberts DS et al. Intraperitoneal cisplatin plus intravenous cyclophosphamide versus intravenous cisplatin plus intravenous cyclophosphamide for stage III ovarian cancer. N Engl J Med 335: 1950–1955, 1996.

Markman M et al. Intraperitoneal chemotherapy with high-dose cisplatin and cytosine arabinoside for refractory ovarian carcinoma and other malignancies principally involving the peritoneal cavity. J Clin Oncol 3: 925–931, 1985.

PAC VERSUS PC

PAC—CISPLATIN-DOXORUBICIN-CYCLOPHOSPHAMIDE

Cisplatin. 50 mg/m² intravenously on day 1.
Doxorubicin. 45 mg/m² intravenously on day 1.
Cyclophosphamide. 600 mg/m² intravenously on day 1.
NOTE: Repeat the cycle every 28 days for 6 cycles. The complete response (CR) rate for the PAC regimen was 41%; the partial response rate was 17%.

PC—CISPLATIN-CYCLOPHOSPHAMIDE

Cisplatin. 50 mg/m² intravenously on day 1.
Cyclophosphamide. 600 mg/m² intravenously on day 1.
NOTE: Repeat the cycle every 28 days for 6 cycles. The CR rate for the PC regimen was 20%; the PR rate was 34%.

Selected Reading

Conte PF et al. A randomized trial comparing cisplatin plus cyclophosphamide versus cisplatin, doxorubicin and cyclophosphamide in advanced ovarian cancer. J Clin Oncol 4: 965–971, 1986.

PACLITAXEL-CISPLATIN

Paclitaxel. 135 mg/m² intravenously over 3 hours on day 1.
Cisplatin. 75 mg/m² intravenously over 1 hour on day 1.
NOTE: Repeat the cycle every 3 weeks. Paclitaxel is always given before cisplatin. This program was superior to cisplatin-cyclophosphamide in a Gynecologic Oncology Group study. Neijt et al used paclitaxel at 175 mg/m² over 3 hours followed by cisplatin 75 mg/m². The trend of many other studies is to use the higher dose of paclitaxel (175 mg/m²), although some investigators have gone to 200, 225, or even 250 mg/m² at the cost of substantially higher toxicity.

Selected Readings

McGuire WP et al. Cyclophosphamide and cisplatin compared with paclitaxel and cisplatin in patients with stage III and stage IV ovarian cancer. N Engl J Med 334: 1–6, 1996.

Neijt JP et al. Exploratory phase III study of paclitaxel and cisplatin versus paclitaxel and carboplatin in advanced ovarian cancer. J Clin Oncol 18: 3084–3092, 2000.

Rowinsky EK et al. Sequences of taxol and cisplatin: a phase I and pharmacologic study. J Clin
    Oncol 9: 1692–1703, 1991.

PACLITAXEL-CARBOPLATIN

Paclitaxel. 175 mg/m^2 intravenously over 3 hours on day 1.
Carboplatin. At AUC 7.5 intravenously on day 1.
*NOTE: Repeat the cycle every 21 days for up to 6 cycles. Meerpohl et al used a
paclitaxel dose of 185 mg/m^2 and carboplatin at AUC 6. Coleman et al used
paclitaxel 175 mg/m^2 and carboplatin at AUC 7.0 to 7.5, while Schink et al used
paclitaxel 150 mg/m^2 and carboplatin at AUC 5.*

Selected Readings

Bookman MA et al. Carboplatin and paclitaxel in ovarian carcinoma: a phase I study of the
    Gynecologic Oncology Group. J Clin Oncol 14: 1895–1902, 1996.
Coleman RL et al. Carboplatin and short-infusion paclitaxel in high-risk and advanced-stage ovarian
    carcinoma. Cancer J Sci Am 3: 246–253, 1997.
Meerpohl HG et al. Paclitaxel combined with carboplatin in the first line treatment of advanced
    ovarian cancer. Semin Oncol 22(6 suppl 15): 7–12, 1995.
Ozols RF. Combination regimens of paclitaxel and platinum drugs as first-line regimens for ovarian
    cancer. Semin Oncol 22(6 suppl 15): 1–6, 1995.
Schink JC et al. Outpatient taxol and carboplatin chemotherapy for suboptimally debulked epithelial
    carcinoma of the ovary results in improved quality of life: an Eastern Cooperative Oncology Group
    phase III study. Cancer J 7: 155–164, 2001.

7

OVARIAN CARCINOMA

PACLITAXEL-CISPLATIN-TOPOTECAN

Paclitaxel. 110 mg/m^2 intravenously by continuous 24-hour infusion on day 1.
Cisplatin. 50 mg/m^2 intravenously in 3 hours on day 2.
Topotecan. 0.3 mg/m^2 intravenously in 30 minutes on days 2 to 6.
*NOTE: Repeat the cycle every 21 days. Use filgrastim (G-CSF) 5 microg/kg/day
subcutaneously starting on day 6. Give paclitaxel first.*

Selected Reading

Herben VMM et al. Phase I and pharmacologic study of the combination of paclitaxel, cisplatin, and
    topotecan administered intravenously every 21 days as first-line therapy in patients with
    advanced ovarian cancer. J Clin Oncol 17: 745–755, 1999.

SINGLE AGENTS

Altretamine. 260 mg/m^2/day orally in divided doses for 14 days of every 28-day cycle
for relapsed disease.

Selected Readings

Rustin GJ et al. Phase II trial of oral altretamine for relapsed ovarian carcinoma: evaluation of
    defining response by serum CA125. J Clin Oncol 15: 172–176, 1997.
Markman M et al. Altretamine (hexamethylmelamine) in platinum-resistant and platinum-refractory
    ovarian cancer: a Gynecologic Oncology Group phase II trial. Gynecol Oncol 69: 226–229, 1998.

CARBOPLATIN

Carboplatin. At AUC of 6 intravenously every 28 days for 6 cycles (Gore et al). There
is clearly no consensus on dosage. The ICON2 study used AUC 5. Ozols used
800 mg/m^2 intravenously every 35 days for 4 cycles. Ten Bokkel Huinink et al used
800 mg/m^2 as did Reed et al and Christian & Trimble. Myelotoxicity was severe in
these studies and filgrastim (G-CSF) was frequently used, but tumor response was

good in patients with platinum-sensitive tumors. In contrast, Bolis et al used carboplatin 300 mg/m^2 and had a reasonable response with less toxicity. Response was poor in platinum-resistant tumors in all of these studies. Carboplatin is less toxic as a single agent than cisplatin and has equal efficacy.

Selected Readings

Bolis G et al. Carboplatin alone vs carboplatin plus epidoxorubicin as second-line therapy for cisplatin- or carboplatin-sensitive ovarian cancer. Gynecol Oncol 81: 3–9, 2001.

Christian MC, Trimble EL. Salvage chemotherapy for epithelial ovarian carcinoma. Gynecol Oncol 55(3 Pt 2): S143–S150, 1994.

Gore M et al. Randomized trial of dose-intensity with single-agent carboplatin in patients with epithelial ovarian cancer. London Gynaecological Oncology Group. J Clin Oncol 16: 2426–2434, 1998.

ICON2. Randomized trial of single-agent carboplatin against three-drug combination of CAP (cyclophosphamide, doxorubicin, and cisplatin) in women with ovarian cancer. ICON Collaborators. International Collaborative Ovarian Neoplasm Study. Lancet 352: 1571–1576, 1998.

Ozols RF. New developments with carboplatin in the treatment of ovarian cancer. Semin Oncol 19(1 suppl 2): 85–89, 1992.

Reed E et al. High-dose carboplatin and recombinant granulocyte-macrophage colony-stimulating factor in advanced-stage recurrent ovarian cancer. J Clin Oncol 11: 2118–2126, 1993.

Ten Bokkel Huinink WW et al. Replacement of cisplatin with carboplatin in combination chemotherapy against ovarian cancer: long-term treatment results of a study of the Gynaecological Cancer Cooperative Group of the EORTC and experience at the Netherlands Cancer Institute. Semin Oncol 19(1 suppl 2): 99–101, 1992.

CISPLATIN

Cisplatin. 100 mg/m^2 intravenously every 21 days for 6 cycles.

Selected Reading

Muggia FM et al. Phase III randomized study of cisplatin versus paclitaxel versus cisplatin and paclitaxel in patients with suboptimal stage III or IV ovarian cancer: a Gynecologic Oncology Group study. J Clin Oncol 18: 106–115, 2000.

DOCETAXEL

Docetaxel. 75 or 100 mg/m^2 intravenously every 3 weeks until toxicity or progression of the tumor.

Selected Reading

Verschraegen CF et al. Docetaxel for patients with paclitaxel-resistant Mullerian carcinoma. J Clin Oncol 18: 2733–2739, 2000.

GEMCITABINE

Gemcitabine. 800 mg/m^2 intravenously once a week for 3 weeks followed by 1 week of rest. Repeat the cycle until toxicity or progression.

Selected Reading

Lund B et al. Phase II study of gemcitabine (2′,2′-difluorodeoxycytidine) in previously treated ovarian cancer patients. J Natl Cancer Inst 86: 1530–1533, 1994.

LIPOSOMAL DOXORUBICIN

Liposomal doxorubicin. 50 mg/m^2 intravenously every 3 weeks. Reduce dose to 40 mg/m^2 in the event of grade 3 or 4 toxicities, or lengthen the cycle interval to 4 weeks (or occasionally 5 weeks).

Selected Readings

Gordon AN et al. Recurrent epithelial ovarian carcinoma: a randomized phase III study of pegylated liposomal doxorubicin versus topotecan. J Clin Oncol 19: 3312–3322, 2001.

Muggia FM et al. Phase II study of liposomal doxorubicin in refractory ovarian cancer: antitumor activity and toxicity modification by liposomal encapsulation. J Clin Oncol 15: 987–993, 1997.

PACLITAXEL

Paclitaxel. 175 mg/m^2 intravenously over 3 hours every 3 weeks until toxicity or progression of disease.

Selected Readings

Eisenhauer EA et al. European-Canadian randomized trial of paclitaxel in relapsed ovarian cancer: high-dose versus low-dose and long versus short infusion. J Clin Oncol 12: 2654–2666, 1994.

TOPOTECAN

Topotecan. 1.5 mg/m^2/day intravenously in 30 minutes for 5 days every 3 weeks. Major toxicity is myelosuppression.

Selected Readings

Creemers GJ et al. Topotecan, an active drug in the second-line treatment of epithelial ovarian cancer: results of a large European phase II study. J Clin Oncol 14: 3056–3061, 1996.

Kudelka AP et al. Phase II study of intravenous topotecan as a 5-day infusion for refractory epithelial ovarian carcinoma. J Clin Oncol 14: 1552–1557, 1996.

OVARIAN GERM CELL CANCER

Ovarian germ cell cancer accounts for about 5% of all ovarian malignancies in the United States. The incidence is much higher in the Orient, where up to 15% of ovarian cancers are of the germ cell type. They are generally classified as dysgerminomas and nondysgerminomas. The latter include embryonal carcinoma, endodermal sinus tumor, choriocarcinoma, mature teratoma, immature teratoma, and mixed germ cell tumor. After surgical removal in stages I, II, and III, even when it is complete, chemotherapy is indicated as adjuvant, except in stage IA grade I immature teratoma and stage IA pure dysgerminoma. Progress of the disease may often be followed with titers of beta-human chorionic gonadotropin (beta-HCG) or alfa-fetoprotein (AFP). Incomplete removal of stage III disease and all stage IV disease requires active chemotherapy. The three most commonly used combinations in order of their efficacy and inverse order of their development are BEP (bleomycin, etoposide, cisplatin), PVB (cisplatin, vinblastine, bleomycin), and VAC (vincristine, dactinomycin, cyclophosphamide). Long-term survival rates with this type of therapy range from 85% for dysgerminoma down to 50% to 70% for the nondysgerminomas.

ADJUVANT VAC—VINCRISTINE-DACTINOMYCIN-CYCLOPHOSPHAMIDE

Vincristine. 1.5 mg/m^2 intravenously on days 1 and 15.

Dactinomycin. 0.35 mg/m^2/day intravenously on days 1 to 5.

Cyclophosphamide. 150 mg/m^2/day intravenously on days 1 to 5.

NOTE: Repeat the cycle every 4 weeks. Gershenson et al gave vincristine on day 1 of each cycle and dactinomycin 0.5 mg/m^2.

OVARIAN GERM CELL CANCER

7

Selected Readings

Gershenson DM et al. Treatment of malignant non-dysgerminomatous germ cell tumors of the ovary with vincristine, dactinomycin and cyclophosphamide. Cancer 56: 2756–2761, 1985.

Williams SD et al. Chemotherapy of advanced dysgerminoma: trials of the Gynecologic Oncology Group (GOG). J Clin Oncol 9: 1950–1955, 1991.

ADJUVANT BEP—BLEOMYCIN-ETOPOSIDE-CISPLATIN

Bleomycin. 20 units/m^2/week intravenously.

Etoposide. 100 mg/m^2/day intravenously on days 1 to 5.

Cisplatin. 20 mg/m^2/day intravenously on days 1 to 5.

NOTE: Three cycles are given over a 9-week period (i.e., every 21 days). Brewer et al used bleomycin 10 to 15 units/m^2/day for 3 days by continuous intravenous infusion, etoposide 100 mg/m^2/day intravenously for 3 days, and cisplatin 100 mg/m^2 intravenously on day 1 and repeated the cycle every 4 weeks for 3 to 6 cycles.

Selected Readings

Brewer M et al. Outcome and reproductive function after chemotherapy for ovarian dysgerminoma. J Clin Oncol 17: 2670–2675, 1999.

Williams S et al. Adjuvant therapy of ovarian germ cell tumors with cisplatin, etoposide and bleomycin: a trial of the Gynecologic Oncology Group. J Clin Oncol 12: 701–706, 1994.

ADVANCED AND RECURRENT: PVB—CISPLATIN-VINBLASTINE-BLEOMYCIN

Cisplatin. 20 mg/m^2/day intravenously on days 1 to 5.

Vinblastine. 12 mg/m^2 intravenously on day 1.

Bleomycin. 20 units/m^2 intravenously weekly.

NOTE: Three or four cycles are given at 3-week intervals.

Selected Reading

Williams SD et al. Cisplatin, vinblastine, and bleomycin in advanced and recurrent ovarian germ-cell tumors. Ann Intern Med 111: 22–27, 1989.

PANCREATIC CARCINOMA

Pancreatic carcinoma is the fifth most common cause of cancer death in the United States. It is an insidious malignancy that causes late symptoms and hence late diagnosis, so that cure is uncommon. In the rare instances when early diagnosis is made, surgical pancreaticodudodenectomy with curative intent may be attempted by those skilled and experienced in performance of this challenging procedure. Although operative mortality rates are much improved, survival is only slightly improved. Adjuvant chemoradiation therapy has prolonged survival in some trials and not in others. Toxicity of the combined modality therapy is severe. Gemcitabine appears to have some activity and has been FDA approved for this cancer. Although several combinations have been reported to have activity greater than single agents, this has not been demonstrated in prospective clinical trials. Many clinicians use single agents or supportive palliative therapy, or enter willing patients into clinical trials.

CAPECITABINE

Capecitabine. 1,250 mg/m^2 orally twice a day (2,500 mg/m^2/day) for 14 days of a 21-day cycle which is repeated until progression or toxicity.

Selected Reading

Cartwright TH et al. Phase II study of oral capecitabine in patients with advanced or metastatic pancreatic cancer. J Clin Oncol 20: 160–164, 2002.

FAC—FLUOROURACIL-DOXORUBICIN-CISPLATIN

5-Fluorouracil. 300 mg/m^2/day intravenously on days 1 to 5.
Doxorubicin. 40 mg/m^2 intravenously on day 1.
Cisplatin. 60 mg/m^2 intravenously on day 1.
NOTE: Repeat the cycle every 35 days.

Selected Reading

Moertel CG et al. A phase II study of combined 5-fluorouracil, doxorubicin and cisplatin in the treatment of advanced upper gastrointestinal adenocarcinomas. J Clin Oncol 4: 1053–1057, 1986.

FAM—FLUOROURACIL-DOXORUBICIN-MITOMYCIN

5-Fluorouracil. 600 mg/m^2 intravenously on days 1, 8, 29, and 36.
Doxorubicin. 30 mg/m^2 intravenously on days 1 and 29.
Mitomycin. 10 mg/m^2 intravenously on days 1 and 29.
NOTE: Repeat the cycle every 8 weeks. Palmer et al gave the 5-fluorouracil orally on days 8 and 36 to save the patient a visit. Although 5-FU is not available in the United States in a tablet or capsule, one may use the liquid preparation intended for intravenous use and simply drink it in a glass of water. However, oral bioavailability is unpredictable. Median survival in the treated group was 33 (range 9–80) weeks compared with 15 (range 1–62) in the untreated control group.

Selected Reading

Palmer KR et al. Chemotherapy prolongs survival in inoperable pancreatic carcinoma. Br J Surgery 81: 882–885, 1994.

FLUOROURACIL-LEUCOVORIN

5-Fluorouracil. 425 mg/m^2/day intravenously for 5 days.
Leucovorin. 20 mg/m^2/day intravenously for 5 days.
NOTE: Repeat the cycle monthly for 6 months. In this randomized study, there was no survival benefit for adjuvant chemoradiotherapy (median survival 15.5 months versus controls 16.1 months), but there was a potential benefit for adjuvant chemotherapy (median survival 19.7 months versus 14.0 months).

Selected Reading

Neoptolemos JP et al. Adjuvant chemoradiotherapy and chemotherapy in resectable pancreatic cancer: a randomised controlled trial. Lancet 358: 1576–1585, 2001.

GEMCITABINE

Gemcitabine. 1,000 mg/m^2 intravenously every week for 7 weeks, then a week of rest, then weekly times 3 every 4 weeks until progression or toxicity.

Selected Reading

Burris HA 3rd et al. Improvements in survival and clinical benefit with gemcitabine as first-line therapy for patients with advanced pancreas cancer: a randomized trial. J Clin Oncol 15: 2403–2413, 1997.

GEMCITABINE-OXALIPLATIN

Gemcitabine. 1,000 mg/m^2 as a 10 mg/m^2/min infusion on day 1.
Oxaliplatin. 100 mg/m^2 as a 2-hour infusion on day 2.
NOTE: Repeat the cycle every 2 weeks for 6 cycles or until progression or unacceptable toxicity.

Selected Reading

Louvet C et al. Gemcitabine combined with oxaliplatin in advanced pancreatic adenocarcinoma: final results of a GERCOR multicenter phase II study. J Clin Oncol 20: 1512–1518, 2002.

G-FLIP—GEMCITABINE-LEUCOVORIN-IRINOTECAN-CISPLATIN

Gemcitabine. 500 mg/m^2 intravenously on day 1.
Irinotecan. 80 mg/m^2 intravenously on day 1.
Leucovorin. 300 mg/m^2 intravenously on days 1 and 2.
5-Fluorouracil. 400 mg/m^2 intravenous bolus on days 1 and 2.
5-Fluorouracil. 600 mg/m^2 as a continuous infusion over 8 hours on day 1 after 5-FU bolus, and on day 2 after cisplatin.
Cisplatin. 50 to 75 mg/m^2 intravenously on day 2 followed by above infusional 5-FU.
NOTE: Repeat the cycle every 2 weeks until disease progression or unacceptable toxicity.

Selected Reading

Kozuch P et al. Irinotecan combined with gemcitabine, 5-fluorouracil, leucovorin, and cisplatin (G-FLIP) is an effective and noncross-resistant treatment for chemotherapy refractory metastatic pancreatic cancer. Oncologist 6: 488–495, 2001.

IRINOTECAN-GEMCITABINE

Gemcitabine. 1,000 mg/m^2 intravenously in 30 minutes on days 1 and 8, each time followed immediately by
Irinotecan. 100 mg/m^2 intravenously in 90 minutes on days 1 and 8.
NOTE: Repeat the cycle every 21 days until progression or unacceptable toxicity.

Selected Reading

Rocha Lima CMS et al. Irinotecan plus gemcitabine induces both radiographic and CA 19-9 tumor marker responses in patients with previously untreated advanced pancreatic cancer. J Clin Oncol 20: 1182–1191, 2002.

PROSTATIC CARCINOMA

Prostatic carcinoma is now the most common cause of cancer in males in the United States and the fourth most frequent cause of all cancer deaths. Although it is true that prostate cancer is found microscopically in most men by age 90 (of those who come to autopsy), it will be the cause of death of an estimated 28,900 men in the United States in 2003. With the wide availability of the prostate-specific antigen test (PSA), earlier diagnosis and therapy increased the 5-year survival rate to 96%. In 1996, approximately 41,000 men died of prostate cancer.

The disease is most frequent in older men with the median at age 72, but it is known to afflict men in their late 40s and early 50s. Therapy is usually surgical under age 65 or 70 in those with localized tumor and no comorbidity. Other alternatives are external beam radiation therapy or brachytherapy with radioactive seed implantation, or watchful waiting in apparently indolent cases. When or whether to treat early-stage disease is still controversial. For advanced or metastatic disease, hormonal therapy is preferred with single agents or combinations that may include aminoglutethimide, bicalutamide, flutamide, goserelin, triptorelin, leuprolide, hydrocortisone, ketoconazole, megestrol, nilutamide, and prednisone. Chemotherapy is used only after hormonal resistance or relapse occurs and may include single agents like docetaxel, estramustine, or paclitaxel, or combinations of chemotherapy drugs with or without hormones. The single agents are described in the individual drug monographs section in Chapter 4.

DOCETAXEL-ESTRAMUSTINE

Estramustine. 280 mg orally 3 times a day is given 1 hour before or 2 hours after meals on days 1 to 5.
Docetaxel. 70 mg/m^2 intravenously on day 2.
NOTE: Patients previously treated with myelosuppressive therapies are given docetaxel 60 mg/m^2. Repeat the cycle every 21 days until progression or toxicity.

Selected Reading
Petrylak DP et al. Phase I trial of docetaxel with estramustine in androgen-independent prostatic cancer. J Clin Oncol 17: 958–967, 1999.

DOCETAXEL-ESTRAMUSTINE-HYDROCORTISONE

Estramustine. 10 mg/kg/day orally (total dose divided and rounded to the nearest capsule size dose) and given 3 times a day on days 1 to 5.
Docetaxel. 70 mg/m^2 intravenously over 1 hour on day 2.
Hydrocortisone. 30 mg orally each morning and 10 mg orally each evening and given continuously.
Dexamethasone. 8 mg orally every 12 hours for 6 doses starting 24 hours prior to the docetaxel dose.
NOTE: Repeat the cycle every 3 weeks.

Selected Reading
Savarese DM et al. Phase II study of docetaxel, estramustine, and low-dose hydrocortisone in men with hormone-refractory prostate cancer: a final report of CALGB 9780. J Clin Oncol 19: 2509, 2001.

ESTRAMUSTINE-CARBOPLATIN-PACLITAXEL

Estramustine. 10 mg/kg/day orally in 3 divided doses (rounded to nearest capsule size dose) 1 hour before or 2 hours after a meal on days 1 to 5.
Paclitaxel. 100 mg/m^2 intravenously over 1 hour on days 3, 10, and 17.
Carboplatin. To AUC 6 given over 30 minutes on day 3 after the paclitaxel.
NOTE: Repeat the cycle every 4 weeks.

Selected Reading
Kelly WK et al. Paclitaxel, estramustine phosphate, and carboplatin in patients with advanced prostate cancer. J Clin Oncol 19: 44–53, 2001.

ESTRAMUSTINE-ETOPOSIDE

Estramustine. 10 mg/kg/day orally in four divided doses.
Etoposide. 50 mg/m^2/day orally in two divided doses.
NOTE: Both drugs given daily for 21 days of every 28-day cycle. In the 1994 report the authors used estramustine in a dose of 15 mg/kg/day but find similar efficacy and

less toxicity at the 10 mg/kg/day dose. Therapy is continued until evidence of disease progression. Watch out for thromboembolic problems and neutropenia.

Selected Readings

Pienta KJ et al. Phase II evaluation of oral estramustine and oral etoposide in hormone-refractory adenocarcinoma of the prostate. J Clin Oncol 12: 2005–2012, 1994.

Pienta KJ et al. A phase II trial of oral estramustine and oral etoposide in hormone-refractory prostate cancer. Urology 50: 401–406, 1997.

ESTRAMUSTINE-PACLITAXEL

Estramustine. 600 mg/m^2/day orally in divided doses.

Paclitaxel. 120 mg/m^2 intravenously by continuous infusion over 96 hours starting on day 1.

NOTE: Repeat the cycle every 3 weeks. In the earlier report paclitaxel was begun on day 2; in the 1997 report, it was started on day 1.

Selected Readings

Hudes GR et al. Paclitaxel plus estramustine in metastatic hormone-refractory prostate cancer. Semin Oncol 22(5 suppl 12): 41–55, 1995.

Hudes GR et al. Phase II trial of 96-hour paclitaxel plus oral estramustine phosphate in metastatic hormone-refractory prostate cancer. J Clin Oncol 15: 3156–3163, 1997.

ESTRAMUSTINE-VINBLASTINE

Estramustine. 600 mg/m^2 orally on days 1 to 42.

Vinblastine. 4 mg/m^2 intravenously weekly for 6 weeks.

NOTE: Repeat the cycle every 8 weeks or until evidence of progression. Seidman et al use 10 mg/kg estramustine. Overall survival was the same with vinblastine alone.

Selected Readings

Hudes GR. Phase II study of estramustine and vinblastine, two microtubule inhibitors, in hormone-refractory prostate cancer. J Clin Oncol 10: 1754–1761, 1992.

Hudes GR et al. Vinblastine versus vinblatine plus oral estramustine phosphate for patients with hormone-refractory prostate cancer: A Hoosier Oncology Group and Fox Chase Network phase III trial. J Clin Oncol 17: 3160–3166, 1999.

Seidman AD et al. Estramustine and vinblastine: use of prostate specific antigen as a clinical trial end point for hormone refractory prostate cancer. J Urol 147: 931–934, 1992.

GOSERELIN-FLUTAMIDE

Goserelin. 3.6 mg subcutaneously every 28 days.

Flutamide. 250 mg orally three times a day.

NOTE: A goserelin preparation of 10.8 mg for injection every 90 days is available.

Selected Readings

Denis LJ et al. Goserelin acetate and flutamide versus bilateral orchiectomy: a phase III EORTC study (30853). Urology 42: 119–130, 1993.

Jurincic CD et al. Combined treatment (goserelin plus flutamide) versus monotherapy (goserelin alone) in advanced prostate cancer: a randomized study. Semin Oncol 18(suppl 6): 21–25, 1991.

KETOCONAZOLE-HYDROCORTISONE

Ketoconazole. 400 mg orally 3 times a day.

Hydrocortisone. 20 mg orally each morning and 10 mg each evening.

NOTE: This therapy is meant to be given after withdrawal of antiandrogen therapy with flutamide or bicalutamide. If primary gonadal deprivation is due to an LHRH agonist, it may be continued. It is important to dose between meals and to avoid H-2 blockers, sucralfate, and antacids because ketoconazole requires an acid environment for absorption. Do not allow use of astemizole (Hismanal®) or terfenadine (Seldane®) when using ketoconazole.

Selected Reading
Small EJ et al. Simultaneous antiandrogen withdrawal and treatment with ketoconazole and hydrocortisone in patients with advanced prostate carcinoma. Cancer 80: 1755–1759, 1997.

LEUPROLIDE-FLUTAMIDE
Leuprolide. 1 mg/day subcutaneously daily or 7.5 mg every 28 days.
Flutamide. 250 mg orally three times a day.
NOTE: Leuprolide depot preparations are now available with 22.5 mg for injection every 90 days and 30 mg every 120 days.

Selected Readings
Benson RC Jr et al. National Cancer Institute study of luteinizing hormone-releasing hormone plus flutamide versus luteinizing hormone-releasing hormone plus placebo. Semin Oncol 18(suppl 6): 26–28, 1991.
Crawford ED et al. A controlled trial of leuprolide with and without flutamide in prostatic carcinoma. N Engl J Med 321: 419–424, 1989.
Eisenberger MA et al. Prognostic factors in stage D2 prostate cancer: important implications for future trials, results of a cooperative intergroup study (INT 0036). Semin Oncol 21: 613–619, 1994.

LHRH-ANALOGUE-BICALUTAMIDE
Goserelin acetate. 3.6 mg total subcutaneously every 28 days.
Bicalutamide. 50 mg/day orally,
OR
Leuprolide acetate. 7.5 mg total intramuscularly every 28 days.
Bicalutamide. 50 mg/day orally.
NOTE: Goserelin as 10.8 mg for injection every 90 days is available and leuprolide as a 22.5-mg dose every 90 days or 30 mg every 120 days.

Selected Reading
Schellhammer P et al. A controlled trial of bicalutamide versus flutamide, each in combination with luteinizing hormone–releasing hormone analogue therapy in patients with advanced prostate cancer. Urology 45: 745–752, 1995.

MITOXANTRONE-PREDNISONE
Mitoxantrone. 12 mg/m^2 intravenously on day 1.
Prednisone. 5 mg orally twice a day.
NOTE: Mitoxantrone is given every 21 days and prednisone daily. Watch for neutropenia and cardiac toxicity. Do not exceed total cumulative lifetime mitoxantrone dose of 140 mg/m^2. Kantoff et al used mitoxantrone 14 mg/m^2 and substituted hydrocortisone 30 mg orally in the morning and 10 mg in the evening for the prednisone.

Selected Readings
Kantoff PW et al. Hydrocorisone with or without mitoxantrone in men with hormone-refractory prostate cancer: results of the Cancer and Leukemia Group B 9182 study. J Clin Oncol 17: 2506–2513, 1999.

Tannock I et al. Chemotherapy with mitoxantrone and prednisone or prednisone alone for symptomatic hormone-resistant prostate cancer: a Canadian randomized trial with palliative end points. J Clin Oncol 14: 1756–1764, 1996.

RENAL CELL CARCINOMA

Renal cell carcinoma is an adenocarcinoma that arises from the parenchyma of the kidney and is associated with a loss of heterozygosity of 3p13-26 and the familial Lindau–von Hippel disease (associated loss of a tumor-suppressor gene involving the short arm of chromosome 3). A causative relationship has also been found with tobacco use and less directly but still significantly with analgesic abuse, obesity, and asbestos exposure. Stage I lesions have a high cure rate. If the tumor has not penetrated the renal capsule, local recurrence is rare. Biological response modifiers have shown encouraging responses in patients with metastatic disease. Interferon-alfa and interleukin-2 (IL-2) result in some responses and a few of the IL-2 responses are of long duration, but the therapy is very toxic. Whether low-dose IL-2 is as efficacious as high-dose is controversial. Combinations of IL-2 and interferon-alfa have been used clinically with some minor success. No cytotoxic chemotherapy has demonstrated clear responses. Early reports of responses to thalidomide are intriguing. At this point in time, it is advisable to have patients with renal cell carcinoma enter into an experimental protocol so that better treatments can be developed and the existing promising agents can be compared with each other in controlled clinical trials. Worthwhile treatment is now available for this disease. Clinicians must sort out the better approaches while trying to develop new and improved therapies.

HIGH-DOSE INTRAVENOUS INTERLEUKIN-2 (ALDESLEUKIN)

Aldesleukin. 600,000 or 720,000 international units (IU)/kg intravenously every 8 hours for 5 days as tolerated.
NOTE: A second identical cycle of treatment is scheduled following 5 to 9 days of rest and another cycle can be repeated every 6 to 12 weeks in responding patients. Maximum support is necessary including pressors. Overall response rate is about 14% with complete responses (CR) of 5%, but some of those with a CR have long disease-free periods, occasionally measured in years.

Selected Reading

Fyfe G et al. Results of treatment of 255 patients with metastatic renal cell carcinoma who received high-dose recombinant interleukin-2 therapy. J Clin Oncol 13: 688–696, 1995.

LOW-DOSE INTRAVENOUS INTERLEUKIN-2 (ALDESLEUKIN)

Aldesleukin. 72,000 international units (IU)/kg intravenously every 8 hours for 5 days as tolerated.
NOTE: After 7 to 10 days, retreat with a second identical cycle of therapy. Those patients who are stable or responding to treatment in 5 or 6 weeks receive another course (2 cycles) of therapy. Overall response rate is 15% with 7% CRs. The high-dose group in this study had 20% ORR and 3% CRs.

Selected Reading

Yang JC et al. Randomized comparison of high-dose and low-dose intravenous interleukin-2 for the therapy of metastatic renal cell carcinoma: an interim report. J Clin Oncol 12: 1572–1576, 1994.

LOW-DOSE SUBCUTANEOUS INTERLEUKIN-2 (ALDESLEUKIN)

Aldesleukin. 18 million international units (MIU) subcutaneously daily for 5 days per week. In subsequent weeks the dose is reduced to 9 MIU for the first 2 days of each 5-day week and the total cycle is 6 weeks.

NOTE: After a 3-week rest period, treatment may be repeated in patients who had a response or stable disease.

Selected Reading

Sleijfer DT et al. Phase II study of subcutaneous interleukin-2 in unselected patients with advanced renal cell cancer on an outpatient basis. J Clin Oncol 10: 1119–1123, 1992.

INTERFERON-ALFA

Interferon-alfa. 5 million international units (MIU) subcutaneously 3 times a week with progressively increasing doses each week as tolerated.

NOTE: In the second week 10 MIU is given 3 times and in the third week and thereafter, a maximum of 15 MIU is given as tolerated. If depression develops, interferon should be discontinued.

Selected Reading

Tsavaris N et al. Treatment of renal cell carcinoma with escalating doses of alfa-interferon. Chemotherapy 39: 361–366, 1993.

SUBCUTANEOUS INTERLEUKIN-2 (ALDESLEUKIN) AND INTERFERON-ALFA

Aldesleukin. 20 MIU/m^2 subcutaneously 3 times a week in weeks 1 and 4. In weeks 2, 3, 5, and 6, give 5 MIU/m^2 subcutaneously 3 times a week.

Interferon-alfa. 6 MIU/m^2 subcutaneously once a week in weeks 1 and 4. In weeks 2, 3, 5, and 6, give 6 MIU/m^2 subcutaneously 3 times a week.

NOTE: Doses may need to be modified for toxicity. If depression develops, interferon should be discontinued.

Selected Reading

Atzpodien J et al. Multi-institutional home-therapy trial of recombinant human interleukin-2 and interferon alfa-2 in progressive metastatic renal cell carcinoma. J Clin Oncol 13: 497–501, 1995.

THALIDOMIDE

Thalidomide. 100 mg orally every night until disease progression or unacceptable toxicity.

NOTE: Escalating doses may be gradually tested as tolerated.

Selected Reading

Eisen T et al. Continuous low-dose thalidomide: a phase II study in advanced melanoma, renal cell, ovarian and breast cancer. Br J Cancer 82: 812–817, 2000.

SOFT TISSUE SARCOMA

Sarcoma is a relatively uncommon tumor with a heterogeneous and complex histology and classification. Sarcoma pathology is a field of its own. Generally, small, low-grade tumors can be surgically resected with a high cure rate. Large tumors (greater than 5 cm) are usually high grade, spread to lymph nodes and distant sites (most often lung), and have a poor prognosis. Nonetheless, some of these tumors are amenable to limb-sparing combined-modality therapy with neo-adjuvant radiation with or without chemotherapy followed by surgery with long-term survival. If the metastases (usually lung) are isolated and can be resected, cure may be possible.

AD—DOXORUBICIN-DACARBAZINE

Adequate Marrow
Doxorubicin. 60 mg/m^2 intravenously on day 1.
Dacarbazine. 250 mg/m^2/day intravenously on days 1 to 5.
Inadequate Marrow
Doxorubicin. 45 mg/m^2 intravenously on day 1.
Dacarbazine. 200 mg/m^2/day intravenously on days 1 to 5.
NOTE: Repeat the cycle every 21 days.

Selected Reading
Gottlieb JA et al. Adriamycin used alone and in combination for soft tissue and bony sarcomas. Cancer Chemother Rep 6: 271–282, 1975.

CY-VA-DIC—CYCLOPHOSPHAMIDE-VINCRISTINE-DOXORUBICIN-DACARBAZINE

Cyclophosphamide. 500 mg/m^2 intravenously on day 1.
Vincristine. 1 mg/m^2 intravenously on days 1 and 5 (maximum 1.5 mg).
Doxorubicin. 50 mg/m^2 intravenously on day 1 only.
Dacarbazine. 250 mg/m^2 intravenously on days 1 to 5.
NOTE: Repeat cycle every 21 days. Bramwell et al used vincristine 1.4 mg/m^2 intravenously on day 1 and dacarbazine 400 mg/m^2/day on days 1 to 3.

Selected Readings
Bramwell V et al. Adjuvant CYVADIC chemotherapy for adult soft-tissue sarcoma – reduced local recurrence but no improvement in survival: a study of the European Organization for Research and Treatment of Cancer Soft Tissue and Bone Sarcoma Group. J Clin Oncol 12: 1137–1149, 1994.
Yap BS et al. Cyclophosphamide, vincristine, Adriamycin, and DTIC (CYVADIC) combination chemotherapy for the treatment of advanced sarcomas. Cancer Treat Rep 64: 93–98, 1980.

DOXORUBICIN

Doxorubicin. 75 mg/m^2 intravenously.
NOTE: Repeat the cycle every 21 days as tolerated to maximum dose of 450 mg/m^2 or progression of disease. There was no statistically significant difference in response rate with doxorubicin with or without ifosfamide nor as compared to CYVADIC.

Selected Reading
Santoro A et al. Doxorubicin versus CYVADIC versus doxorubicin plus ifosfamide in first-line treatment of advanced soft tissue sarcomas: a randomized study of the European Organization for Research and Treatment of Cancer Soft Tissue and Bone Sarcoma Group. J Clin Oncol 13: 1537–1545, 1995.

DOXORUBICIN-IFOSFAMIDE

Doxorubicin. 75 mg/m^2 intravenously on day 1.
Ifosfamide. 5,000 mg/m^2 intravenously as a continuous 24-hour infusion on day 1.

Mesna. 2,500 mg/m^2 mixed with the ifosfamide and 1,250 mg/m^2 over 12 hours following it.
GM-CSF. 250 microg/m^2/day subcutaneously beginning 24 hours after ifosfamide up to 14 days.
NOTE: The GM-CSF is discontinued once the WBC count equals or exceeds 10,000/microL. Therapy is continued for seven cycles or two cycles beyond a complete response, whichever comes first.

Selected Reading

Steward WP et al. Granulocyte-macrophage colony stimulating factor allows safe escalation of the dose-intensity of chemotherapy in metastatic adult soft tissue sarcomas: a study of the European Organization for Research and Treatment of Cancer Soft Tissue and Bone Sarcoma Group. J Clin Oncol 11: 15–21, 1993.

7

SOFT TISSUE SARCOMA

DOXORUBICIN-DACARBAZINE-IFOSFAMIDE

Doxorubicin. 15 mg/m^2 per day as a continuous infusion on days 1 to 4 (total dose is 60 mg/m^2 infused over 96 hours).
Dacarbazine. 250 mg/m^2 per day as a continuous infusion on days 1 to 4 (total dose is 1,000 mg/m^2 infused over 96 hours).
Ifosfamide. 2,000 mg/m^2 per day as a continuous infusion on days 1 to 3 (total dose is 6,000 mg/m^2 infused over 72 hours).
Mesna. 2,500 mg/m^2 per day as a continuous infusion on days 1 to 4 (total dose is 10,000 mg/m^2 infused over 72 hours).
NOTE: Repeat the cycle every 21 days if WBC count exceeds 3,000/microL and platelet count exceeds 100,000/microL.

Selected Reading

Antman K et al. An intergroup phase III randomized study of doxorubicin and dacarbazine with or without ifosfamide and mesna in advanced soft tissue and bone sarcomas. J Clin Oncol 11: 1276–1285, 1993.

IFOSFAMIDE-(MESNA)-ETOPOSIDE

Etoposide. 100 mg/m^2/day intravenously on days 1 to 5.
Ifosfamide. 1,800 mg/m^2/day intravenously on days 1 to 5.
NOTE: Etoposide is administered over a 1-hour period, followed immediately by ifosfamide and the loading dose of mesna (360 mg/m^2) mixed together and given over a 1-hour span. Subsequently, mesna is given intravenously over 3 hours and then by bolus infusions over a period of 15 minutes every 3 hours for 6 doses at hours 5, 8, 11, 14, 17, and 20. Mesna doses after hour 5 were given orally; all earlier doses were intravenous. After four cycles, sites of residual metastatic disease in responding patients were treated with either surgery or radiation therapy to consolidate the response and achieve a complete remission. A total of 12 chemotherapy cycles at 3-week intervals was the planned goal.

Selected Reading

Miser JS et al. Ifosfamide with mesna uroprotection and etoposide: an effective regimen in the treatment of recurrent sarcomas and other tumors of children and young adults. J Clin Oncol 5: 1191–1198, 1987.

MAID—MESNA-DOXORUBICIN-IFOSFAMIDE-DACARBAZINE

Mesna. 2,500 mg/m^2/day intravenously on days 1 to 4.
Doxorubicin. 20 mg/m^2/day intravenously on days 1 to 3.
Ifosfamide. 2,500 mg/m^2/day intravenously on days 1 to 3.

Dacarbazine. 300 mg/m^2/day intravenously on days 1 to 3.

NOTE: All drugs are administered by continuous infusion; doxorubicin is mixed with dacarbazine, and ifosfamide is mixed with mesna. Repeat the cycle every 21 days. Antman et al use slightly different doses of ifosfamide and dacarbazine.

Selected Readings

Antman K et al. An intergroup phase III randomized study of doxorubicin and dacarbazine with or without ifosfamide and mesna in advanced soft tissue and bone sarcomas. J Clin Oncol 11: 1276–1285, 1993.

Elias A et al. Response to mesna, doxorubicin, ifosfamide, and dacarbazine in 108 patients with metastatic or unresectable sarcoma and no prior chemotherapy. J Clin Oncol 7: 1208–1216, 1989.

TESTICULAR AND EXTRAGONADAL GERM CELL CANCER

Testicular and extragonadal germ cell cancer is the most common cancer in males between 15 and 35. It accounts for 1% of cancers in males, is highly treatable, and usually curable. Tumors are generally designated as seminoma or nonseminomatous. Pure seminomas (normal alfa-fetoprotein [AFP]) are very radiation-sensitive, and stages I and II traditionally were treated with radiation, whereas stage III tumors are curable with combination chemotherapy. Some groups are reconsidering this and treating stage II seminoma with chemotherapy. Nonseminomatous stage I is treated with resection and careful observation and small-volume stage II tumors are treated with resection, retroperitoneal lymph node dissection (RPLND), and careful observation or, in cases at increased risk, with chemotherapy. Bulky stage II and all stage III tumors are treated with combination chemotherapy. In poor-prognosis disease, four courses of BEP are usually given. For refractory or recurrent disease, high-dose therapy with stem cell support is used at major centers. See Chapter 10.

BEP—BLEOMYCIN-ETOPOSIDE-CISPLATIN

Cisplatin. 20 mg/m^2/day intravenously over a period of 15 to 30 minutes on days 1 to 5.

Bleomycin. 30 units intravenously on days 2, 9, and 16.

Etoposide. 100 mg/m^2 intravenously over a 30-minute period on days 1 to 5.

NOTE: Normal saline (100 mg/hour) is given on the days of cisplatin therapy. Watch for hypotension if etoposide is given too rapidly. Patients receive 3 or 4 cycles at 3-week intervals on schedule, regardless of the granulocyte count. The dose of etoposide is reduced 20% for patients who received previous radiotherapy or had granulocytopenia and fever after an earlier course. A later paper showed equivalent efficacy with less toxicity using 3 cycles instead of 4.

Selected Readings

Einhorn LH et al. Evaluation of optimal duration of chemotherapy in favorable-prognosis disseminated germ cell tumors: a SECSG protocol. J Clin Oncol 7: 387–391, 1989.

Williams SD et al. Treatment of disseminated germ-cell tumors with cisplatin, bleomycin, and either vinblastine or etoposide. N Engl J Med 316: 1435–1440, 1987.

CEB—CARBOPLATIN-ETOPOSIDE-BLEOMYCIN

Carboplatin. At AUC 5 intravenously on day 1.

Etoposide. 120 mg/m^2/day intravenously on days 1 to 3.

Bleomycin. 30 units intravenously on days 2, 9, and 16.

NOTE: Repeat the cycle every 21 days for a total of 4 cycles. Diphenhydramine is given concomitantly with each dose of bleomycin to prevent febrile reactions. Carboplatin dose is adjusted to nadir WBC and platelet counts as described in report by Horwich et al.

Selected Readings

Bajorin DF et al. Randomized trial of etoposide and cisplatin versus etoposide and carboplatin in patients with good-risk germ cell tumors: a multi-institutional study. J Clin Oncol 11: 598–606, 1993.

Horwich A et al. Effectiveness of carboplatin, etoposide and bleomycin combination chemotherapy in good-prognosis metastatic testicular nonseminomatous germ cell tumors. J Clin Oncol 9: 62–69, 1991.

ETOPOSIDE-CISPLATIN

Cisplatin. 20 mg/m^2/day intravenously on days 1 to 5.
Etoposide. 100 mg/m^2/day intravenously on days 1 to 5.
NOTE: Repeat the cycle every 3 weeks for 4 cycles, depending on stage and retroperitoneal lymph node dissection results. Consider surgery if there is radiologic evidence of residual disease after 4 cycles.

Selected Reading

Bosl GJ et al. A randomized trial of etoposide and cisplatin versus vinblastine + bleomycin + cisplatin + cyclophosphamide + dactinomycin in patients with good prognosis germ cell tumors. J Clin Oncol 6: 1231–1238, 1988.

ICE—IFOSFAMIDE-CISPLATIN-ETOPOSIDE

Cisplatin. 20 mg/m^2/day intravenously on days 1 to 5.
Etoposide. 100 mg/m^2/day intravenously on days 1 to 5.
Ifosfamide. 1,200 mg/m^2/day intravenously on days 1 to 5.
Mesna. 200 mg/m^2 by IV bolus 30 minutes before and 4 and 8 hours after each dose of ifosfamide.
NOTE: Repeat the cycle every 3 weeks.

Selected Reading

Harstrick A et al. Cisplatin, etoposide, and ifosfamide salvage therapy for refractory or relapsing germ cell carcinoma. J Clin Oncol 9: 1549–1555, 1991.

OXALIPLATIN FOR SALVAGE THERAPY

Oxaliplatin. 60 mg/m^2 intravenously on days 1, 8, and 15.
OR

Oxaliplatin. 130 mg/m^2 intravenously on days 1 and 15.
NOTE: Repeat the cycle every 4 weeks as tolerated or until disease progresses. This regimen is only for salvage therapy.

Selected Reading

Kollmannsberger C et al. Activity of oxaliplatin in patients with relapsed or cisplatin-refractory germ cell cancer: a study of the German Testicular Cancer Study Group. J Clin Oncol 20: 2031–2037, 2002.

PACLITAXEL-GEMCITABINE

Paclitaxel. 110 mg/m^2 intravenously on days 1, 8, and 15.
Gemcitabine. 1,000 mg/m^2 intravenously on days 1, 8, and 15.

NOTE: Repeat the cycle every 4 weeks for 6 cycles.

Selected Reading

Hinton S et al. Phase II study of paclitaxel plus gemcitabine in refractory germ cell tumors (E9897): a trial of the Eastern Cooperative Oncology Group. J Clin Oncol 20: 1859–1863, 2002.

PVB—CISPLATIN-VINBLASTINE-BLEOMYCIN

Cisplatin. 20 mg/m^2/day intravenously on days 1 to 5.
Vinblastine. 0.15 mg/kg/day intravenously on days 1 and 2.
Bleomycin. 30 units intravenously on day 2 and then weekly for 12 consecutive weeks.
NOTE: Repeat the cycle of cisplatin and vinblastine every 3 weeks for a total of 4 cycles.

Selected Reading

Stoter G et al. High-dose versus low-dose vinblastine in cisplatin-vinblastine-bleomycin combination chemotherapy of non-seminomatous testicular cancer: a randomized study of the EORTC Genitourinary Tract Cancer Cooperative Group. J Clin Oncol 4: 1199–1206, 1986.

VAB VI—VINBLASTINE-DACTINOMYCIN-BLEOMYCIN-CYCLOPHOSPHAMIDE-CISPLATIN

Induction
Cyclophosphamide. 600 mg/m^2 intravenously on day 1.
Vinblastine. 4 mg/m^2 intravenously on day 1.
Dactinomycin. 1 mg/m^2 intravenously on day 1.
Bleomycin. 30 units intravenous bolus on day 1.
Completion of cycle
Bleomycin. 20 units/m^2/day intravenously by continuous infusion for 3 days (total dose 60 units/m^2 as a continuous infusion over 72 hours).
Cisplatin. 120 mg/m^2 intravenously on day 4.
NOTE: Repeat the cycle every 3 or 4 weeks for 2 additional cycles, except that bleomycin is omitted from the third cycle.

Selected Reading

Vugrin D et al. VAB-6 combination chemotherapy in disseminated cancer of the testis. Ann Intern Med 95: 59–61, 1981.

VEIP—VINBLASTINE-IFOSFAMIDE-CISPLATIN

Cisplatin. 20 mg/m^2/day intravenously for 5 days on days 1 to 5.
Ifosfamide. 1,200 mg/m^2/day intravenously for 5 days on days 1 to 5.
Vinblastine. 0.11 mg/kg/day intravenously for 2 days on days 1 and 2.
Mesna. 120 mg/m^2 as an initial IV bolus and then 1,200 mg/m^2/day by continuous IV infusion for 5 days on days 1 to 5.
NOTE: Repeat the cycle every 3 weeks for 4 cycles.

Selected Reading

Motzer RJ et al. Salvage chemotherapy for patients with germ cell tumors. The Memorial Sloan-Kettering Cancer Center experience (1979–1989). Cancer 67: 1305–1310, 1991.

VIP—ETOPOSIDE-IFOSFAMIDE-CISPLATIN

Etoposide. 75 mg/m^2/day intravenously on days 1 to 5.
Ifosfamide. 1,200 mg/m^2/day intravenously on days 1 to 5.

Mesna. 400 mg intravenously before the day-1 ifosfamide dose and then
1,200 mg/day by continuous IV infusion on days 1 to 5 (120 hours).
Cisplatin. 20 mg/m^2/day intravenously on days 1 to 5.
NOTE: Repeat the treatment every 21 days.

Selected Reading

Loehrer PJ et al. Salvage therapy in recurrent germ cell cancer: ifosfamide and cisplatin plus either
vinblastine or etoposide. Ann Intern Med 109: 540–546, 1988.

VPV—VINBLASTINE-CISPLATIN-ETOPOSIDE

Vinblastine. 8 mg/m^2 intravenously on day 1.
Cisplatin. 120 mg/m^2 intravenously on day 3.
Etoposide. 50 mg/m^2/day intravenously on days 2 to 5.
NOTE: Repeat the cycle every 3 weeks for a total of 4 cycles.

Selected Reading

Wozniak J et al. A randomized trial of cisplatin, vinblastine, and bleomycin versus vinblastine, cisplatin, and etoposide in the treatment of advanced germ cell tumors of the testis: a Southwest
Oncology Group Study. J Clin Oncol 9: 70–76, 1991.

THYMOMA (MALIGNANT)

Malignant thymoma is a rare tumor that is slow-growing and frequently diagnosed
as an incidental finding of chest radiography. The term is generally restricted to
neoplasms of the thymic epithelial cells and excludes pure lymphomas of the
organ. Verification of malignancy is often difficult and is based on the presence of
invasion of the tumor capsule, surrounding tissue, or metastasis. Myasthenia gravis
is associated in about 30% of thymoma patients, but its presence is not an
adverse prognostic factor in terms of eradication of the tumor. Therapy is surgical if
the tumor is localized, and recurrence is only 2% if it is encapsulated. If the tumor
is invasive, the recurrence rate is 40%, and radiation therapy is given locally. For
metastatic disease, chemotherapy is used in combinations.

ADOC—DOXORUBICIN-CISPLATIN-VINCRISTINE-CYCLOPHOSPHAMIDE

Doxorubicin. 40 mg/m^2 intravenously on day 1.
Vincristine. 0.6 mg/m^2 intravenously on day 3.
Cyclophosphamide. 700 mg/m^2 intravenously on day 4.
Cisplatin. 50 mg/m^2 intravenously on day 1.
NOTE: Repeat the cycle every 3 weeks.

Selected Readings

Fornasiero A et al. Chemotherapy of invasive or metastatic carcinoma: report of 11 cases. Cancer
Treat Rev 68: 1205–1210, 1984.
Fornasiero A et al. Chemotherapy for invasive thymoma: a 13 year experience. Cancer 68: 30–33,
1991.

BAPP—BLEOMYCIN-DOXORUBICIN-CISPLATIN-PREDNISONE

Bleomycin. 12 units/m^2 intravenously on day 1.
Doxorubicin. 50 mg/m^2 intravenously on day 1.
Cisplatin. 50 mg/m^2 intravenously on day 1.
Prednisone. 40 mg/m^2/day orally on days 1 to 5.

NOTE: *Repeat the cycle every 4 weeks to a total cumulative dose of 540 mg/m^2 of doxorubicin and 175 units of bleomycin.*

Selected Reading

Chahinian AP et al. Treatment of invasive or metastatic thymoma: report of eleven cases. Cancer 47: 1752–1761, 1981.

CEE—CISPLATIN-ETOPOSIDE-EPIRUBICIN

Cisplatin. 75 mg/m^2 intravenously on day 1.
Etoposide. 120 mg/m^2/day intravenously on days 1, 3, and 5.
Epirubicin. 100 mg/m^2 intravenously on day 1.
NOTE: *Repeat the cycle every 3 weeks for 3 cycles, and then perform surgery followed by radiation therapy with 4,600 to 6,000 cGy.*

Selected Reading

Macchiarini P et al. Neo-adjuvant chemotherapy, surgery, and postoperative radiation therapy for invasive thymoma. Cancer 68: 706–713, 1991.

CISPLATIN-ETOPOSIDE

Cisplatin. 60 mg/m^2 intravenously on day 1.
Etoposide. 120 mg/m^2/day intravenously on days 1 to 3.
NOTE: *Repeat the cycle every 3 weeks for 6 or more cycles.*

Selected Reading

Giaccone G et al. Cisplatin and etoposide combination chemotherapy for locally advanced or metastatic thymoma: a phase II study of the EORTC Lung Cancer Cooperative Group. J Clin Oncol 14: 814–820, 1996.

COLP—CYCLOPHOSPHAMIDE-VINCRISTINE-LOMUSTINE-PREDNISONE

Cyclophosphamide. 1,000 mg/m^2 intravenously on day 1.
Vincristine. 1.3 mg/m^2 intravenously (maximum 2 mg) on day 1.
Lomustine. 70 mg/m^2 orally on day 1.
Prednisone. 40 mg/m^2/day orally on days 1 to 7.
NOTE: *Repeat the cycle every 4 weeks.*

Selected Reading

Daugaard G et al. Combination chemotherapy for malignant thymoma. Ann Intern Med 99: 189–190, 1983.

PAC—CISPLATIN-DOXORUBICIN-CYCLOPHOSPHAMIDE

Cisplatin. 50 mg/m^2 intravenously on day 1.
Doxorubicin. 50 mg/m^2 on day 1.
Cyclophosphamide. 500 mg/m^2 intravenously on day 1.
NOTE: *Repeat the cycle every 21 days for up to 8 cycles. Adequate hydration and antiemetics are essential.*

Selected Reading

Loehrer PJ et al. Cisplatin plus doxorubicin plus cyclophosphamide in metastatic or recurrent thymoma: final results of an intergroup trial. J Clin Oncol 12: 1164–1168, 1994.

THYROID CARCINOMA

Thyroid carcinoma is responsible for 1% of all cancers in the United States and is the most common endocrine malignancy. It is seen more often in women than men and in patients who had head and neck radiation in childhood. It is now being seen in a 100-fold or more increase in children in the area around Chernobyl after the nuclear reactor release of radiation. Generally, well-differentiated tumors (papillary or follicular) are highly treatable and usually curable. Poorly differentiated cancers (medullary or anaplastic) are less common but are aggressive, metastasize early, and have a poor prognosis.

The recommended therapy for localized disease, depending on histology, is total thyroidectomy (some advocate lobectomy in stage I papillary cancer) plus exogenous thyroid suppression, and in some cases 131-iodine ablation. Regional (stage III) involvement with nodal metastases requires total thyroidectomy, involved node removal or radical neck dissection, and 131-iodine ablation if the tumor demonstrates adequate uptake of the isotope. If not, then external beam radiation is used. Distant metastases are treated with 131-iodine ablation if uptake is adequate. If not, then external beam radiation is given to control local disease, and patients are considered for an investigational chemotherapy protocol or a chemotherapy regimen in the literature. Combinations are usually used, but their efficacy has not been demonstrated in prospective randomized trials.

BAP—BLEOMYCIN-DOXORUBICIN-CISPLATIN

Bleomycin. 30 units/day intravenously by continuous infusion on days 1 to 3.
Doxorubicin. 60 mg/m^2 intravenously on day 5.
Cisplatin. 60 mg/m^2 intravenously on day 5.
NOTE: Repeat the cycle every 3 or 4 weeks. Usual antiemetic and hydration and maximum tolerated dose guidelines all apply.

Selected Reading

De Besi P et al. Combined chemotherapy with bleomycin, Adriamycin, and platinum in advanced thyroid cancer. J Endocrinol Invest 14: 475–480, 1991.

DOXORUBICIN-CISPLATIN

Doxorubicin. 60 mg/m^2 intravenously on day 1.
Cisplatin. 40 mg/m^2 intravenously on day 1.
NOTE: The dose of doxorubicin was adjusted for hematological or hepatic dysfunction. Repeat the cycle every 3 weeks to a total dose of 550 mg/m^2 of doxorubicin or until evidence of failure of therapy.

Selected Reading

Shimaoka K et al. A randomized trial of doxorubicin versus doxorubicin plus cisplatin in patients with advanced thyroid carcinoma. Cancer 56: 2155–2160, 1985.

DMBV—DOXORUBICIN-MELPHALAN-BLEOMYCIN-VINCRISTINE

Doxorubicin. 40 mg/m^2 intravenously on day 1.
Melphalan. 6 mg/m^2/day orally on days 3 to 6.
Bleomycin. 15 units/m^2 intramuscularly on day 15.
Vincristine. 1 mg/m^2 intravenously on day 15.
NOTE: Repeat the cycle every 28 days.

Selected Reading

Durie BGM et al. High risk thyroid cancer: prolonged survival with early multimodality therapy. Cancer Clin Trials 4: 67–73, 1981.

ADDITIONAL NOTE

In compiling this list of protocols, many fine regimens were omitted. In some cases, those omitted may be superior to some included. Since the compilation was completed, many additional useful protocols have been published, and more will be forthcoming every week. Again, we urge clinicians to check the original reference before using any of these protocols. For economy of space, we have omitted most cautions as to premedication, hydration, need for cytokines, antiemetics, laxatives, etc. We presume that prescribing oncologists are familiar with and have institutional guidelines for this.

ETHICAL CONSIDERATIONS IN CANCER

Healthcare in the United States is in a very difficult period. There is a Medicare system for the elderly, a Medicaid system for the severely indigent or disabled, a managed care system for most workers, and 40 million people with no health insurance (primarily the working poor). Nonetheless, healthcare professionals are expected to give everyone the very best care that is available to anyone. Physicians are asked to do more with fewer resources, and are burdened with time-consuming paperwork that does not contribute to patient welfare.

8

MANAGED CARE

Managed care was advertised as a means to reduce the costs of healthcare for the nation, reduce waste, maintain the quality of care, and return the cost savings to society or to the individuals insured. In most areas, managed care has restricted access to care, especially to necessary hospitalization and to consultation by specialists. This leads to a negation of the physician-patient relationship and the obligation of the physician to make the welfare of the patient the prime consideration. The imperative of abiding by the physician-patient covenant was restated by the American College of Physicians, the American Board of Internal Medicine, and numerous other societies (Cassel, 1996; Crawshaw et al, 1995).

It must be remembered that "the physician-patient relationship is the cornerstone for achieving, maintaining, and improving health" (Emanuel & Dubler, 1995). Indeed, the physician is a therapeutic agent when there is a good physician-patient bond, and the disruption of that relationship by closed panels is contrary to good medical care. Patients are not well served when the insurer treats physicians as economic cost centers to be moved around, substituted, or excluded simply for a perceived cost-saving benefit to the insurer.

Hospitals are feeling the restrictions of managed care as acutely as physicians (Anders, 1994). It is clear to hospital administrators that managed care is a misnomer – it is not concerned with care but with cost. As a result, many hospitals have had to drastically reduce the number of professional nurses on their staffs and substitute unlicensed assistant personnel. Some clinics are being closed, equipment maintenance is being deferred, purchases of newer state-of-the-art equipment are on "hold," and the numbers of full-time medical staff (pathologists, radiologists, anesthesiologists) are being reduced by attrition or by discharging personnel and replacing them with independent vendors at market-negotiated rates.

MEDICAL PROFESSIONALISM

One of the consequences of managed care and the federal government treating medicine as a business, is that many physicians have come to regard it as a business instead of an honored profession. In the past two decades, many business leaders, attorneys, accountants, clergy, and, more recently, physicians have subscribed to the doctrine enunciated by Michael Douglas' character in the motion picture *Wall Street*, that "greed is good." We need to remind everyone that greed is NOT good, especially for professionals. The professional is supposed to put the welfare of the client (patient) above his/her own. We need to remember the Hippocratic Oath (Davey, 2001) and the Prayer of Maimonides, which reads, in part:

> The eternal providence has appointed me to watch over the life and health of Thy creatures. May the love for my art actuate me at all time; may neither avarice nor miserliness, nor thirst for glory or for a great reputation engage my mind; for the enemies of truth and philanthropy could easily deceive me and make me forgetful of my lofty aim of doing good to Thy children. May I never see in the patient anything but a fellow creature in pain. Grant me the strength, time and opportunity always to correct what I have acquired, always to extend its domain; for knowledge is immense and the spirit of man can extend indefinitely to enrich itself daily with new requirements. Today he can discover his errors of yesterday and tomorrow he can obtain a new light on what he thinks himself sure of today. Oh, God, Thou hast appointed me to watch over the life and death of Thy creatures; here I am ready for my vocation and now I turn unto my calling.

> *(Oath of Maimonides, 2002; Moses Maimonides 1135–1204 was a physician and rabbi)*

CONFLICTS OF INTEREST

The degree to which we have strayed from these principles is evident in our conflicts of interest which are, in part, responsible for our loss of the public trust (Chabner, 2002). One only has to read the daily newspapers to be reminded of the loss of the ethical and moral compass of our society in general. Illegal behavior is common, and some of its practitioners are being prosecuted as criminals, e.g., corporate executives who file false reports, accountants who certify them as correct, and lawyers who recommend shredding the falsified documents; legislative representatives and executive appointees who solicit and accept bribes; scientists who falsify research data; and physicians who engage in Medicare fraud. On another level, we are being drawn into financial relations with insurers and pharmaceutical companies that undermine our commitments to the welfare of our patients and to society.

In just one year, the New England Journal of Medicine (NEJM) addressed some of these issues including "Medical professionalism – focusing on the real issues" (Rothman, 2000), "Is academic medicine for sale?" (Angell, 2000), "Protecting research subjects – what must be done?" (Shalala, 2000), and "In whose best interest? Breaching the academic-industrial wall" (Martin & Kasper, 2000). Although they lamented the loss of integrity and trust due to these conflicts of interest, two years later the editors of the NEJM abandoned its high-minded policy that authors of reviews and editorials "will not have any financial interest in a company (or its competitor) that makes a product discussed in the article" (Drazen & Curfman, 2002). It modified its policy with the single word "significant." Under the new policy, the authors "will not have any significant financial interest..." What does that mean? The author is disqualified by having received more than $10,000 in the preceding two years from a company whose drug is mentioned. The editors have come to this sorry state of abandoning their ethical constraints because they are having trouble finding authors for reviews and editorials who do not have major conflicts of interest. Authors of original articles or special articles may have any degree of conflict of interest as long as it is stated. A group of journal editors have called attention to the influence of pharmaceutical companies in influencing research and journal reports (Davidoff et al, 2001).

In response to this question, the Executive Council of the Association of American Medical Colleges (AAMC) adopted new guidelines (Kelch, 2002) to prevent such conflicts (Task Force, 2001). Their definition of "significant" is $10,000 in the preceding year or the anticipation of that sum or more in the coming year. The origin of the figure is in the code of Federal Regulations – Title 42, which defines the eligibility of applicants for Public Health Service grants and their responsibility for promoting objectivity in research (Code). It is not clear why receiving $9,999 from a pharmaceutical company or a device manufacturer would not constitute a worrisome conflict of interest.

Another problem that cries for correction is the disconnection between abstracts presented at meetings and their publication in peer-reviewed journals. In reviewing the abstracts in the annual Proceedings of the American Society of Clinical Oncology (ASCO) from 1989 to 1998, Krzyzanowska et al (2002) noted that only 78% of clinical trial reports were ever followed by a full journal article. The probability of publication was 52% for positive studies and 39% for negative trials. Hillner (2002) has pointed out that "the foundation of evidence-based medicine is that randomized controlled clinical trials (RCTs) should guide clinical care. RCTs are usually the culmination of a translation research chain of pilot studies that assess the feasibility and safety of a new approach." Delay or failure to publish these studies are a disservice to science, to medical care, and most of all to the patients who were the subjects of the studies and the patients who may potentially benefit from the information generated by the studies. Krzyzanowska et al (2002) are more blunt. They conclude that "failure to publish the results of clinical trials breaks the agreement that investigators have made with study participants and funding agencies, and is a form of scientific misconduct."

COMMUNITY PRACTICE

Private practice physicians are increasingly being compromised by relationships with pharmaceutical companies. Chren & Landefeld (1994) found that physicians who received gifts or money from drug companies were more likely to request additions to their hospital drug formulary to favor the company providing the largesse. At a conference jointly sponsored by the FDA, NIH, CDC, and HHS entitled "Conflicts of Interest and Human Subject Protection," it was revealed that individual medical practitioners, and more especially group practices, are now doing clinical trials for drug companies (Wolfe, 2000). Some of these physicians are the same ones who declined to participate in NCI cooperative group studies and university studies either because they claimed a lack of qualification or of time. Strange how the extra remuneration has increased their qualification and time. Some practitioners are recruiting patients for clinical trials and getting a "finder's fee." Other physicians or groups of physicians even advertise their services to Health Experimentation Corporations (HECs). Some of them put their private patients into HEC studies and collect a professional fee from the patient (or insurer) and a much larger payment from the HEC or drug company. Whose interest can be expected to be paramount? There have been newspaper and television reports of physicians who conduct clinical trials for HECs or pharmaceutical companies and have altered the data to produce more positive reports in order to get more contracts to do more clinical trials because they are much more remunerative than ordinary patient care. Greed is a powerful force!

For many years, physicians have been visited by pharmaceutical representatives to inform them of new products or of new indications of older products, or just to suggest the superiority of their company's product over the competition. Often, to gain the attention of physicians, they have come bearing gifts, invitations to expensive dinners and free travel to highly desirable tourist destinations to attend mini-teaching sessions or special meetings. Most physicians have accepted something, even if it was only a pen, a sandwich, or a book. Now some of the largest pharmaceutical companies are advertising their drugs directly to patients on nationwide television and bypassing the physician. The enormous costs of these practices are passed on to the patient and the taxpayer in higher drug prices. Although the representatives of the drug industry claim that the high drug prices represent the costs of research, reports in newspapers derived from Security and Exchange Commission documents indicate that marketing and lobbying costs greatly exceed research costs in most pharmaceutical companies. The public is demanding, and Congress is considering, how to lower drug costs, and physicians need to participate in this endeavor to enhance the welfare of patients, who sometimes have to choose between buying medication or buying food.

LOOKING TOWARD THE FUTURE

To counter the erosion of morality and the loss of public trust in physicians, the American Board of Internal Medicine Foundation, the America College of Physicians – American Society of Internal Medicine Foundation, and the European Federation of Internal Medicine issued a joint Charter on Medical Professionalism (Sox, 2002). They say many of the things that we said in this chapter in the last edition and many of the things that we wrote in an earlier draft, but they do it with greater authority. Accordingly, we quote portions of the document.

> *Professionalism is the basis of medicine's contract with society. It demands placing the interests of patients above those of the physician, setting and maintaining standards of competence and integrity, and providing expert advice to society on matters of health. The principles and responsibilities of medical professionalism must be clearly understood by both the profession and society. Essential to this contract is public trust in physicians, which depends on the integrity of both individual physicians and the whole profession.*
>
> *At present, the medical profession is confronted by an explosion of technology, changing market forces, problems in health care delivery, bioterrorism, and globalization. As a result, physicians find it increasingly difficult to meet their responsibilities to patients and society. In these circumstances, reaffirming the fundamental and universal principles and values of medical professionalism, which remain ideals to be pursued by all physicians, becomes all the more important.*
>
> *The medical profession everywhere is embedded in diverse cultures and national traditions, but its members share the role of healer, which has roots extending back to Hippocrates. Indeed, the medical profession must contend with complicated political, legal, and market forces. Moreover, there are wide variations in medical delivery and practice through which any general principles may be expressed in both complex and subtle ways. Despite these differences, common themes emerge and form the basis of this charter in the form of three fundamental principles and as a set of definitive professional responsibilities.*

FUNDAMENTAL PRINCIPLES

Principle of primacy of patient welfare. This principle is based on a dedication to serving the interest of the patient. Altruism contributes to the trust that is central to the physician-patient relationship. Market forces, societal pressures, and administrative exigencies must not compromise this principle.

Principle of patient autonomy. Physicians must have respect for patient autonomy. Physicians must be honest with their patients and empower them to make informed decisions about their treatment. Patients' decisions about their care must be paramount, as long as those decisions are in keeping with ethical practice and do not lead to demands for inappropriate care.

Principle of social justice. The medical profession must promote justice in the health care system, including the fair distribution of health care resources. Physicians should work actively to eliminate discrimination in health care, whether based on race, gender, socio-economic status, ethnicity, religion, or any other social category.

A SET OF PROFESSIONAL RESPONSIBILITIES

Commitment to professional competence...

Commitment to honesty with patients...

Commitment to patient confidentiality...

Commitment to maintaining appropriate relations with patients...

Commitment to improving quality of care...

Commitment to improving access to care...

Commitment to a just distribution of finite resources...

Commitment to scientific knowledge...

Commitment to maintaining trust by managing conflicts of interest. *Medical professionals and their organizations have many opportunities to compromise their professional responsibilities by pursuing private gain or personal advantage. Such compromises are especially threatening in the pursuit of personal or organizational interactions with for-profit industries, including medical equipment manufacturers, insurance companies, and pharmaceutical firms. Physicians have an obligation to recognize, disclose to the general public, and deal with conflicts of interest that arise in the course of their professional duties and activities. Relationships between industry and opinion leaders should be disclosed, especially when the latter determine the criteria for conducting and reporting clinical trials, writing editorials or therapeutic guidelines, or serving as editors of scientific journals.*

Commitment to professional responsibilities. *As members of a profession, physicians are expected to work collaboratively to maximize patient care, be respectful of one another, and participate in the processes of self-regulation, including remediation and discipline of members who have failed to meet professional standards. The profession should also define and organize the educational and standard-setting process for current and future members. Physicians have both individual and collective obligations to participate in*

*these processes. These obligations include engaging in internal assessment
and accepting external scrutiny of all aspects of their professional
performance.*

We could not have said it better.

REFERENCES

Anders G. Required surgery: health plans force even elite hospitals to cut costs sharply. Wall Street J March 8, 1994.

Angell M. Is academic medicine for sale? N Engl J Med 342: 1516–1517, 2000.

Cassel CK. The patient-physician covenant: an affirmation of Asklepios. Ann Intern Med 124: 604–606, 1996.

Chabner BA. The trust factor. The Oncologist 7: 94–95, 2002.

Chren MM, Landefeld CS. Physicians' behavior and their interactions with drug companies. A controlled study of physicians who requested additions to a hospital formulary. JAMA 271: 684–689, 1994.

Code of Federal Regulations, Title 42 – Public Health, Research for which PHS funding is sought. (Accessed July 11, 2002 at http://grants2.nih.gov/grants/compliance/42_CFR_50_Subpart_F.htm.)

Crawshaw R et al. Patient-physician covenant. JAMA 273: 1553, 1995.

Davey LM. The Oath of Hippocrates: an historical review. Neurosurgery 49: 554–566, 2001.

Davidoff F et al. Sponsorship, authorship, and accountability. Ann Intern Med 135: 463–466, 2001.

Drazen JM, Curfman GD. Financial associations of authors. N Engl J Med 346: 1901–1902, 2002.

Emanuel EJ, Dubler NN. Preserving the physician-patient relationship in the era of managed care. JAMA 273: 323–328, 1995.

Hillner BE. Trends in published cancer clinical trial reports 1990–2000. Proc Am Soc Clin Oncol 21: 244a, 2002.

Kelch RP. Maintaining the public trust in clinical research. N Engl J Med 346: 285–287, 2002.

Krzyzanowska MK, Pintile M, Tannock I. Burying of unwanted results: a survey of more than 500 large randomized clinical trials presented at ASCO meeetings to determine the probability and causes of failure to publish. Proc Am Soc Clin Oncol 21: 244a, 2002.

Martin JB, Kasper DL. In whose best interest? Breaching the academic–industrial wall. N Engl J Med 343: 1646–1649, 2000.

Oath of Maimonides (Accessed July 11, 2002 at http://www.fordham.edu/halsall/source/rambam-oath.html.)

Rothman DJ. Medical professionalism – focusing on the real issues. N Engl J Med 342: 1284–1286, 2000.

Shalala D. Protecting research subjects – what must be done? N Engl J Med 343: 808–810, 2000.

Sox HC. Medical professionalism in the new millennium: a physician charter – project of the ABIM Foundation, ACP–ASIM Foundation, and European Federation of Internal Medicine. Ann Intern Med 136: 243–246, 2002.

Task Force on Financial Conflicts of Interest in Clinical Research: Protecting subjects, preserving trust, promoting progress – policy and guidelines for the oversight of individual financial interests in human subjects research. Washington, DC: Association of American Medical Colleges, December 2001. (Accessed July 11, 2002, at http://www.aamc.org/members/coitf/.)

Wolfe SM. Human experimentation for profit, Public Citizen Health Research Group. Health Letter 16(9): 10–12, 2000.

CANCER PAIN MANAGEMENT

Patients understand that we cannot cure all cancer. What they do not understand is why we do not control their pain adequately. The lay press has frequent articles emphasizing this failure. They are variously headlined: from "The tragedy of needless pain" (Melzack, 1990) in the *Scientific American*, to "Misunderstood opioids and needless pain" (Brody, 2002) in the *New York Times,* to "Pain free forever" with subheadings "Who'll stop the pain" and "after years of being stung by doctors' indifference, pain patients are fighting back for the treatment they need" (Heavey, 2002) in *AARP Modern Maturity*, said to be America's largest circulation magazine. Are they telling doctors something that we as oncologists do not know? What do we find when we take a look at the evidence in the peer-reviewed literature?

The SUPPORT study and the HELP study (Lynn et al, 1997; SUPPORT principal investigators, 1995) surveyed the care of dying patients in five teaching (university or university-affiliated) hospitals in the United States. Among other findings, they noted that 50% of conscious patients had moderate to severe pain. After active intervention to alert the staff to the problem and teach them how to respond, a resurvey showed no improvement. An Australian study (Yates et al, 2002) noted that 48% of cancer patients in four separate hospitals reported pain in the preceding 24 hours and 56% of them reported this pain to be "distressing, horrible or excruciating." Another study (Schumacher et al, 2002) showed that our training of patients and families for pain control at home is insufficient. As a result, many cancer patients, perhaps most, fear severe intractable pain even more than death. The physician and the healthcare team are able to cure cancer sometimes and prolong life frequently, but must relieve pain and suffering always. The public perception is that cancer patients are frequently in great pain, and some are reluctant to seek medical attention because of fear of pain. Too often, physicians and nurses do not fully understand the nature and proper treatment of pain in the cancer patient (Portenoy, 1993), which is quite different from the management of acute postoperative or post-traumatic pain (Sinatra et al, 1992).

UNDERESTIMATING NEED

Although 60% to 80% of cancer patients have moderate to severe pain at some time before death, a large proportion of them receive inadequate amounts of analgesics. The Eastern Cooperative Oncology Group (ECOG) study of pain management (Von Roenn et al, 1993) showed that only 50% of physicians believed that pain control was good or very good in their treatment center and 86% believed that most cancer patients in the United States are undermedicated for their pain. The problems were identified as poor pain assessment (69%), patient reluctance to report pain (49%), and patient reluctance to take medication or physician reluctance to give medication (46%). Some people wonder whether the major problem is physician ignorance and indifference and a focus on treating the tumor and not the whole patient.

The Joint Commission on Accreditation of Health Care Organizations (JCAHO), since January 2001 has taken a closer look at pain control. For continued accreditation, institutions and programs must develop and use tools that measure and record the patients' pain. They must also record methods of pain treatment and educate their staff on the principles of pain assessment and management. In order for this pain initiative to work, physicians, nurses, nurses' aides, and the entire healthcare team will have to revise their thinking about pain management. It will also be important to teach patients and their families to report pain and request analgesia. Pain is not punishment, nor is suffering a measure of courage. Poor pain management may delay recovery, affect the quality of life, and lead to depression. Honest and open discussion with the healthcare team is important since pain is not always obvious.

ASSESSMENT OF PAIN

The initial treatment of pain should be to both eliminate the cause and relieve the symptoms (Foley, 1999). The cause of the pain must be determined by carefully evaluating each complaint. Obtain a complete history, including the site, character, and intensity of the pain. Perform a physical examination with emphasis on the site of the pain and on a neurological examination. Obtain a psychosocial assessment of the patient. Complete an appropriate diagnostic workup to determine the cause of the pain. In those cancer patients who do have prolonged pain, it may be caused by one of the following mechanisms:

- partial or complete obstruction of a blood supply by tumor, leading to venous engorgement or arterial ischemia
- compression of the nerves, roots, or trunks by tumor or by metastatic fracture of bones adjacent to the nerves
- infiltration of the nerves, nerve roots, or nerve endings and blood vessels by tumor
- obstruction of a viscus by tumor
- infiltration and tumefaction in tissue enclosed by fascia or periosteum
- necrosis, infarction, or inflammation because of tumor.

In addition to establishing the cause of the pain, assessment should include documentation of how pain is manifested behaviorally and symptomatically. Nevertheless, one cannot always verify a patient's statement of pain with a physiological sign. In chronic pain, a patient's pain expression may be minimized as a result of adaptive behavioral responses. A written pain history should include descriptions of onset, location, duration, intensity, radiation, relieving and aggravating factors, and the cognitive response to pain.

To improve the systematic assessment of pain, a variety of scales are frequently used to help the patient convey to the healthcare professional the degree of suffering that needs to be relieved. Three types of scales are popular:

- a visual analogue scale as a continuum (Box 9-1)
- a numeric rating scale (Box 9-2)
- a categorical scale with verbal descriptors (Table 9-1).

BOX 9-1

VISUAL ANALOGUE SCALE

No		Most
pain		pain

BOX 9-2

NUMERIC RATING SCALE

0	1	2	3	4	5	6	7	8	9	10

0 = No pain   10 = Worst pain imaginable

TABLE 9-1
CATEGORICAL SCALE

0	1	2	3	4	5
No pain	Mild	Discomforting	Distressing	Intense	Excruciating
	Annoying	Troublesome	Miserable	Horrible	Unbearable
	Nagging	Grueling	Agonizing	Dreadful	Torturing
		Numbing	Gnawing	Vicious	Crushing
		Nauseating		Cramping	Tearing

Pain is what the patient says it is. Neither pain nor the patient experiencing the pain can be fitted into a clear-cut category with a predictable response. Indeed, the most helpful evaluations of severity of pain and pain relief come from patients themselves.

Concern about drug addiction, by healthcare professionals and patients, is understandable and appropriate. Although drug abuse is a national problem, it is important to discriminate between personalities who have psychological instability that influences them to abuse drugs and become addicted, and patients who have physical symptoms that require interventions. Development of addiction is rare in medical patients who have pain and who have no history of addiction. Fear of such a rare phenomenon is not an adequate basis for withholding appropriate doses of opioids from cancer patients (Porter & Jick, 1980). It is important to understand the differences between addiction, physical dependence, and tolerance because they are frequently confused. According to a consensus agreement approved on February 2001 by the Boards of Directors of the American Academy of Pain Medicine, the American Pain Society, and the American Society of Addiction Medicine, the appropriate definitions are:

Addiction is a primary, chronic, neurobiologic disease, with genetic, psychosocial, and environmental factors influencing its development and manifestations. It is characterized by behaviors that include one or more of the following:

- impaired control over drug use
- compulsive use
- continued use despite harm
- craving.

Physical dependence is a state of adaptation that is manifested by a drug-class-specific withdrawal syndrome that can be produced by abrupt cessation, rapid dose reduction, decreasing blood level of the drug, and/or administration of an antagonist.

Tolerance is a state of adaptation in which exposure to a drug induces changes that result in diminution of one or more of the drug's effects over time.

Public and professional appreciation of the inadequate use of available drugs and techniques for pain relief led to a decade of attempts to educate physicians, nurses, and the laity in how to manage cancer pain. The World Health Organization published its guidelines and popularized its WHO analgesic ladder (Figure 9-1) in 1986, and a revised second edition in 1996 (Stjernsward et al, 1996). Other guidelines worth consulting are those of the American Pain Society (1999), the Ad Hoc Committee on Cancer Pain of the American Society of Clinical Oncology (1992), the National Comprehensive Cancer Network Practice Guidelines in Oncology (NCCN, 2001), and the Agency for Health Care Policy and Research (1994). The last can be obtained from the NCI Cancer Information Service by calling 1-800-4-CANCER. Also available from the same source are a *Patient Guide*, a *Quick Reference Guide for Clinicians*, and an *Acute Pain Management Guide for Clinicians*. The ACS (American Cancer

9

ASSESSMENT OF PAIN

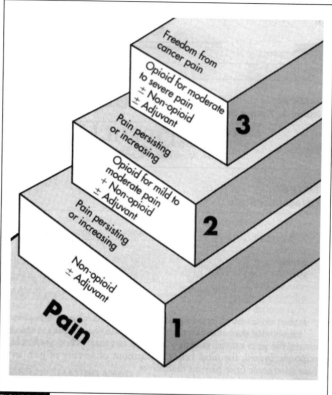

FIGURE 9-1

The WHO three-step analgesic ladder. (From Cancer Pain Relief, 2nd edition. World Health Organization, 1996.)

Society, 2001) publishes a 358-page *Guide to Pain Control* for the use of cancer patients and their families. Physicians should use these professional guides in their practice and should make the patient guides available to their patients who suffer from pain.

USING ANALGESICS FOR MILD PAIN

All pain is best relieved by removing the underlying cause (Fischer, 1984) with hormones or chemotherapy, surgery, or radiation. If that is not possible, however, and if the patient is ambulatory and the pain is mild, it may respond to simple analgesics such as aspirin, acetaminophen, diflunisal, choline magnesium trisalicylate, salsalate, or a nonsteroidal anti-inflammatory drug (NSAID) (Table 9-2). Although aspirin is the standard against which all other analgesics for mild pain have been compared, there is a tendency to avoid aspirin in many patients because of its propensity to cause gastrointestinal (GI) hemorrhage and because it interferes with platelet aggregation and hemostasis. Acetaminophen is a commonly used mild analgesic. Except for inflammatory conditions or bone pain, acetaminophen is as potent as aspirin but with fewer and more tolerable side effects. However, overdosage can be toxic or even fatal, particularly for small children. Acetaminophen does not inhibit platelet aggregation and has a duration of action of 3 to 4 hours. It should not be dosed in excess of 4,000 mg a day, including the amounts in combination preparations. Three long-acting salicylates that have less GI toxicity than aspirin are available. Choline magnesium trisalicylate does not appear to interfere with platelet function at all, and diflunisal and salsalate exhibit only transient and reversible platelet inhibition. The drugs are generally given in the doses listed in Table 9-2 and may be escalated somewhat if necessary. These doses, if taken at bedtime, will usually last through the night.

NSAIDs are helpful in controlling mild pain in general and moderate pain caused by inflammation or bone metastases. This reaction appears to involve, at least in part, an effect on prostaglandins. NSAIDs have a ceiling of effectiveness and doses above that ceiling will not increase pain relief but will add toxicity. Aspirin and other NSAIDs should be used with caution when administering low-dose methotrexate and should not be used at all with high-dose methotrexate.

Ibuprofen and naproxen are available as generics and, in lower doses, are available over the counter without a physician's prescription. In some cases, a long-acting preparation is desirable, but this must be used cautiously because the toxicity as well as the benefits will be prolonged. Most NSAIDs are Cox-1 inhibitors and can produce GI hemorrhage and prolonged bleeding times; they should be used with extreme caution in patients with renal disease, a history of peptic ulcers, or a bleeding tendency. Cox-2 inhibitors, for example celecoxib and rofecoxib, have a lower incidence of GI symptoms and platelet problems and have a relatively long duration of activity. They do not interfere with platelet aggregation when used in standard doses.

USING ANALGESICS FOR MODERATE PAIN

When the cancer patient does not achieve adequate relief with nonopioids, a stronger analgesic is used, such as an opioid like codeine, 65 mg alone or in combination with aspirin or acetaminophen. Some medium-strength opioids like dihydrocodeine and hydrocodone are available only in combinations. It is rational to use such combinations because opioids act centrally and aspirin and acetaminophen act peripherally (Twycross & Lack, 1990). Tramadol 50 mg is equivalent to 60 mg of codeine and frequently effective. Oxycodone 5 mg is available as a single agent and in combination with aspirin or acetaminophen, and as a controlled-release preparation, OxyContin. The latter has been used to treat moderate and severe pain when a longer-acting preparation is needed, since it provides 8- to 12-hour pain relief. Patients should be advised to keep all their drugs in a secure location, but especially OxyContin, to be sure it is not diverted to addicts, who also have an illness that is very difficult to treat. Addicts with bona fide cancer pain should receive analgesics under the supervision of a pain specialist knowledgeable in the therapy of both pain and addiction.

Pentazocine is an agonist-antagonist drug with moderate analgesic effects that at one time was considered nonaddictive and potent. Greater experience has demonstrated substantial side effects, including sedation, drowsiness, nausea, vomiting, blurring of vision, respiratory depression (Catalano, 1985), and, in older patients, a propensity to produce central nervous system (CNS) disturbances, including hallucinations, vertigo, and bad dreams. Like the other agonist-antagonist drugs (i.e., nalbuphine and butorphanol, and the partial agonist buprenorphine), it can also cause

TABLE 9-2

SELECTED ORAL ANALGESICS FOR MILD OR MODERATE PAIN: COMPARATIVE DOSES

Drug	Common brand name	Duration of analgesia (hr)	Usual starting oral dose (mg)	Frequency (hr)	Anti-inflammatory	Platelet problems	Significant adverse effects
Aspirin	Many	3–5	650	4	Yes	Yes	GI, renal
Acetaminophen	Tylenol	3–4	650	4	No	No	Hepatic
Sodium salicylate	Generic	3–4	650	3–6	Yes	No	GI
Diflunisal	Dolobid	8–12	500	12	Yes	Mild	GI
Choline magnesium trisalicylate	Trilisate	8–12	1,000–1,500	8	Yes	No	Tinnitus
Salsalate	Disalcid	16	750–1,000	12	Yes	Mild	Tinnitus
Ibuprofen	Motrin	3–5	400–600	6	Yes	Yes	GI
Fenoprofen	Nalfon	4–5	300–600	6	Yes	Yes	GI
Diclofenac	Voltaren	4–6	50	8	Yes	Yes	GI
Flurbiprofen	Ansaid	6–8	50–100	12	Yes	Yes	GI
Ketoprofen	Orudis	5–7	25–60	6–8	Yes	Yes	GI
Naproxen	Naprosyn	8	250	6–8	Yes	Yes	GI
Naproxen sodium	Anaprox	8	275	6–8	Yes	Yes	GI

Indomethacin	Indocin	3–4	25	8	Yes	Yes	GI, CNS
Tolmetin	Tolectin	3–4	200–400	8	Yes	Yes	GI
Sulindac	Clinoril	7	150	12	Yes	Yes	GI
Meclofenamate	Meclomen	8	50–100	6–8	Yes	Yes	GI
Etodolac	Lodine	4–12	200–400	6–8	Yes	Yes	GI
Celecoxib	Celebrex	12	100–200	12	Yes	No	GI
Rofecoxib	Vioxx	24	12.5–25	12–24	Yes	No	GI
Nambumetone	Relafen	24	1,000	24	Yes	No	GI
Ketorolac	Toradol	4–7	10	4–6	Yes	Yes	Constipation, CNS
Codeine	Many	3–5	32	2–3	No	No	Constipation, CNS
Hydrocodone	Many	3–4	5	3–4	No	No	Constipation, CNS
Oxycodone	Roxicodone	3–6	5	3–6	No	No	CNS
Tramadol	Ultram	4–6	50–100	6	No	No	CNS

GI, Gastrointestinal; CNS, central nervous system.

9

withdrawal symptoms if given to a patient receiving long-term opioid analgesics. These drugs are NOT recommended for treatment of cancer pain because they block the analgesic effects of opioids, they have an analgesic ceiling, and they may precipitate psychotomimetic effects.

Meperidine (demerol, pethidine, and others) is one of the most popular analgesics and is widely used, but it should NOT be used for cancer pain. Its duration of action is short, and it is usually used in doses that are ineffective. Its toxic metabolite, normeperidine, can accumulate, especially when renal function is impaired, and can cause CNS stimulation that may lead to anxiety, tremors, myoclonus, or generalized seizures. When used with a monoamine oxidase (MAO) inhibitor, meperidine has been known to cause severe seizures and some deaths. Meperidine is frequently used intravenously to relieve shaking chills associated with transfusion reactions and with IL-2 and amphotericin.

Three decades ago, undertreatment of medical inpatients with opioid analgesics was called to professional attention (Marks & Sachar, 1973). It was noted that 32% of patients receiving opioid analgesics remained in severe pain and 41% in moderate distress. The opioid used was overwhelmingly meperidine, the dose prescribed by physicians was lower than recommended, and the dose delivered by nurses was less than ordered. For oral use oxycodone alone or in combination with acetaminophen or tramadol or a NSAID is recommended. First-line parenteral opioid analgesics of choice are morphine and hydromorphone. Meperidine parenterally should be restricted to the following usage:

- Treatment (or prevention in patients with known history) of drug-induced or blood-product-induced rigors, or the treatment of shivering post-anesthesia. The recommended dose for this in adults is 12.5 mg–50 mg slow intravenous push every 15–20 minutes until symptoms are controlled and then every 3–4 hours as needed for symptom control.
- Pre-procedural analgesia/sedation for gastrointestinal or obstetrical procedures. The recommended dose in adults is 25 mg–100 mg slow intravenous push, titrated to effect. Doses greater than 50 mg require heightened sedation monitoring.
- Treatment of post-obstetrical surgery pain. Meperidine PCA (patient-controlled analgesia) may be used for up to 24 hours postoperatively, although the superiority of morphine over meperidine in PCA is clear (Plummer et al, 1997).
- Treatment of visceral or spastic pain related to gastrointestinal (primarily biliary) or genito-urinary surgery when first-line opioids, in adequate doses, have failed. The recommended dose is 50 mg–100 mg slow intravenous push every 2–3 hours for no more than 48 hours, and not to exceed 600 mg in 24 hours.
- Management of acute episodes of pain for patients with documented allergy to morphine and when fentanyl is not appropriate. We note that most opioids cause histamine release, while **_anaphylactic and other true allergic reactions are rare_**. Patients with local reactions (redness, swelling at the injection site, mild rash, or itching) to opioids should be premedicated with a parenteral antihistamine (e.g. hydroxyzine, diphenhydramine) and be monitored for signs and symptoms of anaphylaxis. Gastrointestinal symptoms (nausea, vomiting) and CNS (dizziness, sedation) effects are not allergic reactions. True allergies consist of angioedema or extensive urticaria with bronchospasm and/or wheezing. Patients with a documented history or presentation of these symptoms with morphine (or a morphine-class opioid) can be treated with fentanyl (available as a generic injection of 50 microg/ml). When fentanyl is inappropriate, meperidine may be used.

USING OPIOIDS FOR SEVERE PAIN

Opioids are used in the management of severe pain. After more than 1,000 years, there is no better group of drugs for this purpose than the opiates derived from the *Papaver somniferum* plant, more commonly known as the poppy. Morphine is the standard to which all other narcotic drugs are compared (Table 9-3), and so far there is none that is better overall. Morphine is effective, relatively inexpensive, and available as an oral, intramuscular, subcutaneous, rectal, intravenous, or intrathecal preparation. It is available in tablets, capsules, and oral liquid preparations, immediate- or controlled-release preparations, and in parenteral form in several strengths.

Whenever practical, opioids should be given orally for chronic pain. It is important to give adequate doses on a regular schedule. Use of prn dosing (as required) leads to peaks and valleys of analgesia, whereas regular preventive therapy results in a lower total daily dose of opioid with better pain control. The as-needed schedule leads to anxiety about pain, results in overutilization and habituation, and is not recommended.

Morphine is not absorbed as well by the oral route as some other opioids. As an initial dose, the equianalgesic dose of morphine, oral:parenteral, is 6:1, but with subsequent doses and chronic usage, it is closer to 3:1 or 2:1. A starting oral dose of 15–30 mg for an average-size individual (5–10 mg in a debilitated elderly or low-body-mass individual) every 4 hours is recommended, with escalation of the dose

TABLE 9-3
OPIOIDS FOR MODERATE TO SEVERE PAIN: APPROXIMATE EQUIANALGESIC DOSES

Drug	Brand name	Parenteral dose (mg)	Oral dose (mg)	Duration of analgesia (hr)	Plasma half-life (hr)
Morphine	Generic	10	30	2–4	2–3
Controlled-release Morphine	MS Contin, Kadian, Oramorph SR, Avinza	—	30–90	12–24	—
Hydromorphone	Dilaudid	1.5	7.5	3–4	2–3
Oxymorphone	Numorphan	1	5 (rectal)	3–6	2–3
Methadone **	Dolophine	10	20	4–8	15–150
Levorphanol	Levo-Dromoran	2	4	3–6	12–15
Meperidine#	Demerol	75–100	300	2–4	2–3
Fentanyl	Duragesic	0.1	0.05/hr patch	1–2*	1.5–3*
Oxycodone	Roxicodone, OxyIR	—	20–30	3–6	2–4
Controlled-release oxycodone	OxyContin	—	20–30	8–12	—
Ketorolac†	Toradol	30	10	4–7	5
Codeine	Generic	130	200	2–4	2–3

*Intravenously; **For use only by specialist; #Not recommended for cancer pain.
†Nonopiate, nonsteroidal anti-inflammatory inhibitor; use 60 mg initially, then 30 mg every 6 hours.

if pain relief is inadequate or recurs before 4 hours are over. Once the total daily dose has been determined using immediate-release morphine and verified over an additional 24 hours, sustained-release morphine (e.g., MS Contin®, Oramorph-SR®, Kadian®, or Avinza®) may be substituted. The 24-hour dose is divided into two doses given every 12 or 24 hours depending on the preparation used. An extra dose of immediate-release morphine (10% of the total daily dose) can be given every hour or two for breakthrough pain, which is defined as "a transitory exacerbation of pain that occurs on a background of otherwise stable pain in a patient receiving chronic opioid therapy" (Portenoy & Hagen, 1990). If this becomes frequent, the dose may be added to the calculation of the 12-hour or 24-hour sustained-release medication. The 24-hour duration preparations seem to require less frequent amendment. Nausea and vomiting usually respond to an antiemetic. The superiority of this approach and the improvement in the quality of life of cancer patients has been documented (Warfield, 1993). A transdermal preparation of fentanyl (Duragesic®) is available in patches that release the analgesic over 72 hours. Patients usually reach a steady state in 12 hours and then maintain that level of analgesia for 72 hours. Thus, a new patch has to be applied every 3 days. The patches come in four strengths: 25, 50, 75, and 100 microg/hr.

When morphine is not desired for some reason, hydromorphone or levorphanol can be used in the equianalgesic doses as indicated in Table 9-3. It is important to be familiar with several pain drugs because tolerance between opioids is not complete. In patients in whom pain is difficult to control, some authors recommend rotation of opiates (Indelicato & Portenoy, 2002; Mercadante et al, 2001; Ripamonti et al, 1998), but conversions are difficult and require great experience because there is some controversy over the relative equianalgesic doses of these drugs (Anderson et al, 2001; Abrahm, 2000). It is recommended that one use the opioid equianalgesic dose chart (Table 9-3) for a first estimate of the dose of the new drug equianalgesic to the old drug. For patients who develop tolerance to most opioids, an oral transmucosal fentanyl citrate (Actiq®) is available (see product brochure).

Methadone is favored by many because it is long-acting. However, a switch to methadone from another opioid is often accompanied by a greater than expected potency of the methadone. Hence, when switching, reduce the equianalgesic dose by 75% to 90%. Although this drug is often desirable, there is danger of long-term accumulation. With a plasma half-life of 15 to 150 hours and with an analgesic effect of only 4 or 8 hours, methadone accumulation can lead to progressively higher drug levels in plasma until a peak is reached, at which time the patient may be lethargic or comatose. When a long-acting opioid like methadone is necessary, it is probably best to enlist the help of a pain specialist or a respected pain clinic with special experience with this drug.

Opioids predictably produce constipation to which patients do not develop tolerance. Therefore, patients need to be educated to use a stool softener like docusate and a laxative like a senna preparation on a regular basis and to add bulk or fiber to their diet when possible to prevent constipation. If obstipation occurs, then the use of bisacodyl, milk of magnesia, mineral oil, lactulose, citrate of magnesia, or a phosphosoda enema may be necessary on a regular basis. If fecal impaction occurs, disimpaction must be done before taking additional oral laxatives (Levy, 1996).

Increased analgesic effect and decreased sedation have been reported with the use of 5 to 10 mg of methylphenidate with breakfast and 5 mg with lunch. Decreased nausea and vomiting may be achieved with prophylactic use of prochlorperazine, haloperidol, thiethylperazine, lorazepam, or metoclopramide.

SPECIAL PROBLEMS: BONE PAIN AND NEUROPATHIC PAIN

These are two pain situations that are commonly experienced by patients with cancer that require special consideration. Osteolytic or osteoblastic metastases can both cause somatic pain, which is often a dull ache that is fairly well localized and is felt on weight bearing or at night. It is usually constant, gradually progressive in intensity, and exacerbated by different positions or movement. The most common metastatic sites involve bones of the pelvis, vertebrae, ribs, femur and skull. The most common primary sites are breast, lung, and prostate. Bone metastases are associated with edema and inflammation so that nociceptors are activated and sensitized by chemical mediators of the inflammatory response such as prostaglandins (PG), bradykinin, and potassium (Berger & Koprowski, 2002).

Relief of bone pain is most immediately possible with NSAIDs with or without opioids, depending on the severity and response. NSAIDs reduce edema and lead to a reduction in PG synthesis and a reduction in PG-induced pain sensitization and have a direct effect on spinal nociceptive processing. However, NSAIDs, as previously noted, have a "ceiling" to analgesic effect beyond which higher doses produce additional toxicity but no further pain relief, whereas opioids have no "ceiling" doses and one increases the dose of opioid until pain relief is achieved within the limits of collateral toxicity.

Since NSAIDs are not necessarily cross-reactive between groups, failure with one may be followed by success with another if the patient's pain is not severe. If it is severe, an opioid should be added to the pain regimen immediately. When treating bone pain, early relief can usually be achieved with external-beam radiation therapy. More lasting, but later, relief can be provided by the use of the radioactive isotopes strontium-89 or samarium-153. Symptomatic improvement in bone pain has also been reported with pamidronate (Glover et al, 1994) and zoledronic acid (Berenson et al, 2001).

Neuropathic pain usually follows the injured nerve path and is described as tightness, burning, or lancinating. Pain caused by injury to peripheral or central neural structures results in aberrant somatosensory processing of those sites, and may be induced by prolonged nerve compression, surgical nerve transsection, irradiation, or some chemotherapy agents (cisplatin, paclitaxel, vincristine, and others). It may present as trigeminal neuralgia, post-herpetic neuralgia, post-glossopharyngeal neuralgia, or post-traumatic neuralgia. Its response to opioids and NSAIDs is often incomplete and requires the addition of adjuvants like tricyclic antidepressants (amitriptyline, imipramine, nortriptyline, desipramine) or anticonvulsants (gabapentin, phenytoin, carbamazepine, sodium valproate, clonazepam). Other useful agents include baclofen, mexiletine, ketamine, and dextromethorphan.

ADDITIONAL MEASURES FOR PAIN CONTROL

In some circumstances, the pharmacological approaches to pain control already described may not provide adequate relief. Additional therapeutic approaches are then used. Patient-controlled analgesia with a variety of devices permits patients to treat their pain by directly activating doses of IV opioids (Bruera & Schoeller, 1992; Citron et al, 1992). Although this therapy is popular for inpatients, it is being supplanted by fentanyl patches and sustained-release morphine for outpatient use because of the greater convenience of the patches and pills and the lesser cost compared with an ambulatory pump and its servicing. Transcutaneous electrical nerve stimulation is often helpful in reducing pain, especially back pain.

Epidural and intrathecal administration of narcotics can produce localized selective analgesia without motor blockade (Smith et al, 2002). This avoids the side effects of systemic therapy. The infusions can be simplified with an implanted reservoir or with an exterior epidural catheter for self-administration. Various noninvasive procedures may be employed to help control the pain itself or to relieve the emotional distress caused by the pain. Some alternative techniques are intrinsically successful and they also have the added benefit of helping the patient regain some sense of control in a situation plagued by feelings of helplessness.

Coping mechanisms used to reduce the intensity of pain include heat, cold, distraction, hypnosis, imagery, position change, massage, and exercise. Distraction techniques that include watching television, praying, and reading provide relief for some patients who use these techniques. Position change may be beneficial in many cases. Less frequently used methods include exercise, massage, nonopioid medications, and specific foods.

Invasive neurosurgical analgesic interventions may be employed for refractory pain, uncontrolled pain, or pain not controlled well enough with pharmacological interventions. These procedures should only be considered after thorough evaluation by a pain specialist or pain clinic.

PEARLS TO REMEMBER

1. Believe the patient's complaint of pain.
2. Take a careful history of the pain complaint.
3. Perform a careful medical, psychological, and neurological examination.
4. Order and personally review the appropriate diagnostic studies.
5. Individualize the approach to the patient.
6. Consider the full range of available therapeutic options.
7. Refer to the equianalgesic table when switching opioids or routes of administration.
8. Reassess the patient's response to therapy.
9. Do not be easily dissuaded from providing adequate doses of opiates for pain relief.
10. Do not worry about addiction in the terminally ill cancer patient with pain.

REFERENCES

Abrahm JL. A Physician's Guide to Pain and Symptom Management in Cancer Patients. Baltimore, Johns Hopkins University Press, 2000.

Ad Hoc Committee on Cancer Pain of the American Society of Clinical Oncology. Cancer pain assessment and treatment curriculum guidelines. J Clin Oncol 10: 1976–1982, 1992.

Agency for Health Care Policy and Research. Management of Cancer Pain: Clinical Practice Guidelines. Rockville, MD, US Dept of Health and Human Services, 1994.

American Cancer Society. Guide to Pain Control. Atlanta, American Cancer Society, 2001.

American Pain Society. Principles of Analgesic Use in the Treatment of Acute Pain and Cancer Pain, 4th ed. Skokie, IL, American Pain Society, 1999.

Anderson R et al. Accuracy in equi-analgesic dosing: conversion dilemmas. J Pain Symptom Manage 21: 397–406, 2001.

Berenson JR et al. Zoledronic acid reduces skeletal-related events in patients with osteolytic metastases: a double-blind randomized dose-response study. Cancer 91: 1191–1200, 2001.

Berger AM, Koprowski C. Bone pain: assessment and management. In Berger AM, Portenoy RK, Weissman DE, eds. Principles and Practice of Palliative Care and Supportive Oncology. Philadelphia, Lippincott Williams & Wilkins, 2002.

Brody J. Misunderstood opioids and needless pain. New York Times, January 22, F-8, 2002.

Bruera E, Schoeller T. Patient-controlled analgesia in cancer pain. In DeVita VT Jr, Hellman S, Rosenberg SA, eds. Principles and Practice of Oncology. PPO Updates 6: 1–7, 1992.

Catalano RB. Pharmacology of analgesic agents used to treat cancer pain. Semin Oncol Nurs 1: 126–140, 1985.

Citron ML et al. Patient-controlled analgesia for cancer pain: long term study of inpatient and outpatient use. Cancer Invest 10: 335–341, 1992.

Fischer DS. Hormonal and chemical therapy. In Twycross RG, ed. Pain Relief in Cancer. Clin Oncol 3: 55–74, 1984.

Foley KM. Advances in cancer pain. Arch Neurol 56: 413–417, 1999.

Glover D et al. Intravenous pamidronate disodium treatment of bone pain in patients with breast cancer: a dose seeking study. Cancer 74: 2949–2955, 1994.

Heavey B. Pain free forever. AARP Modern Maturity July/August: 64–70, 2002.

Indelicato RA, Portenoy RK. Opioid rotation in the management of refractory cancer pain. J Clin Oncol 20: 348–352, 2002.

Levy MH. Pharmacologic treatment of cancer pain. N Engl J Med 335: 1124, 1996.

Lynn J et al. Perceptions by family members of the dying experience of older and seriously ill patients. Ann Intern Med 126: 97–106, 1997.

Marks RM, Sachar EJ. Undertreatment of medical inpatients with narcotic analgesics. Ann Intern Med 78: 173–181, 1973.

Melzack R. The tragedy of needless pain. Sci Am 262: 27–33, 1990.

Mercadante S et al. Switching from morphine to methadone to improve analgesia and tolerability in cancer patients: a prospective study. J Clin Oncol 19: 2898–2904, 2001.

NCCN. Practice Guidelines in Oncology—v.1.2001 (Accessed August 6, 2002 at http://nccn.org)

Plummer JL et al. Morphine patient-controlled analgesia is superior to meperidine patient-controlled analgesia for postoperative pain. Anesth Analg 84: 794–799, 1997.

Portenoy RK. Cancer pain management. Semin Oncol 20(2 suppl 1): 19–36, 1993.

Portenoy RK, Hagen NA. Breakthrough pain: definition, prevalence and characteristics. Pain 41: 273–281, 1990.

Porter J, Jick H. Addiction rare in patients treated with narcotics. N Engl J Med 302: 123, 1980.

Ripamonti L et al. Switching from morphine to oral methadone in treating cancer pain: what is the equi-analgesic dose ratio? J Clin Oncol 16: 3216–3221, 1998.

Schumacher KL et al. Putting cancer pain management regimens into practice at home. J Pain Symptom Manage 23: 369–382, 2002.

Sinatra RS et al. Acute Pain: Mechanisms and Management. St. Louis, Mosby, 1992.

Smith TJ et al. Randomized clinical trial of an implantable drug delivery system compared with comprehensive medical management for refractory cancer pain: impact on pain, drug-related toxicity, and survival. J Clin Oncol 20: 4040–4049, 2002.

Stjernsward J, Colleau SM, Ventafridda V. The World Health Organization Cancer Pain and Palliative Care Program, past, present, and future. J Pain Symptom Manage 12: 65–72, 1996.

SUPPORT Principal Investigators. A controlled trial to improve care for seriously ill hospitalized patients. JAMA 274: 1591–1598, 1995.

Twycross RG, Lack SA. Therapeutics in Terminal Cancer. Edinburgh, Churchill Livingstone, 1990.

Von Roenn JH et al. Physician attitudes and practice in cancer pain management: a survey from the Eastern Cooperative Oncology Group. Ann Intern Med 119: 121–126, 1993.

Warfield C. Guidelines for routine use of controlled-release oral morphine sulfate tablets. Semin Oncol 20(2 suppl 1): 36–47, 1993.

World Health Organization. Cancer Pain Relief. Geneva, World Health Organization, 1986, and 2nd edition, 1996.

Yates PM et al. Barriers to effective cancer pain management: a survey of hospitalized cancer patients in Australia. J Pain Symptom Manage 23: 393–405, 2002.

HIGH-DOSE CHEMOTHERAPY WITH STEM CELL SUPPORT

Human blood stem cell transplantation is now considered standard therapy for some of the more aggressive hematological malignancies and some hereditary disorders. Early attempts at transplantation from one individual to another had variable success, depending on the relationship of the individuals, because of the incomplete knowledge of human histocompatibility typing and the immunology of the human leukocyte antigen (HLA). This chapter discusses bone marrow transplantation (BMT) and hematopoietic stem cell transplantation (HSCT) in cancer therapy.

There are two major approaches to HSCT: allogeneic and autologous. Allogeneic transplants involve the transfer of donor bone marrow (BM) or peripheral blood stem cells (PBSCs) or umbilical cord blood (UCB) from one individual to another. When the donor is an identical twin, it is called a syngeneic transplant. The earliest successful transplants were of this type.

ALLOGENEIC TRANSPLANTATION

The preferred transplant arrangement is for a BM or PBSC transfer from a six-antigen HLA-matched donor. Graft-versus-host disease (GVHD) and a graft-versus-malignancy effect may still be quite potent because of differences in minor histo-compatibility antigens between the donor and the patient. When no family match is possible, a search through volunteer donor registries may reveal a suitable match.

For children, and increasingly for adults, UCB transplants are being sought through several cord blood banks. UCB has several advantages compared to adult stem cells, as follows:

- UCB cells are enriched in primitive stem cells, which gives them a proliferative advantage that may compensate for the relatively low number of cells in a single cord blood unit.
- UCB cells are immunologically naïve, produce fewer cytokines and less severe or no acute GVHD.
- They are easily obtained with an absence of risk for mothers and donors, they have a decreased risk of transmitting infections, particularly cytomegalovirus (CMV) and human immunodeficiency virus (HIV), and they can be stored fully tested and HLA-typed. Thus stored in the frozen state, they are available for immediate use.

Cord blood transplantation is discussed at length in a recent monograph (Cohen et al, 2000). One of the great advantages of public UCB banks is that they can serve a greater diversity of ethnic populations.

INDICATIONS FOR ALLOGENEIC TRANSPLANTATION

Approximately 15,000 allogeneic transplants were performed in 1998, and 36,000 autologous transplants were reported to the International Bone Marrow Transplant Registry (IBMTR, 2000) and the numbers are increasing year by year. A carefully documented international experience through the records of the IBMTR and peer-reviewed published reports of many centers has clarified the major indications for allo-geneic transplants for a multitude of nonmalignant hematopoietic diseases, metabolic disorders, immunodeficiencies, and malignant diseases, but we will discuss only the malignant diseases. The documentation and bibliographic citations are most easily accessed in the chapters in several recent compilations (Armitage & Antman, 2001; Atkinson, 2000; Ball et al, 2000; Buchner et al, 1999; Thomas et al, 1999; Weiss, 2001). Allogeneic transplantation for cancer, with a few exceptions, is used in hematopoietic malignancies.

In acute lymphoblastic leukemia (ALL) of childhood, cure is achieved in the majority of patients with standard therapy. The results with standard chemotherapy for adults with ALL are less successful. Allogeneic transplantation is used in primary refractory disease, and in first complete remission (CR) in patients with high-risk disease (e.g., Philadelphia chromosome positive), and in second CR if a good donor is available. If there is no good donor, then high-dose chemotherapy (HDCT) with an autologous bone marrow transplant (ABMT) may be attempted.

Chronic lymphocytic leukemia (CLL) is usually an indolent disease of the elderly with a prolonged survival, but most of those with CLL die of it or its complications. There is not a great deal of experience with the use of transplantation in CLL, although, based on theoretical considerations, it should be an effective modality of therapy. Most studies have been done with allogeneic transplants in younger patients with a relatively good performance status and the disease-free survivals have been relatively good, but there are not many long-term follow-up studies. In older patients, greater comorbidity and mortality rates associated with the transplantation have been high and the indications for HDCT are not clear. Similarly, ABMT has been used with mixed results and clearly more information is needed in carefully controlled studies. We would consider HDCT with HSCT as an investigational procedure in CLL.

In acute myelocytic leukemia, allogeneic transplantation is indicated for primary refractory disease and all patients with unfavorable cytogenetics and for patients with relapse after standard chemotherapy. For the younger patient with a sibling-matched donor, most clinicians would also recommend an allogeneic transplant in first CR. Autologous transplantation may be used for older patients and those without a suitable donor.

Allogeneic transplantation is the only known curative therapy for chronic myelocytic leukemia (CML). CML has the best outcome when the patient is still in the chronic phase, and young. In accelerated phase or blast phase CML, results are not as good and there is a higher treatment-related mortality. Imatinib mesylate has largely replaced the use of interferon-alfa and hydroxyurea and busulfan. It may also change the situation in regard to transplantation in a way that it is too early to predict.

The original intent of allogeneic transplantation was to eradicate the patient's hematopoietic malignancy and the marrow that produced it, to impair the recipient patient's immune system so that it would not reject the donor graft, and to create space in the marrow cavity for a new marrow with no malignant cells and a new immune system. A welcome surprise was the important role of the graft-versus-leukemia (GVL) or graft-versus-lymphoma (also designated GVL in the appropriate other circumstance) as a potentially curative modality, and another indication for allogeneic transplantation. In many cases the graft-versus-malignancy response may be potent enough to reduce the intensity of the conditioning (preparative) regimen. As a result, the current approach to nonablative chemotherapy as adoptive immunotherapy is being actively evaluated, and preparative regimens have been published (Chakraverty et al, 2002; Childs et al, 1999, 2000; Giralt et al, 1997; Khouri et al, 1998, 2001; Michallet et al, 2001; Slavin et al, 1998; Spitzer et al, 2000; Spitzer, 2000).

AUTOLOGOUS TRANSPLANTATION

In contrast, autologous transplantation is simply a procedure to replace a marrow with the patient's own saved BM or PBSCs following high-dose chemotherapy. Destruction of the malignant tumor is best achieved with drugs that exhibit a dose-response effect, that are cell-cycle independent, and with hematological toxicity as their major side effect. The alkylating agents are the drugs most often used for this purpose (Table 10-1). However, the plant alkaloids etoposide, teniposide, and paclitaxel have been tried in combination with alkylating agents and show promise in several regimens. The plant antibiotics mitoxantrone and mitomycin, and the antimetabolites cytarabine, fludarabine, and cladribine, have also been combined in a few successful combinations of HDCT. Dose escalation continues until nonhematological toxicity becomes dose-limiting.

With HDCT and BMT or PBSCT (most centers are using PBSCT), the main dose-limiting nonhematological toxicities (Table 10-2) become the ultimate dose-limiting toxicity (DLT). In selecting preparative HDCT regimens, one must be mindful of the patient's associated disease, the patient's prior chemotherapy and radiation therapy (if any), and potential subsequent therapy that may be planned (e.g., avoid carmustine, busulfan, and cyclophosphamide if post-transplant radiation therapy to the lung area is likely). The list of HDCT preparative regimens in this chapter represents a selection from a large group of published trials (Antman et al, 1992; Cohen & Krigel, 1995; Shapiro et al, 1997; Treleaven & Wiernik, 1995). The list is not meant to suggest that these are necessarily the best, but they do seem to be those that are more frequently used at this time. Each is used for a particular neoplasm but under some circumstances is equally suitable for other cancers. The best regimen has not yet been identified; perhaps it has not even been developed. New and better drugs may be forthcoming.

TABLE 10-1

CYTOTOXIC DRUGS USED IN HEMATOPOIETIC TRANSPLANTATION

Drug	Typical standard dose in combination	Typical transplant dose in combination
ALKYLATING AGENTS		
Cyclophosphamide	1,000 mg/m^2	7,500 mg/m^2
Ifosfamide	4,000 mg/m^2	18,000 mg/m^2
Thiotepa	15 mg/m^2	800 mg/m^2
Melphalan	16 mg/m^2	60 mg/m^2
Busulfan	4 mg/day	16 mg/kg
Carmustine	150 mg/m^2	450 mg/m^2
Cisplatin	60 mg/m^2	165 mg/m^2
Carboplatin (AUC)	5–7 mg/ml/min	12–32 mg/ml/min
PLANT ALKALOIDS		
Etoposide	300 mg/m^2	2,400 mg/m^2
Paclitaxel	175 mg/m^2	775 mg/m^2
PLANT ANTIBIOTICS		
Mitoxantrone	12 mg/m^2	75 mg/m^2
Mitomycin	10 mg/m^2	90 mg/m^2

TABLE 10-2

DOSE-LIMITING NONHEMATOLOGICAL TOXICITY

Toxicity	Drugs
Pulmonary fibrosis and pneumonitis	Carmustine, busulfan, cyclophosphamide, cytarabine
Cystitis	Cyclophosphamide, ifosfamide, etoposide
Myocarditis	Cyclophosphamide, mitoxantrone, paclitaxel
Nephrotoxicity	Cisplatin, ifosfamide, carmustine, carboplatin, cyclophosphamide
Ototoxicity	Cisplatin, carboplatin
Hepatotoxicity and veno-occlusive disease	Carboplatin, mitomycin, carmustine, busulfan, etoposide, cytarabine
Mucositis	Thiotepa, melphalan, etoposide, mitoxantrone, busulfan, paclitaxel, cytarabine
Neurological	Ifosfamide, cytarabine, busulfan, carmustine
Peripheral neuropathy	Carboplatin, paclitaxel, cisplatin, etoposide

10

AUTOLOGOUS TRANSPLANTATION

INDICATIONS FOR AUTOLOGOUS TRANSPLANTATION

HDCT with HSCT has been demonstrated to be effective in most hematopoietic tumors. In Hodgkin's disease (HD), approximately two-thirds of patients are cured with standard therapy. In patients who relapse or fail to achieve remission, there is a role for HDCT with ABMT or PBSCT that may be curative (Argiris et al, 2000; Mink & Armitage, 2001). Allogeneic HSCT carries a higher treatment-related mortality and is generally used only after failure of HDCT with autologous PBSCT or ABMT.

The treatment of non-Hodgkin's lymphoma (NHL) at present depends on the histologic type and aggressiveness as well as on the extent of disease spread. The cure rate of advanced aggressive NHL is in the range of 30% to 50%. For relapsed aggressive NHL, there is ample evidence of its efficacy (Gianni et al, 1997; Haioun et al, 2000; Mink & Armitage, 2001; Philip et al, 1995; Santini et al, 1998). An international consensus conference on aggressive NHL concluded that HDCT was appropriate therapy in first or subsequent relapse whether the patient's BM was positive or negative so long as it was chemotherapy-sensitive (Shipp et al, 1999). There was no evidence to indicate that total body irradiation (TBI) was superior to HDCT and there was no HDCT preparative regimen that was demonstrably superior to others. The preferred mobilization technique is a combination of the appropriate chemotherapy regime for the particular tumor type followed by filgrastim for a few days to obtain sufficient PBSCs. As yet there is no demonstrated role for purging of autologous BM or PBSCs.

The treatment of multiple myeloma has been difficult and cure remains elusive. Nonetheless, a consensus seems to be evolving that survival appears to be longer with autologous PBSCT in appropriately selected patients as compared to optimal standard-dose chemotherapy (Attal et al, 1996; Barlogie et al, 1999; Bensinger et al, 1996; Cunningham et al, 1994; Fermand et al, 1998; Imrie et al, 2002; Moreau et al, 2002; Vesole et al, 1999). Previous exposure to alkylating agents may reduce the stem cell pool and the ablity to mobilize and harvest sufficient stem cells, especially if melphalan, busulfan, mustargen, carmustine, or lomustine have been used. Radiation therapy may also reduce the stem cell pool. Conditioning regimens may be HDCT alone or with TBI. Moreau et al (2002) concluded that 200 mg/m^2 melphalan is a less toxic and at least as effective a conditioning regimen when compared with 800 cGy TBI with 140 mg/m^2 melphalan. Tandem transplants have been evaluated (Barlogie et al, 1999; Vesole et al, 1994) but there is no firm scientific evidence for the superiority of tandem transplants and they should only be conducted within a clinical trial.

Although patients with advanced germ cell tumors have a high cure rate, between 20% and 30% of patients with disseminated disease fail to achieve a durable complete response with standard chemotherapy (Motzer et al, 2000). For those patients with a gonadal primary who relapse after a response to first-line therapy, there is a high likelihood of response to conventional dose salvage therapy. However, patients with an incomplete response to first-line therapy or an extragonadal primary site need to be considered for clinical trials that include a dose-intensive regimen with PBSCT. Such patients are potentially curable (Broun et al, 1992; Lotz et al, 1995).

Despite the fact that most epithelial ovarian malignancies are relatively sensitive to chemotherapy with frequent partial responses and some complete responses, late diagnosis and advanced disease result in a limited number of cures. Studies of HDCT with HSCT (Legros et al, 1997; Stiff et al, 1997) indicate that the best outcome of HDCT is seen in those with minimal residual disease that was responsive to initial chemotherapy. Increased disease-free survival and overall survival have been reported in selected patients, but the experience is limited and HDCT with HSCT for epithelial ovarian carcinoma is currently considered investigational.

Metastatic breast cancer is generally considered incurable with standard chemotherapy, so attempts were made to improve the outcome using HDCT with autologous transplantation. Although it had been suggested that the use of ABMT should be confined to well-designed, randomized, controlled trials (Fischer, 1998; Henderson et al, 1988), only a few prospective randomized trials were done. Many oncologists and patients elected not to enter a clinical trial, based on the assumption that the results with ABMT would be better, and were treated with HDCT and ABMT. As insurance companies were reimbursing for transplants for breast cancer, many university and community hospitals began to set up transplantation units. In Europe, it has been suggested, "many centers now consider high-dose chemotherapy an easy way to balance budgets" (Gianni, 1997).

The only randomized prospective trial in the literature (Bezwoda et al, 1995) had been reported as showing the superiority of an HDCT regimen with ABMT or PBSCT in achieving increased CRs, increased duration of response, and increased duration of survival in women with metastatic breast cancer. *At the time, it was not known that the study of Bezwoda et al (1995) was not only "poorly designed and unconvincing," it was blatantly fraudulent.* In 1999, Bezwoda reported a highly statistically significant improved relapse-free survival and overall survival for women with breast cancer treated with his prior HDC regimen and a control group treated with CAF (cyclophosphamide, doxorubicin [adriamycin], and fluorouracil), a different control regimen than that in the 1995 paper. These results were so enticing that a delegation of physician-scientists went to the University of Witwatersrand in Johannesburg, South Africa, to review his results. They were stunned to find that he could produce only some of the records of the patients given HDCT and very few of the records of the control group (Weiss et al, 2000, 2001). An investigation by the University of Witwatersrand concluded that the studies were fraudulent and represented scientific misconduct and the studies were officially withdrawn from the literature. In contrast, several studies in peer-reviewed journals have reported no relapse-free or overall survival advantage with HDCT (Bergh et al, 2000; Hortobagyi et al, 2000; Rodenhuis et al, 1998; Stadtmauer et al, 2000). The use of four-cycle HDCT with HSCT showed no improvement compared with single-course HDCT (Hu et al, 2000). The substantial number of published uncontrolled studies gave an overly optimistic impression of the therapy. Currently there are no data to support the use of HDCT with ABMT or PBSCT in the treatment of breast cancer outside of a clinical trial. The lesson to be learned is that new therapies need to be evaluated with scientific rigor before we accept them as standard care for our patients.

CURRENT STATUS

HDCT with ABMT or PBSCT has been used in the treatment of a variety of malignancies (Box 10-1). Critical to its success is the appropriate selection of an HDCT program. In selecting an HDCT regimen, it is generally important to demonstrate that the tumor is still inherently drug-sensitive to standard (induction) drug therapy because those tumors that are not inherently drug-sensitive have a low rate of response and/or short duration of response to HDCT with ABMT or PBSCT. There should also be an expectation that the tumors selected for HDCT with ABMT or PBSCT are potentially curable (e.g., germ cell tumors, leukemias, lymphomas) or at least highly responsive (e.g., multiple myeloma). Other tumors that may be treated with HDCT and HSCT should be approached as part of a well-designed clinical trial. Needless to say, these brief summaries of complex regimens should not be used without reviewing the original reports, and they should be administered only by individuals adequately trained and in institutions that have the appropriate facilities and a cadre of trained oncology/transplantation nurses. As in the previous edition of this book, the HDCT regimens are listed in a chapter at some distance from the compilations of standard dose chemotherapy regimens in order to heighten the awareness of the differences in dose ranges (Table 10-1) and to avoid the potential problems of lethal overdosing.

10

CURRENT STATUS

BOX 10-1

NEOPLASMS TREATED WITH HIGH-DOSE CHEMOTHERAPY UNDER SPECIAL AND APPROPRIATE CIRCUMSTANCES

LEUKEMIAS

Acute myeloblastic leukemia	Myelodysplastic syndromes
Acute lymphoblastic leukemia	Acute myelofibrosis
Chronic myelogenous leukemia	

LYMPHOPROLIFERATIVE DISORDERS

Hodgkin's lymphoma
Non-Hodgkin's lymphoma
Multiple myeloma

SOLID TUMORS

Germ cell tumors
Testicular carcinoma

UNDER INVESTIGATION

Breast cancer	Astrocytomas, gliomas
Chronic lymphocytic leukemia	Osteosarcoma
Lung cancers	Ewing's sarcoma
Melanoma	Ovarian carcinoma
Neuroblastoma	

REFERENCES

Antman K et al. Dose-intensive therapy in breast cancer. Bone Marrow Transplant 10(suppl 1): 67–73, 1992.

Argiris A, Seropian S, Cooper DL. High-dose BEAM chemotherapy with autologous peripheral blood progenitor-cell transplantation for unselected patients with primary refractory or relapsed Hodgkin's disease. Ann Oncol 11: 665–672, 2000.

Armitage JO, Antman KH, eds. High-Dose Cancer Therapy, 3rd ed. Philadelphia, Lippincott Williams & Wilkins, 2001.

Atkinson K, ed. Clinical Bone Marrow and Blood Stem Cell Transplantation, 2nd ed. Cambridge, UK, Cambridge University Press, 2000.

Attal M et al. A prospective, randomized trial of autologous bone marrow transplantation and chemotherapy in multiple myeloma. N Engl J Med 335: 91–97, 1996.

Ball ED, Lister J, Law P, eds. Hematopoietic Stem Cell Therapy. New York, Churchill Livingstone, 2000.

Barlogie B et al. Total therapy with tandem transplants for newly diagnosed multiple myeloma. Blood 93: 55–65, 1999.

Bensinger WI et al. Allogeneic marrow transplantation for multiple myeloma: an analysis of risk factors on outcome. Blood 88: 2787–2793, 1996.

Bergh J et al. Tailored fluorouracil, epirubicin, and cyclophosphamide compared with marrow-supported high-dose chemotherapy as adjuvant treatment for high-risk breast cancer: a randomised trial. Scandinavian Breast Group 9401 study, Lancet 356: 1384–1391, 2000.

Bezwoda WR. Randomized, controlled trial of high-dose chemotherapy (HD-CNVp) versus standard dose (CAF) chemotherapy for high-risk, surgically treated, primary breast cancer [abstract]. Proc ASCO 18: 2a, 1999.

Bezwoda WR, Seymour L, Dansey RD. High-dose chemotherapy with hematopoietic rescue as primary treatment for metastatic breast cancer: a randomized trial. J Clin Oncol 13: 2483–2489, 1995.

Broun ER et al. Long-term outcome of patients with relapsed and refractory germ cell tumors treated with high-dose chemotherapy and autologous bone marrow rescue. Ann Intern Med 117: 124–128, 1992.

Buchner TH et al, eds. Transplantation in Hematology and Oncology. Berlin, Springer-Verlag, 1999.

Chakraverty R et al. Limiting transplantation-related mortality following unrelated donor stem cell transplantation by using a nonmyeloablative conditioning regimen. Blood 99: 1071–1078, 2002.

Childs R et al. Engraftment kinetics after nonmyeloablative allogeneic peripheral blood stem cell transplantation: full donor T-cell chimerism precedes alloimmune responses. Blood 94: 3234–3241, 1999.

Childs R et al. Regression of metastatic renal-cell carcinoma after nonmyeloablative allogeneic peripheral-blood stem cell transplantation. N Engl J Med 343: 750–758, 2000.

Cohen SBA, Gluckman E, Rubinstein P, Madrigal JA, eds. Cord Blood Characteristics: Role in Stem Cell Transplantation. London, Martin Dunitz, 2000.

Cohen SC, Krigel RL. High-dose therapy with stem-cell infusion in lymphoma. Semin Oncol 22: 218–229, 1995.

Cunningham D et al. High-dose melphalan for multiple myeloma: long-term follow-up data. J Clin Oncol 12: 764–768, 1994.

Fermand J-P et al. High-dose therapy and autologous peripheral blood stem cell transplantation in multiple myeloma: up-front or rescue treatments? Results of a multicenter sequential randomized clinical trial. Blood 92: 3131–3136, 1998.

Fischer DS. Need randomized clinical trials, not litigation. J Clin Oncol 16: 1237–1238, 1998.

Gianni AM. High-dose chemotherapy and autotransplants: a time for guidelines. Ann Oncol 8: 933–935, 1997.

Gianni AM et al. High-dose chemotherapy and autologous bone marrow transplantation compared with MACOP-B in aggressive B-cell lymphoma. N Engl J Med 336: 1290–1297, 1997.

Giralt S et al. Engraftment of allogeneic hematopoietic progenitor cells with purine analog-containing chemotherapy: harnessing graft-versus-leukemia without myeloablative therapy. Blood 89: 4531–4536, 1997.

Haioun C et al. Survival benefit of high-dose therapy in poor-risk aggressive non-Hodgkin's lymphoma: final analysis of the prospective LNH87-2 protocol – a Groupe d'Etude des Lymphomes de l'Adulte study. J Clin Oncol 18: 3025–3030, 2000.

Henderson IC, Hayes DF, Gelman R. Dose-response in the treatment of breast cancer: a critical review. J Clin Oncol 6: 1501–1515, 1988.

Hortobagyi GN et al. Randomized trial of high-dose chemotherapy and blood cell autografts for high-risk primary breast cancer. J Natl Cancer Inst 92: 225–233, 2000.

Hu WW et al. Four-cycle high-dose therapy with hematopoietic support for metastatic breast cancer: no improvement in outcomes compared with single course high-dose therapy. Biol Blood Marrow Transplant 6: 58–69, 2000.

IBMTR. Newsletter 7: 3–10, 2000.

Imrie K et al. The role of high-dose chemotherapy and stem-cell transplantation in patients with multiple myeloma: a practice guideline of the Cancer Care Ontario Practice Guidelines Initiative. Ann Intern Med 136: 619–629, 2002.

Khouri IF et al. Transplant-lite: induction of graft-versus-malignancy using fludarabine-based nonablative chemotherapy and allogeneic blood progenitor-cell transplantation as treatment for lymphoid malignancies. J Clin Oncol 16: 2817–2824, 1998.

Khouri IF et al. Nonablative allogeneic hematopoietic transplantation as adoptive immunotherapy for indolent lymphoma: low incidence of toxicity, acute graft-versus-host disease, and treatment-related mortality. Blood 98: 3595–3599, 2001.

Legros M et al. High-dose chemotherapy with hematopoietic rescue in patients with stage III to IV ovarian cancer: long-term results. J Clin Oncol 15: 1302–1308, 1997.

Lotz JP et al. High-dose chemotherapy with ifosfamide, carboplatin, and etoposide combined with autologous bone marrow transplantation for the treatment of poor-prognosis germ cell tumors and metastatic trophoblastic disease in adults. Cancer 75: 874–885, 1995.

Michallet M et al. Allogeneic hematopoietic stem-cell transplantation after nonmyeloablative preparative regimens: impact of pretransplantation and posttransplantation factors on outcome. J Clin Oncol 19: 3340–3349, 2001.

Mink SA, Armitage JO. High-dose therapy in lymphomas: a review of the current status of allogeneic and autologous stem cell transplantation in Hodgkin's disease and non-Hodgkin's lymphoma. The Oncologist 6: 247–256, 2001.

Moreau P et al. Comparison of 200 mg/m^2 melphalan and 8 Gy total body irradiation plus 140 mg/m^2 as conditioning regimens for peripheral blood stem cell transplantation in patients with newly diagnosed multiple myeloma: final analysis of the Intergroupe Francophone du Myelome 9502 randomized trial. Blood 99: 731–735, 2002.

Motzer RJ et al. Sequential dose-intensive paclitaxel, ifosfamide, carboplatin, and etoposide salvage therapy for germ cell tumor patients. J Clin Oncol 18: 1173–1180, 2000.

Philip T et al. Autologous bone marrow transplantation as compared with salvage chemotherapy in relapses of chemotherapy-sensitive non-Hodgkin's lymphoma. N Engl J Med 333: 1540–1545, 1995.

Rodenhuis S et al. Randomised trial of high-dose chemotherapy and haemopoietic progenitor-cell support in operable breast cancer with extensive axillary lymph-node involvement. Lancet 352: 515–521, 1998.

Santini G et al. VACOP-B versus VACOP-B plus autologous bone marrow transplantation for advanced diffuse non-Hodgkin's lymphoma: results of a prospective randomized trial by the non-Hodgkin's Lymphoma Cooperative Study Group. J Clin Oncol 16: 2796–2802, 1998.

Shapiro TW, Davison DB, Rust DM. Stem Cell and Bone Marrow Transplantation. Boston, Jones and Bartlett, 1997.

Shipp MA et al. International Consensus Conference on High-Dose Therapy with Hematopoietic Stem Cell Transplantation in Aggressive Non-Hodgkin's Lymphomas: report of the jury. J Clin Oncol 17: 423–428, 1998.

Slavin S et al. Nonmyeloablative stem cell transplantation and cell therapy as an alternative to conventional bone marrow transplantation with lethal cytoreduction for the treatment of malignant and nonmalignant hematologic diseases. Blood 91: 756–763, 1998.

Spitzer TR. Nonmyeloablative allogeneic stem cell transplant strategies and the role of mixed chimerism. The Oncologist 5: 215–223, 2000.

Spitzer TR et al. Intentional induction of mixed chimerism and achievement of antitumor responses after nonmyeloablative conditioning therapy and HLA-matched donor bone marrow transplantation for refractory hematologic malignancies. Biol Blood Marrow Transplant 6: 309–320, 2000.

Stadtmauer EA et al. Conventional-dose chemotherapy compared with high-dose chemotherapy plus autologous hematopoietic stem-cell transplantation for metastatic breast cancer. N Engl J Med 342: 1069–1076, 2000.

Stiff PJ et al. High-dose chemotherapy with autologous transplantation for persistent/relapsed ovarian cancer: a multivariate analysis of survival for 100 consecutively treated patients. J Clin Oncol 15: 1309–1317, 1997.

Thomas ED, Blume KG, Forman SJ, eds. Hematopoietic Cell Transplantation. Malden, MA, Blackwell Scientific, 1999.

Treleaven J, Wiernik P, eds. Color Atlas and Text of Bone Marrow Transplantation. St. Louis, Mosby-Wolfe, 1995.

Vesole DH et al. High-dose therapy for refractory multiple myeloma: improved prognosis with better supportive care and double transplants. Blood 84: 950–956, 1994.

Vesole DH et al. High-dose melphalan with autotransplantation for refractory multiple myeloma: results of a Soutwest Oncology Group phase II trial. J Clin Oncol 17: 2173–2179, 1999.

Weiss RB, ed. Dose-intensive therapy for adult malignancies. Semin Oncol 26: 1–137, 1999.

Weiss RB et al. High-dose chemotherapy for high-risk primary breast cancer: an on-site review of the Bezwoda study. Lancet 355: 944–945, 2000.

Weiss RB, Gill GG, Hudis CA. An on-site audit of the South African trial of high-dose chemotherapy for metastatic breast cancer and associated publications. J Clin Oncol 19: 2772–2777, 2001.

HIGH-DOSE CHEMOTHERAPY PREPARATIVE REGIMENS FOR USE WITH BONE MARROW OR PERIPHERAL BLOOD STEM CELL TRANSPLANTATION

LEUKEMIAS

BUCY—BUSULFAN-CYCLOPHOSPHAMIDE

Busulfan. 4 mg/kg/day in divided doses orally on days −7, −6, −5, and −4.
Cyclophosphamide. 60 mg/kg/day intravenously on days −3 and −2.

NOTE: Now that intravenous busulfan is available, most institutions give 0.8 mg/kg busulfan intravenously over 2 hours in place of each 1 mg/kg of the previous oral dose. All patients with leukemia are given methotrexate intrathecally (10 mg/m^2 but not more than 12 mg total). Allogeneic bone marrow is infused on day 0. Use of mesna should be considered.

Selected Readings

O'Donnell MR et al. Busulfan/cyclophosphamide as conditioning regimen for allogeneic bone marrow transplantation for myelodysplasia. J Clin Oncol 13: 2973–2979, 1995.

Tutschka PJ et al. Bone marrow transplantation for leukemia following a new busulfan and cyclophosphamide regimen. Blood 70: 1382–1388, 1987.

BUVP—BUSULFAN-ETOPOSIDE

Busulfan. 1 mg/kg every 6 hours orally on days −7, −6, −5, and −4.
Etoposide. 60 mg/kg intravenously over 6 to 10 hours on day −3.

NOTE: Autologous bone marrow was treated in vitro with 100 microg/mL 4-hydroper-
oxy-cyclophosphamide and infused on day 0. Etoposide phosphate is more soluble
than etoposide and is used in its place mg for mg. Now that intravenous busulfan is
available, most institutions give 0.8 mg/kg busulfan intravenously over 2 hours in
place of each 1 mg/kg of the previous oral dose.

Selected Readings

Chao NJ et al. Busulfan/etoposide: initial experience with a new preparatory regimen for autologous
bone marrow transplantation in patients with acute nonlymphocytic leukemia. Blood 81:
319–323, 1993.
Linker CA et al. Autologous bone marrow transplantation for acute myeloid leukemia using busulfan
plus etoposide as a preparative regimen. Blood 81: 311–318, 1993.

LYMPHOMAS

BEAM—CARMUSTINE-ETOPOSIDE-CYTARABINE-MELPHALAN

Carmustine. 300 mg/m^2/day intravenously on day −6.
Etoposide. 200 mg/m^2/day intravenously on days −5, −4, −3, and −2.
Cytarabine. 400 mg/m^2/day intravenously on days −5, −4, −3, and −2.
Melphalan. 140 mg/m^2 intravenously on day −1.

NOTE: Bone marrow infusion is given on day 0. Carmustine has been given in a dose
of 600 mg/m^2 but caused unacceptable toxicity. It has been used by some in a dose
of 450 mg/m^2 as a compromise dose.

Selected Readings

Gribben JG et al. Successful treatment of refractory Hodgkin's disease by high-dose combination
chemotherapy and autologous bone marrow transplantation. Blood 73: 340–344, 1989.
Mills W et al. BEAM chemotherapy and autologous bone marrow transplantation for patients with
relapsed or refractory non-Hodgkin's lymphoma. J Clin Oncol 13: 588–595, 1995.

BEAC—CARMUSTINE-ETOPOSIDE-CYTARABINE-CYCLOPHOSPHAMIDE

Carmustine. 300 mg/m^2 intravenously on day −6.
Etoposide. 200 mg/m^2/day intravenously on days −5, −4, −3, and −2.
Cytarabine. 100 mg/m^2/day intravenously twice daily on days −5, −4, −3, and −2.
Cyclophosphamide. 35 mg/kg/day intravenously on days −5, −4, −3, and −2.

NOTE: Mesna may be given 50 mg/kg in divided doses on days −5, −4, −3, and
−2. Bone marrow or PBSCT is given on day 0, after 2 days of no chemotherapy.
In the report by Philip et al in Blood (1991) there is a typographical error in Table
2 on p. 1590, indicating that etoposide is given for 6 days. It was given for only 4
days and this is clearly indicated in the final report (Philip et al, 1995). One
should be very careful not to administer this high dose of cyclophosphamide if the
patient has had a significant previous treatment with an anthracycline antibiotic
such as doxorubicin or if the patient has had chest radiation that included the
heart. If so, consider melphalan instead and use the BEAM regimen above.
Etoposide phosphate is more soluble than etoposide and may be substituted for it
mg for mg.

Selected Readings

Philip T et al. Parma international protocol: pilot study of DHAP followed by involved field irradi-
    ation and BEAC with autologous bone marrow transplantation. Blood 77: 1587–1592, 1991.
Philip T et al. Autologous bone marrow transplantation as compared with salvage chemotherapy in
    relapses of chemotherapy sensitive non-Hodgkin's lymphoma. N Engl J Med 333: 1540–1545,
    1995.

CBV—CYCLOPHOSPHAMIDE-CARMUSTINE-ETOPOSIDE

Cyclophosphamide. 1,800 mg/m^2/day intravenously on days −5, −4, −3, and −2.
Carmustine. 100 mg/m^2/day intravenously on days −5, −4, −3, and −2.
Etoposide. 400 mg/m^2/day every 12 hours on days −8, −7, and −6.

*NOTE: Bone marrow is infused on day 0. Reece et al (1991) gave 600 mg/m^2 of
carmustine but noted increased toxicity and a higher early death rate. Jagannath et
al (1989) gave total doses of cyclophosphamide 6,000 mg/m^2 (1,500/day for 4
days), carmustine 300 mg/m^2, and etoposide 900 mg/m^2 (300/day for 3 days). Use
of mesna should be considered for uroprotection. Etoposide phosphate is more soluble than etoposide and may be substituted mg for mg.*

Selected Readings

Demirer T et al. High-dose cyclophosphamide, carmustine, and etoposide followed by allogeneic
    bone marrow transplantation in patients with lymphoid malignancies who had received prior
    dose-limiting radiation therapy. J Clin Oncol 13: 596–602, 1995.
Jagannath S et al. Prognostic factors for response and survival after high-dose cyclophosphamide,
    carmustine, and etoposide with autologous bone marrow transplantation for relapsed Hodgkin's
    disease. J Clin Oncol 7: 179–185, 1989.
Reece DE et al. Intensive chemotherapy with cyclophosphamide, carmustine and etoposide followed
    by autologous bone marrow transplantation for relapsed Hodgkin's disease. J Clin Oncol 9:
    1871–1879, 1991.

ICE—IFOSFAMIDE-CARBOPLATIN-ETOPOSIDE

Ifosfamide. 4,000 mg/m^2/day intravenously on days −6, −5, −4, and −3.
Carboplatin. 600 mg/m^2/day intravenously on days −6, −5, and −4.
Etoposide. 500 mg/m^2/day intravenously on days −6, −5, and −4 in the morning.

*NOTE: Ifosfamide infusion is begun after morning etoposide. Mesna uroprotection is
essential. Bone marrow is infused on day 0. Etoposide phosphate is more soluble
than etoposide and may be substituted mg for mg.*

Selected Reading

Wilson WH et al. Phase I and II study of high-dose ifosfamide, carboplatin, and etoposide with autolo-
    gous bone marrow rescue in lymphomas and solid tumors, J Clin Oncol 10: 1712–1722, 1992.

CBVP—CYCLOPHOSPHAMIDE-CARMUSTINE-ETOPOSIDE-CISPLATIN

Cyclophosphamide. 1,800 mg/m^2/day intravenously on days −6, −5, −4, and −3.
Carmustine. 500 mg/m^2 intravenously on day −2.
Etoposide. 2,400 mg/m^2 continuous IV infusion for 34 hours beginning on day −7.
Cisplatin. 50 mg/m^2/day intravenously on days −7, −6, and −5.

*NOTE: Doses are calculated on the basis of the lower value of ideal or actual body
weight. Bone marrow is infused on day 0. Adequate hydration is essential before,*

during, and after therapy. Use of mesna should be considered for uroprotection. Etoposide phosphate is more soluble than etoposide and may be substituted mg for mg.

Selected Reading

Reece DE et al. Intensive therapy with cyclophosphamide, carmustine, etoposide 6 cisplatin, and autologous bone marrow transplantation for Hodgkin's disease in first relapse after combination chemotherapy. Blood 83: 1193–1199, 1994.

MULTIPLE MYELOMA

TBC—THIOTEPA-BUSULFAN-CYCLOPHOSPHAMIDE

Thiotepa. 250 mg/m^2/day intravenously on days –9, –8, and –7.
Busulfan. 1 mg/kg orally every 6 hours for 12 doses on days –6, –5, and –4.
Cyclophosphamide. 60 mg/kg/day intravenously on days –3 and –2.

NOTE: Mesna 250 mg/m^2 is given 30 minutes before and every 4 hours for six doses after each cyclophosphamide infusion. Bone marrow infusion is given on day 0 preceded by methylprednisolone 100 mg IV and diphenhydramine 50 mg IV. Now that intravenous busulfan is available, most institutions give 0.8 mg/kg busulfan intravenously over 2 hours in place of each 1 mg/kg of the previous oral dose.

Selected Reading

Dimopoulos MA et al. Thiotepa, busulfan, and cyclophosphamide: a new preparative regimen for autologous marrow or blood stem cell transplantation in high-risk multiple myeloma. Blood 82: 2324–2328, 1993.

DOUBLE-DOSE MELPHALAN AND SECOND TRANSPLANT

Melphalan. 100 mg/m^2/day intravenously on days –3 and –2.

NOTE: Both bone marrow and peripheral blood stem cells are infused on day 0. On day 11, start daily subcutaneous injections of GM-CSF 250 microg/m^2 until granulocyte counts are greater than 2,000/microL on 3 successive days. Many centers complete the therapy at this point. At the University of Arkansas, in some patients, three to six months later, a second autotransplant is given, usually using the same melphalan preparative regimen. However, for the second regimen, some patients were given total doses of busulfan 14 mg/kg and cyclophosphamide 120 mg/kg.

Selected Reading

Vesole DH et al. High-dose therapy for refractory multiple myeloma: improved prognosis with better supportive care and double transplants. Blood 84: 950–956, 1994.

GERM CELL TUMORS

PICE—PACLITAXEL-IFOSFAMIDE-CARBOPLATIN-ETOPOSIDE

Treatment on this protocol consisted of two cycles of paclitaxel plus ifosfamide given 14 days apart followed by three cycles of carboplatin and etoposide with PBSC support given at 14- to 21-day intervals. The authors summarize their treatment plan as follows:

Cycle 1:

target day 1:	*Paclitaxel* 200 mg/m^2 intravenously over 24 hours.
target days 2–4:	*Ifosfamide* 2,000 mg/m^2/day intravenously over 4 hours with mesna protection.
target days 11–13:	*Leukapheresis no. 1.*

Cycle 2:

target day 1:	*Paclitaxel* 200 mg/m^2/day intravenously over 24 hours.
target days 2–4:	*Ifosfamide* 2,000 mg/m^2/day intravenously over 4 hours with mesna protection.
target days 11–13:	*Leukapheresis no. 2* (if needed).

Cycles 3, 4, 5:

target days 1–3:	*Carboplatin* intravenously dosed to AUC (range 12 to 32 – see original article) divided over 3 days given by 1-hour bolus or 20-hour infusion.
	Etoposide 400 mg/m^2/day intravenously each of 3 days.
target day 5:	*Stem cell infusion.*

NOTE: This is a complex regimen and there is no substitute for intense study of the original article and extensive experience with this kind of therapy.

Selected Readings

Motzer RJ et al. Sequential dose-intensive paclitaxel, ifosfamide, carboplatin, and etoposide salvage therapy for germ cell tumor patients. J Clin Oncol 18: 1173–1180, 2000.

ASSESSMENT AND MANAGEMENT OF ORGAN SYSTEM TOXICITY

Systemic cancer therapy can produce a wide range of toxicity to normal cells. This chapter will review the most common side effects, and strategies to prevent, minimize, or manage treatment-related toxicity. Bone marrow suppression (anemia, neutropenia, thrombocytopenia) and gastrointestinal, dermatological, renal, pulmonary, cardiac, neurological, and gonadal toxicities will be discussed.

BONE MARROW SUPPRESSION

ANEMIA

The etiology of anemia in the cancer patient is multifactorial and includes blood loss, diminished or absent nutritional stores, marrow infiltration by tumor, cumulative marrow suppression associated with prior treatment, anemia of chronic disease, decreased erythropoietin production, and direct effects of cytotoxic drugs. The relationship between platinum-based therapies and the risk of anemia is strongly established, but other chemotherapy agents, such as altretamine, cytarabine, docetaxel (especially with higher doses), paclitaxel, and topotecan, are also associated with a higher risk for anemia. Symptoms associated with even mild to moderate anemia can negatively affect the person's energy level, functional ability, mood, and overall quality of life (Gillespie, 2002). Severe anemia is associated with greater functional deficits and an increase in distressful physical symptoms (e.g., dyspnea, dizziness, headaches, tachycardia). A thorough laboratory assessment with a complete blood count, including a reticulocyte count, serum ferritin, iron, total iron-binding capacity, vitamin B12, folate, Coombs' test and erythropoietin level, is recommended to identify the cause of the anemia (Preston & Cunningham, 1998). Laboratory values combined with the underlying cause of the anemia and the patient's symptom profile will enable the clinician to choose an appropriate therapy. Red blood cell transfusion or human recombinant erythropoietin are the treatment options.

The decision to transfuse should be based on the patient's symptoms in concert with laboratory data. Generally, transfusion support is indicated for an acute need, such as blood loss or symptom severity that warrants prompt intervention, or for those patients who have failed to respond to epoetin alfa. For the average adult, one RBC transfusion raises the hemoglobin by 1 g/dL and the hematocrit by 3% (Snyder, 1997). Subjective improvement in anemia-associated symptoms following transfusion generally occurs but not universally. Epoetin alfa is approved for the treatment of anemia associated with cancer chemotherapy for nonmyeloid malignancies (Chapter 5). Multiple studies have demonstrated that epoetin alfa increases hemoglobin, decreases symptoms, especially fatigue, increases functional ability, decreases the need for transfusion support, and improves quality of life (Cella & Bron, 1999; Gillespie, 2002) for patients on platinum- and nonplatinum-based therapies (Littlewood et al, 2001). The approved manufacturer's dosing recommendation is 150 units/kg three times per week, but studies have demonstrated that 40,000 units once weekly produce similar results, specifically increased hemoglobin levels, decreased transfusion requirements, and improvements in functional status, fatigue, and quality of life (Gabrilove et al, 2001). In addition, epoetin alfa has been reported to improve hemoglobin levels and quality of life in patients with cancer-related anemia not on chemotherapy (Quirt et al, 2001). Epoetin alfa is indicated for patients on chemotherapy with a hemoglobin less than 10 g/dL. Since not all patients will benefit, patients should be monitored and assessed at regular intervals for response and decisions to continue or discontinue epoetin alfa therapy. Reassessment at four weeks after initiation of therapy is recommended. If, at that time, the hemoglobin fails to rise more than 0.5 g/dL and the ferritin level is greater than 400 mg/ml, a response is unlikely. Some clinicians prefer to continue therapy for another four weeks with or without a dose increase. If the hemoglobin rise remains less than 1 g/dL, epoetin alfa therapy should be discontinued. Darbopoetin alfa is a new erythropoiesis-stimulating agent that differs somewhat biochemically from epoetin alfa although its action is similar. It is currently approved for the treatment of anemia in chronic renal failure and in patients with cancer. Trials in patients with cancer have reported similar response rates compared to epoetin alfa but with an added advantage of less frequent dosing, specifically every week or every two weeks (Glaspy et al, 2001).

NEUTROPENIA

The inverse relationship between the degree and duration of neutropenia and risk of infection reported by Bodey et al in 1966 has remained unchanged (Alexander & Pizzo, 1999). Neutropenia is defined as an absolute neutrophil count (ANC) less than 500 cells/mm^3 or a count of less than 1000 cells/mm^3 with a predicted decrease to 500 cells/mm^3 (Hughes et al, 2002). Patients with an ANC <100 cells/mm^3 or those with prolonged neutropenia (>7 days) are at significantly higher risk for serious infection (Rolston, 2000).

Afebrile Neutropenia

For afebrile neutropenic patients, the goal is to prevent infectious complications or detect infection at the earliest possible stage and promptly intervene. Assessment, prevention, and early detection are collaborative activities shared by healthcare providers, the patient, and the patient's family or support persons. Patient and family education should include an explanation of the function of white blood cells; meaning of nadir; instructions for temperature taking; signs and symptoms of infection (Box 11-1); hygiene practices emphasizing hand washing; identification and assessment of high-risk areas for infection; care of access devices; avoidance of exposure to persons with communicable or infectious illnesses; and specific directions for access to their healthcare system 24 hours a day, 7 days a week.

Interventions by healthcare providers to reduce the risk of infection in neutropenic patients have included prophylactic antibiotics and administration of colony-stimulating factors (CSFs). Current evidence does not support the routine use of CSFs in afebrile neutropenic patients unless the patient is at high risk, defined as ≥40% predicted febrile neutropenic risk based on the known chemotherapy regimen (Ozer et al, 2000). However, the use of CSFs may be indicated in special circumstances that are associated with an increased risk of febrile neutropenia because of bone marrow compromise or comorbidity. Examples include pre-existing disease-related neutropenia, previous radiation to large areas of bone marrow, recurrent febrile neutropenia with similar dose chemotherapy, extensive prior chemotherapy, or active tissue infection. The routine use of prophylactic antibiotics in patients with afebrile neutropenia is not recommended (Hughes et al, 2002). Two exceptions to this general guideline include administration of trimethoprim-sulfamethoxazole for immunosuppressed patients at risk for *P. carinii* pneumonitis, and antifungal (fluconazole) and antiviral

---

BOX 11-1

SIGNS AND SYMPTOMS OF INFECTION

INSTRUCT THE PATIENT AND FAMILY ABOUT THE FOLLOWING SIGNS AND SYMPTOMS OF INFECTION

- Temperature greater than 38°C (100.4°F)
- Chills
- Inflammation
- Rash
- Increased respiration
- General malaise
- Tenderness
- Swelling
- Headache
- Inability to bend head forward
- Urinary frequency with or without pain
- Cough with or without sputum

(acyclovir or gancyclovir) prophylaxis for patients under-going allogeneic stem cell transplant.

Fever and Neutropenia

Fever is defined as a single temperature greater than 101°F (38.3°C) or a persistent fever greater than or equal to 100.4°F (38.0°C) (Alexander & Pizzo, 1999). The development of fever in a neutropenic patient represents an urgent clinical problem requiring prompt assessment and intervention. More than half of all patients will not exhibit any other signs or symptoms of infection. Initial assessment should include a careful history and physical examination, complete blood count, chemistry profile (especially liver and renal function), urinalysis, and blood cultures. For patients with central venous access devices (VAD), two sets of blood cultures are recommended despite some controversy (Hughes et al, 2002; Mermel et al, 2001; Moran & Camp-Sorrell, 2002). One culture should be drawn peripherally and one from the device, unless there is an obvious port pocket infection in an unaccessed implanted VAD (Viale, 2002). Cultures of other sites and the need for a chest x-ray should be based on clinical suspicion and the patient's symptoms. Urgent care and emergency personnel in the patient's healthcare system must be well educated and fully under-stand the critical nature of febrile neutropenia in oncology patients. Prompt initiation of empiric antibiotic therapy is essential, but assessment of individual patient risk should be done prior to making the decision for antibiotics; specifically, is the patient low or high risk and is there an indication for gram-positive coverage (i.e., vancomycin) (Hughes et al, 2002). Low risk for severe infection is associated with but not limited to ANC >100 cells/mm^3, normal hepatic and renal function, normal chest x-ray, short duration of neutropenia, no comorbidities, no catheter-related infection, temperature <39°C, normotensive, and disease that is in partial or complete remission.

Choice of antibiotics is influenced by the ever changing environment, individual institution susceptibility patterns, emergence of resistant organisms, and the individual patient characteristics and risk. General guidelines based on current evidence, however, can guide empiric therapy in the cancer patient (Figure 11-1). Risk stratification should occur at the outset as well as 3–5 days after initiation of therapy. Assessment of risk helps determine subsequent antibiotic therapy and would be based on whether the fever has resolved, specific organisms identified by cultures, overall status of the patient, the

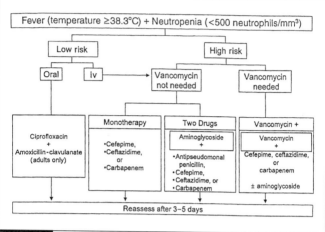

FIGURE 11-1

Algorithm for initial management of febrile neutropenia. (Used with permission. From Hughes, WT et al. 2002 guidelines for the use of antimicrobial agents in neutropenic patients with cancer. Clin Infect Dis 34:730–751, 2002.)

degree of neutropenia, and the projected duration of neutropenia. Use of antiviral agents is not recommended unless there is laboratory or clinical indication of viral disease. Although there is some renewed interest, the use of granulocyte transfusions remains experimental (Hughes et al, 2002). The use of CSFs is not recommended for the management of uncomplicated fever and neutropenia, defined as a fever lasting less than 10 days and the absence of pneumonia, cellulitis, abscess, sinusitis, hypotension, multiorgan dysfunction, invasive fungal infections, or advanced or progressive malignancy (Ozer et al, 2002). In contrast, CSFs are recommended as adjuncts for patients who undergo autologous or allogeneic peripheral blood stem cell transplantation.

Nonpharmacological Prevention and Management of Infection

Twenty years ago, Pizzo and Schimpff (1983) identified four general principles to prevent or minimize the risk of infection in the patient with cancer: bolstering the host defense mechanisms, preserving the body's natural barriers of defense, reducing environmental organisms, and minimizing the endogenous microflora of the patient as a source of infection. These general principles remain relevant today and provide the foundation for essential care practices that are adjunct to antimicrobial therapy but also make independent contributions to reducing infection risk and degree of infectious complications. Preserving the body's natural barriers of defense for the neutropenic patient includes maintaining the integrity of mechanical barriers (skin and mucous membranes) and supporting the integrity of the intestinal mucosa. Hand washing is a simple but critical intervention for healthcare providers, patients, and family members to reduce infection risk. In addition, it is recommended that nails be kept clean and short. Artificial nails of healthcare workers have been found to have a greater number of pathogens, especially gram-negative bacilli and yeasts, compared to workers with natural nails (Hedderwick et al, 2000) and they persist at much higher levels even after hand washing with antimicrobial soap or alcohol-based gel (McNeil et al, 2001). Therefore, the use of artificial nails by healthcare workers should be discouraged, especially for high-risk populations. Other interventions to promote mechanical barrier integrity include:

- avoidance of injections whenever possible
- strategies to prevent skin breakdown
- avoidance of bladder catheterization unless absolutely necessary (if necessary, intermittent catheterization is preferred over an indwelling catheter)
- perineal and rectal care guidelines (stress the importance of good personal hygiene, cleanliness, lubrication, and prevention of cross-contamination from sexual activity; avoid enemas, rectal thermometers, and rectal medications; prevent constipation with laxatives and stool softeners)
- daily baths
- cleansing of puncture sites with iodophor solution twice a day until healed
- oral care after meals and before bed or more frequently depending on level of risk.

Supporting the integrity of the intestinal mucosa and preventing infection also encompass the principle of minimizing the patient's endogenous flora as a source of infection. Despite many years of research with low microbial or "neutropenic" diets, there is little evidence demonstrating a reduction in morbidity or infectious complications, especially in low or moderate risk patients with neutropenia. For these patients, instruction on safe food handling is adequate. For patients at higher risk, such as dose-intense therapy or high-dose therapy with peripheral blood stem cell therapy (PBSCT), a low bacterial diet is prudent including restricting: raw or unpasteurized milk or milk products, raw or undercooked meats, fish, eggs, poultry, tofu, lox; aged cheese; hot chili pepper; cheese-based salad dressing; unwashed raw fruits and vegetables; unpasteurized fruit and vegetable juices; and unpasteurized beer or beer with raw uncooked brewer's yeast (Rust et al, 2000).

Interventions to reduce environmental organisms are applicable to the patient's home environment, but the risk of infection is greater in the hospital setting and is related to nosocomial infection and the number of personnel who are in contact with the patient. Suggested guidelines for care of the **hospitalized** neutropenic patient include the following:

- **Wash hands frequently and thoroughly;** this is the single most important measure in preventing infection. Use clean, disposable gloves with each patient.
- Place patient in a private room.
- Teach patients to avoid persons with viral or contagious illnesses; screen visitors for contagious diseases. Personnel who are ill, particularly with a respiratory or viral infection, should avoid direct patient care. Patients should avoid contact with persons recently vaccinated with live or attenuated virus vaccines.
- Do not allow stagnant water, fresh flowers, plants, humidifiers, or vaporizers in the patient's room; change water pitcher every day; avoid use of bar soap.
- Clean and disinfect equipment before patient contact and after each use with solution of one part bleach to nine parts water.
- Use a separate stethoscope for the patient and disinfect after each use.

THROMBOCYTOPENIA

Thrombocytopenia (platelet count of less than 100,000/mm^3) is reported as a potential or actual dose-limiting side effect for standard doses of carboplatin, dacarbazine, fluorouracil, lomustine, mitomycin, thiotepa, and trimetrexate.

Carmustine, fludarabine, lomustine, mitomycin, streptozocin, and thiotepa exhibit delayed-onset thrombocytopenia and have a cumulative dose effect. Increased risk of bleeding is the most significant outcome of a reduced platelet count. A moderate risk of bleeding exists when the platelet count falls to less than 50,000 cells/mm³, and major risk is associated with platelet counts less than 10,000 cells/mm³. Clotting and platelet disorders that are drug- or illness-related can contribute to serious bleeding problems. Several categories of drugs are known to influence platelet function, but of greatest concern are the anti-inflammatory drugs (aspirin and nonsteroidal anti-inflammatory drugs) and anticoagulants. It is also important to review with the patient any use of complementary or alternative therapies (CAM). These may independently interfere with platelet function or cause an additive and/or synergistic effect when combined with other drugs. As an example, ginko biloba is known to inhibit platelet-activating factor (Glisson et al, 1999). References to check CAM products should be readily available in all clinical settings. Careful assessment of the patient for potential signs and symptoms of bleeding is indicated. The skin, mucous membranes, and fundi are important areas to assess. Clinical manifestations include increased bruising, petechiae, purpura (most frequently found on lower extremities, in skin creases, and along scratch marks), oozing from mucosal surfaces, and hypermenorrhea. The stool, urine, and vomitus should be tested for blood in patients at high risk for bleeding. To prevent or minimize bleeding in patients with a moderate to severe risk, the following guidelines for practice are recommended. Intramuscular injections should be avoided unless there is absolutely no alternative. If given, pressure should be maintained on the site for at least five minutes to avoid hematoma formation.

- Avoid trauma.
- Decrease the patient's level of activity.
- Avoid drugs that alter platelet function or clotting.
- Monitor the platelet count regularly and anticipate nadir. Treatment should be modified according to the laboratory values, degree of risk, and patient symptoms.
- Surgical procedures, bone marrow biopsies, spinal taps, and parenteral injections are relatively contraindicated in the thrombocytopenic patient. Invasive procedures that are deemed essential should be done with trepidation, and platelet coverage should be planned ahead of time and availability confirmed. If a parenteral injection is necessary, a small-gauge needle should be used for intravenous or subcutaneous administration.
- Pressure should be applied for at least five minutes with a pressure bandage for all IV injections, venipunctures, and bone marrow procedures.
- Patients should avoid blowing their noses and sneezing. For shaving, an electric razor is recommended. Blood pressure should be taken only when necessary.

Any sites of actual bleeding that develop in a patient should be kept clean, and measures should be taken to encourage clot formation. Ice application, nasal packing, or topical epinephrine may be necessary to stop epistaxis. Absorbable gelatin sponge (Gelfoam) or liquid thrombin applied to the site may be helpful in controlling bleeding gums.

Management of Moderate to Severe Thrombocytopenia with Platelet Transfusions

Platelet transfusions can reduce or eliminate fatal consequences of bleeding in patients at high risk because of thrombocytopenia. The usual dose of platelets is 4 to 6 units of random donor platelets or 1 unit of single donor apheresis platelets. A rise in the platelet count of 5,000 to 10,000/microL can be expected from a transfusion of random donor platelets, assuming that there are no underlying factors that would influence platelet, survival. Post-transfusion platelet counts are recommended (Shiffer et al,

2001), especially when platelet refractoriness is suspected. To determine if the platelet increment is appropriate for the body size of the patient and the amount of platelets transfused, the following formula can be used (Snyder, 1997):

$$CCI = \frac{[\text{Post-transfusion platelet count}] - [\text{Pretransfusion platelet count}]}{\text{Total platelets transfused} \times 10^{-11}} \times BSA$$

Note: CCI, corrected count increment; platelet count is in micro/L; BSA, body surface area in m^2

Measured at 1 to 4 hours after a platelet transfusion, a CCI ≥ 7500 would indicate that platelets are surviving appropriately. Unfortunately, platelet transfusions are also associated with a wide range of negative side effects such as allergic transfusion reactions and alloimmunization. Thus, there must be prudent decisions regarding indications and use of platelet transfusions. The American Society of Clinical Oncology has proposed clinical practice guidelines for platelet transfusions (Schiffer et al, 2001) and stress that these recommendations are meant to guide practice and not to take the place of physician judgment related to individual patients (Table 11-1).

In an attempt to reduce or eliminate the need for platelet transfusions, a biological agent was explored. Interleukin-11 (Oprelvekin) was approved by the FDA in 1997 (see Chapter 5), and reduces the need for platelet transfusions. However, it is associated with a wide range of cardiopulmonary side effects and less serious, but

TABLE 11-1

SUMMARY HIGHLIGHTS OF ASCO'S CLINICAL PRACTICE GUIDELINES FOR PLATELET TRANSFUSIONS

Indication	Guideline
Platelet product	Use random donor pooled platelets unless histocompatible platelets are needed, then use single donor platelets.
Prophylactic platelet transfusion: acute leukemia and hematopoietic cell transplant	A threshold of 10,000/microL is recommended for asymptomatic patients. Transfusions at levels above this threshold are indicated for patients with complicating clinical conditions.
Prophylactic transfusions: solid tumors	A threshold of 20,000/microL is recommended for patients with bladder cancer receiving aggressive therapy and those with necrotic tumors. For all others, a threshold of 10,000/microL is recommended.
Surgical or invasive procedures	A platelet count of 40,000/microL to 50,000/microL is deemed sufficiently safe to perform invasive procedures in the absence of coagulation problems.
Prevention of alloimmunization with leukoreduced blood products	Recommended for patients with AML from time of diagnosis; consider for all other patients.

Data from: Shiffer CA, Anderson KC, Bennet CL, et al. Platelet transfusion for patients with cancer: clinical practice guidelines of the American Society of Clinical Oncology. J Clin Oncol, 19: 1519–1538, 2001.

predictable, conjunctival irritation (Rust, 1999). The side-effect profile has significantly limited enthusiasm for its routine use in clinical practice.

GASTROINTESTINAL TOXICITY

NAUSEA, VOMITING, AND ANTIEMETIC THERAPY

Clinical practice and patient outcomes have been dramatically influenced by advances in the understanding of the physiology of chemotherapy-induced nausea and vomiting, the role of serotonin in the process, and the development and clinical application of serotonin antagonists.

Nausea, vomiting, and retching are conceptually separate terms and it is important to define them in language that is understood by the patient and family for accurate assessment (Rhodes et al, 1995). Nausea is an unpleasant sensation that is difficult to describe, but the term usually refers to a vague uneasiness or discomfort located in the epigastrium, throat region, or diffusely throughout the abdomen. It is characterized by a revulsion to food and is commonly referred to as "feeling sick to your stomach." Mild nausea may be relieved by eating, but moderate to severe nausea may prevent normal food intake and interfere with an individual's ability to carry on normal activities. Retching is a rhythmic, spasmodic movement involving the chest, diaphragm, and abdominal muscles that occurs before vomiting or alternately with vomiting. Vomiting is the forceful expulsion of the contents of the stomach, duodenum, or proximal jejunum through the mouth or nose, accompanied by somatic changes. Vomiting can be objectively measured or assessed by self-report but nausea is usually subjectively reported. Quantitative measurements of subjective ratings of nausea and vomiting are needed to document the patient's response and for re-evaluation and management of subsequent treatments. Likert-type or visual analogue scales for assessment are user-friendly, quick to complete, and practical for clinical and home settings. Such scales help discriminate among symptoms and identify patterns, as well as capture the level of perceived symptom distress. Monitoring the patient's weight and nutritional intake provides additional clinical parameters to assess, especially for patients who are not fully protected against treatment-induced nausea and vomiting.

Patterns of Nausea and Vomiting

There are three patterns of nausea and vomiting associated with chemotherapy: acute, delayed, and anticipatory. Acute nausea and vomiting occurs within the first 24 hours of treatment. The incidence and severity of nausea and vomiting are related to the emetogenic potential of the drug (Table 11-2), dose, route of administration, schedule, infusion rate, time of day the drug is given, patient characteristics, and combination of drugs. Knowledge of the onset and duration of symptoms of individual drugs (Table 11-3) and patterns for combination drug therapy is also essential for planning appropriate antiemetic therapy.

Delayed nausea and vomiting is defined by timing, specifically, development of symptoms 24 hours after treatment. Delayed nausea and vomiting is associated with cisplatin and highly emetogenic noncisplatin therapy (e.g., cyclophosphamide, anthracyclines, carboplatin) and may last from one to seven days. Delayed or residual nausea and vomiting occurs even when antiemetics are effective in preventing acute symptoms within the first 24 hours. Persistent nausea is more common than vomiting after treatment. It is unclear if persistent nausea responds less well to antiemetic treatment or whether it is underassessed and undermanaged.

Anticipatory nausea and vomiting is the experiencing of one or both of these symptoms before receiving another chemotherapy treatment. It is a conditioned or learned

TABLE 11-2

EMETIC POTENTIAL OF CHEMOTHERAPY DRUGS AS SINGLE AGENTS

Very high (> 90%)	High (60–90%)	Moderate (30–60%)	Low (10–30%)
Carmustine*	Azacitidine	Altretamine	Cytarabine
Cisplatin	Carboplatin	Daunorubicin	Docetaxel
Cyclophosphamide*	Carmustine	Doxorubicin	Etoposide
Cytarabine*	Cyclophosphamide	Epirubicin	5-Fluorouracil
Mechlorethamine	Dacarbazine	Idarubicin	Gemcitabine
Melphalan*	Dactinomycin	Ifosfamide	Irinotecan
Streptozocin	Lomustine	Mitomycin	Paclitaxel
		Mitoxantrone	Thiotepa
		Oxaliplatin	Topotecan
		Plicamycin	
		Procarbazine	

*High dose.

TABLE 11-3

EMETIC DURATION POTENTIAL OF ANTINEOPLASTIC AGENTS

Agent	Onset emesis (hr)	Duration emesis (hr)
Bleomycin	3–6	1–4
Carboplatin	1–6	6–24
Carmustine*	2–4	4–12
Cisplatin*	1–4	12–20
Cyclophosphamide*	4–8	4–36
Cytarabine high dose	1–3	3–8
Cytarabine standard dose	6–12	3–5
Dacarbazine	1–6	6–24
Dactinomycin	2–5	4–24
Daunorubicin	1–3	4–24
Docetaxel	4–8	1–2
Doxorubicin	1–3	4–24
Etoposide	3–8	1–4
Ifosfamide	2–3	4–24
Irinotecan	2–6	6–12
Lomustine	3–6	6–12
Mechlorethamine	0.5–2	2–24
Methotrexate*	4–12	3–12
Mitomycin	1–2	3–4
Mitoxantrone	2–6	6–24
Paclitaxel	4–8	1–2
Procarbazine	24–27	Varies
Streptozocin	2–6	12–24

*Dose-related; potential for emesis increases with higher doses. Modified from: ASHP. ASHP therapeutic guidelines on the pharmacologic management of nausea and vomiting in adult and pediatric patients receiving chemotherapy or radiation therapy or undergoing surgery. Am J Health Syst Pharm 56: 729–764, 1999.

response to previous effects from therapy and associated environmental stimuli. Approximately 20% to 65% of patients will develop anticipatory symptoms, with nausea occurring much more commonly (24% to 65%) than vomiting (9% to 18%) (Coons et al, 1987; Morrow, 1984; Nerenz et al, 1986). Factors associated with anticipatory nausea and vomiting are moderate to severe postchemotherapy nausea and vomiting, increased anxiety levels, history of motion sickness, increased number of chemotherapy courses, and younger age (Eckert, 2001). Precipitating environmental factors include odors such as rubbing alcohol, certain substances and colors referable to particular cytotoxic drugs, personnel involved in drug administration, tastes, the drive to the office or hospital, anxiety about the potential success of venipuncture, and the actual physical treatment setting.

Pharmacological Therapy

General principles for successful antiemetic therapy for chemotherapy-induced nausea and vomiting include:

- aggressive therapy for chemotherapy-naïve patients
- adequate duration of coverage with antiemetics for the predicted risk period of symptoms
- appropriate selection of agents and dosing according to the emetic potential of the chemotherapy
- consideration of nonpharmacological therapy such as distraction, meditation, or relaxation.

Management of nausea and vomiting is dependent on knowledge of the underlying physiological processes, emetogenic potential of the drug (Table 11-2), the onset and duration of nausea and vomiting of chemotherapy drugs (Table 11-3), the pharmacology and the spectrum of activity of the antiemetic drugs (Table 11-4) and the use of adjunct drugs.

Therapy to prevent acute nausea and vomiting should be chosen based on emetogenic risk of the chemotherapy. For highly and moderately emetogenic chemotherapy, a serotonin antagonist with dexamethasone is recommended (Box 11-2). The serotonin antagonists provide complete responses in 40–60% of patients and the addition of dexamethasone increases that response rate another 20–30%. The efficacy and side-effect profile of the serotonin antagonists are similar, and appropriate oral dosing produces equivalent responses to intravenous dosing (Bender et al, 2002). Because the efficacy of the serotonin antagonists is similar, it is recommended that the choice of which agent to use should be based on acquisition cost (Gralla et al, 1999). Oral dosing is less costly (nursing time and drug cost) than intravenous dosing and practice guidelines assist in cost effectiveness (Engstrom et al, 1999; Goldsmith & Wodinsky, 1999). However, choosing which drug and which route must include an evaluation of the potential financial burden to the patient, based on cost and reimbursement practices, as well as implications for the practice setting.

For moderately emetogenic therapy (30% to 60% risk) a serotonin antagonist with dexamethasone is also recommended (ASHP, 1999). For low-risk emetogenic chemotherapy, dexamethasone, metoclopromide, or prochlorperazine are recommended (Box 11-2). There are other antiemetics available (e.g., butyrophenones and the cannabinoids) but they are of low therapeutic efficacy and are not indicated as first-line therapy (Gralla et al, 1999).

Breakthrough emesis, that is, nausea or vomiting despite optimal prophylactic pretreatment and/or delayed therapy, is an unfortunate reality that may occur in nearly a third or quarter of patients treated. Although there is little evidence to guide

TABLE 11-4
ACTIONS OF ANTIEMETICS

Drug type	Mechanism of action	Type of nausea controlled
Antihistamines	Act in neural pathways originating in the labyrinth	Motion sickness, Meniere's syndrome, vestibular sensitivity from narcotics, pregnancy-induced nausea, some postanesthetic vomiting
Benzodiazepines	Act centrally by depressing cerebral cortex or vomiting center	Nausea and vomiting with anxiety component, pregnancy-induced nausea, and postanesthetic vomiting
Anticholinergic drugs	Depress conduction in the vestibular cerebellar pathways and decrease excitability of labyrinth receptors	Little antiemetic activity, but scopolamine is of some value in motion sickness
Dopamine inhibitors, phenothiazines, butyrophenones	Reduce the effect of dopamine in the CTZ and in high doses may suppress the vomiting itself; potent inhibitor of the CTZ by blocking synaptic transmission of dopamine	All types of nausea and vomiting, excluding motion sickness. Suggested activity with some chemotherapy-induced vomiting
Cannabinoids	Unknown Cerebral cortex?	Some activity with low emetogenic chemotherapy
Corticosteroids	Unknown Inhibition of enkephalins? Inhibition of prostaglandins?	Effective alone and in combination with other antiemetic drugs
Metoclopramide	Same as phenothiazines; also a 5-HT_3 inhibitor; may inhibit GI-induced nausea and vomiting	Most effective in prevention of delayed nausea/vomiting; for acute prevention, effective for moderate/low emetogenic drugs
Serotonin antagonists	Binds to type 3 serotonin receptor 5-HT_3	Most effective for acute nausea and vomiting
NK-1 receptor antagonists	Antagonist of substance P at NK-1 receptor site	Appears most effective in preventing delayed nausea/vomiting; may enhance prevention of acute emesis

CTZ, Chemoreceptor trigger zone; 5-HT_3, 5-hydroxytryptamine, type 3; GI, gastrointestinal.

management of breakthrough symptoms, it is recommended that an agent from another pharmacological class be added and antiemetic doses should be evaluated to insure that the patient has/will receive the maximum effective dose (ASHP, 1999). Agents used for breakthrough include chlorpromazine, prochlorperazine, methylprednisolone, lorazepam, metoclopramide, dexamethasone, and haloperidol (ASHP, 1999). Droperidol is no longer recommended for routine use because of serious QTc

---

> **BOX 11-2**
>
> ## PREVENTION OF ACUTE NAUSEA AND VOMITING
>
> ##### HIGH TO MODERATE EMETIC POTENTIAL (30% TO >90%)
> Recommendation: Serotonin (5HT$_3$) antagonist and corticosteroid
>
> ##### SEROTONIN (5HT$_3$) ANTAGONISTS
>
> | | |
> |---|---|
> | Dolesetron (Anzemet®) | 100 mg IV or PO |
> | Granisetron (Kytril®) | 1 mg IV or 2 mg PO |
> | Ondansetron (Zofran®) | 8 mg IV or 16 mg PO |
>
> ##### CORTICOSTEROID
>
> | | |
> |---|---|
> | Dexamethasone (Decadron®) | 20 mg IV |
> | Methylprednisolone (Medrol®) | 40–125 mg IV |
>
> ##### LOW EMETOGENIC POTENTIAL (10% TO 30%)
> Recommendation: Corticosteroid, metoclopramide or prochlorperazine, or combination of corticosteroid and antiemetic
>
> ##### CORTICOSTEROID
>
> | | |
> |---|---|
> | Dexamethasone (Decadron®) | 8–20 mg IV or PO |
>
> ##### ANTIEMETIC DRUG
>
> | | |
> |---|---|
> | Metoclopramide (Reglan®) | 20–40 mg IV or PO |
> | Prochlorperazine (Compazine®) | 10–20 mg IV or PO |

prolongation (YNHH, 2002). In addition, to further reduce the risk of breakthrough emesis or delayed emesis, new combinations need to be explored such as a serotonin antagonist, prochlorperazine, and dexamethasone, which provided a complete response in 84% of patients who received high-dose cisplatin therapy (Hesketh et al, 1997).

Highly emetogenic chemotherapy is associated with delayed symptomatology, and treatment beginning on day 2 and extending for 3 to 4 days is recommended (Box 11-3). An exception to that recommendation may be cisplatin. Delayed emesis associated with cisplatin may actually begin some 16 hours after therapy (ASHP, 1999) and antiemetic coverage before or at this time should be strongly considered with a non-serotonin antagonist. Pharmacological data suggest that initiation of a delayed regimen at 24 hours (day 2) for nonplatinum regimens is appropriate. However, patients should be carefully assessed for symptoms between day 1 and 2 to determine the most appropriate delayed regimen for subsequent cycles. A delayed regimen should also be prescribed for patients who develop residual symptoms, which may occur after several cycles of drugs or with lower emetogenic chemotherapy. Prochlorperazine, metoclopramide, a serotonin antagonist, dexamethasone, or the combination of any one of those antiemetics with dexamethasone have been reported as delayed regimens. Dexamethasone is clearly effective in the prevention of delayed symptoms (Ioannidis et al, 2000). Short duration use of dexamethasone is not associated with adrenal insufficiency but patients at higher risk for hyperglycemia should be monitored (Gralla et al, 1999). The combination of a corticosteroid and an antiemetic is superior to either alone. The pathophysiology of delayed emesis is unknown but appears to be mediated by serotonin-independent mechanisms. The serotonin antagonists have been very successful in preventing acute emesis, but evidence to support their ability to prevent delayed symptoms is mixed with reported superiority to placebo but equal or less efficacy compared to dopamine antagonists. These data support the use of antiemetic drugs with different mechanisms of action for prevention of delayed

---

BOX 11-3

REGIMENS FOR PREVENTING DELAYED NAUSEA AND VOMITING

HIGHLY EMETOGENIC CHEMOTHERAPY

Recommendation: Corticosteroid plus metoclopramide or corticosteroid plus 5HT$_3$
  antagonist*

Dexamethasone (Decadron®)	8 mg bid days 1–2; 4 mg bid days 3–4**
Metoclopramide (Reglan®)	20–40 mg tid-qid days 1–4
Prochlorperazine (Compazine®)	10 mg bid days 1–4
5HT$_3$ antagonists:	
Ondansetron (Zofran®)	8 mg bid-tid days 1–4

MODERATELY EMETOGENIC CHEMOTHERAPY

Recommendation: Corticosteroid plus metoclopramide or corticosteroid plus 5HT$_3$
  antagonist*

Dexamethasone (Decadron®)	4–8 mg bid days 1–2
Metoclopramide (Reglan®)	20–40 mg bid-qid days 1–2
Prochlorperazine (Compazine®)	10 mg bid days 1–2
5HT$_3$ antagonist	
Ondansetron(Zofran®)	8 mg bid day 1–2

LOW EMETOGENIC CHEMOTHERAPY

Recommendation: No delayed therapy

*Evidence for efficacy for delayed nausea and vomiting with the combination prochlorperazine and
dexamethasone is weak (ASHP, 1999).

**Some clinicians prefer to taper dexamethasone over days 2–4.

11

GASTROINTESTINAL TOXICITY

symptoms, such as metoclopramide or prochlorperazine, although there is less strong
evidence to recommend the phenothiazines (ASHP, 1999). A corticosteroid is
recommended as first-line therapy and a combination of a corticosteroid and
antiemetic is superior for highly and moderately emetogenic chemotherapy. The lower
cost of metoclopramide combined with similar efficacy favors this combination over
the serotonin antagonists (Gralla et al, 1999).

A new class of agents, neurokinin-1 (NK-1) antagonists, are now in phase III trials
(Rittenberg, 2001). Substance P is found in the gastrointestinal tract and vagal nerves
and is thought to play a role in emesis. Antagonists to substance P act selectively at
the NK-1 receptor. Animal data suggested this hypothesis to be true and activity has
been confirmed with the NK-1 antagonist, MK-869, in four trials in patients on
chemotherapy (Campos et al, 2001; Cocquyt et al, 2001; Navari et al, 1999; Van
Belle et al, 2002). The following conclusions can be drawn from these studies:

- MK-869 as monotherapy with/without dexamethasone is less effective than
  serotonin antagonists/dexamethasone combination for acute nausea and
  vomiting.
- MK-869 appears to enhance the response rate (complete protection) of the
  combination of a corticosteroid and serotonin antagonist.
- For prevention of delayed nausea and vomiting, MK-869 provided superior
  protection compared to placebo.

This new class of antiemetic agents offers hope to the challenge of managing nausea
and vomiting, especially delayed symptoms.

Adjuncts to antiemetic regimens have commonly included a benzodiazepine and an antihistamine. While neither has any antiemetic activity, other properties have determined them to be somewhat useful in selected patients. The benzodiazepine drugs vary somewhat in their pharmacological spectrum, but as a class they are effective as a sedative, hypnotic, anxiolytic drug, muscle relaxant, and preanesthetic. Lorazepam is the most commonly prescribed drug for its sedative and antianxiety effects and its ability to reduce extrapyramidal reactions. Prior to the approval of serotonin antagonists, high doses of metoclopramide were commonly used and there was a need to manage potential and actual extrapyramidal effects. Today, there is little need for this except perhaps in younger patients on the phenothiazines. Thus, there is currently little or no indication to use antihistamines in antiemetic regimens, but the role of lorazepam to reduce anxiety remains an important adjunct for selected patients.

Anticipatory nausea and vomiting are strongly associated with post-treatment emesis, and therefore adequate control of acute post-treatment nausea and vomiting is critical. Once anticipatory symptoms develop, combining drugs with amnesic and antianxiety properties, such as lorazepam, might be useful. Behavioral treatment using progressive muscle relaxation and guided imagery instituted before chemotherapy can reduce anxiety levels and may have a role in reducing, or preventing these conditioned responses (Eckert, 2001).

Nonpharmacological Approaches to Nausea and Vomiting

Despite research efforts and advances in antiemetic therapy, drug therapy has failed to effectively control chemotherapy-induced nausea and vomiting in some patients. Many alternative approaches to drug therapy have been explored, including massage, distraction with music or art, and behavioral therapy (e.g., hypnosis, progressive muscle relaxation, biofeedback, systemic desensitization). It is hoped that continued research in this area will define the future role and benefit of behavioral treatment for chemotherapy-induced nausea and vomiting.

ANOREXIA AND TASTE CHANGES

Anorexia is simply the loss of appetite, although patients often may describe it in much stronger statements, such as "I can't stand the thought of food." Anorexia is the major cause of decreased dietary intake, and many factors contribute to this common patient symptom (Figure 11-2). The duration of anorexia in a patient depends on the underlying cause. Transient anorexia is commonly associated with emotional distress, such as the initial diagnosis or diagnosis of a recurrence. This short-term anorexia is less likely to affect the patient's nutritional status as significantly as the anorexia associated with treatment or advanced disease, which is often chronic.

Changes in taste sensation and aversions to certain foods and food odors contribute to a decreased appetite in the cancer patient. Taste abnormalities include increased and decreased thresholds to sweet, sour, salty, and bitter tastes; a general loss of taste for food; metallic taste after drug therapy; and aversions to specific foods or liquids. For patients who experience a loss of sense of taste, a variety of simple interventions can be helpful such as sucking on sour candies, using aroma to improve appeal of food, use of plastic utensils if food tastes metallic, and chewing sugar-free gum (Grant & Kravits, 2000; Sherry, 2002). Interventions for anorexia include pharmacological (e.g., steroids, megestrol) and nonpharmacological approaches, specifically dietary counseling, symptom management, psychosocial support, and nutritional support. The importance of eating despite anorexia

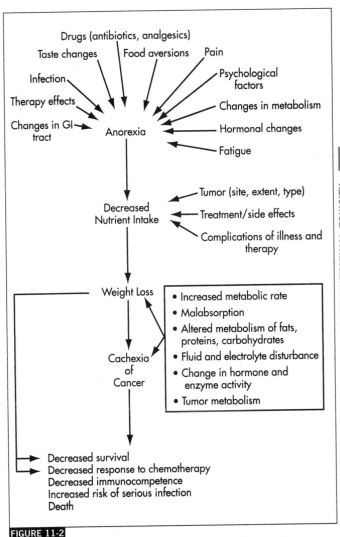

FIGURE 11-2

Factors contributing to malnutrition in the cancer patient. GI, Gastrointestinal.

should be emphasized, with food intake identified as a component of the treatment plan. Persuasion should never be used, nor should anger be shown with the patient for not eating. Approaches often need to be discussed and reinforced with the family members.

ORAL MUCOSITIS

Oral mucositis is estimated to occur in approximately 40% of patients who receive standard-dose chemotherapy and in some 60–70% of patients treated for hematological malignancies. High-dose therapy with/without stem cell transplantation, new drugs, and curative radiation approaches have prompted renewed interest in prevention and management of oral mucositis over the past five years (Berger & Eilers, 1998; Kostler et al, 2001; Larson et al, 1998; Miller & Kearney, 2001; Wilkes, 1998; Wojtaszek, 2000). Interest in gaining a better biological understanding of the process to explain clinical variability and design more targeted interventions has led to a new hypothesis for the development and resolution of mucositis. A four-phase model has been proposed (Peterson, 1999; Sonis, 1998).

Inflammatory/Vascular Phase

Cytokines are released, which cause local tissue damage and initiate an inflammatory response that results in increased vascularity.

Epithelial Phase

Well-known effect of drugs on rapidly dividing oral epithelial cells, resulting in reduced renewal, atrophy, and ulceration. It is thought that the locally produced cytokines enhance the tissue destruction, leading to the atrophic and ulcerative changes.

Ulcerative/Bacterial Phase

Typically occurs 7–10 days after chemotherapy and usually concurrent with neutropenia. Tissue erosion occurs and secondary bacterial colonization which likely leads to further cytokine release and further local tissue injury.

Healing Phase

Resolution of neutropenia, epithelial renewal and proliferation, and local microbial flora is re-established.

Risk factors for the development of oral mucositis include poor oral hygiene, poorly fitting dental appliances, nutritional status, type of malignancy, specific chemotherapy drugs, pre-existing oral conditions (e.g., periodontal disease, dental caries), smoking, and alcohol consumption. Routine dental hygiene procedures are recommended before chemotherapy, and dental work should be performed for existing problems such as periodontal disease, extensive dental caries, or defective dental restorations. The cell-cycle-specific agents are more likely to produce this toxicity, with antibiotics and antimetabolites as major offenders. The drugs most frequently associated with mucositis are dactinomycin, daunorubicin, docetaxel, paclitaxel, doxorubicin, 5-fluorouracil, methotrexate, raltitrexed, and with high-dose therapy using busulfan, etoposide, melphalan, and thiotepa. The occurrence and severity of mucositis are influenced by dose, schedule of drugs, combination drug therapy, and impairment of renal and hepatic function.

Prevention and Treatment

The goal of oral care for the patient at risk or with mucositis is to maintain the integrity of the oral mucosa, prevent secondary infection, provide pain relief, and maintain dietary intake. Assessment of the oral mucosa is a critical component before, during, and after therapy. Consistency of how assessments are performed, the criteria used, and documentation is more important than which assessment tool is used. However, it is strongly recommended that providers in each clinical site choose an assessment method or tool in order to provide continuity of assessments (Miller & Kearney, 2001).

Dental hygiene practices and instructions for oral self-examination with a mirror should be reviewed with each patient. Preventive oral care should begin at the start of treatment in an attempt to prevent or minimize oral complications, which can result in costly hospitalizations, pain, and compromised nutrition (Wilkes, 1998). The toothbrush is the most effective instrument for mechanical cleansing and plaque removal. Brushing is recommended after meals and before bed, with a nonirritating fluoride toothpaste (Miller & Kearney, 2001). For proper brushing, the toothbrush is held at a 45-degree angle at the junction of the tooth and gum. With a back-and-forth motion, ten strokes are used for each two teeth. If the patient has dental prostheses, they should be brushed and placed in water until rinsing and cleansing of the oral cavity is completed. A foam toothbrush can be substituted for a toothbrush during the ulcerative phase or if the patient is symptomatically thrombocytopenic.

Rinsing and flossing provide additional cleansing activity and aid in removal of food particles. Commercial mouthwashes are generally contraindicated because of the alcohol content and subsequent drying effect on the oral mucosa. The alcohol content of some common mouthwashes ranges from 9% to 27%. Patient education should include reminding patients and family members to check labels for content. Sodium chloride 0.9% solution, which is isotonic, nonirritating, and inexpensive, is preferred. Unwaxed dental floss should be wrapped around the side of the tooth and carefully brought into the space between the tooth and gum with a gentle up-and-down motion three or four times. Flossing straight up and down should be avoided since that will injure the gum and is relatively contraindicated in patients with severe mucositis, neutropenia, and thrombocytopenia.

Performance of routine systematic oral care is a primary intervention and its value in preventing and minimizing the incidence and severity of oral mucositis and oral complications **cannot be overemphasized** (Kostler et al, 2001; Larson et al, 1998; Miller & Kearney, 2001; Wojtaszek, 2000). Patients at risk for mucositis should perform oral care after meals and before bedtime. For those with evidence of mucositis, oral care is recommended every 2 hours, and **every hour** for patients with severe mucositis, on oxygen therapy, and those with oral infections (Miller & Kearney, 2001). In addition to meticulous oral care, a wide variety of agents (topical and systemic) have been investigated in attempts to prevent or manage oral mucositis (Table 11-5). Many agents have no research-based data supporting their use despite widespread clinical use. Yet, there are data demonstrating efficacy for other agents (e.g., cryotherapy for 5-fluorouracil) that fail to be implemented routinely in practice.

DIARRHEA

Diarrhea in cancer patients may be related to a number of causes, such as anxiety, a change in diet, medication, infection, radiation, tumor, obstruction, and chemotherapy. The GI tract is susceptible to chemotherapy toxicity because of the rapid turnover of the mucosal cells, particularly with cell-cycle-specific agents. Diarrhea has been observed in as many as 75% of patients who receive chemotherapy. The agents most commonly associated with diarrhea are capecitabine, cytarabine, dactinomycin, 5-azacitidine, 5-fluorouracil (especially in high dose or in combination with leucovorin or oxaliplatin), hydroxyurea, irinotecan, methotrexate, mitotane, raltitrexed (Tomudex), and topotecan. For pharmacological management, loperamide is often the treatment of choice, starting at 4 mg for the first dose, followed by 2 mg after each loose stool, up to 12 mg or more per day (Mercadante, 2002). Despite initial pharmacological

TABLE 11-5

REVIEW OF INTERVENTIONS FOR PREVENTION AND MANAGEMENT OF ORAL MUCOSITIS*

Therapy	Evidence/comments
Oral Protectants	
Routine oral hygiene	Effective in reducing incidence and severity
Cryotherapy	Effective – consistent results across studies (5FU).
Allopurinol	+/– study results; overall deemed not effective
Leucovorin	Negative study results
Glutamine	+/– study results; further research warranted
Vitamin E	Suggested benefit; further research warranted
Mouthwashes	
Saline	Isotonic, nonirritating, inexpensive; effective
Sodium bicarbonate	Good cleanser for debris; unpleasant taste
Chlorhexidine	+/– study results; data do not support routine use
Hydrogen peroxide	Not recommended
Multiagent antibacterial washes	Modest reduction in mucositis; as prophylaxis, recommended only for patients at high risk
Mouth Coating Agents	
Sucralfate	+/– study results; data not consistently supportive
Kaopectate	Clinical evidence only
Magnesium hydroxide	Short-term clinical effect; will dry out mucosa if not fully rinsed out
Multiagent mixtures (coating plus analgesics)	Lack of research base to support efficacy
Antiviral Prophylaxis	
Acyclovir	No impact on incidence or severity
Antifungal Prophlaxis	
Clotrimazole	Effective
Fluconazole	Effective
Multiagent amphotericin B rinse	+/– but not recommended due to side-effect profile
Anti-inflammatory	
Chamomile, betamethasone, benzydamine	No trials in chemotherapy; only tested in radiation
Local Anesthetics	
Xylocaine 2% viscous, dyclonine hydrocholride, ulcerase	Short term relief (20 minutes–1 hour); clinical evidence
Saliva Substitutes/Stimulants	Provide comfort; do not have antibacterial properties of normal saliva

*Data from: Kostler WJ et al. Oral mucositis complicating chemotherapy and/or radiotherapy: options for prevention and treatment. CA Cancer J Clin 51: 290–315, 2001. Miller M & Kearney N. Oral care for patients with cancer. Can Nurs 24: 241–254, 2001. Wilkes JD. Prevention and treatment of oral mucositis following chemotherapy. Semin Oncol 25: 538–551, 1998. Wojtaszek C. Management of chemotherapy-induced stomatitis. Clin J Oncol Nurs 4: 263–270, 2000.

management, some patients may report prolonged or severe diarrhea. Persistent diarrhea requires intervention to minimize complications of dehydration, electrolyte imbalance, weakness, decreased caloric intake, and weight loss. For refractory diarrhea related to chemotherapy or graft-versus-host disease (GVHD), octreotide has been successful (Mercadante, 2002).

Nonpharmacological supportive care recommendations include: eat a low-residue diet high in protein and calories; eliminate irritating or stimulating foods and beverages (e.g., whole-grain products, fried or greasy foods, fresh fruits, vegetables, products containing caffeine, and citrus juices); eat foods and drink liquids high in potassium (e.g., baked potato, asparagus, bananas, Gatorade, and Kool-aid); drink at least 3,000 mL of noncarbonated fluid each day (bouillon, apple or grape juice, noncarbonated beverages, and Gatorade); avoid cola drinks (Weizman, 1986); eat small, frequent meals; avoid extremes in food temperature; and avoid milk and milk products; restart milk intake slowly after symptoms subside. For comfort, suggest that the patient use local heat to abdomen to minimize discomfort caused by cramping; rest to conserve energy; take a warm-water sitz bath; and consider topical applications of an anesthetic or ointment on the rectal area to enhance comfort and promote healing (e.g., Tucks®, Desitin®, Benzocaine®, A+D ointment®).

CONSTIPATION

Constipation is defined as the infrequent, difficult passage of hard, dry stool. Symptoms include excessive straining, sensation of incomplete evacuation, abdominal cramping, discomfort with or without distention, and a feeling of fullness or pressure in the rectum. Prevention is the major therapeutic goal. Assessment should include a dietary history, age, usual elimination patterns, history of bowel alterations and management, mobility, and drugs. Decreased mobility, older age, diuretics, anticholinergics, phenothiazines, antidepressants, iron preparations, laxative abuse, low-fiber diet, depressed mood, ignoring of the body's signal to defecate, opioids, and hemorrhoids are potential causes of constipation. High-risk factors for the patient with cancer include opioids, immobility, older age, decreased oral intake, metabolic abnormalities (hypercalcemia, hypokalemia, hypomagnesemia), and chemotherapy with vinca alkaloids. Opioid analgesics predictably produce constipation, and the effect is dose-related.

Dietary changes and a bulk laxative are usually insufficient, and a prophylactic bowel program is needed for any patient receiving narcotic medication (Mercadante, 2002). The senna compounds, anthraquinone cathartics that stimulate the longitudinal peristalsis in the colon, have been shown to regularly prevent or reverse opioid-induced constipation. Senokot® dosing varies from one to two tablets every day up to four tablets twice daily. For patients who need a stool softener, Senokot-S® includes the standardized senna concentrate and a stool softener, dioctyl sodium sulfosuccinate. Although there is great individual variety, the general goal should be a bowel movement every 2 to 3 days. If no bowel movement occurs after that time, a more aggressive approach is indicated, such as saline laxatives, sorbitol, lactulose, or suppositories (Hawkins, 2000), with careful monitoring for potential impaction. Protecting the integrity of the rectal mucosa of the patient who is leukopenic or thrombocytopenic is a priority, and a prophylactic bowel regimen is essential to prevent the need for suppositories or enemas, which are contraindicated in this patient population.

Nonpharmacological guidelines for prevention and management of constipation include the following (Gross, 1998): increase fiber in the diet (e.g., vegetables, fruits, nuts, raisins, and bran); add prunes or prune juice to the diet; drink adequate amounts of fluid daily – at least eight glasses; engage in light exercise; plan a regular time every day, about 20 minutes, to sit on the toilet or commode, uninterrupted, in an attempt to defecate; drink hot liquids that may stimulate bowel activity; use bulk producers (Metamucil®, Mitrolan®), a stool softener, or both; and consider laxative use for patients who do not respond to these measures.

DERMATOLOGICAL TOXICITY

Antineoplastic therapy can produce both local and systemic dermatological toxicities. Local toxicity occurs in the tissues surrounding the site of drug administration and is described by a variety of venous and cutaneous responses: phlebitis, urticaria, pain, erythema, vein discoloration, and tissue necrosis secondary to extravasation of a drug.

Systemically, hair loss is the most common manifestation, but erythematous rashes, pruritus, dermatitis, and hyperpigmentation are reported with chemotherapy toxicity. Although most cutaneous reactions are short-lived and associated with minimal physical morbidity, nurses and physicians must be alert to potential reactions, keep the patient informed, institute prompt interventions, and continually assess for potential psychological morbidity associated with alterations in body image.

ALOPECIA

The actual experience of complete or nearly complete hair loss has often been described by patients as the most devastating side effect of chemotherapy. Hair is an integral part of physical appearance, and its loss may negatively affect self-image, body image, coping skills, and social interactions (McGarvey et al, 2001). The degree of distress may be minimized by adequate preparation for the loss, possible interventions, and ongoing support from healthcare professionals and family members.

Hair loss from chemotherapy is reversible. Many times hair begins to regrow despite continued therapy, and it is not unusual for new hair to reappear two to three months later. Hair growth during treatment can be explained by a certain percentage of the hair being in the telogen or resting phase when the initial insult from chemotherapy was received. Drugs mainly affect growing hairs (anagen phase), which accounts for 85% of the hair follicles on the human scalp (Paus & Cotsarelis, 1999). Since the anagen phase is approximately three months for scalp hair, it is common not to see hair regrowth for three to five months.

Chemotherapeutic agents most frequently associated with hair loss are cyclophosphamide, doxorubicin, dactinomycin, daunorubicin, docetaxel, etoposide, idarubicin, ifosfamide, irinotecan, mechlorethamine, paclitaxel, topotecan, and vincristine. Drugs described as less frequently associated because of a lower incidence and/or a lesser degree of alopecia include bleomycin, carmustine, epirubicin, 5-fluorouracil, methotrexate, melphalan, mitomycin, mitoxantrone, teniposide, and vinorelbine. High-dose alkylating-agent therapy is also associated with a very predictable complete hair loss risk.

Nurses, physicians, and pharmacists should make every effort to provide accurate information and support to patients at risk for hair loss. Patients are shocked when they experience hair loss unexpectedly, and the purchase of a wig or head covering before loss of more than 50% of hair occurs, may decrease the distress. Interventions to help maximize patient adjustment and minimize the distress associated with hair loss include the following:

- explain to the patient the rationale for the occurrence of alopecia, the relative incidence, and the degree of hair loss expected specific to the chemotherapy drug(s) prescribed

- encourage the patient to express emotions regarding the information provided
- reiterate the fact that hair regrows and that changes in color or texture may occur (e.g., curly or gray)
- discourage the use of dryers, hot rollers, and curling irons, since they may facilitate increased hair loss
- protect the head from the sun with a hat or sunscreen for complete or nearly complete alopecia
- maintain scalp cleanliness and conditioning after total alopecia
- suggest the use of wigs, colorful scarves, and hats.

Every attempt should be made to provide culturally appropriate recommendations. Explore insurance coverage for the use of wigs as prosthetic devices for the head; encourage purchasing wigs before total hair loss occurs and provide information about supportive programs such as the "Look Good, Feel Better Program."

DRUGS WITH POTENTIAL FOR LOCAL TISSUE TOXICITY

Potential local toxic effects from chemotherapeutic drugs range from transient local discomfort during administration to severe tissue necrosis with potential damage to tendons and nerves. Chemotherapeutic drugs have been described as irritants, vesicants, and those associated with acute local reactions such as erythema, phlebitis, urticaria, and pain. An irritant is a drug that often produces a local venous response with or without a skin reaction. Complaints of tenderness along the vein and burning are common and may be accompanied by erythema. These symptoms are usually short-lived, subsequent tissue damage is uncommon, and necrosis does not occur. A vesicant is a drug that produces an irritant reaction so severe that plasma escapes from the extracellular space, blisters are formed, and tissue destruction results. Drugs have been described as vesicants by degree (i.e., severe, moderate), as a potential vesicant, or as having vesicant properties.

Rudolph and Larson (1987) suggest classifying drugs according to their tissue nucleic acid binding affinity. Drugs that do not bind to DNA cause tissue damage immediately, but are either inactivated or quickly metabolized and follow the normal healing process. Drugs that bind to DNA also produce immediate tissue damage, but in contrast, they remain in the tissues, resulting in long-term injury (Table 11-6). This proposed concept, supported by laboratory data, demonstrates that anthracycline levels can persist in the tissues for several months and supports the clinical observations of lack of spontaneous healing, progressive ulceration, delayed skin reactions, recall phenomena, and the necessity of complete surgical excision for cure (Argenta & Manders, 1983; Duray et al, 1986; Wood & Ellerhorst-Ryan, 1984).

EXTRAVASATION PREVENTION

Extravasation is the escape of a chemotherapeutic drug from a vessel to the surrounding tissues, either by leakage or direct infiltration. The onset of symptoms may occur immediately or several days to weeks after drug administration. Immediate symptoms commonly described are discomfort, burning, and erythema. Pain, edema, induration, ulceration, and necrosis often occur later.

For peripheral drug administration, the risk of extravasation can be minimized by prudent site selection, good venipuncture technique, and careful drug administration. Cancer patients at high risk for complications from chemotherapy administration include those with pre-existing vascular disease, malnutrition, small or fragile veins, previous chemotherapy, recent skin testing, combination chemotherapy, axillary lymphadenectomy, and prior radiation to potential infusion sites.

TABLE 11-6

LOCAL TISSUE INJURY OF SELECTED CHEMOTHERAPEUTIC DRUGS

Long-term injury	Short-term injury
Dactinomycin	Carmustine
Daunorubicin	Cisplatin
Doxorubicin	Etoposide
Epirubicin	5-Fluorouracil
Idarubicin	Mechlorethamine
Mitomycin	Plicamycin
	Vinblastine
	Vincristine
	Vinorelbine

The general principle in site selection is to choose an area that will offer the best protection to tendons and nerves and cause the least loss of function if extravasation occurs. Generally, one should avoid areas of recent chemotherapy administration and prior irradiation, and extremities with lymphedema or prior axillary dissection. Venipuncture sites that are 24 hours old or less should be noted and infusion sites distal to these avoided. An area in the forearm, preferably the upper part of the forearm, is the optimal site because of the presence of extensive soft tissue. The dorsum of the hand and joints are not recommended because of the potential damage to tendons and neurovascular structures, the potential for contractures or functional loss, and the difficulty posed by these sites for successful surgical interventions (Camp-Sorrell, 1998). The antecubital fossa is recognized for its large veins that often are easily accessible, but it is the least favorable alternative because important arteries and veins are located there. Extravasation may be more difficult to detect there because of the amount of subcutaneous tissue, resulting in a greater concentration of drug infiltration and subsequent functional loss of a major joint temporarily, or perhaps permanently, from contractures.

Central venous access devices are extremely common in practice. While there may be substantial benefits to central access, the risk of extravasation is not eliminated. Backflow caused by fibrin sheath formation, needle dislodgment from port reservoir, and catheter damage or malposition, have been causative factors in drug extravasation (Camp-Sorrell, 1998; Mayo & Pearson, 1995). The guidelines used to ensure patency of central devices serve as the basis for proceeding with drug administration, especially regarding the ability to withdraw blood. If a blood return is not established, a chest radiograph or dye study is indicated before administration of a vesicant. These studies will confirm catheter placement and identify any fibrin sheath formation that may cause potential backtracking of the drug.

EXTRAVASATION MANAGEMENT

Early recognition of an extravasation may help prevent serious toxicity. Signs and symptoms of an infiltration include slowing or cessation of IV flow, increased resistance when administering the drug, patient complaints, swelling or erythema, and poor or no blood return. Once an extravasation is recognized, delay because of lack of knowledge or policy about treatment can affect the outcome. It is important to have a written protocol established for the staff to treat extravasation immediately and with consistency. The following guidelines should be followed if an extravasation is suspected:

1. Stop the infusion.
2. Disconnect intravenous tubing and attempt to aspirate residual medication from the access needle.
3. For all drugs except the vinca alkaloids: during the first 24 to 48 hours, apply ice for 15 to 20 minutes at least 4 times a day and elevate the extremity if it is a peripheral site (Rudolph & Larson, 1987).
4. For the vinca alkaloids, apply heat.
5. Consider an antidote, although most research on antidotes is drawn from animal data and efficacy in humans has not been definitely established (Camp-Sorrell, 1998). Hyaluronidase and local heat are recommended by the manufacturer for the vinca alkaloids; for all other drugs, standard practice is the application of ice (Brown et al, 2001). Local injection of steroids has been proposed but no definitive advantage to healing has been established. Clinical reports on the benefits are even lacking for the clinically accepted instillation of one-sixth molar sodium thiosulfate for mechlorethamine infiltration.
6. Document the incident. Documentation records for venipuncture sites and reactions provide valuable information and legal protection (Boyle & Engelking, 1996). Photograph the site if possible.
7. Follow the patient closely for at least 2 weeks, carefully observing the site. This should include an early consultation with a plastic surgeon and, if symptoms are present, with a physical therapist.

VENOUS REACTIONS

Local venous and cutaneous reactions can be acute or occur weeks after treatment. Burning, pain, erythema, tenderness along the vein, urticaria, and pruritus are common immediate reactions, whereas thrombosed veins, persistent phlebitis, hyperpigmentation of veins, or discoloration of affected tissues may be observed weeks to months after drug administration.

The anthracyclines are associated with local urticaria, streaking erythema, pain, and complaints of a stinging sensation, commonly referred to as a flare reaction. These reactions occur in probably less than 20% of patients treated, are transient, and usually resolve within 1 to 2 hours (Curran et al, 1990). Reconstitution with an isotonic diluent, slowing the rate of administration, and dilution of the drug concentration with the IV solution may minimize or prevent recurrence of flare reactions with subsequent doses. Carmustine and dacarbazine often produce significant burning and discomfort. Placing ice along the venous pathway above the insertion site and adequate dilution of the drug may provide some pain relief. Vinorelbine produces venous irritation, reported as tenderness along the vein and erythema, in about one-third of patients (Brogden & Nevidjon, 1995). This can be reduced by administering the drug over 6 to 10 minutes rather than a 20- to 30-minute infusion (Rittenberg et al, 1995). It is also recommended that a flush of 75–125 mL IV solution after vinorelbine may reduce the incidence of phlebitis (Brown et al, 2001).

SYSTEMIC DERMATOLOGICAL EFFECTS

Skin changes not caused by extravasation of chemotherapeutic drugs include dermatitis, nail changes, hyperpigmentation, urticaria, acral erythema, photosensitivity reactions, and radiation-enhancing reactions. Many of these cutaneous reactions are

TABLE 11-7

DERMATITIS ASSOCIATED WITH CHEMOTHERAPEUTIC DRUGS

Chemotherapeutic drug	Type of reaction
Aminoglutethimide	Erythematous maculopapular rash
Azacitidine	Pruritic rash (rare)
Bleomycin	Rash, urticaria, erythematous swelling, hyperkeratosis
Carboplatin	Rash (rare)
Carmustine	Transient facial and neck flush, rash, pruritus
Cetuximab	Acneiform rash
Chlorambucil	Occasional dermatitis
Cytarabine	Rash
Dacarbazine	Transient facial and neck flush
Dactinomycin	Acneiform rash, folliculitis
Daunorubicin	Rash, urticaria
Doxorubicin	Local erythemia, urticaria, and pruritus along vein
Epirubicin	Dermatitis
Erlinotib	Acneiform rash
Floxuridine	Rash, pruritus (rare)
5-Fluorouracil	Dermatitis
Gefitinib	Acneiform rash
Leuprolide	Erythema, skin rash
Hydroxyurea	Rash
Isotretinoin	Dry skin, pruritus, exfoliation
Methotrexate	Rash, urticaria
Mitomycin	Rash, photosensitivity
Pentostatin	Rash, dry skin
Plicamycin	Dermatitis, facial flushing
Procarbazine	Facial flushing associated with alcohol intake, skin rash, photosensitivity
Raltitrexed	Rash, pruritus
Tomudex	Rash
Tretinoin	Dry skin, pruritus, mild exfoliation
Trimetrexate	Rash (dose-limiting)
Troxacitabine	Skin rash, pruritus

self-limited, lasting only for the duration of therapy. Rash formation and erythema can occur with a variety of chemotherapy drugs (Table 11-7). Nail changes during chemotherapy include pigmentation, brittleness, and slowed growth (Table 11-8). Pigmentation is the most frequent change and seems to affect dark-skinned patients more commonly than Caucasian patients. Drug-induced hyperpigmentation of the skin and mucous membranes (Table 11-9) can be focal or diffuse and generally resolves with time, although occasionally it may be permanent.

Acral erythema is a syndrome of demarcated, tender erythematous plaques, on the soles of the feet and palms of the hands of patients, which can range from mild to extremely painful. This toxicity, also referred to as palmar-plantar erythrodysesthesia syndrome, has been associated with cyclophosphamide, cytarabine, docetaxel, doxorubicin, liposomal doxorubicin, capecitabine, etoposide, 5-fluorouracil, hydroxyurea, lomustine, mercaptopurine, methotrexate, mitotane, paclitaxel, suramin, and vinblastine (Koppel & Boh, 2001). The patient initially may complain of tingling

TABLE 11-8
NAIL CHANGES

Drug	Effect
Bleomycin	Nail loss
Cyclophosphamide	Hyperpigmentation
Doxorubicin	Hyperpigmentation
5-Fluorouracil	Nail cracking and loss
Hydroxyurea	Brittle nails
Paclitaxel	Hyperpigmentation, cracking, loss

TABLE 11-9
PIGMENTATION CHANGES ASSOCIATED WITH CHEMOTHERAPY

Drug	Pigmentation change
Bleomycin	Linear hyperpigmented streaks across the trunk, hyperpigmentation over small joints
Busulfan	Generalized skin darkening, hyperpigmentation
Carmustine	Hyperpigmentation after erythema
Cyclophosphamide	Hyperpigmentation in sun-exposed areas (nails, teeth, gingivae)
Dactinomycin	Hyperpigmentation
Doxorubicin	Oral mucosa hyperpigmentation
5-Fluorouracil	Photosensitivity, hyperpigmentation
Methotrexate	Photosensitivity, hyperpigmentation
Thiotepa	Hyperpigmentation (areas occluded by bandages)

sensations of the hands and feet that generally progress to swelling, pain, tenderness to touch, intense erythema with blanching between joints, and finally, desquamation (Coyle & Wenhold, 2001). Management is focused on pain relief (systemic and local measures), elevation of extremities, and prevention of infection.

RENAL TOXICITY

Major risk factors for renal toxicity in patients with cancer include nephrotoxic chemotherapy drugs, age, nutritional status, concurrent use of other nephrotoxic drugs, and pre-existing renal dysfunction. Of the major risk factors for nephrotoxicity, impaired renal function is a significant one. Repeated courses of nephrotoxic drugs may result in decreased renal function demonstrated by subclinical or clinically obvious renal impairment. High-dose therapy may result in a greater incidence of, and more severe, renal toxicity. Acute renal failure and hemolytic uremic syndrome are potentially serious and fatal complications (Long, 2002). Drugs with a high risk for renal toxicity include azacitidine, cisplatin, ifosfamide, methotrexate (high dose), mitomycin, plicamycin, and streptozocin (Weiss, 2001). Carboplatin is significantly less nephrotoxic than cisplatin, but if administered in high doses (e.g., stem cell transplant) or given with other nephrotoxic drugs, it has the potential to contribute to renal damage.

Before initiating therapy with any potentially renal-toxic drug, it is essential to assess renal function and evaluate risk factors. Plasma concentrations of blood urea nitrogen (BUN) and creatinine are common assessment parameters, but their use is very limited because damage to the kidney may be quite significant before elevations in serum levels are detected (Lydon, 1989). The most reliable method to assess renal function that will reflect glomerular function with reasonable accuracy is a urinary creatinine collection. A 24-hour collection of urine for creatinine clearance is recommended to monitor patients and alter drug doses to prevent or minimize renal toxicity. Patient teaching about the urine-collection process and the need for adequate hydration is essential. Written instructions should be provided and translated into appropriate languages for the population served. Inadequate or inaccurate collections may result in erroneous values with unexpected toxicities, delays in treatment, and alterations in planned hospitalizations (Table 11-10).

BLADDER TOXICITY

Hemorrhagic cystitis is associated with ifosfamide and cyclophosphamide, and an increased incidence of bladder carcinoma has been associated with prolonged use of these drugs. Standard doses of cyclophosphamide, especially with oral administration, produce bladder toxicity in less than 10% of patients (Patterson & Reams, 1992). High-dose cyclophosphamide, like its structural analogue ifosfamide, presents a major risk for the development of hemorrhagic cystitis. Contact of the bladder wall with toxic metabolites, primarily acrolein, produces mucosal erythema, inflammation, ulceration, necrosis, diffuse small-vessel hemorrhagic oozing, and a reduced bladder capacity (Stillwell & Benson, 1988). Symptoms include hematuria (microscopic or gross) and dysuria. The uroprotective agent 2-mercaptoethane sulfonate sodium (mesna) acts by binding to acrolein to result in a nontoxic thioether. The use of mesna and hydration with ifosfamide or high-dose cyclophosphamide significantly reduces the incidence of bladder toxicity. If hemorrhagic cystitis develops, discontinuation of treatment with the drug and vigorous hydration are indicated. Depending on the degree of toxicity, bladder irrigation, fulguration, and in rare instances cystectomy may be warranted (Stillwell & Benson, 1988).

CARDIOPULMONARY TOXICITY

PULMONARY TOXICITY

Chemotherapy drugs can directly or indirectly produce lung-tissue damage. Regardless of a direct or indirect action, the resulting toxicity is damage to both endothelial and epithelial cells (pneumocytes). The clinical presentations of pulmonary toxicity associated with chemotherapy fall into four major patterns:

- acute pneumonitis
- pulmonary fibrosis
- hypersensitivity pneumonitis
- noncardiogenic pulmonary edema.

Drugs associated with acute pneumonitis include bleomycin, carmustine, gemcitabine, methotrexate, mitomycin, procarbazine, and the vinca alkaloids, and those that pose a risk for the development of pulmonary fibrosis include bleomycin, carmustine, cyclophosphamide, methotrexate, and mitomycin (Davies et al, 2002). Bleomycin can be used as a prototype for the pattern of pneumonitis and fibrosis (Kriesman & Wolkove, 1992). Symptoms include dyspnea, nonproductive cough, fatigue, and weight loss and may occur acutely but more commonly over a period of several weeks. On physical examination, findings may include tachycardia, tachypnea, or diffuse rales. Chest radiography often shows pulmonary infiltrates and a diagnostic work-up is indicated to rule out an infectious etiology. Treatment includes discontinuation of the suspected causative chemotherapy drug and administration of corticosteroids.

Hypersensitivity pneumonitis has been associated with azathioprine, bleomycin, methotrexate, and procarbazine (Cooper & Matthay, 1987). Symptoms of dyspnea, cough, chills, myalgia, and headache are reported with physical findings of fever, pulmonary crackles, and a skin rash in up to half of patients. The chest radiograph shows diffuse infiltrates, and a pleural effusion may be present. Treatment is discontinuation of treatment with the drug and administration of corticosteroids. The outcome of treatment is generally good, although the condition can be potentially life-threatening. Noncardiogenic pulmonary edema is associated with an acute onset of respiratory symptoms and is likely related to capillary leak syndrome. Drugs associated with this uncommon toxicity include cytarabine, cyclophosphamide, methotrexate, mitomycin, and teniposide (Cooper & Matthay, 1987). Docetaxel is associated with fluid retention, which may result in pulmonary edema, or pleural effusion.

The four patterns described are not exclusive categories, and many patients will exhibit symptoms and histological findings representative of more than one type of toxicity. For example, methotrexate represents a drug with a broad range of pulmonary toxicity: endothelial injury, capillary leak, pulmonary edema, and pulmonary fibrosis (Kriesman & Wolkove, 1992). Symptoms may be acute and precipitate acute respiratory distress syndrome or may be gradual, with their onset varying from days to years. Recovery generally occurs, although fatal cases of pulmonary fibrosis have been reported (van der Veen et al, 1995).

CARDIAC TOXICITY

Cardiomyopathy is the most common chemotherapy-associated cardiac toxicity. Myocardial ischemia, pericarditis, arrhythmias, miscellaneous electrocardiogram (ECG) changes, and angina occur much less frequently. The anthracyclines have the highest consistent risk for cardiomyopathy, which is cumulative dose-response related. However, there is sufficiently strong evidence that high-dose cyclophosphamide, 5-fluorouracil, and amsacrine also pose an increased risk for cardiac damage and somewhat weaker evidence (case reports) for docetaxel, etoposide, ifosfamide (high dose), losoxantrone, and mitoxantrone (Davies et al, 2002). Cardiac effects of anthracycline therapy can be acute, subacute, or late-onset. Acute effects (arrhythmias, ECG changes, sinus tachycardia) occur within hours of bolus administration, are transient, and do not appear to be related to dose, schedule, or future development of cardiomyopathy. Subacute anthracycline cardiomyopathy may present during or weeks to months after therapy, but most commonly occurs within one year of treatment (Shan et al, 1996).

Late-onset cardiac toxicity (more than one to five years after treatment) increases with length of follow-up and occurs in previously asymptomatic patients, emphasizing the need for continued assessment of cardiac function in long-term survivors. Observed abnormalities include arrhythmias, left ventricular dysfunction, decreased ejection fraction, fractional shortening on echocardiogram, and cardiac failure. The cumulative anthracycline drug dose and mediastinal radiation are the two most significant risk factors. Age (young children, older adults), concurrent chemotherapy (with increased risk of cardiac toxicity), pre-existing cardiac disease, schedule of

TABLE 11-10

ALTERATIONS IN RENAL FUNCTION OF SELECTED CHEMOTHERAPEUTIC DRUGS

Drug	Alteration	Risk factors	Abnormalities	Management
Cisplatin	Damage to proximal and distal tubules Decreased renal tubular reabsorption	Concurrent use of other nephrotoxic drugs Existing renal dysfunction	Azotemia ↑BUN ↑Serum creatinine ↑Uric acid ↓Creatinine clearance ↓Serum magnesium ↓Serum calcium Proteinuria ↓Potassium	Prevention: hydration (2–3 L) and diuresis (>100 mL/hr) Magnesium supplement Supportive: electrolyte replacement, dose adjustment, discontinuation of drug therapy
Cyclophosphamide	SIADH	High dose and hydration with free water (i.e., D₅W)	Hyponatremia ↓Urine output ↑Urine osmolality ↓Serum osmolality	Prevention: monitor electrolytes, hydration with normal saline Supportive: discontinue drug therapy
Ifosfamide	Proximal tubular defect	High-dose administration Existing renal dysfunction	↑BUN ↑Serum creatinine ↓Creatinine clearance Proteinuria	Prevention: adequate hydration, monitor for early signs of toxicity; may be reversible
Methotrexate	Injury to proximal and distal convoluted tubules	High-dose therapy Dehydration Existing renal dysfunction Concurrent use of other nephrotoxic drugs Existing effusions or ascites Prior treatment with cisplatin	↑BUN ↑Serum creatinine ↓Creatinine clearance Hematuria Azotemia Oliguria Hypokalemia Aminoaciduria Electrolyte abnormalities	Prevention (high dose): hydration, adequate urine output, alkalinization to maintain pH ≥ 7.0 Supportive: hydration Administer leucovorin if serum methotrexate levels are elevated (see Chapter 4)

Drug	Effect	Risk Factors	Findings	Prevention/Supportive
Mitomycin	Mild, reversible renal insufficiency; Hemolytic-uremic syndrome (uncommon)	Prolonged therapy; Cumulative doses >60–100 mg	↑BUN; ↑Serum creatinine; ↓Platelets; Anemia; Proteinuria; Hematuria; Hypertension	Prevention: none; Supportive: ? plasma pheresis
Nitrosoureas	Glomerular and tubular damage	Cumulative doses ≥1.2 g/m^2	↑BUN; ↑Serum creatinine	Prevention: adjust dose for renal impairment; Supportive: monitor cumulative dose and renal function
Plicamycin	Damage to proximal and distal tubules	Daily schedule with cumulative doses 25–50 microg/kg	↑BUN; ↑Serum creatinine; Proteinuria; Azotemia; ↓Serum electrolytes	Prevention: avoid high doses; monitor for early signs of toxicity
Streptozocin	Damage to renal tubules	Doses >1–1.5 g/m^2/wk; Concurrent use of other nephrotoxic drugs; Existing renal dysfunction	↑BUN; ↑Serum creatinine; Proteinuria; ↓Creatinine clearance; Glucosuria; Hypokalemia; Renal tubular acidosis; Hypophosphatemia	Prevention: monitor early signs of toxicity; protein, amino acids in urine, phosphate, potassium in serum; Adequate hydration

SIADH, Syndrome of inappropriate antidiuretic hormone; D_5W, 5% dextrose in water.

11

TABLE 11-11

SUMMARY OF ASCO GUIDELINES FOR THE USE OF CARDIOPROTECTANT, DEXRAZOXANE*

Disease/Drug indication	Recommendation
Metastatic breast cancer	Begin at a cumulative dose of 300 mg/m^2 of doxorubicin; monitor frequently
Adjuvant therapy breast cancer	Not recommended
Other cancers	Caution in use where doxorubicin has been shown to improve survival
Other anthracyclines	May be considered for women with advanced breast cancer who are responding to epirubicin and for whom continuation of epirubicin is indicated
High-dose anthracycline therapy	Insufficient data
Patients with cardiac risk factors	Insufficient data

*Schucter LM et al. 2002 update of recommendations for the use of chemotherapy and radiotherapy protectants: clinical practice guidelines of the American Society of Clinical Oncology. J Clin Oncol, 20: 2895–2903, 2002.

administration (e.g., bolus versus continuous), and individual sensitivity may contribute to the overall risk of developing cardiac complications. The concurrent use of trastuzumab with an anthracycline and cyclophosphamide is associated with a risk of cardiac dysfunction (Seidman et al, 2002), but any cardiac sequelae related to sequential use is not yet known.

The primary management strategy of anthracycline cardiac toxicity is prevention and early detection. Patients should be assessed prior to treatment and monitored during and after therapy. Multigated blood pool imaging (MUGA) or echocardiogram are the standard noninvasive methods to assess cardiac function. Long-term follow-up monitoring is also recommended based on the risk of cardiac toxicity over time (Shan et al, 1996).

Management of chemotherapy-induced cardiac dysfunction is conventional therapy for heart failure. Because of the limited value of this intervention in the face of existing cardiac disease, prevention of cardiac toxicity has been a focus for clinicians and researchers. Use of the cardioprotectant, dexrazoxane, represents the primary preventive approach and recommendations for its use are given in Table 11-11. For patients who are treated with dexrazoxane, they should receive it at a ratio of 10:1 to the doxorubicin dose and it is recommended that it be administered 15 to 30 minutes prior to doxorubicin as a slow intravenous push or short intravenous infusion (Schucter et al, 2002). An optimal dose ratio for epirubicin has not yet been determined. Frequent cardiac monitoring is strongly recommended for patients who receive dexrazoxane and doxorubicin (e.g., performed at the cumulative dose of 400 mg/m^2 and then every 50 mg/m^2 of doxorubicin after a cumulative dose of 500 mg/m^2).

NEUROLOGICAL TOXICITY

Encephalopathy, peripheral neuropathy, cerebellar syndromes, autonomic neuropathy, and cranial nerve toxicity represent the range of neurological complications associated with systemic drug treatment (Box 11-4). Symptoms may be transient and mild or severe with significant dysfunction. Dose, route of administration, age of the patient, hepatic and renal function, prior and/or concomitant use of other neurotoxic drugs, and concurrent use of cranial or CNS radiotherapy can each influence the incidence rate and severity of neurological symptoms associated with selected chemotherapy drugs.

Acute encephalopathies and cerebellar syndromes are serious CNS toxicities, but they are fairly limited to a few drugs and select patient populations. In contrast, peripheral neuropathy is associated with several commonly prescribed chemotherapeutic

---

BOX 11-4

NEUROTOXICITY ASSOCIATED WITH CYTOTOXIC DRUGS

ACUTE MYELOPATHY

Intrathecal cytarabine
Intrathecal methotrexate
Intrathecal thiotepa

AUTONOMIC NEUROPATHY

Cisplatin	Vincristine
Paclitaxel	Vinorelbine
Procarbazine	Vindesine
Vinblastine	

CEREBELLAR SYNDROMES

Altretamine	5-Fluorouracil
Cytarabine	Procarbazine

CRANIAL NERVE TOXICITY

Carmustine	Vinblastine
Cisplatin	Vincristine
5-Fluorouracil	Vindesine
Ifosfamide	

ENCEPHALOPATHY (CEREBRAL)

L-Asparaginase	Fludarabine
Azacitidine	5-Fluorouracil
Busulfan (high dose)	Ifosfamide
Carmustine	Mitotane
Cisplatin	Pentostatin
Cladribine	PALA
Cyclophosphamide	Procarbazine
Cytarabine (high dose)	Methotrexate

PERIPHERAL NEUROPATHY

Altretamine	Paclitaxel
Azacitidine	Procarbazine
Carboplatin	Suramin
Cisplatin	Teniposide
Cytarabine	Thiotepa (high dose)
Docetaxel	Vinblastine
Etoposide	Vincristine
Fludarabine	Vindesine
Oxaliplatin	Vinorelbine

11

NEUROLOGICAL TOXICITY

TABLE 11-12
COMMON CHEMOTHERAPY AGENTS ASSOCIATED WITH PERIPHERAL NEUROPATHY

Agent	Injury/Risk factors
Cisplatin	Loss of vibration and proprioceptor function; loss of proximal deep tendon reflexes, sensory alterations; ± Lhermitte's sign; autonomic neuropathy
	Increased risk >300 mg/m^2
Docetaxel Paclitaxel	Injury to large and small fibers but predominantly affect large nerve fibers. Loss of deep tendon reflexes, proximal and distal extremity weakness; loss of vibratory sense; autonomic neuropathy
	Docetaxel: Risk increased with single dose >100 mg/m^2 and increased risk of severity level with cumulative doses >400 mg/m^2
	Paclitaxel: Risk increased with single dose >175 mg/m^2 and increased with cumulative dosing (no threshold established)
Oxaliplatin	Two distinct syndromes (Wilson et al, 2002):
	Acute: dysesthesias of hands, feet, perioral; jaw tightness, pharyngo-laryngo-dysesthesia, enhanced by cold exposure.
	Chronic: Sensory neuropathy in small and large nerve fibers similar to cisplatin; estimated 10–15% risk with cumulative doses 780–850 mg/m^2 (Wilkes, 2002)
Vincristine	Injury to large and small nerve fibers but > small fibers; loss of deep tendon reflexes; lower extremity weakness; autonomic neuropathy
	Increased risk with increasing total cumulative dose

agents and occurs predictably with cisplatin, docetaxel, paclitaxel, oxaliplatin, and vincristine (Table 11-12) (Rowinsky et al, 1993; Siegal & Haim, 1990; Weiss, 2001; Wilkes, 2002; Wilson et al, 2002).

Mild distal sensory paresthesias are tolerable for most patients, but more severe sensory alterations (i.e., painful paresthesias, loss of deep tendon reflexes, sensory ataxia, perceptual alterations) can significantly alter a patient's functional ability, comfort, and overall quality of life (Rowinsky et al, 1993). Physical and subjective assessments of the patient's distress and perceived functional impairment are critical to therapeutic decisions and plan of care. The only effective therapy is discontinuation of the causative chemotherapy agent. And even when therapy is discontinued, symptoms have been reported to persist for months or years after treatment. Pharmacological therapy with tricyclic antidepressants (e.g., amitriptyline) and anticonvulsants (e.g., gabapentin) has been evaluated with some relief of symptom distress, but the side-effect profile of these agents limits their acceptability (Brant, 1998; Morello et al, 2000; Woolf & Mannion, 1999). Amifostine has been evaluated as a neuroprotectant but there are insufficient data to indicate its use at this time (Schucter et al, 2002). Data from animal studies with glutamine as a protectant suggest that it may have a role and should be evaluated in patients who receive cisplatin or paclitaxel (Boyle et al, 1999).

GONADAL TOXICITY

Gonadal dysfunction as a consequence of treatment with alkylating agents was reported in the early 1970s, and these drugs remain the most significant gonadal toxins. High-dose therapy, especially in transplantation, results in more predictable and irreversible gonadal toxicity. Several decades ago, patients with Hodgkin's disease, because of their age and curability potential, were the major focus for evaluating chemotherapy effects on fertility and sexuality (Chapman et al, 1979a,b). The underlying malignancy appears to be an important factor, particularly for males diagnosed with Hodgkin's disease. Gonadal dysfunction, observed as impotence and inadequate sperm counts, has been reported before initiation of therapy. Assessment of pretreatment gonadal function is very important in predicting outcome and for counseling patients regarding fertility options after completion of therapy (Sweet et al, 1996). Healthcare providers need to be knowledgeable about gonadal preservation, discuss options, and offer the opportunity before therapy (Schover et al, 2002a,b).

More recently, the widespread use of adjuvant chemotherapy and hormonal therapy in premenopausal women with breast cancer has shifted the focus to concerns about late effects of premature chemotherapy-induced menopause on survivors (Ganz et al, 1998; Goodwin et al, 1999; Knobf, 2001, 2002). The incidence of drug-induced premature menopause is 65% to 75%, and even with shorter anthracycline/alkylating agent combinations, nearly half of women over the age of 40 years will become irreversibly menopausal (Lower et al, 1999; Moore et al, 1999). Furthermore, younger women who either maintain their menses or who experience irregular menses will enter menopause at an earlier than expected age. Menopausal symptoms include vasomotor symptoms of hot flushes and night sweats, sleep disturbances, atrophic vaginal changes, mood and cognitive changes, and potential alterations in risk for osteoporosis and heart disease.

Options for fertility preservation in women have been less successful than in men. Hormonal protection is controversial; cryopreservation of oocytes raises concerns about superovulation and oocytes do not freeze well; and the most recent idea of cryopreservation of ovarian tissue is experimental. Insemination using donor eggs, surrogate carriers, or adoption provide alternative options for a young woman with premature induced menopause who wishes to have children.

In addition to chemotherapy, there is a wide variety of symptoms associated with hormonal therapies, including diminished or lost libido, hot flushes, mood changes, and vaginal discharge in women, and hot flushes, changes in libido, gynecomastia, and impotence in men. These are important side effects related to quality of life and should be assessed and managed according to the patient's perceived distress. Sexuality and sexual relationships are an important part of life and nurses and physicians need to be more assertive in assessing, managing, and referral for counseling and intervention (Shell, 2002).

POTENTIAL TERATOGENIC EFFECTS OF THERAPY

The decision to treat a pregnant woman requires significant discussion between the woman, her partner, and the physician, addressing each individual chemotherapy agent and its potential for fetal harm should be addressed. Thalidomide and alkylating agents are known to be teratogenic (Colvin, 2001). Fetal malformations have been reported in women who were treated with alkylating agents in the first trimester of pregnancy, but not if the woman was treated during the second or third trimester. Most chemotherapy agents are considered pregnancy category D or X, implying that they may cause fetal harm.

GONADAL TOXICITY

REFERENCES

Bone marrow suppression

Alexander SW, Pizzo PA. Current consideration in the management of fever and neutropenia. Current Clin Topics Infect Dis 19: 160–180, 1999.

Bodey GP et al. Quantitative relationships between circulating leukocytes and infection in patients with acute leukemia. Ann Intern Med 64: 328–340, 1966.

Cella D, Bron D. The effect of epoetin alfa on quality of life in anemic cancer patients. Cancer Pract 7: 177–182, 1999.

Gabrilove JL et al. Clinical evaluation of once-weekly dosing of epoetin alfa in chemotherapy patients: improvements in hemoglobin and quality of life are similar to three-times weekly dosing. J Clin Oncol 19: 2875–2882, 2001.

Gillespie TW. Effects of cancer-related anemia on clinical and quality of life outcomes. Clin J Oncol 6: 206–211, 2002.

Glaspy JA et al. Randomized active-controlled phase I/II dose-escalation study of NESP administered weekly and every two weeks in patients with solid tumors. Proc Am Soc Clin Oncol 20: 387a, (abstract # 1546), 2001.

Glisson J, Crawford R, Street S. The clinical applications of ginko biloba, St. John's wort, saw palmetto and soy. Nurs Pract 24: 28–49, 1999.

Hedderwick SA et al. Pathogenic organisms associated with artificial fingernails worn by healthcare workers. Infect Control Hosp Epidemiol 21: 505-509, 2000.

Hughes WT et al. 2002 guidelines for the use of antimicrobial agents in neutropenic patients with cancer. Clin Infect Dis 34: 730–751, 2002.

Littlewood TJ et al. Effects of epoetin alfa on hematologic parameters and quality of life in cancer patients receiving nonplatinum chemotherapy: results of a randomized double-blind placebo-controlled trial. J Clin Oncol 19: 2865–2874, 2001.

McNeil SA et al. Effect of hand cleansing with antimicrobial soap or alcohol based gel on microbial colonization of artificial fingernails worn by health care workers. Clin Infect Dis 32: 367–372, 2001.

Mermel IA et al. Guidelines for the management of intravascular catheter-related infection. Clin Infect Dis 32: 1249–1272, 2001.

Moran AB, Camp-Sorrell D. Maintenance of venous access devices in patients with neutropenia. Clin J Oncol Nurs 6: 126–130, 2002.

Ozer H et al. 2000 update of recommendations for the use of hematopoietic colony-stimulating factors: evidence-based, clinical practice guidelines. J Clin Oncol 18: 3558–3585, 2000.

Pizzo PA, Schimpff SC. Strategies for the prevention of infection in the myelosuppressed cancer patient. Cancer Treat Rep 67: 223–234, 1983.

Preston FA, Cunningham RS. Clinical Guidelines for Symptom Management in Oncology. New York, Clinical Insights Press, 1998.

Quirt I et al. Epoetin alfa therapy increases hemoglobin levels and improves quality of life in patients with cancer-related anemia who are not receiving chemotherapy and patients with anemia who are receiving chemotherapy. J Clin Oncol 19: 4126–4134, 2001.

Rolston KV. Prediction of neutropenia. Int J Antimicr Agents 16: 113–115, 2000.

Rust DM et al. Nutritional issues in patients with severe neutropenia. Sem Oncol Nurs 16: 152–162, 2000.

Shiffer CA et al. Platelet transfusion for patients with cancer: clinical practice guidelines of the American Society of Clinical Oncology. J Clin Oncol 19: 1519–1538, 2001.

Snyder E. Blood transfusion therapy for the cancer patient. In: Fischer DS, Knobf MT, Durivage H, eds: The Cancer Chemotherapy Handbook. St. Louis, Mosby-Yearbook, 1997, pp 553–563.

Viale PH. To draw or not to draw: drawing blood cultures from a potentially infected port site. Clin J Oncol Nurs 6: 232, 2002.

Gastrointestinal toxicity

ASHP. ASHP therapeutic guidelines on the pharmacologic management of nausea and vomiting in adult and pediatric patients receiving chemotherapy or radiation therapy or undergoing surgery. Am J Health Syst Pharm 56: 729–764, 1999.

Bender CM et al. Chemotherapy-induced nausea and vomiting. Clin J Oncol Nurs 6: 94–102, 2002.

Berger AM, Eilers J. Factors influencing oral cavity status during high dose antineoplastic therapy: a secondary data analysis. Oncol Nurs Forum 25: 1623–1629, 1998.

Campos D et al. Prevention of cisplatin-induced emesis by the oral neurokin-1 antagonist, MK-869, in combination with granisetron and dexamethasone or with dexamethasone alone. J Clin Oncol 19: 1759–1767, 2001.

Cocquyt V et al. Comparison of L-758-298, a prodrug for the selective NK-1 antagonist, L-754-030, with ondansetron for the prevention of cisplatin-induced emesis. Eur J Cancer 37: 835–842, 2001.

Coons HL et al. Anticipatory nausea and emotional distress in patients receiving cisplatin-based chemotherapy. Oncol Nurs Forum 14: 31–35, 1987.

Eckert RM. Understanding anticipatory nausea. Oncol Nurs Forum 28: 1553–1558, 2001.

Engstrom C et al. The efficacy and cost effectiveness of new anti-emetic guidelines. Oncol Nurs Forum 26: 1453–1458, 1999.

Goldsmith M, Wodinsky H. Controlling costs using evidence-based guidelines: 5-HT$_3$ antagonists as a model. Managed Care and Cancer (May/June), 20–24, 1999.

Gralla RJ et al. Recommendations for the use of anti-emetics: evidence based, clinical practice guidelines. J Clin Oncol 17: 2971–2994, 1999.

Grant M, Kravits K. Symptoms and their impact on nutrition. Semin Oncol Nurs 16: 113–121, 2000.

Gross J. Functional alterations – bowel. In Johnson BL, Gross J, eds. Handbook of Oncology Nursing, 3rd ed. Boston, Jones and Bartlett, 1998, pp 545–556.

Hawkins R. Diarrhea. In: Camp-Sorrell D, Hawkins RA, eds. Clinical Manual for the Oncology Advanced Practice Nurse. Pittsburgh, Oncology Nursing Press, 2000, pp 339–342.

Hesketh PJ et al. Improved control of high-dose-cisplatin induced acute emesis with the addition of prochlorperazine to granisetron/dexamethasone. Cancer J Sci Am 3: 180–183, 1997.

Ioannidis JP, Hesketh PJ, Lau J. Contribution of dexamethasone to control of chemotherapy-induced nausea and vomiting: a meta-analysis of randomized evidence. J Clin Oncol 18: 3409–3422, 2000.

Kostler W et al. Oral mucositis complicating chemotherapy and/or radiotherapy: options for prevention and treatment. CA Cancer J Clin 51: 290–315, 2001.

Larson PJ et al. The PRO-SELF Mouth Aware program: an effective approach for reducing chemotherapy-induced mucositis. Cancer Nurs 21: 263–268, 1998.

Mercadante S. Diarrhea, malabsorption and constipation. In: Berger A, Portenoy R, Weissman DE, eds. Principles and Practice of Palliative and Supportive Oncology, 2nd ed. Philadelphia, Lippincott, Williams and Wilkins, 2002, pp 233–249.

Miller M, Kearney N. Oral care for patients with cancer: a review of the literature. Cancer Nurs 24: 241–254, 2001.

Morrow GR. Clinical characteristics associated with the development of anticipatory nausea and vomiting in cancer patients undergoing chemotherapy treatment. J Clin Oncol 2: 1170–1176, 1984.

Navari RM et al. Reduction of cisplatin-induced emesis by a selective neurokin-1 receptor antagonist. N Engl J Med 340: 190–195, 1999.

Nerenz DR et al. Anxiety and drug taste as predictors of anticipatory nausea in cancer chemotherapy. J Clin Oncol 4: 224–233, 1986.

Peterson D. Research advances in oral mucositis. Curr Opin Oncol 11: 261–272, 1999.

Rhodes VA et al. Nausea, vomiting and retching: management of the symptom experience. Semin Oncol Nurs 11: 256–265, 1995.

Rittenberg CN. A new class of anti-emetic agents on the horizon. Clin J Oncol Nurs 6: 103–104, 2001.

Rust DM et al. Oprelvekin: an alternative treatment for thrombocytopenia. Clin J Oncol Nurs 3: 57–62, 1999.

Sherry VW. Taste alterations among patients with cancer. Clin J Oncol Nurs 6: 73–77, 2002.

Sonis SS. Mucositis as a biological process: a new hypothesis for the development of chemotherapy induced stomatotoxicity. Oral Oncol 34: 39–43, 1998.

Van Belle S et al. Prevention of cisplatin-induced acute and delayed emesis by the selective neurokin-1 antagonists, L-758,298 and MK-869. Cancer 94: 3032–3041, 2002.

Weizman Z. Cola drinks and rehydration in acute diarrhea (letter). N Engl J Med 315: 768, 1986.

Wilkes JD. Prevention and treatment of oral mucositis following cancer chemotherapy. Semin Oncol 25: 538–551, 1998.

11

REFERENCES

Wojtaszek C. Management of chemotherapy-induced stomatitis. Clin J Oncol Nurs 4: 263–270, 2000.
Yale New Haven Hospital: Pharmacy alert, January 28, 2002.

Dermatological toxicity

Argenta LC, Manders EK. Mitomycin C extravasation injuries. Cancer 51: 1080–1082, 1983.
Boyle DM, Engelking C. Vesicant extravasation: myths and realities. Oncol Nurs Forum 22: 57–67, 1996.
Brogden JM, Nevidjon B. Vinorelbine tartrate (Navelbine): drug profile and nursing implications of a new vinca alkaloid. Oncol Nurs Forum 22: 635–646, 1995.
Brown KA et al. Chemotherapy and biotherapy guidelines and recommendations for practice. Oncology Nursing Society, Pittsburgh, PA, 2001.
Camp-Sorrell D. Developing extravasation protocols and monitoring outcomes. J IV Nurs 21: 232–239, 1998.
Coyle C, Wenhold V. Painful blistered hands and feet. Clin J Oncol Nurs 5: 230–232, 2001.
Curran CF, Luce JK, Page JA. Doxorubicin-associated flare reactions. Oncol Nurs Forum 17: 387–389, 1990.
Duray PH, Cuono CB, Madri JA. Demonstration of cutaneous doxorubicin extravasation by rhodamine filtered fluorescence microscopy. J Surg Oncol 31: 21–25, 1986.
Koppel R, Boh EE. Cutaneous reactions to chemotherapeutic agents. Am J Med Sci 321: 327–335, 2001.
Mayo DJ, Pearson DC. Chemotherapy extravasation: a consequence of fibrin sheath formation around venous access devices. Oncol Nurs Forum 22: 675–680, 1995.
McGarvey EL et al. Psychological sequelae and alopecia among women with cancer. Cancer Pract 9: 283–289, 2001.
Paus R, Cotsarelis G. The biology of hair follicles. N Engl J Med 341: 491–497, 1999.
Rittenberg CN, Gralla RJ, Rehmeyer TA. Assessing and managing venous irritation associated with vinorelbine tartrate (Navelbine). Oncol Nurs Forum 22: 707–710, 1995.
Rudolph R, Larson DL. Etiology and treatment of chemotherapeutic agent extravasation injuries: a review. J Clin Oncol 5: 1116–1126, 1987.
Wood H, Ellerhorst-Ryan JM. Delayed adverse skin reactions associated with mitomycin-C administration. Oncol Nurs Forum 11: 14–18, 1984.

Renal toxicity

Long S. Management of renal failure. In: Berger A, Portenoy RK, Weissman DE, eds. Principles and Practice of Palliative and Supportive Oncology. 2nd ed. Philadelphia: Lippincott Williams and Wilkins, 2002, pp 477–491.
Lydon J. Assessment of renal function in the patient receiving chemotherapy. Cancer Nurs 12: 133–143, 1989.
Weiss RB. Nephrotoxicity. In: DeVita VT, Hellman S, Rosenberg SA, eds. Principles and Practice of Oncology, 6th ed. Philadelphia: Lippincott Williams and Wilkins, 2001, pp 2968–2970.

Bladder toxicity

Patterson WP, Reams GP. Renal toxicities of chemotherapy. Semin Oncol 19: 521–528, 1992.
Stillwell TJ, Benson RC. Cyclophosphamide-induced hemorrhagic cystitis. Cancer 61: 451–457, 1988.

Cardiopulmonary toxicity

Cooper JA, Matthay R. Drug-induced pulmonary disease. Dis Mon 33: 61–120, 1987.
Davies MA, Schultz MZ, Murren JK. Cardiopulmonary toxicity of cancer therapies. In: Berger A, Portenoy RK, Weissman DE, eds. Principles and Practice of Palliative and Supportive Oncology, 2nd ed. Philadelphia: Lippincott Williams and Wilkins, 2002, pp 413–440.
Kriesman H, Wolkove N. Pulmonary toxicity of antineoplastic therapy. Semin Oncol 19: 508–520, 1992.
Schucter LM et al. 2002 update of recommendations for the use of chemotherapy and radiotherapy protectants: clinical practice guidelines of the American Society of Clinical Oncology. J Clin Oncol 20: 2895–2903, 2002.

Seidman A et al. Cardiac dysfunction in the trastuzumab clinical trials experience. J Clin Oncol 20: 1215–1221, 2002.

Shan K, Lincoff M, Young JB. Anthracycline-induced cardiotoxicity. Ann Intern Med 125: 47–58, 1996.

van der Veen MJ et al. Fatal pulmonary fibrosis complicating low dose methotrexate therapy for rheumatoid arthritis. J Rheumatol 22: 1766–1768, 1995.

Neurological toxicity

Boyle FM, Wheeler HR, Shenfield GM. Amelioration of experimental cisplatin and paclitaxel neuropathy with glutamate. J Neurol Oncol 41: 107–116, 1999.

Brant JM. Cancer-related neuropathic pain. Nurs Pract Forum 9: 154–162, 1998.

Morello CM et al. Gabapentin vs amitriptyline for the treatment of peripheral neuropathy. Arch Intern Med 160: 1040–1041, 2000.

Rowinsky EK et al. Clinical toxicities encountered with paclitaxel (Taxol). Semin Oncol 20(4 suppl 3): 1–15, 1993.

Schuster LM et al. 2002 update of recommendations for the use of chemotherapy and radiotherapy protectants: clinical practice guidelines of the American Society of Clinical Oncology. J Clin Oncol 20: 2895–2903, 2002.

Siegal T, Haim N. Cisplatin-induced peripheral neuropathy. Cancer 66: 1117–1123, 1990.

Weiss RB. Neurotoxicity. In: DeVita VT, Hellman S, Rosenberg SA, eds. Principles and Practice of Oncology, 6th ed. Philadelphia: Lippincott Williams and Wilkins, 2001, pp 2964–2968.

Wilkes G. New therapeutic options in colon cancer: focus on oxaliplatin. Clin J Oncol Nurs 6: 131–137, 2002.

Wilson RH et al. Acute oxaliplatin-induced peripheral nerve excitability. J Clin Oncol 20: 1767–1774, 2002.

Woolf CJ, Mannion RJ. Neuropathic pain: aetiology, symptoms, mechanisms and management. Lancet 353: 1959–1964, 1999.

Gonadal toxicity

Chapman RM, Sutcliffe SB, Malpas JS. Cytotoxic-induced ovarian failure in women with Hodgkin's disease. I. Hormone function. JAMA 242: 1877–1881, 1979a.

Chapman RM, Sutcliffe SB, Malpas JS. Cytotoxic-induced ovarian failure in women with Hodgkin's disease. II. Effects on sexual function. JAMA 242: 1882–1884, 1979b.

Ganz PA et al. Life after breast cancer: understanding women's health related quality of life and sexual functioning. J Clin Oncol 16: 501–514, 1998.

Goodwin P et al. Risk of menopause during the first year after breast cancer diagnosis. J Clin Oncol 17: 2365–2370, 1999.

Knobf MT. The menopausal symptom experience in young mid-life women with breast cancer. Cancer Nurs 24: 201–210, 2001.

Knobf, MT. Carrying on: the experience of premature menopause in women with early stage breast cancer. Nurs Res 51: 9–17, 2002.

Lower EE et al. The risk of premature menopause induced by chemotherapy for early breast cancer. J Women's Health & Gender Based Med 8: 949–954, 1999.

Moore HCF, Mick R, Fox KR. An associated incidence of chemotherapy related amenorrhea (CRA) following adjuvant doxorubicin and cyclophosphamide (AC) for early stage breast cancer. Proc Am Soc Clin Oncol 18: 83a(abstract # 313), 1999.

Schover L et al. Knowledge and experience regarding cancer, infertility and sperm banking in younger male survivors. J Clin Oncol 20: 1880–1889, 2002a.

Schover L et al. Oncologists' attitudes and practices regarding banking sperm before cancer treatment. J Clin Oncol 20: 1890–1897, 2002b.

Shell JA. Evidence-based practice for symptom management in adults with cancer: sexual dysfunction. Oncol Nurs Forum 29: 53–68, 2002.

Sweet V, Servy EJ, Karow AM. Reproductive issues for men with cancer: technology and nursing management. Oncol Nurs Forum 23: 51–58, 1996.

Teratogenic

Colvin OL. Antitumor alkylating agents. In: DeVita VT, Hellman S, Rosenberg SA, eds. Cancer Principles and Practice, 6th ed. Philadelphia: Lippincott Williams & Wilkins, 2001, pp 363–376.

APPENDIX

TABLE A-1
CALCULATION OF BODY SURFACE AREA*

Mostellar	Du Bois	Haycock
a. BSA (m^2) = $\sqrt{\dfrac{height \times weight}{3600}}$	BSA (m^2) = $(wt^{0.425}) \times (ht^{0.725}) \times$ 0.007184	BSA (m^2) = $(wt^{0.5378}) \times (ht^{0.3964}) \times$ 0.024265
b. BSA (m^2) = $\sqrt{\dfrac{height \times weight}{3131}}$		

From: Mostellar RD. Simplified calculation of body-surface area. N Engl J Med 317: 1098, 1987.
Du Bois D, Du Bois EF. A formula to estimate the approximate surface area if height and weight be known. Arch Intern Med 17: 863–871, 1916. Haycock GB, Schwartz GJ, Wisotsky DH. Geometric method for measuring body surface area: a height-weight formula validated in infants, children, and adults. J Pediatr 93: 62–66, 1978.
*BSA = Body surface area; m^2 = meters squared; ht = height in centimeters (except as noted in Mostellar formula b where height is in inches); wt = weight in kilograms (except as noted in Mostellar formula b where weight is in pounds).

TABLE A-2
CALCULATION OF BODY SURFACE AREA IN ADULT AMPUTEES*

Body parts	Women (%)	Men (%)
Hand plus five fingers	2.65	2.83
Lower part of arm	3.80	4.04
Upper part of arm	5.65	5.94
Foot	2.94	3.15
Lower part of leg	6.27	5.99
Thigh	12.55	11.80

NOTE: Dose reductions may not be necessary in all amputee patients. Metabolism and clearance of a drug does not necessarily change in amputee patients. Use professional judgment when deciding to reduce drug doses.
From: Colangelo PM et al. Two methods for estimating body surface area in adult amputees. Am J Hosp Pharm 41: 2650–2655, 1984.
*BSA (m^2) = BSA − [(BSA) × (%BSA$_{part}$)], where BSA is body surface area, m^2 is meters squared, and BSA$_{part}$ is body surface area of amputated body part.

TABLE A-3
IDEAL BODY WEIGHT CHARTS*

	Height (cm)	Weight (kg)	Height (cm)	Weight (kg)	Height (cm)	Weight (kg)
Males						
	145	51.9	159	59.9	173	68.7
	146	52.4	160	60.5	174	69.4
	147	52.9	161	61.1	175	70.1
	148	53.6	162	61.7	176	70.8
	149	54.0	163	62.3	177	71.6
	150	54.5	164	62.9	178	72.4
	151	55.0	165	63.5	179	73.3
	152	55.8	166	64.0	180	74.2
	153	56.1	167	64.6	181	75.0
	154	56.6	168	65.2	182	75.6
	155	57.2	169	65.9	183	76.5
	156	57.9	170	66.6	184	77.3
	157	58.6	171	67.3	185	78.1
	158	59.3	172	68.0	186	78.9
Females						
	140	44.9	150	50.4	160	56.2
	141	45.4	151	51.0	161	56.9
	142	45.9	152	51.5	162	57.6
	143	46.4	153	52.0	163	58.3
	144	47.0	154	52.5	164	58.9
	145	47.5	155	53.1	165	59.5
	146	48.0	156	53.7	166	60.1
	147	48.6	157	54.3	167	60.7
	148	49.2	158	54.9	168	61.4
	149	49.8	159	55.5	169	62.1

Modified from Jellife DB. The Assessment of the Nutritional Status of the Community. Geneva, World Health Organization, 1986.

*Ideal body weight for height. This table corrects the 1960 Metropolitan Standards to nude weight without shoe heels.

TABLE A-4
PERFORMANCE SCALE (KARNOFSKY AND ECOG)

ECOG		Karnofsky	
0	Fully active, able to carry on all pre-disease performance without restriction.	100%	Normal, no complaints, no evidence of disease.
		90%	Able to carry on normal activity; minor signs or symptoms of disease.
1	Restricted in physically strenuous activity but ambulatory and able to carry out work of a light or sedentary nature, (e.g., light housework, office work).	80%	Normal activity with effort; some signs or symptoms of disease.
		70%	Cares for self; unable to carry on normal activity or to do active work.
2	Ambulatory and capable of all self-care but unable to carry out any work activities; up and about more than 50% of waking hours.	60%	Requires occasional assistance, is mostly able to care for him/herself.
		50%	Requires considerable assistance and frequent medical care.
3	Capable of only limited self-care, confined to bed or chair more than 50% of waking hours.	40%	Disabled, requires special care and assistance.
		30%	Severely disabled, hospitalization indicated; death not imminent.
4	Completely disabled; cannot carry on any self-care; totally confined to bed or chair.	20%	Very sick, hospitalization necessary; active supportive treatment necessary.
		10%	Moribund, fatal processes progressing rapidly.
5	Dead	0%	Dead

Modified from Karnofsky DA et al. The use of the nitrogen mustards in the palliative treatment of carcinoma with particular reference to bronchogenic carcinoma. Cancer 1: 634–656, 1948; Oken MM et al. Toxicity and response criteria of the Eastern Cooperative Oncology Group. Am J Clin Oncol 5: 649–655, 1982; and Zubrod GC et al. Appraisal of methods for the study of chemotherapy in man: comparative therapeutic trial of nitrogen mustard and triethylene thiophosphoramide. J Chron Dis 11: 7–33, 1960.

TABLE A-5

METHODS USED TO CALCULATE CREATININE CLEARANCE*

Calculated from a timed urine collection

$$\text{Creatinine Clearance} = \frac{(\text{Urine Creatinine})}{\text{Serum Creatinine}} \times \frac{(\text{Urine Volume})^\dagger}{\text{Time}}$$

Estimated from age, weight, serum of creatinine
Cockcroft and Gault method[‡]:

$$\text{Creatinine Clearance}_{men} = \frac{[(140 - age) \times (\text{Lean Body Wt.})]}{(\text{Serum Creatinine}) \times 72}$$

$$\text{Creatinine Clearance}_{women} = 0.85 \times \text{Creatinine Clearance}_{men}$$

Jeliffe method[§]: (For an individual with BSA of 1.73 m^2)

$$\text{Creatinine Clearance} = \frac{100}{(\text{Serum Creatinine})} - 12$$

*Units used in calculations are as follows: creatinine clearance (mL/min); age (yr); serum creatinine (mg/dL); time (min); urine creatinine (mg/dL); weight (kg); urine volume (mL).
[†]Time = duration of urine collection; 24 hours = 1440 minutes; 12 hours = 720 minutes; 8 hours = 480 minutes; less than 20% variability with 8, 12, and 24-hour collection times.
(From Baumann TJ et al. Minimum urine collection periods for accurate determination of creatinine clearance in critically ill patients. Clin Pharm 6: 393–398, 1987.)
[‡]From Cockcroft DW, Gault MH. Prediction of creatinine clearance from serum creatinine. Nephron 16: 31–41, 1976.
[§]From Jeliffe RW. Estimation of creatinine clearance when urine cannot be collected. Lancet 1: 975–976, 1971.
BSA = Body surface area.

TABLE A-6

TEMPERATURE CONVERSION

Fahrenheit	Celsius (Centigrade)
94	34.4
95	35.0
96	35.5
97	36.1
98	36.6
98.6	37.0
99	37.2
100	37.7
101	38.3
102	38.8
103	39.4
104	40.0
105	40.5
106	41.1
107	41.6

INDEX

Note: Drugs are indexed under the generic name; Cross-references are provided from alternative names, even when target entry is directly above/below.